Clinical Psychiatry for Medical Students

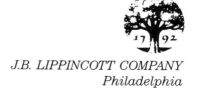

J.B. LIPPINCOTT COMPANY
Philadelphia

Clinical Psychiatry for Medical Students

Second Edition

Edited by

Alan Stoudemire, M.D.

Professor of Psychiatry and Behavioral Sciences
Director, Medical Student Education in Psychiatry
Department of Psychiatry and Behavioral Sciences
Emory University School of Medicine
Atlanta, Georgia

45 Contributors

Acquisitions Editor: Richard Winters
Sponsoring Editor: Jody Schott
Production Service: Chernow Editorial Services, Inc.
Indexer: Melanie Belkin
Cover Designer: Tom Jackson
Production Manager: Janet Greenwood
Production Coordinator: Mary Kinsella
Compositor: Circle Graphics
Printer/Binder: R.R. Donnelley & Sons, Crawfordsville

Second Edition

6 5 4 3 2 1

Library of Congress Cataloging-in-Publication Data

Clinical psychiatry for medical students/edited by Alan Stoudemire;
  with 45 contributors. − − 2nd ed.
      p.   cm.
  Companion v. to: Human behavior/edited by Alan Stoudemire. 2nd
ed. c1994.
  Includes bibliographical references and index.
  ISBN 0-397-51338-0
  1. Psychiatry.   I. Stoudemire, Alan.   II. Human behavior.
  [DNLM: 1. Mental Disorders.   2. Psychophysiologic Disorders. WM
100 C641 1994]
RC454.C539 1994
616.89 − − dc20
DNLM/DLC
for Library of Congress   93-34226
                                                                            CIP

The authors and publisher have exerted every effort to ensure that drug selection and dosage set forth in this text are in accord with current recommendations and practice at the time of publication. However, in view of ongoing research, changes in government regulations, and the constant flow of information relating to drug therapy and drug reactions, the reader is urged to check the package insert for each drug for any change in indications and dosage and for added warnings and precautions. This is particularly important when the recommended agent is a new or infrequently employed drug.

Accompanying text:
Human Behavior: An Introduction for Medical Students, Second Edition
Edited by Alan Stoudemire, M.D.

This book is dedicated to Susan, Anna, and Will

Disease in man is never exactly the same as disease in an experimental animal, for in man the disease at once affects and is affected by what we call the emotional life. Thus, the physician who attempts to take care of a patient while he neglects this factor is as unscientific as the investigator who neglects to control all the conditions that may affect his experiment. The good physician knows his patients through and through, and his knowledge is bought dearly. Time, sympathy and understanding must be lavishly dispensed, but the reward is to be found in that personal bond which forms the greatest satisfaction of the practice of medicine. One of the essential qualities of the clinician is interest in humanity, for the secret of the care of the patient is in caring for the patient.

Francis Peabody, *The Care of the Patient,*
Journal of the American Medical Association, 88:882, 1927

Contributors

David B. Abrams, *Ph.D.*

Professor of Psychiatry and Human Behavior
Brown University School of Medicine
Providence, Rhode Island

David Bienenfeld, *M.D.*

Associate Professor and Vice Chair of Psychiatry
Wright State University School of Medicine
Dayton, Ohio

Jerry L. Carter, *M.D.*

Assistant Professor of Psychiatry and Internal Medicine
Medical College of Pennsylvania
Allegheny Campus
Pittsburgh, Pennsylvania

Dennis S. Charney, *M.D.*

Professor of Psychiatry
Yale University School of Medicine
New Haven, Connecticut

CDR Alberto Diaz, Jr., *M.D., USNR*

Assistant Professor in Psychiatry
Uniformed Services University of the Health Sciences
29 Palms, California

Karl Doghramji, *M.D.*

Associate Professor of Psychiatry and Human Behavior
Jefferson Medical College
Philadelphia, Pennsylvania

William R. Dubin, M.D.

    Professor of Psychiatry
    Temple University School of Medicine
    Philadelphia, Pennsylvania

Mina K. Dulcan, M.D.

    Osterman Professor of Child Psychiatry
    Head, Department of Child Psychiatry
    Children's Memorial Hospital
    Chief, Division of Child and Adolescent Psychiatry
    Northwestern University Medical School
    Chicago, Illinois

Peter J. Fagan, Ph.D.

    Associate Professor of Medical Psychology
    Johns Hopkins University School of Medicine
    Baltimore, Maryland

Eugene W. Farber, Ph.D.

    Assistant Professor of Psychiatry and Behavioral Sciences
    Emory University School of Medicine
    Atlanta, Georgia

David G. Folks, M.D.

    Professor and Chair
    Creighton-Nebraska Department of Psychiatry
    Creighton University School of Medicine
    and University of Nebraska College of Medicine
    Omaha, Nebraska

Charles V. Ford, M.D.

    Professor of Psychiatry and Behavioral Neurobiology
    University of Alabama at Birmingham School of Medicine
    Birmingham, Alabama

Allen Frances, M.D.

    Professor and Chair, Department of Psychiatry
    Duke University Medical Center
    Durham, North Carolina

Richard J. Goldberg, M.D., F.A.P.A.

    Professor of Psychiatry and Medicine
    Brown University School of Medicine
    Providence, Rhode Island

Michael G. Goldstein, M.D.

    Associate Professor of Psychiatry and Human Behavior
    Brown University School of Medicine
    Providence, Rhode Island

Barrie J. Guise, Ph.D.

Clinical Psychologist
Lenox Hill Hospital
New York, New York

Robert Hales, M.D.

Clinical Professor of Psychiatry
University of California, San Francisco
San Francisco, California

Carl A. Houck, M.D.

Assistant Professor of Psychiatry
University of Alabama at Birmingham School of Medicine
Birmingham, Alabama

Mark E. James, M.D.

Assistant Professor of Psychiatry and Behavioral Sciences
Emory University School of Medicine
Atlanta, Georgia

Nadine J. Kaslow, Ph.D.

Associate Professor of Psychiatry
Emory University School of Medicine
Atlanta, Georgia

Roger G. Kathol, M.D.

Professor of Internal Medicine and Psychiatry
University of Iowa College of Medicine
Iowa City, Iowa

John H. Krystal, M.D.

Assistant Professor of Psychiatry
Yale University School of Medicine
New Haven, Connecticut

James L. Levenson, M.D.

Professor of Psychiatry, Medicine, and Surgery
Medical College of Virginia
Richmond, Virginia

Steven T. Levy, M.D.

Professor of Psychiatry and Behavioral Sciences
Emory University School of Medicine
Atlanta, Georgia

Rosalind M. Mance, M.B.B.S.

Assistant Professor of Psychiatry and Behavioral Sciences
Emory University School of Medicine
Atlanta, Georgia

Deborah B. Marin, M.D.

Assistant Professor of Psychiatry
Mount Sinai School of Medicine
New York, New York

Michael G. Moran, M.D.

Associate Professor of Psychiatry
University of Colorado School of Medicine
Denver, Colorado

William D. Murphy, Ph.D.

Associate Professor of Psychiatry
University of Tennessee College of Medicine
Memphis, Tennessee

Linda M. Nagy, M.D.

Assistant Professor of Psychiatry
Yale University School of Medicine
New Haven, Connecticut

Philip T. Ninan, M.D.

Associate Professor of Psychiatry and Behavioral Sciences
Emory University School of Medicine
Atlanta, Georgia

Emile D. Risby, M.D.

Assistant Professor of Psychiatry and Behavioral Sciences
Emory University School of Medicine
Atlanta, Georgia

Samuel Craig Risch, M.D.

Professor of Psychiatry and Behavioral Sciences
Medical College of South Carolina
Charleston, South Carolina

Laurie Ruggiero, Ph.D.

Assistant Professor of Psychology
University of Rhode Island
Kingston, Rhode Island

Chester W. Schmidt, Jr., M.D.

Associate Professor of Psychiatry
Johns Hopkins University School of Medicine
Baltimore, Maryland

Elizabeth D. Schwarz, M.D.

Department of Psychiatry
University of Tennessee College of Medicine
Memphis, Tennessee

Edward K. Silberman, M.D.

Clinical Professor of Psychiatry
Jefferson Medical College
Philadelphia, Pennsylvania

Jonathan M. Silver, M.D.

Associate Professor of Clinical Psychiatry
Columbia University College of Physicians and Surgeons
New York, New York

Alan Stoudemire, M.D.

Professor of Psychiatry and Behavioral Sciences
Emory University School of Medicine
Atlanta, Georgia

Robert M. Swift, M.D., Ph.D.

Associate Professor of Psychiatry
Brown University School of Medicine
Providence, Rhode Island

Robert J. Ursano, M.D.

Professor and Chair, Department of Psychiatry
Uniformed Services University of the Health Sciences
Bethesda, Maryland

Randon D. Welton, M.D.

Senior Resident in Psychiatry
Wright State University School of Medicine
Dayton, Ohio

Thomas A. Widiger, Ph.D.

Professor of Psychology
University of Kentucky College of Arts and Sciences
Lexington, Kentucky

Joel Yager, M.D.

Professor of Psychiatry and Biobehavioral Sciences
Associate Chair for Education of Psychiatry
University of California at Los Angeles School of Medicine
Los Angeles, California

William R. Yates, M.D.

Associate Professor of Psychiatry
University of Iowa College of Medicine
Iowa City, Iowa

Stuart C. Yudofsky, M.D.

D. C. and Irene Ellwood Professor and Chairman
Department of Psychiatry and Behavioral Sciences
Baylor College of Medicine
Houston, Texas

Foreword

There are many reasons why physicians should be knowledgeable about clinical psychiatry. First, individuals who are experiencing emotional distress usually seek help initially not from mental health professionals but from their personal physicians. Since psychological distress is often accompanied by stress-related symptoms such as headaches, indigestion, loss of appetite, fatigue, and insomnia, it is often the task of the physician to ascertain when such physical complaints actually represent "masked" psychiatric illness. Conservative estimates have established that approximately 20–25% of office visits to primary care physicians are primarily for psychiatrically-related reasons.

It is well-known, however, that primary care physicians, as well as other medical and surgical subspecialists, frequently overlook or minimize the psychiatric problems of their patients. Misdiagnosis of psychiatric illness can lead to prolonged and unnecessary suffering, disability, and excessive health care expenditures. Early recognition and prompt treatment of psychiatric conditions that initially present in the general medical setting would result not only in better medical and psychological care for patients but would also result in the elimination of misdirected medical expenses in the form of unnecessary laboratory testing and surgical procedures.

The first task for medical students in gaining the knowledge and skills necessary to care for the psychiatric and emotional needs of their patients is to develop the ability to properly recognize psychiatric illness in the medical setting. A major goal of this text is to assist future physicians in that task. In this spirit, special emphasis has also been placed on practical treatment strategies suitable for the medical setting as well as the indications for psychiatric referral.

While this text emphasizes practical aspects of diagnosis and treatment, recent research that has yielded many exciting discoveries in detecting the neurochemical basis of the major psychiatric disorders is also discussed. State-of-the-art scientific information is provided on advances in areas such as genetics, neuroimaging, psychopharmacology, and other neurobiological aspects of psychiatric disorders. The text, however, strives toward an integrated biopsychosocial model in understanding the etiology of psychiatric disorders and considers biological, psychological, and social factors in the development of treatment strategies.

Dr. Stoudemire has organized a superb second volume of this text and is very well qualified to do so based on his experience as both an educator and clinician. He has served as Director of Medical Student Education in Psychiatry at Emory University School of Medicine for a number of years, and has developed first hand knowledge of medical students' interests and needs regarding clinical psychiatry. Dr. Stoudemire also founded and has served as Director of the Medical-Psychiatry Unit at Emory University Hospital for a number of years, a nationally recognized program designed to treat patients with combined medical and psychiatric illness. This position has enabled him to interact on a daily basis with physicians in many other specialties and, thereby, to see what they most want and need to learn about psychiatry to be better able to care for their patients. From these experiences, Dr. Stoudemire distilled the framework of this textbook, which specifically focuses on the basic clinical psychiatric knowledge and skills needed by medical students for their future careers regardless of their clinical specialty.

Dr. Stoudemire then assembled a group of chapter authors from across the country who meet two criteria. First, they are skilled psychiatric educators with a great deal of personal experience teaching medical students. Second, they have up-to-date scientific knowledge of their topic and have refined their ideas on their topic by teaching and receiving feedback from medical students. The result is a rare combination of new and exciting psychiatric knowledge that is clearly, concisely, and practically discussed at the level of medical students in their clinical years. This also makes this text a superb overview for first or second year psychiatry residents and residents in primary care disciplines. A number of psychiatrists preparing for the written and oral specialty Board examinations also have told me this text served as a well-organized and -edited, crisply reasoned, and up-to-date review of major psychiatric topics.

I hope the physicians who care for me and my family and friends in future years are well-grounded in the basic biopsychosocial and psychiatric knowledge, skills, and physicianly attitudes embodied in this excellent text.

Troy L. Thompson II, M.D.
The Daniel Lieberman Professor and Chair
Department of Psychiatry and Human Behavior
Jefferson Medical College and Hospital
Philadelphia, Pennsylvania

Preface

It is the fundamental premise of this text that psychiatric illness must be understood, evaluated, and treated in a multidimensional manner. Hence, biological, psychological, and sociological factors are all considered to be potentially important in evaluating and treating psychiatric illness. While it will be noted in the introductory chapter on assessment that the amount of attention given to any particular area will vary depending on the clinical situation, the complexity of psychiatric illness requires that a comprehensive assessment of the patient be performed to facilitate accurate diagnosis and effective treatment.

Recent developments in descriptive and biological psychiatry have provided physicians with more exact methods of diagnosis as well as psychopharmacologic treatments that are often dramatically effective. Some psychiatrists, while acknowledging the importance of recent developments in the classification of psychiatric disorders and biologic treatments, have been concerned that the importance of understanding developmental and experiential aspects of the patient's life and the role of psychotherapy in treatment may be being neglected in the process. A fundamental premise that has guided the development of this text is that multiple perspectives (biological, psychological, sociological) must be simultaneously integrated in research and clinical practice to fully understand and effectively treat psychiatric disorders. While controversy still reigns as to which *forms* of treatment are most effective for certain disorders and to what the relative contribution of psychological and biological factors is in determining disease vulnerability, clinicians should strive to understand patients and their illnesses in the context of their developmental life experiences and their current interpersonal relationships. Those who still argue the "nature vs. nurture" issue are fundamentally missing the point: Elements of both almost always influence vulnerability to emotional illness and need to be considered in treatment. A new generation of psychiatrists is gradually emerging who will be able to fully integrate both the perspectives of developmental psychology and biological understanding of the etiology and treatment of psychiatric disorders. It is this integrated psychobiologic paradigm in research and clinical practice that forms the future for psychiatry. While the complete scientific integration of psychoanalytic, behavioral, sociological and biological theories is not yet possible, the inability to do so is primarily the result of our insufficient understanding of the etiology of psychiatric illness.

As will be noted in the first chapter, this text will advocate a structured approach to psychiatric diagnosis within the matrix of the biopsychosocial model. In addition, as will be discussed in Chapter 2, the importance of understanding the patient's developmental life experiences and quality of their interpersonal relationships is considered to be of crucial importance in personality formation, vulnerability or resistance to stress, as well as susceptibility and adaptability to both medical and psychiatric illness. Comprehensive patient care must be based on assessing and treating each patient from the biological, psychological, and social perspectives.

This text is unique in that it deals with the major clinical psychopathological syndromes from this perspective as well as specifically addressing, in the second half of the text, the practical management of the common psychiatric disorders encountered in medical and surgical practice. These latter chapters are all written by clinicians who have extensive experience in working with physicians in medical settings, so readers should find them both precise and practical. In addition, Chapter 16 addresses the major childhood psychiatric disorders that are likely to be encountered in family and pediatric practice and emphasizes their diagnosis and treatment.

Finally, it should be noted that this text provides only an overview and covers the essential aspects of clinical psychiatry that are most pertinent for medical students. Each chapter is followed by an annotated bibliography of recommended references that students are referred to for more extensive reading, and a general reading list if provided. It should also be noted that this text is best used when it is preceded by reading the companion volume to this series, *Human Behavior: An Introduction for Medical Students*, which covers the fundamental principles of human behavior in health and illness using the biopsychosocial model and a psychobiological perspective.

It is hoped that in using and studying this text students will gain some appreciation of the exciting developments that have evolved in psychiatry and will be able to use this knowledge in providing excellent integrated medical and psychiatric care to their patients.

A NOTE REGARDING DSM-IV

Every effort has been made to make this text current with the Diagnostic and Statistical Manual of Mental Disorders, 4th edition (DSM-IV), which is due to be published in the Spring of 1994. Since this text was prepared and edited prior to the official publication of the final draft of DSM-IV, the diagnostic criteria used were those published in the DSM-IV Draft Criteria published in March, 1993. Certain changes in the names of certain diagnoses, as well as in the diagnostic criteria, may have been made in the final (1994) published version of DSM-IV. Students should refer to the final version of DSM-IV for final verifications of the names and criteria for diagnostic categories, although any inconsistencies with the semi-final draft published in March, 1993 are anticipated to be minor. The editor would like to thank the American Psychiatric Association and the American Psychiatric Association Press for their cooperation in granting permission for the preliminary criteria for DSM-IV to be published in several parts of this text.

Alan Stoudemire, M.D.

Acknowledgments

This text could not have been completed without the tireless dedication, loyalty, and effort of my administrative assistant, Lynda Mathews. Her contribution to this book is greatly appreciated.

Thanks are also extended to the students and faculty of Emory University School of Medicine as well as those of other medical schools. Their suggestions regarding the first edition of this text have, I hope, resulted in a more complete and refined second edition.

The contributors to this textbook are all dedicated clinicians and researchers who represent the very best in academic psychiatry. It has been a pleasure and a privilege to work with them. Their dedication to patient care and medical education will be evident in the quality of the chapters contained herein.

Recommended Textbooks

Diagnostic and Statistical Manual of Mental Disorders, 4th ed. Washington, DC. American Psychiatric Association, 1994.

> This is the "bible" of descriptive psychiatry. It contains epidemiological and descriptive data of the major psychiatric disorders.

Kaplan HI, Sadock BJ (eds): Comprehensive Textbook of Psychiatry, 6th ed, Vols 1 and 2. Baltimore, Williams & Wilkins, 1994

> This is an encyclopedic textbook that covers all areas of psychiatry. Detailed and comprehensive, it should be primarily used as a reference source.

Michels R (ed): Psychiatry, Vols 1–III. Philadelphia, JB Lippincott, 1993

> This is an excellent and comprehensive textbook of clinical psychiatry. Published in three volumes, the chapters are lucid, well edited, and are kept fresh by a subscription process that periodically updates the material.

Nicholi AM Jr (ed): New Harvard Guide to Psychiatry, 2nd ed. Cambridge, MA, Belknap Pres sof Harvard University Press, 1988

> This is an excellent overview of clinical psychiatry that is very readable and practical for a medical student audience. Chapters that are especially strong are those on the biological aspects of depression, the genetic aspects of schizophrenia, and the chapters on psycho-dynamic and psychoanalytic theory by Meissner, Vaillant, and Nemiah.

Stoudemire A, Fogel BS (eds): Psychiatric Care of the Medical Patient. New York, Oxford University Press, 1993

> This comprehensive textbook is a detailed reference on the psychiatric disorders as encountered in medically ill patients. It contains detailed information regarding diagnosis, psychotherapy, and psychopharmacologic modifications that are required in treating psychiatric disorders in the medically ill.

Talbott J, Hales RE, Yudofsky S (eds): Textbook of Psychiatry, 2nd ed. Washington, DC, American Psychiatric Press, 1994

> This is an excellent textbook of clinical psychiatry that is eminently readable and practical. The chapters will provide a somewhat more expanded discussion of the psychopathological syndromes contained in this text.

Yudofsky SC, Hales RE (eds): Textbook of Neuropsychiatry. Washington, DC. American Psychiatric Press, 1992

> This is a clearly written and practical guide to neuropsychiatric disorders.

Contents

1

Psychiatric Assessment, DSM-IV, and Differential Diagnosis

William R. Yates,
Roger G. Kathol, and
Jerry Carter

During the past 20 years, advances in psychiatric research have led to a better understanding of mental and emotional disorders. This improved knowledge has modified the approach to evaluating and treating patients with psychiatric conditions. This chapter focuses on how to perform a basic and practical evaluation of psychiatric problems. It provides a method of psychiatric evaluation, useful in both the psychiatric and medical setting, that increases the likelihood that the most effective treatment will be given.

The *biopsychosocial* approach currently is advocated as the best paradigm of psychiatric assessment (Fink, 1988). Using a model of assessment based on general systems theory, this approach suggests that equal emphasis be given to the evaluation of the psychological, social, and biological factors impacting on the patient's clinical presentation. In the clinical setting, however, the importance of each of these areas of assessment varies depending on the emotional or behavioral difficulty with which the patient presents. For example, in a patient experiencing marital problems where neither spouse has interfering medical difficulties, the psychological assessment (the patient's view of his or her role in the relationship, the patient's expectations of the marriage, the patient's ultimate life goals) and social assessment (the relationship with the spouse, the causes of conflicts, family member influences, economic constraints) would receive greater attention than the biological assessment. Thus, therapeutic intervention directed toward the psychological and social realms would receive the most emphasis, unless a concurrent medical illness in one of the family members was a primary cause of the crisis. Alternatively, if a patient is delirious, biological factors (underlying medical differential diagnosis, likelihood of improvement, or complications with various interventions) become paramount.

As in all areas of medicine, students learn to balance their evaluations to best explore the complaints and needs of the patient. The astute clinician develops skills in each area of assessment and incorporates them when the clinical situation dictates.

In this introductory chapter, a biopsychosocial approach using a structured system of psychiatric diagnosis will be presented for patient assessment. In addition, the importance of understanding patients in light of both their present and past experiences will be emphasized. Students are referred to the companion volume to the text on human behavior for background information and substantiated evidence for the biopsychosocial model of human disease and illness (Stoudemire, 1994). Chapter 2 of this text will discuss the practical aspects of the biopsychosocial model as it relates to psychodynamic and psychosocial assessment of patients.

VALUE OF A DIAGNOSIS

Although many psychiatrists spend a good deal of their time assisting *normal* patients in their adjustment to *normal* life experiences, the main reason for psychiatric evaluation is the identification of mental and emotional disorders. To do this effectively, clinicians must develop a basic understanding of what constitutes "abnormal" behavior.

During medical training, students and residents learn to differentiate the normal human condition from the abnormal. When is the liver enlarged? When is a cardiac murmur clinically significant? How high does the alkaline phosphatase level have to go before further diagnostic testing is needed? Implicit in the answers to these questions is an understanding of what is "normal." In most medical disciplines, the distinction between normal and abnormal has been quantified. Laboratory tests list a "normal range," which indicates an acceptable deviation from the mean for a control population. Alternatively, the presence of certain findings indicates abnormality. Examples would include fungating skin lesions or rales in the chest, which are uniformly absent in normal individuals.

One of the most perplexing but seldom asked questions in psychiatry is, "What constitutes normal emotions and behavior?" Without an answer to this question, is it possible to define the "abnormal"? In one experimental study, Rosenhan (1979) reported that nonpsychiatrically ill "pseudopatients," who faked having heard the words "hollow," "thud," and "empty" for several days, presented themselves for psychiatric evaluation. The pseudopatients were diagnosed as having schizophrenia, in remission, during 11 of 12 inpatient encounters at independent hospitals. One must question if so few symptoms, which cause no incapacity and resolve spontaneously and immediately after the initial evaluation, are sufficient to label a person schizophrenic with its attendant personal, social, legal, and economic repercussions.

Although there are diverse opinions on what constitutes "normalcy," most consider it to be defined by behavior that falls within a commonly recognized "standard" within a given culture. Aberrant behavior can be identified by this method, although the reliability of such an approach, especially in mild conditions, is limited by the United States's cultural diversity (ethnic—white, black, Asian; religious—Hari Krishna, Jehovah's Witness, fundamentalist; organizational—Ku Klux Klan, motorcycle gangs) and by the cultural background, personal biases, and norms of the person performing the examination. Essentially, what is deemed "normal" ends up being that which is not too different from the accepted cultural and behavioral norms of the evaluator!

Mere recognition of those with "abnormal" behavior is insufficient for diagnosing a psychiatric disorder. That would be equivalent to calling a jockey who races horses and a person who plays center on a basketball team medically ill because they fall at the extremes of the bell-shaped curve for height. Yet doctors often consider those who do not conform to their concept of appropriate behavior psychologically unstable.

Despite the difficulty in specifying abnormal emotions and behavior, there are clearly individuals who are *functionally impaired* as a result of emotion, thought, or behavior. Few would argue that a delirious or profoundly depressed patient represents a variant of normal behavior. *It is, in fact, impairment of function that distinguishes "eccentric behavior" from psychiatric illness.* As with all other medical disorders, psychiatric *disease* includes conditions associated with pain, disability, death, or an increased liability to these states (Robins and Guze, 1970).

A disease is more than just a *descriptor* of conditions causing human suffering. Perhaps more importantly, it is a *predictor*. Consistent and reliable identification of syndromes with specific symptoms and signs allows documentation of the condition's cause, the mode of transmission, family involvement, the age of onset, the natural course of the symptoms, and the treatments that might alter the ultimate outcome. One of the primary objectives of the rapidly changing editions of the *Diagnostic and Statistical Manual of Mental Disorders-IV* (DSM-IV) (American Psychiatric Association, in press [1994]) is categorization of incapacitating aberrant behavior (see Chapter 1 Appendix). Reliable identification using this "cookbook" approach can improve our ability to study these predictive factors. This nomenclature system has been a major advance in psychiatric diagnosis during the past 20 years.

The following case study will be presented and then used throughout the chapter as a teaching example of the correct way to perform a medical/neurological assessment (which includes the mental status examination) in a patient with psychiatric symptoms and as an example of use of the DSM-IV classification scheme. Readers should study it carefully, because reference to this case will be made throughout the first part of this chapter. Reasons for the therapeutic intervention will be provided at the conclusion of the chapter.

A CASE STUDY

Patient Identification
RH is a 57-year-old alcoholic man admitted to the emergency room who is drowsy and somewhat combative after being brought from a boarding house by the police.

Chief Complaint
"Bugs crawling on my skin and the mob is after me."

History of Present Illness

The patient was marginally responsive and was unable to say why he was brought to the hospital. He had been drinking his usual fifth of whiskey until 2 days before admission when "the mob stole" his social security check and he had no money for liquor. Since then he had "holed up" in his room and "nearly starved to death." He refused to give more history for fear that it might have "repercussions."

After the patient gave reluctant permission, the family was contacted. They stated that the patient had been drinking since the age of 13 and had been hospitalized on numerous occasions for alcohol-related problems. Volumes of hospital charts on the patient confirmed this information. He had binged since age 16 and had been drunk nearly every day, except when in treatment, since his mid-30s. His first blackout occurred at age 22, "the shakes" had predictably come on with abstinence of greater than 18 hours for many years, and he had had several episodes of "the DTs." There was no history of withdrawal seizures, however. Short periods of enforced sobriety occurred when the patient was hospitalized for hemorrhaging gastric ulcers. Numerous alcohol rehabilitation programs failed to change his drinking habits.

The family kept track of the patient because "he was a good man when he wasn't drinking," but they didn't want him home because he was abusive during periods of inebriation and was arrested frequently for public intoxication. He had not had a job for many years and had a strong family history for alcoholism. When he was feeling remorseful about his effect on his family, he became despondent and talked of killing himself, but he had never attempted suicide. His suicidal tendencies did not occur during periods of abstinence.

Medical and Psychiatric History

The patient had a 120-pack-a-year smoking history and had been treated for hypertension, which was unsuccessful due to noncompliance. He had been given benzodiazepines in an apparent attempt to help curb his drinking, but he denied nervousness or panic attacks in the absence of alcohol intoxication or during withdrawal. He had numerous alcohol-related injuries and sequelae. His history did not include abuse of controlled substances or over-the-counter medication. He was prone to fighting while under the influence but had no difficulty with the law when sober.

Developmental/Social History

The patient was the only son in a family of four. There were no known problems with gestation, delivery, or reaching developmental milestones. His childhood was disturbed by frequent fights between his parents, mainly over his father's drinking. He was raised largely by his mother, who was nurturing and attentive to his needs until he was in high school, when he began getting into trouble with authorities. He was suspended and eventually expelled for drinking on school premises, when he had "run-ins" with his teachers. While in school he had a close group of friends, was reasonably successful in organized sports, and participated in extracurricular activities. After holding numerous small jobs, he spent 3 years in military service and received a general discharge. He was married at age 23, when he was working as a laborer in a steel mill, and had two daughters. After 14 years of marriage, the patient's wife divorced him because "it was apparent that nothing was going to change." Since then, the patient had lived in numerous places on social security and provided little in the way of child support.

Family History

The patient's father, paternal uncle, and paternal and maternal grandfathers were alcoholics. One paternal aunt saw doctors nearly all the time for health problems. Deaths in the family were mainly due to liver and heart problems. There were no other family illnesses.

Review of Systems

Unable to be obtained.

Physical Examination

The patient was disheveled, cachectic, and had poor hygiene. Blood pressure was 160/94 mm/Hg. Pulse was 98 and regular. Respirations were 20 and unlabored. Temperature was 36.2°C. The skin revealed profuse sweating, several ecchymoses, palmar erythema, and numerous spider angiomata, but no jaundice. There was a recent bruise on the patient's forehead. Poor compliance prevented observation of the patient's fundi. The heart examination revealed no murmurs or rubs, and there were diffuse pulmonary rhonchi. The liver was enlarged and tender. No ascites could be demonstrated. Stool was brown and positive for occult blood. Cranial nerves were "grossly intact," and the patient could move all extremities. There was no strabismus. The patient was tremulous and responsive to pinching in all extremities. Deep tendon reflexes were 1+ and symmetrical, while the plantar response was downgoing bilaterally. Gait was unsteady, and the patient refused to tandem walk.

Mental Status Examination

The mental status examination revealed the patient to be drowsy, uncooperative, and intermittently agitated. His speech was slurred and coherent but his responses to questions were appropriate only occasionally. He remained silent and lying flat with eyes closed when not pressed to respond but lashed out when shaken. His mood was angry and distrustful. Affect was exaggerated but appropriate to the stimulus. He denied thoughts of harming himself or others but stated that he sure would protect himself if anyone "came at him." The patient's statements were understandable but laced with concerns about being imprisoned and tortured (by the mob). He had difficulty maintaining a coherent train of thought. Complaints of the floor crawling with snakes or other repulsive animals and feeling bugs under his skin were frequent. The patient *could not maintain attention long enough for full assessment of cognitive function with the Mini–Mental State Examination.*

Screening Laboratory

The patient's sodium, magnesium, and calcium levels were low, and his liver enzymes and amylase levels were elevated. B_{12} was normal, but folate was low. There was a macrocytic anemia and thrombocytopenia; however, bleeding parameters were normal. Blood alcohol level was 2 mg/ dl (intoxicated 50 to 100 mg/dl). Urine screen for other drug abuse was negative. Chest X-ray and electrocardiogram were normal.

Hospital Course

The patient initially required large doses of chlordiazepoxide for alcohol withdrawal. This was tapered during the first 9 days of his hospital stay with gradual resolution of the changes in mental state. Sodium, magnesium, and calcium levels returned to normal with replacement and adequate nutrition. Thiamine and multivitamins were given. When the patient became less paranoid and confused, he scored 29/30 on the Mini–Mental State Examination. Elevated amylase levels returned toward normal spontaneously, and blood in the stool disappeared after treatment of alcoholic gastritis documented by endoscopy.

The patient expressed remorse for his drinking behavior and promised to attend Alcoholics Anonymous (AA) meetings when released from the hospital. Contact was made with AA during his hospitalization. He demonstrated no evidence of depression when his withdrawal symptoms had resolved. After 3.5 weeks of treatment, he was preparing for discharge when he had a grand mal seizure. Electroencephalogram demonstrated diffuse slowing with increased prominence on the right. Computed tomography of the head revealed a large right frontoparietal subdural hematoma. The hematoma was surgically evacuated, and the patient was discharged to his boarding house 6 weeks later with the intent to initiate alcohol outpatient treatment. An AA sponsor was contacted to ensure the patient's participation in outpatient treatment.

HISTORY, PHYSICAL EXAMINATION, AND LABORATORY ASSESSMENT IN THE PSYCHIATRIC EVALUATION

Psychiatric evaluations can be conveniently divided into those that take place in the *psychiatric* setting (inpatient psychiatric hospital, outpatient psychiatry clinic, psychiatry consultation service, or other situations in which the patient expects to see a psychiatrist for possible psychiatric problems) and those that take place in the *medical* (nonpsychiatric) setting. In the first situation, patients are referred or are being treated specifically for psychiatric problems. In the second instance, the patient's principal problem probably is nonpsychiatric in nature, but psychiatric factors could be involved. Because misconceptions exist about what constitutes an appropriate psychiatric evaluation in these two situations, they will be addressed separately.

Psychiatric Evaluation in a Psychiatric Setting

The principal features of the psychiatric evaluation are the *psychiatric history* and the *mental status examination*. These establish the presence of a psychiatric syndrome. A medical history, physical examination, and laboratory assessment also are included in psychiatric evaluations, although little emphasis is placed on their role during medical training when patients are assumed to have "primarily psychiatric problems." *Because 30 to 50% of psychiatric inpatients and outpatients have medical disease concurrent with their psychiatric symptoms (LaBruzza, 1981), 5 to 30% of which either actually cause or exacerbate the psychiatric problem, it is inappropriate for psychiatrists or medical students to neglect the medical part of the evaluation in patients with psychiatric symptoms.*

It is not reasonable to expect psychiatrists to complete a medical history and a physical examination every time they see a patient, just as it is not logical for primary care physicians to perform complete psychiatric examinations on all the patients they see. In two studies, medical findings in 45% of psychiatric patients led to reconsideration of the psychiatric diagnosis, and in 6 to 9% they led to a *major* alteration in the approach to treatment (Hoffman, 1982; Chandler and Gerndt, 1988). *It is therefore essential to include the physical examination as an integral part of the psychiatric evaluation in all first-time inpatients and outpatients being appraised for a psychiatric disease.* This point is particularly true when the risk for a metabolic or neurologic component is high, such as in patients over 50 years old, in those with atypical psychiatric presentations or adverse (or no) responses to treatment for disorders in which improvement should be expected, or in patients with known or suspected underlying medical conditions that could contribute to their symptoms.

Psychiatric Evaluation in the Medical Setting

Medical students are usually taught psychiatric evaluation in *psychiatric* settings. In most medical centers, little or no instruction is given for initiating psychiatric questions in patients seen in primarily medical settings, despite the fact that 80% of patients with psychiatric conditions are seen by primary care specialists (Regier et al., 1978). Medical students frequently are indoctrinated with the idea that "nonpsychiatric patients shouldn't be asked embarrassing psychiatric questions." The end result of this advice is that, in their future practices, psychiatric problems in many if not most of their primary care patients are overlooked.

Psychiatrists have little difficulty asking patients referred for psychiatric evaluation personal and confidential questions. That, after all, is what psychiatrists are trained to do. Medical patients, however, come to see nonpsychiatric physicians for "physical" problems. To embark on a series of psychological questions usually is unexpected and may be viewed initially by the patient as an invasion of privacy unless the reasons for the questions are explained or the patient can be led to see a possible connection to the presenting complaint or general condition. The patient also may be both relieved and reassured that the physician is interested in him or her "as a person" and may use the opportunity to express worries and emotional and psychological distress.

Because psychiatric questions are not asked routinely in the medical setting, psychiatric illness frequently remains undetected, or, alternatively, a psychiatric illness may be presumptively diagnosed without just cause. The prevalence of mental illness, the availability of effective treatments for many psychiatric disorders, and the harm of inappropriate diagnosis make it imperative that all physicians develop the skills for initiating psychiatric evaluations. Nothing can replace specific psychiatric questions in documenting the presence or absence of a psychiatric disorder.

Psychiatric Interviewing

The psychiatric interview is an interaction between patient and physician designed to assess psychiatric status or to provide treatment of an emotional or behavioral problem. During the first interview, patients typically describe their perception of the difficulty. The physician clarifies the chief complaint and enhances the patient's history by observing the patient's behavior during the interaction (*infra vide*) and listening to the patient's responses to open-ended questions. During this encounter, the physician should establish a rapport, if possible, by being honest and straightforward during the interview, by showing empathy for the patient's condition or situation, and by demonstrating his or her willingness and ability to improve the patient's problem.

Ideally, when the patient is coherent, the patient and physician arrive at a general understanding of the nature of the problem and agree on the form and duration of treatment. This approach clearly and unambiguously defines the limits of the relationship, the goals, and the expectations of each party. Such an approach is particularly important when working with patients with certain psychiatric disorders. For instance, patients with psychotic disorders or borderline/antisocial personality disorders often distort, misinterpret, or manipulate what is said; thus, initial clarification and guidelines are necessary.

Certain critical ingredients are important during the initial interview. First, *adequate time* should be set aside for the interview. This entails not only time to obtain the necessary information to make a diagnosis but also time to initiate the interview on a personal note. Patients can then feel that you are seeing and treating them as individuals. Second, if possible, steps should be taken to ensure that there are no interruptions. Third, the patient should be put at ease. Such details as providing adequate space for patient movement, equal eye level of the examiner and patient, the presence or absence of other support personnel or the patient's acquaintances, and limiting noise can make significant differences in the patient's willingness to share pertinent information about problems. Fourth, note-taking should be limited, especially if it makes the patient feel uncomfortable. These simple, seemingly inconsequential details can affect not only the type of behavior demonstrated and information obtained during the initial interview but also the course of treatment. Finally, if the situation permits, the physician should usually *sit down* when speaking to the patient and avoid standing over and shifting around him or her when standing at their bedside.

There are some who consider the psychiatric interview to be different and distinct from the interview performed in primary care. In fact, considerable importance is given to observing behavior and obtaining data related to psychiatric issues during the general medical history-taking process (Bates and Hoekelman, 1983). The primary care physician, however, is usually dealing with signs and symptoms of medical conditions in the absence of psychiatric involvement. Therefore, observations such as the color of the patient's skin, the rapidity of his or her breathing, and the coarseness of a tremor take on greater clinical importance. When complaints in the primary care setting point to a psychiatric problem, nonpsychiatric physicians, like psychiatrists, merely need to extend their observations to include mood, behavior, and thought processes. Additional questions to confirm or deny the presence of a psychiatric syndrome complete the history. There is no magic in this as long as the basics about psychiatric syndromes and symptoms are known.

A good deal of emphasis in psychiatry is placed on the interpretation of answers to questions or manifest behaviors. When a patient who obviously looks depressed because of poor eye contact, tearfulness, apparent fatigue, latency of response, or stooped posture says he or she does not feel sad (essentially denying being depressed), how should this be handled? It is best to take what the patient says at face value initially and try to make sense of it in relation to the remainder of the clinical picture before suggesting that the patient is unable to identify emotions, is unable to report accurately, is lying, or is massively denying. It is just as possible that the patient with the symptoms described above is suffering from anemia or cancer.

Psychiatric interviews are designed to be predominantly diagnostic or therapeutic, but elements of both are often contained in initial evaluations. Primarily diagnostic interviews detect and characterize psychiatric illness. Interviews arranged to follow the course of psychiatric illness or response to therapy might also be considered partly diagnostic because they provide a steady flow of information that allows for ongoing assessment of the patient's condition. Therapeutic interviews involve the use of psychotherapeutic techniques. These are primarily intended to provide treatment in the form of support, reassurance, and exploration of the patient's past history and current stresses to facilitate expression of painful feelings and to provide insight.

The form of psychotherapy employed may influence the nature of patient questioning beyond that required to make a DSM-IV diagnosis. For example, the cognitive therapist might pursue details regarding the manner in which one deals with current life problems, whereas the psychoanalyst or psychodynamically oriented psychiatrist might be interested in details regarding one's perceptions of, and emotional reactions to, historical life events. These forms of therapy and special interview techniques will be covered elsewhere in this text (see Chapter 17).

In addition to gathering historical data narrated by the patient, the physician derives diagnostic data by observing and assessing the patient's appearance, behavior, and various aspects of mental functioning during the interview process. Thus, in addition to assessing the *content* of the patient's history, the psychiatrist routinely looks beyond the narrative to assess the patient's mental apparatus that perceives, formulates, and elaborates the history and the behavior that emanates from it. This will provide objective data in a manner analogous to the physical examination of the internist. For example, patients with major depression frequently demonstrate poor eye contact, stooped posture, latency of response, and psychomotor retardation. When a patient presents with a history that corresponds with the clinical picture, an initial diagnosis can be made with more confidence.

The importance of documenting information from both the history (including history provided by the patient's family) and direct observation of the patient is essential because signs and symptoms during the interview may be limited. For instance, there are medical conditions that show no evidence of disease on physical examination (e.g., migraine headache), just as there are patients with certain psychiatric conditions who may demonstrate completely normal mental function and behavior during the examination (e.g., alcohol dependence, eating disorders, sexual disorders, and so forth). The reverse is also true for patients with dementia, who may have no idea that problems exist, although their behavior may demonstrate the opposite.

One means of acquiring more accurate information as well as a better understanding of the mental and emotional state is to perform the interview using open-ended, unstructured questions. Many medical and psychiatric interviews resemble interrogations, with rapid-fire questions that require yes or no answers and leave almost no chance for the patient to elaborate on his or her own perception of the problem, much less express painful emotions or experiences. Avoiding leading questions allows patients to provide an unbiased account of their perception of the problem. Contextually accurate information is obtained by following the patient's lead with questions directed at clarifying or enlarging on historical items. As the interview progresses, it may become increasingly structured and specific to fill in details and to complete the history, as detailed in following sections.

Many physicians are afraid of open-ended, unstructured questions because time constraints do not allow the luxury that questioning during numerous hour-long psychotherapy sessions provides. For this reason, psychiatric questions are often avoided altogether. Nonetheless, a limited amount of time devoted to this type of questioning is essential for a more accurate diagnostic impression, regardless of time constraints. The accomplished physician develops skill in providing a balance between the open-ended, person-to-person questions and the single-answer questions that are required to make a diagnosis. In this way, critical information from and about the patient can be obtained while controlling interviewing time and maintaining a more predictable schedule.

Factors Affecting the Interview

Patients present to psychiatrists in a variety of situations that greatly influence the form of the interview, the nature of patient–physician interaction, and the overall goals. These situations range from the highly functioning patient presenting for an outpatient evaluation of a moderate depression to the emergency evaluation of a hostile, psychotic patient taken to the emergency room in restraints by police officers, as in the case presented at the beginning of this chapter. In the first situation (moderate depression in an outpatient), one might obtain a meticulous psychiatric and medical history, physical and mental status examination, and screening laboratory evaluation. Such interviews facilitate therapeutic decision making. In the situation of an agitated, medically ill alcoholic, the evaluation would initially include documenting the presence of delirium, performing the physical examination, and admitting the patient for inpatient care. Only later, when information can be obtained from charts, relatives, and the patient, when he or she becomes better controlled, will a comprehensive, accurate understanding of the case become possible.

Other factors also may influence the ability to conduct a thorough psychiatric interview. For instance, some patients may be so fatigued from medical illness that they require a concise interview. Alternatively, some patients refuse to cooperate. Often this can be a clue to their diagnosis, as in the case of a patient with borderline personality or paranoid disorder. In such cases, additional information from the patient's doctor, nursing personnel, or descriptions in the chart can provide valuable insight into the nature and cause of the patient's difficulties and lead perhaps to more effective management. Thus, the skilled interviewer must be flexible and ever mindful of not only the details of a patient's psychiatric condition but also the interwoven social, legal, and medical factors that complicate psychiatric assessment and intervention.

Specific Interview Situations

Although each patient is unique, necessitating a flexible and individualized interview style, many psychiatric disorders influence aspects of the interview in a manner that is predictable and characteristic of that disorder. Thus, the following comments are not intended to offer a "cookbook" approach to these patients but rather offer suggestions in the interpretation and planning of specific interview situations.

The Depressed Patient

A prominent feature of severe depression is the tendency for all perceptions to be colored by bleakness and pessimism. When the history is taken, therefore, it is essential to keep in mind that many descriptions presented by the patient in a negative light by way of his depressed state may actually be more positive or at least neutral. For example, it is common for depressed patients to think that they are going bankrupt or doing terrible things to family and friends. Information from other sources may reveal that the situation is not nearly so dismal.

Depressed patients are often in desperate need of hope and reassurance. They may repeatedly ask whether they are a bad person or if they can be helped. Nonetheless, when reassurance is provided, it may be received with quiet skepticism and generally results in only temporary relief.

Depressed persons often have their own ways of accounting for suffering. For example, they may be convinced that they are being justly punished by God for transgressions. Such beliefs may become delusional in psychotic depressions, such as when patients think they have committed the "unforgivable" sin; think they, or the world, no longer exists (nihilism); or think they are riddled with cancer (somatic). Explaining that such ideas are the result of depression and will go away with treatment offers momentary hope but is unlikely to alter their opinion until improvement occurs.

The Psychotic Patient

The term *psychosis* includes a broad range of clinical presentations unified by loss of contact with reality and the presence of delusions or hallucinations. Such presentations range from the patient who appears to function normally (with the exception of a well-circumscribed paranoid delusional system) to the acutely disorganized, agitated, vividly hallucinating patient. The severity of the patient's thought disorder and degree of departure from reality will determine the structure of the interview. The former patient may be able to provide a history that is complete and reliable with the exception of issues relating to the delusional system. When the patient discusses these beliefs, details should be sought regarding the nature and extent of the delusions and how the patient makes sense of them. These details, as well as the degree of conviction in the delusional beliefs, can be followed to assess the course of and response to treatment. When delusions are persecutory in nature, the patient may be reluctant or unwilling to provide information or even consent to be interviewed for fear that the interviewer is an agent of the persecutory process. Such was the situation in the case presented earlier.

When a patient is floridly psychotic, the interview may involve little more than observing the patient as findings are noted. Interacting with such patients often provides stimulation that may make evidence of psychosis more apparent. In addition to grossly distorting reality, acutely psychotic patients are often very frightened. Both of these factors can result in unpredictable and, rarely, even violent behavior. While such patients should be treated with kindness and understanding, necessary precautions must be taken. *Florid psychosis should not deter the physician from performing the physical examination or laboratory assessment, although special care and techniques may be required. These are essential to rule out a neurologic, metabolic, or toxic cause for the psychosis.* (See also Chapters 4, 5, and 19.)

The Hostile Patient

When assessing a hostile patient, interviewers must take whatever precautions are necessary to ensure their safety. The initial step is identification of the potentially violent patient. Clues include a previous history of violent behavior such as that often seen in patients with antisocial personality disorder, alcoholism, and substance abuse; a paranoid psychosis; and a person who is angry and threatening violence, even in the absence of a psychiatric disorder.

One sensitive indicator of whether the situation is becoming dangerous is your emotional response to the patient's behavior, that is, your "gut level" reaction. If the interviewer feels uncomfortable or fearful of the patient, precautions should be taken *immediately* to ensure safety. If concern is minimal, precaution may involve nothing more than sitting between the patient and an open door or making sure other personnel are nearby. When the index of concern is higher, one or several security officers—without guns—may be stationed in the interview area or be used to restrain the patient if needed during the interview. Such precautions are often a relief to confused, psychotic, or agitated patients because they provide the situation with structure and absolve patients of the necessity of making decisions at a time when they may not be in control of their actions. Chapter 19 on emergency psychiatry also discusses special considerations in interviewing violent and hostile patients.

The Somatic Patient

Many psychiatric disorders manifest somatic symptoms in which a medical disorder is not readily found. These include conversion disorder, hypochondriasis, somatization disorder, and nonspecific complaints associated with anxiety or depression. Such complaints, however, may just as likely be the result of medical disease too early in onset to diagnose due to insensitivity of the physical examination and laboratory tests; a medical problem more benign than the evaluation needed to diagnose it; or merely the patient's attempt to receive attention. Care must be taken, therefore, in diagnosing somatoform disorders (see Chapter 9).

A convenient way to categorize patients with unexplained somatic complaints is to determine whether the complaints are *single or multiple*. If the somatic complaint is single, the evaluation should proceed until a physical cause has been reasonably excluded *and* a psychiatric cause is deemed possible. This may entail no more than a careful history with a brief physical examination, but occasionally it requires more extensive testing.

If the complaints are multiple and somatization disorder is a possibility, then symptoms must be *seriously listened to*, but only objective evidence of disease on basic evaluation should lead to further workup. At the first evaluation, time should be taken to obtain a directed history about the main complaint and each complaint with a potentially dangerous cause. A complete physical examination and basic laboratory evaluation (if not already done) are required. Records from prior physicians and hospitals are particularly helpful and should be obtained before further workup unless eminent problems are evident. Any objective finding on the physical examination or laboratory evaluation should prompt further investigation or treatment after the nature and extent of previous evaluations have been delineated. It should also be noted that some patients have a very limited "psychological vocabulary," and when in emotional distress communicate their feelings predominately in physical or somatic terms. This trait has been called *somatothymic* and is a very common form of "affective language" in many cultures worldwide and in certain types of patients in the United States (Stoudemire, 1991a & b). This concept is discussed further in Chapter 9.

In patients with multiple somatic complaints, the physician should place particular emphasis on the terms of agreement regarding specific responsibilities of physician and patient. The physician should agree to evaluate symptoms when deemed appropriate and to follow the patient at regular intervals to assess change. The patient should allow the physician adequate time to complete the evaluation and should seek no other medical evaluations unless consent is first obtained from the physician. This approach will not guarantee ease in caring for such patients but may result in the development of rapport and trust, which are essential if the patient's suffering is to be eased and the pursuit of evaluations slowed. The diagnosis and management of patients with chronic somatic complaints is further discussed in Chapter 9.

The Psychiatric History

Many psychiatric patients make the process of obtaining an accurate history a challenge for a variety of reasons. First, they may have illnesses, such as dementia or delirium, that prevent them from revealing details related to the onset and type of symptoms that brought them to the physician's attention. Second, they may wish to hide salient facts related to their difficulties because of embarrassment, mistrust, or outright deception. Third, they may present with symptoms that follow a variable pattern or are difficult to describe. It is for these reasons that *obtaining additional information from a second or, preferably, a third and fourth source, such as family members, friends, or police,* as well as scrutinizing available information in the patient's records, is *critical* to assure that the correct diagnosis is made and appropriate treatment is given. Table 1–1 outlines the main sections of the psychiatric history. Important factors related to each part of the psychiatric history are enumerated below.

Identifying Information

Chief Complaint

Often the patient's chief complaint differs from the examining physician's perception of the problem. In this situation the primary problem that the patient perceives should be addressed first while the "real" problem waits. In this way the patient is indirectly told that his or her complaint is important, thus creating an alliance in trying to clarify and relieve both the perceived and the "real" problem.

History of Present Illness

As with any medical evaluation, clarification of the chief psychiatric complaint lies at the heart of the psychiatric history. Pertinent information includes

Table 1–1 **The Psychiatric History**

Identifying Information
   Sociodemographic Summary
Chief Complaint
History of Present Illness
   Extended Information About Chief Complaint
   Onset
   Duration/Course
   Precipitants
   Exaggerating and Alleviating Factors
Psychiatric Review of Systems
   Psychological Symptom Inventory
   Review of Major DSM-IV Psychiatric Diagnostic Symptoms
Medical History
Personal/Family History of Psychiatric Disorders and Treatment
Personal History
   Prenatal/Birth History
   Childhood
   Adolescence
   Adulthood
     Educational
     Occupational
     Interpersonal/Social
     Sexual (Table 1–2)
     Habits—Alcohol, other Drugs

an accurate description of the difficulty, the mode of onset and duration, the course of the symptoms (steady, intermittent, progressively worse), exacerbating and alleviating factors (medication, position, time of day), and factors such as recent deaths or illnesses in the family, marital or family relationship problems, financial or legal problems, medical illness, problems at work, or intractable social problems where the patient feels unable to cope, possibly associated with the onset and continuation of the symptoms. These details relevant to the chief complaint are supplemented with pertinent features from the past medical and psychiatric history, past personal history, family history, sexual history, and review of systems. The objective in obtaining this information is to typify the difficulty that the patient is experiencing, to establish whether it warrants psychiatric diagnosis, and to consider ways in which the problem might be alleviated, whether or not a psychiatric disease is present.

Information obtained in this data-gathering section of the interview is coupled with observations made during the interaction with the patient that constitutes part of the mental status examination. It is important that the patient's history and clinical presentation be consistent with the psychiatric condition under consideration; otherwise, alternative explanations should be explored. As might be recalled in the study by Rosenhan alluded to earlier using "fake" patients presenting with complaints of hearing "hollow," "thud," and "empty" (auditory hallucinations?), there was neither a syndrome picture (early age of onset, chronic deteriorating clinical course, and so forth) nor other past or present clinical signs (thought disorder, blunted affect, ambivalence, anhedonia) that suggested schizophrenia as a primary diagnostic entity.

Review of Systems

One of the principal ways in which unexplained somatic complaints are identified is through a review of the symptoms the patient has experienced. The review of systems also serves as a means of reviewing potential medical causes for the principal complaint of the patient. Frequently it will uncover a problem that has a direct and pertinent relation to the chief complaint. Each positive finding on the review of systems should be understood well enough to know whether further investigation is needed. Such investigation may include anything from a spot physical examination to an invasive X-ray procedure.

In medical settings, most patients with psychiatric problems initially present with *physical* symptoms (such as in depression). Physical symptoms of anxiety and depression may be mixed with symptoms of concurrent underlying medical illness as well, thus further complicating the clinical assessment. For example, somatic symptoms associated with depression include sleep fragmentation (usually early morning awakening with an inability to get back to sleep), headaches, constipation, physical fatigue, decreased appetite, weight loss, and gastrointestinal distress.

Psychophysiological symptoms of anxiety include palpitations, tachycardia, diaphoresis, hyperventilation, diarrhea, urinary urgency and frequency, restlessness, chronic fatigue, insomnia, dry mouth, blurred vision, nausea, vomiting, chest pain, dizziness, choking, difficulty swallowing, headaches, muscle aches, and pain. Patients with schizophrenia will occasionally have bizarre physical sensations such as their brain dissolving or body parts feeling disconnected. Patients with somatoform disorders such as hypochondriasis are preoccupied with physical complaints to an excessive, unrealistic degree. Hence, while somatic complaints are nonspecific, they often constitute a predominant component of the signs and symptoms of psychiatric disorders. Care must be taken, however, since it is all too easy to ascribe a physical complaint to a psychiatric condition when, in fact, it is caused by an underlying medical illness.

Medical History

Any medical history pertinent to the chief complaint is included in the history of the present illness. Such information usually becomes evident during the careful questioning used in delineating the chief complaint. Thus, current medical illnesses, which might be contributing to the symptoms and medications, and familial medical illnesses that are known to be associated with the development of psychiatric symptoms would be enumerated in the history of present illness and their possible association with the current psychiatric condition suggested.

In addition to the review of pertinent physical factors in the history of present illness, other seemingly less-relevant medical or surgical difficulties, allergies, and medications should also be recorded. Even though they may not be helpful in understanding the patient's reason for seeking psychiatric assistance, they frequently become important when assessing the need for additional information concerning the patient's case when deciding on the type of treatment to be given. For instance, in the case of RH, if it had been known that he had a bleeding disorder, then the bruise on his head might have precipitated a more extensive neurologic investigation before the development of the seizure.

Personal and Family History
of Psychiatric Disorders and Treatment

As with the past medical history, pertinent past psychiatric history related to the chief complaint should be included in the history of present illness. *The longitudinal course of psychiatric symptoms and responses to treatment is one of the most important ingredients in making a psychiatric diagnosis.* It is known, for instance, that alcoholism often begins in the teenage years to the 20s, has a fluctuating but progressive course unless the individual maintains prolonged abstinence, and often leads to chronic disability. Had patient RH had a good premorbid history and only started drinking weeks to months before his admission, then the primary diagnosis of alcoholism with alcohol withdrawal delirium (delirium tremens) would have become suspect. Alternative explanations for the drinking behavior and delirium would have been required.

Other factors related to the psychiatric history should be reported under a separate heading. Even though no apparent relation to the current presentation can be shown, they can sometimes provide additional insight into the patient's problem and may alter the course of treatment or investigation. Past suicide attempts should be carefully documented.

Specific questions that delineate the past psychiatric history include the following: First, patients can be asked, using colloquial terms, if they have ever had difficulties with nerves or emotions or whether or not they have ever had a "nervous breakdown." Often patients will not remember or do not think they should reply in the affirmative unless they were hospitalized for the problem. Therefore, patients should be asked whether they have been given medication by a primary physician for "nerves" or emotional problems or whether they have seen a counselor, pastor, psychologist, social worker, or physician for counseling.

Second, patients should be asked if there has ever been a time when they felt they needed help but did not get it. Hence, the history should involve both untreated and formally treated bouts of psychiatric illness. If the patient did get treatment, where did they get it and for how long were they treated? Were they ever hospitalized for a psychiatric problem? If they did get treatment, including medications, what drugs were given and what was their response? Were there any side effects that caused problems?

Third, and perhaps most important, the same questions should be asked of someone who knows the patient well enough to confirm or deny the patient's answers.

A family history of psychiatric illness is crucial, because certain psychiatric disorders have a genetic component (schizophrenia, mood disorders, alcoholism, Alzheimer's disease) (Baron, 1994). In fact, a strong family history of affective disorder can be used to reinforce a diagnostic impression in a patient with an otherwise confusing presentation. It is important to ask about the nature of symptoms, type of treatment (medication or electroconvulsive treatment), response to treatment, complications, and hospitalizations for involved family members. A family history of suicide and violence should also be elicited.

Personal History

The personal history includes information about the patient's relationships, schooling, employment, personal achievements and failings, and goals. As might be expected, each of these areas can impact in a major way on the course and duration of psychiatric symptoms.

A person's prenatal history and development through the various stages of infancy, childhood, and adolescence are the principal areas of interest in the personal development section of the examination. Items such as birth trauma, developmental physical and emotional milestones, illnesses, parental and sibling relationships, important memories, rewards and punishments, exposure to abuse, and the establishment of independence are addressed. Major milestones, frustrations, and problems in childhood and adolescence should be identified, when appropriate, along with the quality of family and peer relationships during each phase of development.

One frequently *unasked* question is whether or not sexual molestation occurred as a child. Patients should be asked about sexual molestation in a frank and straightforward manner, although some tact may be required. For example, one might ask, "Were you ever sexually molested or attacked as a child by anyone—including members of your family?" Most patients harbor severe shame and guilt about incest in particular, requiring special sensitivity to this issue in the session.

When pursuing a psychodynamic understanding of the patient's problems, a chronological picture of the patient's developmental history—including their adult history—should be reconstructed, and events or experiences that may have been psychologically or emotionally traumatic should be noted. Past life experiences that appear to correlate with current life events or stresses should be noted by the examiner and explored with the patient.

Social History

This part of the psychiatric history recounts the patient's educational background and functioning in the school system; encounters with the law; lawsuits or criminal connections; premarital, marital, postmarital, and extramarital relationships; relationships and problems with children; employment (types, frequency of change, reasons for job changes, compensation issues) and fiscal responsibility; military history (assignment and nature of discharge, history of combat experience); and personal goals and expectations. Criminal charges, arrests, convictions, or time served in prison should be carefully addressed, as should the circumstances leading up to the encounter with the law. During the process of gathering this information, the physician can identify areas in the patient's life that might serve as precipitating stresses or recurrent patterns of problematic social relationships. *All social factors of importance to the presenting complaint should be included in the history of present illness, while the remainder are recorded under the personal or social history section of the examination.*

When considering those areas of the social history that may be stresses involved in precipitating the patient's presenting complaint, it should be remembered that life is literally a "series of crises." It is always possible to point to a flat tire, fight with a relative or friend, failed test, or unpaid bill as a potential stressor for the development of symptoms. A means of placing social factors in proper perspective is to establish whether current stressors in relation to other stressors the patient has previously experienced are of sufficient magnitude to influence the patient's ability to cope.

Interpersonal Relationships. Of major importance in the patient's social history is the nature, pattern, and stability of his or her interpersonal relationships, whether they relate to romantic involvements, friendships, occupational relationships, or relationships with authorities. For example, is the patient capable of forming stable relationships based on trust? Is the patient capable of forming close friendships? What is the pattern of the patient's romantic and sexual involvements? How successful have they been in working with peers and for those in authority? Problematic patterns in interpersonal and social relationships often indicate the presence of a personality disorder. One of the cardinal symptoms of a personality disorder is the tendency of the individual to "repeat mistakes" in their interpersonal and social relationships, to fail to learn from experience, and to assign fault to others rather than to accept responsibility for their life difficulties.

The Sexual History. There are occasional situations in which the sexual history is of significant importance in understanding the patient's problem. Certainly basic questions concerning sexual function, such as whether the patient is sexually active, what the sexual preference is, and whether there is concern about a venereal disease, should always be asked, because most persons cannot be expected to volunteer such information. When the problem involves potential difficulty within relationships, sexual deviancy, or other problems that may influence sexual function, then more detailed information may be necessary. Because this area of questioning is highly personal, the physician may encounter more resistance than in other areas of the examination. As the doctor–patient relationship becomes better established, however, patients will often become more willing to talk about such matters. Details of a comprehensive sexual history are listed in Table 1–2 and are also discussed in Chapter 14. Physicians should focus on various parts of the history as the clinical situation dictates.

Alcohol and Substance Dependency/Abuse. Obtaining a substance-abuse history should be of paramount importance in the history given the prevalence of alcoholism and drug abuse in our society. Use of alcohol, cocaine, marijuana, stimulants, sedative-hypnotics, analgesic opiates, and sleeping pills should be rigorously investigated, including age at first use, frequency of use, amount, and complications in the inter-personal, occupational, medical, and legal spheres that may have resulted. A history of the results of intoxication, withdrawal, and "bad trips" should be explored. The use of caffeine (coffee, tea, soft drinks, chocolate) is almost always overlooked by examiners, even though caffeine may be addicting and is associated with a withdrawal syndrome. The use of tobacco products—perhaps the most lethal substance abused in our

Table 1–2 Basic Sexual History
(Modified to Age of Patient and Clinical Circumstances)

Introductory comments about why the interview is being conducted and its routine or special nature given the clinical situation at hand; reassurance about confidentiality
Open-ended question to give the patient an opportunity to voice any areas of special worry or concern regarding the part of the interview or sexual concerns in general
Source of information about sex in growing up
Attitudes of the parents toward sex
Age of onset of puberty
Age of menarche and menstrual history in women
Age of first intense romantic or sexually oriented relationship
History of childhood molestation or incest
History of venereal diseases
Attitudes about masturbation and frequency of masturbation
Age of first intercourse; number of partners
General pattern of attraction to person of the opposite or same sex; general patterns of heterosexuality or homosexuality
Abortions, miscarriages, pregnancies
Method(s) of birth control
Frequency of current sexual activity and its nature
Physical discomfort with sexual activity:
  Men: Problem with arousal or achieving/maintaining erection, ejaculation control
  Women: Problems with arousal, lubrication, achieving orgasm, physical comfort with intercourse
Conflicts in relationship or marriage over sexual matters: frequency, methods of birth control, sexual dysfunction
Medications or illness that seem to negatively affect sexual desire or functioning
Issues regarding decision to avoid or achieve conception and have children
Risk factors for AIDS or other concerns regarding this disease

(From Becker J, Hunter JA: Human sexual development. In Stoudemire A (ed): Human Behavior: An Introduction for Medical Students. 2nd Ed. Philadelphia, JB Lippincott, 1994)

society—should also be documented. Pertinent aspects of the substance use history are also discussed in Chapter 10.

Assimilation of the Psychiatric History

When a psychiatric syndrome is suggested by the information gathered during the psychiatric history, only the beginning of the diagnostic process has been completed. Depressive symptoms, anxiety symptoms, psychosis, and symptoms from most other psychiatric syndromes can, after all, be caused by a spectrum of psychiatric and medical diseases and can even be seen in some normal individuals. For instance, some clinicians automatically think that patients who meet criteria for major depression develop their symptoms in response to a primary psychiatric illness. Medical conditions such as hypothyroidism and cancer are frequently responsible for the production or exacerbation of depression or symptoms that mimic depression. Even patients with other psychiatric conditions, such as somatization disorder or alcoholism, can have a depressive symptom complicating their primary psychiatric condition. It is for these reasons that the psychiatric history should not be limited to the identification of symptom complexes themselves but should incorporate pertinent medical, personal, and social information to complete the assessment. This additional information can have a substantial impact on the approach taken in the patient's treatment.

Preparing Medical Patients for Psychiatric Evaluation

How can a physician lead into psychiatric screening questions without antagonizing the patient? First, it cannot be done in every case. Regardless of how tactful you are, some may be offended at first. Table 1–3 outlines a way to decrease the likelihood of offending medical patients. This approach will often "break the ice" and allow the patients to describe areas in their lives that have been troubling but that they find difficult to discuss. Occasionally these questions will lead to the most dreaded reactions of all: "What! Do you think I'm putting this on?" or "Do you think this is all in my head?" or "Do you think I'm crazy?" In response to this, the patient might be told, "Emotional factors and stress can influence physical symptoms (some people get headaches, some ulcers from stress—the medical problem is real but can be triggered by stress). I routinely ask these and other questions of all my patients so that I can give the best and most appropriate treatment and don't miss anything important." There-

Table 1–3 **Initiating Psychiatric Questions**
in Patients with Nonpsychiatric Complaints

Discuss and define the nonpsychiatric problem with the patient first (it may be related to the emotional problem).

If there is some question about whether the nonpsychiatric complaint is "real," do not challenge the patient with this possibility. You don't have to state that you feel the complaint is or isn't real, but you can acknowledge the patient's perception of its presence.

Ask, "Do you think your symptom(s) is (are) affected by nerves or emotions?" "Do you think that your symptom(s) is (are) related to stress?"

after, additional psychiatric screening questions (Table 1–4) can be asked if circumstances warrant. If screening questions are positive, a more detailed psychiatric history can be obtained.

When Is It Appropriate to Ask Medical Patients Psychiatric Questions?

In many patients, psychiatric illness with or without concurrent medical illness is readily apparent. Presence of a persistent and pervasive depressed mood, frank psychosis, or an agitated confusional state are clear indications to pursue further psychiatric evaluation. Unfortunately, psychiatric illness is often not so apparent. The following indicators are helpful in detecting patients with psychiatric disorders presenting in a subtle or ambiguous manner: (1) nonresponse to treatment in situations in which it is usually effective (particularly true when litigation is pending); (2) multiple somatic complaints not accounted for by known medical conditions or symptoms not conforming to the bounds of anatomy or physiology; (3) a chaotic lifestyle (e.g., unstable relationships, frequent job changes, substance abuse, frequent legal problems, and so forth); (4) a history of "hopping" from one physician to another (doctor shopping); (5) symptoms related to stress, anxiety, or depression; (6) a personal or family history of psychiatric illness; (7) a degree of disability or resultant lifestyle changes out of proportion to symptoms; and (8) suspected or known alcohol and substance abuse. Although none of these indicators is pathognomonic, they suggest the possibility of psychiatric illness.

Table 1–4 **Psychiatric Screening Questions for Patients in the Primary Care Setting**

Depression

"Have you been feeling sad or depressed? Is this accompanied by trouble with sleep or appetite, low energy, or decreased interest in doing things? Do you have feelings of guilt or thoughts of harming yourself?"

Mania

"Do you feel on top of the world? Is this out of proportion to your usual self such that you talk more, don't need as much sleep, your thoughts race, or your enthusiasm gets you into trouble?"

Psychosis

"Have you heard or seen things that others didn't? Do you feel that you have special powers? Have you felt that others were watching or following you? Have you received peculiar or special messages or felt that others knew or controlled your thoughts?"

Alcoholism

"Have others thought you had a drinking problem? Has drinking alcohol caused problems with friends or relatives, caused you to miss work or lose a job, resulted in arrest, or caused health problems? Do you use recreational drugs?"

Anxiety disorder

"Have you had trouble with nervousness, anxiety, or feeling like you are going to panic?"

Anorexia nervosa

"Do you take special measures to keep your weight at its current level?"

Perhaps of equal importance are factors indicating that psychiatric illness should be viewed with a relatively *lower* index of suspicion than other possible causes of the patient's symptoms. This is particularly important because inappropriately labeling a patient's symptoms as "psychiatric" can lead to delay in identifying the correct primary diagnosis. Items in this category include (1) any *objective* finding on physical examination or laboratory evaluation that appears directly related to the symptom; (2) previous emotional *stability* as reflected by work responsibilities, family relationships, and personal endeavors, in a person with questionable "psychiatric" symptoms; (3) an unusual psychiatric presentation of the characteristics of the possible psychiatric syndrome under consideration; and (4) the lack of any acute or chronic stressors in the patient's life. It is in these patients that there is a high risk of labeling the symptoms "psychiatric" when there actually is an underlying medical disease. This brings us to the importance of the physical assessment as part of the evaluation process.

Physical Examination

The physical examination is currently included in 0 to 11% of outpatient psychiatric evaluations and in 4 to 40% of inpatient evaluations (Krummel and Kathol, 1987). Ideally, all psychiatric patients should receive a physical examination. Unfortunately, many psychiatrists, like other medical specialists, logically focus their examination on areas related to their specialty. Few "primary" psychiatric diagnoses can be confirmed by positive findings on the physical examination; thus, it is often bypassed altogether.

Of what importance, then, is the physical examination in the evaluation of psychiatric patients? Unlike many subspecialties in medicine, psychiatry deals with clinical presentations that frequently have as their origin a primary medical disorder that causes the patient's symptoms. The list for major depression alone includes diseases from most organ systems (Hall, 1980). To exclude an underlying medical disorder as a cause of the patient's symptoms, a systematic evaluation is required that traditionally has included a physical examination.

The next obvious question is whether clinical tradition is correct in requiring the performance of a physical examination as a part of the assessment, because most medical diagnoses are made from historical information alone. Hampton, Harrison, Mitchell et al (1975) answered this question when they found that the physical examination confirmed, denied, or narrowed the differential diagnosis arrived at from historical information in 30% of patients in a primary medical setting. In 7.5% it uncovered unexpected yet important findings that led to the diagnosis of a disease that was not necessarily related to the chief complaint. Considering that Chandler and Gerndt (1988) showed similar findings in 224 consecutively examined psychiatric inpatients, the need for a physical examination to confirm or deny medical factors is evident. It is for these reasons that psychiatrists should include a physical examination in psychiatric patients at risk for medical illness co-morbidity. This would include (1) any new patient with a psychiatric disorder, (2) patients older than 50 years of age, (3) patients with an unusual psychiatric presentation or response to treatment,

(4) patients with medical conditions known to cause or exacerbate psychiatric symptoms, and (5) patients with significant complaints from the review of systems.

There are some clinicians who think that adding a neurological examination to the psychiatric interview is sufficient to exclude most underlying medical causes of psychiatric symptoms. Although there are certainly a number of neurologic conditions that can cause behavioral or emotional problems (Taylor, Sierles, and Abrams, 1987), medical illness frequently mimics psychiatric disorders (Chandler and Gerndt, 1988). For this reason, it is important to perform a complete physical examination. Hall, Gardiner, Stickney et al (1980) showed that a cursory physical examination was unreliable in identifying physical changes when they were present; thus, a complete physical is required. When findings are identified, they should be explained and treated along with the psychiatric manifestations accompanying them.

The scope of this chapter does not allow individual treatment of the different sections of the physical examination. These can be reviewed in Bates' (1983) *A Guide to Physical Examination*. A word can be said, however, about the difficulties that are encountered in performing the physical examination in the psychiatric setting. This portion of the psychiatric evaluation is often neglected, only partially because it is not patently pertinent to the presenting complaint. Other factors are also involved. These include (1) worry about missing abnormalities due to lack of experience, (2) no examination facilities, (3) no assistant (or chaperone) for the examination, (4) no reimbursement for the "extra effort," (5) concern that the examination might influence the therapeutic relationship, and (6) dislike for doing physical examinations.

The student should know that, with a little effort in setting up an office or hospital practice, examination facilities and support personnel can be made available. This will enable more frequent physical examinations and thus reduce concern about the quality of the examination. Payment schedules can often be set up to provide fair reimbursement for time used in adding this essential aspect to the remainder of the psychiatric assessment.

Koranyi (1980) showed that physical examination did not adversely affect the therapeutic relationship in over 2000 psychiatric outpatient evaluations. Those who claim transference and countertransference problems due to the physical examination are creating imaginary dragons, because the psychoanalytic/psychodynamic process involves working through these and other psychological conflicts. More likely, those who suggest this reason for avoiding the physical examination are merely rationalizing their dislike of doing them. In some outpatient settings, however, it may be more realistic for the psychiatrist to insist that a physical examination be performed by a family physician or internist as part of the overall evaluation before formal psychiatric treatment proceeds.

Laboratory Assessment

Laboratory assessment, like the physical examination, should be performed in patients at risk for medical co-morbidity (*supra vide*). Screening tests included in an initial evaluation are a complete blood count, electrolytes, blood chemistry screen, and urinalysis. Medication blood levels and urine screen for drug abuse should be included when indicated. In patients over 50 years old, an electrocardiogram and chest X-ray may be added. Depressed and anxious patients should have a thyroid-stimulating hormone (TSH) level drawn, even in the absence of clinical symptoms or signs.

Although there is a great deal of interest in the measurement of other hormones and neurotransmitters in patients with psychiatric disorders, none of these have been found to be useful in diagnostic or therapeutic decision making. Even the dexamethasone suspension test (DST), widely investigated in patients with mood disorders, has some potential value only in predicting who is likely to relapse when it remains positive after successful treatment.

The basic evaluation listed above provides a screen for metabolic or neurologic factors that might be contributing to the psychiatric presentation. This does not replace the need to perform specific laboratory tests when the clinical history dictates. For instance, a chronic schizophrenic patient from a state hospital who presents with a documented 2-month history of weight loss and low-grade fevers even in the absence of "basic" laboratory abnormalities requires further workup to explain the presenting complaints. Just such a case was diagnosed as having tuberculous meningitis on a recent admission to our institution.

Although all diagnostic testing procedures, regardless of complexity and invasiveness, should be considered when the clinical assessment dictates, computed tomography (CT) of the head, magnetic resonance imaging (MRI) of the head, and electroencephalography (EEG) deserve special attention, because they are frequently considered in the evaluation of patients presenting with psychiatric symptomatology. Head CT is a specialized, noninvasive X-ray technique that allows visualization of the anatomy of the head in slices of various thickness. MRI, using an entirely different imaging technique, provides similar slices; however, it has an advantage in that radiation is not involved, the images are not interfered with by bony structures, the images can be obtained in multiple planes, and the differentiation between gray and white matter is better delineated. EEG is the measurement of electrical activity on the surface of the brain. (Use of these techniques in neuropsychiatric assessment is also discussed in Chapter 4.)

There is no simple formula to cover all the indications for these procedures. Simply stated, MRI is the most expensive but the most sensitive test to pick up anatomic pathology. Because the images using this technique are not altered by bony structures and can be obtained in multiple projections, posterior fossa and brain stem abnormalities are better seen with MRI. For these reasons, some authorities consider it the noninvasive test of choice. Some types of pathology can be seen on MRI that cannot be seen on CT. Examples would include strokes within the first 3 to 7 days of occurrence and multiple sclerosis lesions. Basically, all that can be seen on head CT can be seen on MRI, but the cost, accessibility, limits in interpretation, and problems with patient cooperation in lying still during a relatively lengthy period make it unlikely that it will replace head CT completely.

EEG complements MRI and CT but does not replace them. EEG is not a tool that separates normal from abnormal anatomy; rather, it separates normal and abnormal electrical physiology. In some situations, the two can correspond, as is seen with some brain tumors. In others, the EEG may identify changes (epilepsy) while the imaging procedures remain normal, or vice versa.

MRI, CT, and EEG should all be used to detect structural, metabolic, and seizure-related causes of psychiatric syndromes. One study found increased use of MRI, CT, and EEG studies in patients with a mental disorder compared to patients without a mental disorder (Olfson, 1992). Clinical clues about when the EEG, CT, and MRI are more likely to be abnormal are: (1) if there are focal neurological deficits; (2) if there has been a recent and marked change in mental status; (3) if there is a history of substance abuse/alcoholism, head trauma, or other central nervous system (CNS) pathology; (4) if the patient is elderly; and (5) if the patient presents in an atypical fashion and has a history that does not suggest psychiatric involvement. It should be remembered that medicine is based on probability. A certain number of normal tests are necessary to ensure that abnormal tests aren't missed.

The Mental Status Examination

The term *mental status examination* is somewhat misleading, because it suggests a circumscribed period of assessment that takes its turn, as would auscultation of the heart or inspection of the fundi. To the contrary, the skilled interviewer gathers data regarding the multiple facets of mental functioning as they are observed and elicited during the psychiatric interview. For example, performing tests of recent memory imparts little information not already apparent in a patient who provides an accurate, detailed history. In fact, such exercises may convey a sense of rote mechanical detachment rather than empathy and positive regard for the patient. Furthermore, some aspects of the mental status examination, such as judgment, can be better assessed by what brought the patient to your attention than by asking the patient artificial questions.

Not all areas of the mental status examination are adequately covered during the psychiatric interview. These must be addressed more directly with questions specifically formulated to assess mental function or emotional state. In developing a technique that is both thorough and personalized, it is essential to have a clear understanding of each of the mental status parameters.

A rational method of organizing the mental status examination is to follow the order in which findings are apparent during the interview. Appearance, level of consciousness, psychomotor activity, behavior, and general mood state are observed before and also throughout the interview. Speech, thought content and form, orientation, and memory are appraised throughout the interview. Insight and judgment are usually determined at the conclusion of the interview.

This overview of the basic aspects of the mental status examination is intended to provide a guide to the many areas of inquiry that should be evaluated and recorded in the process of patient assessment. Assignment of a formal psychiatric diagnosis requires completely integrating the patient's psychiatric and medical history and laboratory assessment with the findings on mental status examination. Knowledge of how certain signs and symptoms "fit" into certain categories in the current psychiatric nomenclature system determines the diagnosis.

The mental status examination is a systematic method to gather behavioral and psychological data with the understanding that such data is then processed, analyzed, and integrated to determine whether or not a diagnosis of a formal psychiatric disease should be made. The principal features can be found in Table 1–5. Even if the degree and severity of the patient's symptoms do not warrant formal DSM-IV diagnosis, one may nevertheless assess the possible relationship between the symptoms and current stresses to identify a point of therapeutic intervention.

Appearance, Attitude, and Behavior

Any clues regarding the patient's mental functioning and emotional state should be noted. A slovenly appearance, tattered and dirty clothes, pungent body odor, unkempt hair, and dirty hands are often seen in patients with undifferentiated schizophrenia, alcoholism, or dementia. Stooped posture, poor eye contact, tearing, and slow response to questions in a person with an otherwise normal appearance, on the other hand, are more likely to be seen in patients with depression. Other facets of a patient's appearance and behavior include the patient's apparent health (well developed, bedridden), nutritional state (well nourished, emaciated), posture (catatonic, vigilant), mannerisms (tics, hand-wringing), and actions (compulsions, apparent response to hallucinations, random acts). Behavioral and neurological signs and symptoms of intoxication or medication side effects should be noted here as well.

Another aspect of observing behavior is noting the attitude toward the interviewer. For instance, patients who are unusually guarded and suspicious suggest paranoia. Patients who are flattering and ingratiating but then demand special privi-

Table 1–5 **Mental Status Examination Outline**

Appearance, attitude and behavior
   Description of appearance, hygiene
   Attitude toward examiner
   Psychomotor activity
Speech
Mood and Affect
   Subjective and objective mood
   Affect variability and appropriateness
   Presence of Anxiety
   Assessment of Suicidality
Thought and Language
   Production
   Form
   Content (Obsessions/Delusions)
Perceptions
   Hallucinations/Illusions
   Depersonalization
   Derealization
Cognitive Function
   Level of Consciousness
   Orientation
   Concentration
   Memory
   Intelligence
Insight and Judgment

leges or request disability compensation suggest the manipulative behavior of anti-social, histrionic, or borderline personality disorders. Other descriptors of attitudes toward the interviewer include friendly, cooperative, hostile, threatening, seductive, challenging, and competitive. Each provides a clue to normal and abnormal function when coupled with other aspects of the patient's presentation.

Speech

Tone, rate, and volume of speech should be noted. Depressed patients may speak slowly and quietly with effort, whereas the speech of the manic patient is often rapid, pressured, and resists interruption. The speech of an anxious patient may be both rapid and frantically expressive. Intoxicated patients often speak with loud, slurred speech and are disinhibited in *what* they say.

Mood and Affect

Mood describes the *prevailing* emotional state of the patient whereas "affect" generally refers to how the patient's mood is expressed or exuded. The mood may be euthymic (normal mood state), happy, sad, euphoric, suicidal, guilty, bored, anxious, irritable, agitated, panicky, terrified, angry, enraged, or sensual. If affect varies appropriately with the content of the patient's thoughts (becomes bright and warm when discussing close relatives or sad when discussing the death of a friend), the patient is demonstrating a *full* and *appropriate* affect. When the patient is depressed or in a manic euphoria, the affect is characteristically *confined* to that particular range of mood. In some patients with depression or schizophrenia, the affect may be described as *blunted* or *flat* when it is static, regardless of the environmental stimuli. Patients with schizophrenia, and occasionally other conditions, may also demonstrate *inappropriate* affect by laughing or grinning while describing an unfortunate or tragic event. Other descriptors of affect are *superficial, shallow,* or *labile.*

Depressed mood is characterized by general hopelessness, passivity, lifelessness, dysphoria, demoralization, and pessimism. Patients are often irritable, labile, and querulous. Some patients may be profoundly agitated and anxious, whereas others may be quietly apathetic and vegetative. Crying spells may be frequent and uncontrollable. Anhedonia, the inability to experience pleasure and interest in life, is a cardinal symptom of depression. Physical symptoms may also be prominent in depression. In psychotic depression, paranoia and somatic delusions of parasitic infestation or venereal infection may be present. Other symptoms of depression include low self-esteem, feelings of inadequacy, helplessness, guilt, unlovability, worthlessness, excessive self-criticism, and suicidal thoughts. Many if not most patients will initially be presented with physical or somatic complaints as the primary manifestation of their depression (insomnia, headache, G.I. distress, fatigue, loss of appetite and weight, etc.). If persistent and patients display little ability to verbalize their feelings, or are unable to make a connection between somatic complaints and their depression, they may be somatothymic, a condition discussed earlier in this chapter.

In mania, the mood is inappropriately euphoric, giddy, silly, disinhibited, or extremely irritable. Grandiose ideas and schemes as well as an inflated self-image may be observed. Emotional expansiveness and excessive and intrusive gregariousness may be observed with the patient's manic mood.

Anxiety. Components of acute or chronic anxiety are often reported by way of the expression of psychophysiologic symptoms. Subjectively, patients may complain of being tense, nervous, fearful, frightened, anxious, worried, fretful, or unable to relax or sleep. Phobic symptoms may be present, such as circumscribed simple phobias (of snakes or spiders, for example), social phobia, or agoraphobia (fear of being alone or being in open or crowded spaces). Anxiety, as part of an obsessive–compulsive disorder, can lead to severe crippling anxiety usually centered on intrusive thoughts or fears. Patients with posttraumatic stress disorders are often chronically anxious and plagued by nightmares and startle responses and are hypervigilant. Symptoms of anxiety are often mixed with those of depression.

Suicidal and Homicidal Ideation. Detailed questions should be asked about present and past suicidal behavior. Patients should be asked directly if they have had any thoughts of hurting or killing themselves. If such thoughts have occurred, the patient should be asked about his or her plan, the exact methods considered, and how far he or she got with the thoughts or plans. If previous suicide attempts have occurred, their nature, severity, and precipitating cause should be documented, as well as any family history of suicide (assessment of the suicidal patient is further discussed in Chapter 19).

The patient also should be asked if they have had thoughts of hurting others, and if so, what the thoughts have been and how far the planning has progressed. Have they been violent before? Toward whom? And what were the circumstances and consequences? Do they have weapons in their possession or do they have access to them? Have they ever been arrested or incarcerated for violence? Were drugs or alcohol involved? Do they feel in control of their impulses at the current time?

Thought and Language

An impairment in the ability to translate thoughts into symbols or to use symbols in communication (*language disorder*) differs from a *thought disorder* in that the latter implies a compromised ability to organize, coherently associate, and effectively use information and ideas. Both problems are identified during the process of human interaction and usually require the production of speech. Examples of language disorders include aphasias, alexias, and agraphias and are by definition the result of focal brain dysfunction. A screening examination for language disorders includes the evaluation of spontaneous speech, repetition of words and sentences, comprehension of spoken and written language, the ability to produce names of objects on confrontation, and the ability to write. These are all found on the Mini-Mental State Examination discussed at some length in Chapter 4.

Thought is subdivided into *production of thought, form of thought* (thought process), and *content of thought* and can be disordered in several ways.

Disorders of the Production of Thought. This refers to the abundance of thought as evidenced by a person's interactional capabilities. In most situations this is assessed by observation of the patient's verbal communication; however, those with speech impediments or congenital mutism can also demonstrate difficulties in this area through other modalities of communication. *Poverty of thought* is characterized by a decrease in the apparent ability or interest in interacting with the environment and other people. This is seen most frequently in schizophrenia and major depression. In some situations, one's thoughts race ahead of one's ability to communicate them (*flight of ideas*); this is usually seen in mania. *Thought blocking* is characterized by an abrupt cessation of communication before the topic of discussion is completed. The delay that follows may be prolonged, following which patients are often unable to recall the topic. Patients sometimes explain this by stating that their "mind went blank."

Disorders of the Form of Thought. *Form of thought* or *thought process* refers to the manner in which thoughts are connected or associated. Normal thinking is goal-directed, with sequential thoughts having logical connections. The "train of thought" can be easily followed, and the communicant reaches the intended goal. Conditions characterized by abnormalities in thought processing, such as psychotic disorders, may be manifested in several ways (see Table 1–6).

Disorders of Thought Content. Disorders of thought content are often divided into two broad categories—preoccupations and delusions. Preoccupations include phobias, obsessions, and compulsions. A *phobia* is an irrational, pathologic dread of a specific type of stimulus or situation that results in marked anxiety and avoidance of the situation. An *obsession* is a disturbing, persistent, and usually intrusive thought, feeling, or impulse that cannot be eliminated from consciousness. Common obsessions include fear of contamination or of losing control and harming others. Obsessions may involve fear of self-harm or suicide, even though the patient may deny feeling de-

---

Table 1–6 **Disorders of Thought Processing**

Circumstantiality
Marked by tedious and unnecessary details but eventually reaches the point.

Tangentiality
Marked by skirting the question rather than answering it. Connections between subsequent thoughts are apparent, but a goal is never reached.

Loosening of associations
A jumping from subject to subject without apparent connection.

Verbigeration
Conveys little information despite adequate volume of speech due to vagueness, empty repetitions, or obscure phrases.

Word salad
An incoherent collection of words and phrases.

Neologisms
Made-up words that have meaning only for the patient.

Clang associations
Words or phrases connected due to characteristics of the words themselves (rhyming, punning) rather than the meaning they convey.

Echolalia
Repetitive, often playful repetition of the words of others.

pressed or wishing to die. Such suicidal thoughts would be properly included in this portion of the mental status examination. *Compulsions* are irresistible urges to perform meaningless, often ritualistic motor acts, such as handwashing.

Delusions are fixed, false beliefs that have no basis in reality, are not held by one's culture, and from which the patient will not be dissuaded despite evidence to the contrary. Delusions can be mood-congruent with the psychiatric state, such as those of *nihilism* (life or world is ending), *poverty* (all life possessions have been lost), *somatic* distress (a serious illness [cancer] has invaded the body), or *sin* (heinous sins have been committed for which punishment is necessary), as is sometimes seen in depression. Delusions of *grandeur*, in which special powers are claimed, are characteristically found in mania. Delusions also can be incongruent with the prevailing mood, such as delusions of reference (unrelated events apply to oneself) or control (outside force controlling actions). These usually are more characteristic of schizophrenia. Karl Schneider described a group of delusions characterized by externally imposed influences concerning thought, feelings, and somatic function. These are referred to as the "first-rank symptoms of schizophrenia," although they are known to occur in affective psychoses and delirium as well (see Table 1–7). These symptoms also are reviewed in the chapter on schizophrenia (Chapter 5).

Perception

Perceptual disturbance involves disordered processing of sensory information. Hallucinations are perceptions that occur in the absence of actual stimuli. Illusions are

Table 1–7 **Schneider's First-Rank Symptoms of Schizophrenia**

	BELIEF
Thought insertion	An external agency is inserting thoughts into the passive mind.
Thought withdrawal	An external agency is removing thoughts from the passive mind.
Thought broadcasting	Thoughts are audible to others.
Made feelings (passivity feelings)	Feelings being experienced are imposed by an external source.
Made drives (passivity feelings)	Powerful drives (to which the patient usually responds) are being imposed by an external agency.
Made volitional acts (passivity feelings)	Actions are completely under the control of an external influence.
Somatic passivity (passivity feelings)	Bodily sensations are being imposed by an external agency against the will.
Delusional perception	A two-stage phenomenon in which a normally perceived stimulus is followed by a delusional belief regarding the meaning of the stimulus.

Other first-rank symptoms involve specific types of auditory hallucinations.

misinterpretations of existing stimuli. Auditory hallucinations occur most frequently in the psychoses of schizophrenia, mania, or other "functional" disorders. Visual hallucinations occur more frequently than auditory hallucinations in psychotic episodes due to medical, neurologic and toxin-induced disorders (i.e., substance abuse, toxins, and intrinsic brain disease), although visual hallucinations are often associated with primary psychiatric disease. Olfactory and gustatory hallucinations often occur as prodromal symptoms of complex partial seizures. Haptic hallucinations, especially the sensation of bugs crawling on one's skin (formication), frequently occur in delirium induced by sedative withdrawal. There is considerable overlap in these symptoms, however, and none is specific to, or pathognomonic of, the disorders noted.

Paranoid delusions may be highly systematized (such as elaborate systems of observations by the FBI, or CIA plots) or bizarre (Martians peering at one from outer space). Paranoia as an isolated symptom is not specifically diagnostic. It is the nature, duration, *and* severity of the paranoia in the context of the patient's history that relates it to one particular diagnosis or the other. For example, the isolated delusion that one's wife is having an affair in the absence of other signs or symptoms would be diagnosed as delusional disorder. A severely depressed patient who had paranoid delusions of being persecuted would most likely have a major depression with psychotic features; a woman with paranoid delusions of being watched and followed by the CIA, with a longtitudinal course and other more pervasive symptoms of a thought disorder, might be diagnosed as having paranoid schizophrenia; a man with paranoid ideation in the context of amphetamines might be considered to have a substance-induced delusional disorder. Somatic delusions such as feelings of rotting inside, being infected with a venereal disease, or having AIDS may be seen in psychotic depression. Alternatively, general suspiciousness, mistrust, cynicism, and querulousness of others that does not reach overtly delusional proportions may be seen as a trait of a paranoid personality disorder.

Depersonalization refers to feelings that one is falling apart, fragmenting, "not the same," not one's self, becoming unreal, or detached and may be seen in a number of psychiatric disorders—principally anxiety disorders, but also delirious states, including those that are substance induced. Symptoms of *derealization* include the feeling that the world is not real, people are not real, or things are becoming distant, alien, or strange. Both types of symptoms are variations on the same theme and may be seen in CNS disease, such as complex partial epilepsy.

Cognitive Functioning

Level of Consciousness. It is best to describe patients' levels of consciousness by their ability to respond to the environmental stimuli. Extremes include hyperalertness and coma. *Hyperalertness* is characterized by hypervigilance, often with agitation or tremulousness, and is seen most often in mania or delirium. *Alert* describes normal wakefulness and awareness of the environment. *Lethargic* indicates the patient has a tendency to drift into unresponsiveness if left alone but is easily roused to verbal stimulus. *Stupor* reflects the need for continual stimulation to maintain consciousness, and *coma* is characterized by unconsciousness and the absence of response to any stimuli.

Orientation. Orientation assesses awareness of identity, time (day of week, month, exact day of month, year, time of day), place, and situation. Awareness of person usually indicates that a person can remember his or her name. Awareness of time and place involves the ability to provide the correct date and current location, while awareness of situation suggests a grasp of the circumstances surrounding the patient's current plight. In confusional states, the first manifestation of disorientation normally involves time and situation, and these are usually the last to normalize with recovery.

Concentration (Attention). Concentration refers to the ability to direct and sustain attention. Patients with impaired attention require repetition of questions and may be distracted by seemingly inconsequential stimuli. Concentration is formally tested by performance of serial 7s or 3s (counting backward from 100 by 7s or 3s). Alternatively, the patient can be asked to repeat strings of random numbers forward (average normal—seven digits) or in reverse (average normal—five digits). Failure is identified by two unsuccessful attempts at the same number. Gross impairment of concentration (attention) is characteristic of delirium and is usually recognized by the patient's inability to respond to your requests consistently and coherently.

Memory. Tests of memory assess the ability to retrieve and recite information previously stored (retrograde memory) and to form new memories (anterograde memory). Remote memory (usually retrograde) involves remembering events that occurred many years ago, such as the name of a school attended, the nature of previous jobs, and so forth. With disorders of declining intellectual function, this is usually one of the last to be affected. Recent past memory (retrograde and/or anterograde) involves remembering events occurring months ago and may be assessed as the patient provides believable and/or confirmed details of the present illness or events leading up to the assessment.

Inability to form new memories (anterograde) is clinically identified when patients are unable to recall events that have just occurred or people they have just met. Less obvious forms of anterograde memory dysfunction can be assessed by providing the names of three unrelated objects that the patient immediately repeats (immediate recall) and then recalls after 5 minutes (short-term memory). Impairment of immediate recall, especially with repeated attempts, suggests an attention deficit that precludes further anterograde memory testing. Intact immediate recall with impaired recall after 5 minutes suggests impairment of short-term memory.

Isolated deficits in cognitive function are diagnostically nonspecific because they can occur with intellectual decline of varied cause. If identified by the screening tests performed on the mental status examination, they should be further characterized by more formal neuropsychological testing (*infra vide*). Use of the Mini-Mental State Examination, a structured approach to assessing memory, is discussed in Chapter 4 and will also be discussed in Chapter 3 on psychological assessment. Further discussion of cognitive assessment is deferred to those chapters.

Intelligence. Some observations may be made about the patient's general education level and the ability to learn, integrate, and process new information. Formal education level does not necessarily indicate intelligence, because intelligence, most basically, is an assessment of the individual's ability to learn new information, process that information, and solve problems. Individuals with relatively little or no formal education can be quite intelligent. On the other hand, a person who has completed his or her doctorate would not be expected to function in the range of those with borderline intellectual function. Formal psychological testing may be needed, especially in children or where mental retardation is expected, to assess the patient's intelligence level accurately (see also Chapter 3 on psychological testing).

Insight and Judgment

Insight refers to awareness of factors influencing one's situation. When a patient has a psychiatric illness, insight refers to the appreciation that an illness or psychiatric difficulty is occurring, recognition of its impact on the ability to function, and awareness of the need to take steps to correct it. The most meaningful method of assessing insight is to gather data about these factors throughout the history. The presence or absence of insight has profound impact on adjustment to illness, compliance with treatment, and consequent level of function. Thus, an estimation of a patient's insight is helpful in planning an effective treatment strategy.

The patient's capacity for self-observation and demonstration of empathy are also measures of insight that are helpful in assessing the presence of a personality disorder. Patients with a personality disorder are often egocentric, tend to blame others for their problems, and resist self-examination to determine their personal contribution to their difficulties in life.

Empathy refers to the ability to identify with the feelings of others and to "feel with them." It is also a measure of consideration for the feelings, welfare, and rights of others. Patients with some personality disorders (antisocial, paranoid, narcissistic, and borderline personality disorders) often show a lack of empathy for others and exploit other people for their own gratification. Traits found in personality disorder and details about their diagnosis are discussed in Chapter 6.

Judgment refers to a person's ability to handle finances; manage day-to-day activities; and avoid danger, including exposure to heat, cold, malnutrition, and crime. Insight into factors influencing a person's well-being must be present before options and priorities can be weighed and judgment exercised. Standardized methods of assessment, such as asking what a person would do if he or she found a stamped, addressed envelope on the sidewalk, are inadequate for most purposes. It is more helpful to rely on an understanding of the circumstances that led to the patient's seeking psychiatric attention in assessing judgment. For instance, a person walking in the snow with shorts and no shoes would, in the absence of extenuating circumstances, be exhibiting poor judgment. Despite the subjective nature of the assessment, impaired judgment resulting from mental illness or substance dependence that directly or indirectly places the patient or others in danger is a prerequisite for involuntary commitment in many states.

PSYCHOLOGICAL AND NEUROPSYCHOLOGICAL TESTING

The clinical indications and usefulness of psychological and neuropsychological testing are discussed in Chapter 3, but a brief overview of the place of such testing in the general psychiatric assessment will be mentioned here.

Tests of psychological and neuropsychological function complement but do not replace the psychiatric history and mental status examination, just as laboratory and radiologic procedures complement but do not replace the medical history and physical examination. This is a particularly important point, because no standardized test used in clinical practice provides an assessment that allows a psychiatric diagnosis to be made, with the possible exception of dementia. There is a tendency among nonpsychiatrists to use psychological tests, such as the Minnesota Multiphasic Personality Inventory (MMPI) or the General Health Questionnaire (GHQ), to establish whether a psychiatric disorder may be involved in a patient's symptom picture. As will be discussed later, this can lead to inappropriate labeling and ineffective treatment. When correctly used, however, psychological and neuropsychological tests provide an important adjunct to the psychiatric evaluation and treatment plan.

Neuropsychological tests assess cognitive abilities and require the expertise of a psychologist who has received specialized training in their administration and interpretation (a neuropsychologist). *Psychological tests* were developed to identify the presence and frequency of psychological symptoms in various populations. Some psychological tests are easily administered or self-administered and can be readily scored merely by reading a short description of the test. Others are more complex and require skills in the interpretation and quantification of the behaviors being tested. Those with master's degrees or doctorates in psychology usually possess the skills necessary to perform these tests if they choose to emphasize this area in their work. Not all psychologists, however, specialize in giving and interpreting psychological tests, so care should be taken to assure that the person doing the testing has an adequate background and interest.

As is discussed in Chapter 3, psychological and neuropsychological tests are best used to clarify specific important questions during patient assessment and management. Although the multitude of standardized tests cannot be covered in this chapter, four common clinical questions in which psychological and neuropsychological tests can help with clinical decision making will be addressed here: (1) Are psychiatric factors involved in the patient's clinical presentation? (2) Can the severity of the patient's psychiatric symptoms be reproducibly assessed and used to monitor improvement? (3) Does the patient's personality assessment give a clue about psychiatric involvement? and (4) Does the patient have impaired brain function? Because it is impossible to review all the tests that could potentially assist in answering these questions, only a few widely used and well-standardized tests will be discussed. More extensive discussion of these and other tests can be found in the book by van Riezen and Segal (1988). Psychological tests are used to address the first three questions, whereas neuropsychological tests are used in the last.

Screening Tests for Psychiatric Involvement

Are there screening tests that detect the presence of specific psychiatric disorders? *No!* There are, however, self-administered screening questionnaires that can be used before a psychiatric assessment that identify those at risk for psychiatric difficulties. These instruments are best used in primary care outpatient and inpatient settings. Because these tests are often exquisitely sensitive but have limited specificity, it is necessary to be aware of the need for more formalized psychiatric assessment before a diagnosis is considered and treatment for a "psychiatric" condition is instituted.

The General Health Questionnaire (GHQ) is a widely studied self-report instrument validated primarily in nonpsychiatric outpatient populations. A low score on this test predicts that a psychiatric disorder is unlikely and that psychiatric factors are probably not involved in the symptom presentation. High scores suggest the need for further questioning if the presentation of the patient suggests that psychiatric factors may be playing a role. The GHQ can save valuable time in screening new outpatients attending a primary care clinic by alerting the clinician to patients who might require more careful psychiatric evaluation in addition to the medical workup.

Depression is one of the most common psychiatric disorders seen in primary care medical populations. The Center for Epidemiologic Studies-Depression Scale (CES-D) is a self-report questionnaire that has been standardized to identify those at risk for depression in the general population. It lists the presence of a number of depressive symptoms but does not, even when the score is elevated, suggest that a pathological depression is present or that treatment should be administered. The CES-D is a sensitive screen for depression in clinical samples requiring confirmation through clinical evaluation.

The Mini-Mental State Examination (MMSE) screens for deteriorating *cognitive* function and is not a comprehensive psychiatric assessment instrument. This exam is administered by the physician at the bedside and covers a variety of cognitive skills. Unlike the GHQ and screening tests for depression, impaired function (scores of less than 24 or 25 out of 30 in an alert subject) on the MMSE is highly suggestive of cognitive difficulties. More specific neuropsychiatric testing should be done in these patients. The use of the MMSE is addressed in detail in Chapter 4.

Screening for Severity of Illness

One of the most important tasks of the clinician is to establish a baseline level of symptoms and to confirm that the treatment being given results in their reduction. Although the patient interview is the principal means of accomplishing this purpose, several tests that reliably document psychiatric symptoms can improve consistency. Depression severity and change can be monitored with the Beck Depression Inventory (self-report) or the Hamilton Rating Scale for Depression (interviewer-rated). However, these scales should not be used for diagnosis as they can frequently misclassify medically ill patients (Kathol et al, 1990). The Hamilton Rating Scale for Anxiety (interviewer-rated) is available to quantitate symptoms of anxiety. General psychiatric severity can be assessed with the Hopkins Symptoms Checklist 90 (HCL-90) (self-report), whereas psychotic symptoms can be enumerated with the Brief Psychiatric Rating Scale (interviewer-rated). Because the HCL-90 is divided into subscales pertaining to specific areas of psychiatric symptoms, the questions pertinent only to that area can be repeatedly administered during treatment.

Screening with Personality Questionnaires

Although personality disorders have received relatively little rigorous, systematic research attention, there is growing evidence that the presence of personality disorder in patients with other major psychiatric disorders is associated with increased severity and poorer outcome. Additionally, personality disorder may increase the likelihood of contact with health professionals for medical conditions (Reich, 1987).

The Minnesota Multiphasic Personality Inventory (MMPI) is perhaps the most commonly used personality assessment instrument. It has nine clinical scales from which profiles of behavioral patterns are derived and, when originally formulated (1939), was well standardized in a large control population. Two problems arise with the use of the MMPI in current practice. First, the MMPI was standardized when cultural mores were considerably different from today and well before the psychiatric diagnostic system in current use. The importance of this problem is emphasized by the fact that restandardization of the MMPI in a contemporary population showed that there was a 20 to 30% difference in the identification of dysfunction between the old and new standards (Colligan, Osborne, Swenson, Offord, 1983). Despite these findings, which suggest that many patients are being misclassified, few testing centers have switched to the new standards, and the revised MMPI is just beginning to be implemented at the level of the general community practice setting.

Not only are there problems with the use of a dated population standard, but there are also difficulties in the interpretations made based on test results. In the 1940s, interpretation was based on a conceptualization of psychiatric disease very different from that espoused today. The relevance of "standard" (often computer-generated) personality profiles from the MMPI to current psychiatric disorders is uncertain, because they are based on different theoretical constructs. Significant differences can therefore occur between the MMPI results and a diagnosis revealed through clinical interview.

The second major problem with the MMPI is that it is commonly used to assess patients with medical illness. Because the test was standardized in a nonmedically ill control group, using this instrument to determine whether psychiatric factors may be involved in the complaints of patients with real or potential medical illness is inappropriate (Osborne, 1987). Such patients will routinely rate high on the hypochondriacal and depressive scales because a number of the questions in these scales reflect the presence of physical symptoms (real or imagined). Unfortunately, those evaluating patients in whom a functional cause is in the differential are frequently enamored by the fact that the MMPI gives real and reproducible numbers to quantitate psychiatric disturbances while forgetting that the results are of questionable validity. *For this and the reasons listed above, the MMPI is not recommended as a routine adjunct to the clinical interview*, and its use should be limited to special situations.

Screening for Impaired Brain Function

The principal aims of neuropsychological testing are to provide an estimate of the severity of cognitive deficit, to localize the areas of the brain that are impaired, and to assess the degree and estimated duration of functional limitations. The Halstead–Reitan Battery and the Luria–Nebraska Inventory are two extensive test batteries that help answer questions related to the areas above. Unfortunately, the length of testing makes these tests unsuitable in severely ill psychiatric patients. The Wechsler Adult Intelligence Scale–Revised and other briefer screens (Berg, Franzen, Wedding, 1987) of cognitive function now frequently replace the more comprehensive batteries (see Table 1–8). When mental retardation in children is the focus of assessment, specialized age-specific measurements of intelligence can be used. These tests include the Wechsler Intelligence Scale Children–Revised and the Wechsler Preschool and Primary Scale of Intelligence. These tests require the assistance of a neuropsychologist for administration and interpretation. Additionally, the comprehensive neuropsychological batteries can be expensive. Nevertheless, complete neuropsychological batteries may be helpful in defining subtle cognitive deficits and are indicated in some clinical situations, such as in evaluating patients who have sustained severe head injuries or occupational exposure to potential neurologic toxins, patients who may have temporal lobe seizures, or patients with cerebrovascular disease. Comprehensive neuropsychological inventories also can be helpful when legal compensation issues are important or for planning rehabilitation programs. The use of neuropsychological testing is discussed further in Chapter 3.

Table 1–8 **Comprehensive Neuropsychologic Batteries and Specific Function Tests**

NEUROPSYCHOLOGIC BATTERIES	NUMBER OF SECTIONS	COMMENTS
Halstead–Reitan Battery (HRB)	10	Includes MMPI & WAIS. Full test may take several days
Luria–Nebraska Inventory	11	Provides score on 14 measures of cognitive function with t scores
Tests of Specific Function	**Function Tested**	
Wechsler Adult Intelligence Screen-R (WAIS)	Verbal and nonverbal skills	Provides verbal and performance intelligence scores as well as a full-scale IQ
Token Test	Speech	Can be used as a screening test for aphasia
Wechsler Memory Scale	Memory	Seven subtests; provides memory quotient similar to IQ
Wisconsin Card Sort	Abstraction—conceptual shifting	Considered a test of frontal lobe function
Trail-Making Test	Visuomotor tracking	Contains parts A and B; performance decreases with age
Seashore Rhythm Test	Nonverbal auditory	Part of HRB; tests ability to discriminate between two tone groups
Finger-Tapping Test	Motor	Cortical damage slows tapping speed

CLASSIFICATION OF PSYCHIATRIC DISEASE: DSM-IV

As in all medical disciplines, the nature of the information obtained during the diagnostic interview conforms to the classification of illness used. The classification, in turn, should be derived from the ability to consistently identify complexes of signs and symptoms that predict etiology, natural course, family involvement, outcome, and response to treatment of a condition that causes or leads to impairment. DSM-IV reflects the state of the art in classifying psychiatric disease in the United States and, at least in part, stems from three previous classification systems used since the mid-1970s in psychiatric research (the "Feighner criteria" [Feighner et al, 1972] and Research Diagnostic Criteria [Spitzer, Endicott, Robins, 1978]).

DSM-IV uses a signs-and-symptoms, criterion-based approach to psychiatric diagnosis. If certain symptoms are present in sufficient degree and for sufficient duration, then the diagnosis can be made. Those meeting "criteria" are thus more likely to conform to the predictive factors known about the disease being diagnosed. As might be expected, some conditions have greater validity than others. For instance, depression, mania, schizophrenia, panic disorder, alcohol and substance dependency/abuse, and somatization disorder can be reproducibly identified. As a result, definite statements can be made regarding the likely age of onset, sex distribution, familial involvement, course if untreated, and probability of response to certain interventions in those carrying these diagnoses. Other diagnoses, however, such as personality disorder (with the exception of antisocial personality disorder), adjustment disorders, and psychosexual disorders, currently have less predictive value. As more research is performed, these will be further refined or deleted, depending on the findings.

Those who do not meet criteria for diagnosis according to DSM-IV can be diagnosed with "no psychiatric disorder" or the possible/probable distinction for a certain condition. This occurs commonly when DSM-IV is correctly used and does not preclude that such patients be treated. What such diagnoses say is that these patients do not warrant a label with its positive and negative connotations, although a clinical trial may be attempted to see whether symptoms improve.

In an attempt to ensure that information of value in planning treatment and predicting outcome is recorded, DSM-IV uses a multiaxial system of evaluation. Axes I and II comprise mental disorders; Axis III, general medical conditions; Axis IV, psychosocial and environmental problems; and Axis V, global assessment of functioning (GAF).

Axis I diagnoses include clinical syndromes that represent a deterioration from a previous level of functioning, such as schizophrenia, major depression, and substance-abuse disorders. Axis II includes personality disorders. Patients with Axis II diagnoses, in contrast to Axis I, usually have symptoms extending back into the early developmental years. Axis I and II disorders frequently coexist, requiring careful evaluation for Axis I disorders in patients with personality disorder. Physical disorders (Axis III) exacerbate or cause Axis I and II disorders in up to 50% of patients with psychiatric conditions (LaBruzza, 1981). It is therefore very important to document the medical conditions present and assess whether they may be impacting on the psychiatric symptoms.

Although DSM-IV does not identify stress as a major cause of psychiatric disorders, the importance of psychosocial and environmental stressors is noted in Axis IV. Axis V rates the current global assessment of function (GAF) in terms of social, occupational, or academic activity. Ratings of impairment are made on a 0 (most) to 90 (least) scale. An example of the multiaxial patient assessment as it relates to RH is listed in Table 1–9.

V (the letter) codes ("vee" codes) constitute emotional situations not attributable to a mental disorder. Examples include marital problems, uncomplicated bereavement, and so forth, and were described previously as "problems in living." When a patient does not have a psychiatric condition yet seeks emotional support for their personal difficulties, these are used to describe the circumstances in either Axis I or II. V codes allow description of the presenting problem without assigning the patient a psychiatric diagnosis.

Important Diagnostic Issues

Two medical problem-solving principles are important in identifying psychiatric illness (Elstein, Shulman, Sprafka, 1978). First, common diseases are the most likely to be seen and should not be overlooked. Table 1–10 shows that mood disorders, anxiety disorders, alcohol and substance abuse, and adjustment disorders are seen often in several clinical settings. They therefore deserve special attention and consid-

---

Table 1–9 DSM-IV Multiaxial Evaluation for Patient RH

Axis I: Alcohol Dependence
          Alcohol Psychotic Disorder
          Delirium due to multiple etiologies
              Delirium Due to General Medical Conditions
              Alcohol Withdrawal Delirium
Axis II: Diagnosis deferred on Axis II
Axis III: Status post–head trauma
              Subdural hematoma
          Alcoholic cirrhosis of liver
          Alcoholic gastritis
          Pancreatitis
          Hyponatremia
          Hypomagnesemia
          Hypocalcemia
          Macrocytic anemia
          Thrombocytopenia
          Essential hypertension
Axis IV: Psychosocial and Environmental Problems
              Primary support group
              Social environment
              Occupational
Axis V: GAF*: 10

*GAF, global assessment of function.

Table 1–10 **Rank Order of Psychiatric Diagnoses by Site of Encounter**

SURVEY OF OUTPATIENT PHYSICIANS	GENERAL HOSPITAL PSYCHIATRIC CONSULTATION	INPATIENT PSYCHIATRIC SERVICE	COMMUNITY SURVEY
Anxiety disorders	Mood disorders	Mood disorders	Substance abuse
Mood disorders	Adjustment disorders	Schizophrenia	Anxiety disorders
Substance abuse	No psychiatric diagnosis	Substance abuse	Mood disorders
Psychophysiologic disorders	Substance abuse	Delirium, dementia	Antisocial personality
Adjustment disorders	Delirium	Adjustment disorders	Schizophrenia

eration. Second, uncommon problems have increased importance when effective treatment is available. Missing an uncommon problem in this situation can be catastrophic. This frequently happens in patients with reversible organic causes of psychiatric syndromes.

Finally, diagnosis of psychiatric disorders that may be complicated by suicidal or homicidal ideation should not be overlooked. Depression, schizophrenia, substance abuse, and antisocial personality deserve serious attention, because all may endanger the patient or others.

Differential Diagnosis

Identifying the underlying psychiatric problem(s) and the variables that might be impacting on it (them) involves a stepwise process. Initially, the chief complaint and associated symptoms related in the history of present illness will suggest the major DSM-IV diagnostic category (see also Fig. 1–1). Once the principal symptoms or problems are identified, refinements (first differential) are made during the history-taking process to help establish which diagnostic category best describes the clinical situation. Because the end product of this process will influence the treatment or assistance given to the patient, thoroughness is very important.

In the differential diagnosis of primary psychiatric disease, medical factors should be identified at the onset of the evaluation. If they are, then the clinician should aggressively pursue medical, neurologic, or toxic factors before planning a specific psychiatric treatment modality. In some cases this is possible, for such conditions as steroid psychosis or systemic lupus cerebritis (both examples of delirium) are often readily identifiable at the onset, thus facilitating the recognition of the medical nature of the mental symptoms.

Much more often, the patient will present with no evidence or limited evidence of medical conditions that might be related to the psychiatric symptoms. In these circumstances, decisions about the psychiatric syndromes in question are made based on the assumption that symptoms are unrelated to medical illness. For instance, a patient with undiagnosed hypothyroidism who has many symptoms in common with depression (Table 1–11) presents to a primary physician or psychiatrist with complaints of weakness, constipation, crying spells, difficulty sleeping, and weight gain.

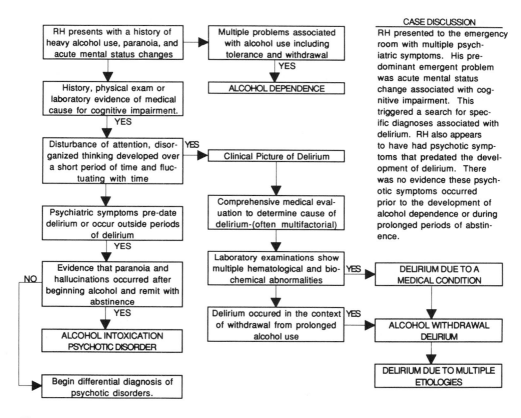

Figure 1–1. *Diagnostic issues in the case of RH*

Because the patient appears depressed and, in fact, has many symptoms of depression, the differential for mood disturbance is entertained. Sure enough, the patient meets all the criteria for a severe single major depressive episode, and yet the underlying problem is hypothyroidism.

This suggests that even after a presumed psychiatric condition is diagnosed, it is often necessary to run through another differential (the second) of conditions that may be causally or casually related to the syndrome. In the case of major depression, for instance, symptoms could be the result of underlying medical conditions, such as endocrine disease, cancer, anemia, hypoxemia, medication reaction, epilepsy, and so forth. It could be the result of stress, such as the death of a loved one. It could be secondary to a preexisting psychiatric condition, such as antisocial personality disorder, alcoholism, and so forth. Or it could be feigned by someone who wants compensation, attention, and so forth.

The reason that this second differential is important in the care of patients is that, depending on the complicating circumstances, major differences may occur in the way the patient is handled. This is illustrated in Table 1–12. DSM-IV lists

Table 1–11 **Comparison of Psychological Symptoms in Hypothyroidism and Depression**

HYPOTHYROIDISM (%)	DEPRESSION
Loss of energy (25–98)	Loss of energy
Weakness (25–95)	Weakness
Poor concentration	Poor concentration
Memory loss (48–66)	Memory loss
Slowed actions (48–91)	Motor retardation
Decreased sex drive	Decreased libido
Constipation (38–61)	Constipation
Insomnia (25–98)	Insomnia
Nervousness (13–58)	Agitation

secondary categories for most symptom groups. For example, depression due to hypothyroidism would be designated "Mood Disorder Due to Hypothyroidism, With Depressive Features."

The psychiatric evaluation as outlined in this chapter helps to perform this function in a time-efficient yet thorough manner. The chief complaint and history of present illness are used to identify the principal difficulty of the patient. The history of present illness helps determine whether a syndrome of behavior is present and how

Table 1–12 **Sample Treatment Strategies in the Treatment of Patients with Depression**

CLINICAL SITUATION	TREATMENT
Primary major depression	Antidepressant medication Cognitive psychotherapy Social support
Depression secondary to hypothyroidism	No antidepressant medication Supportive psychotherapy Reassurance and social support Thyroid replacement Education about when symptoms will resolve
Adjustment disorder with depression in histrionic personality disorder and somatization	No antidepressant medication Supportive psychotherapy Social support
Depression in a patient caught faking the symptoms	Empathic confrontation No antidepressant medication Supportive psychotherapy
Depression two weeks after mother's death	Supportive psychotherapy Social support

typical it is. It also documents the presence of variables that may directly influence the production or continuation of symptoms.

The past medical and psychiatric history, personal and social history, and review of systems uncover information and discrepancies that could have a bearing on the presenting complaints but do not, at first glance, appear to have a relationship. And the physical examination and laboratory assessment confirm or deny suspicions derived from the history about possible medical/neurologic involvement and check for signs of diseases not entertained.

One help in differentiating primary psychiatric disorders from those related to the secondary conditions noted is to have a good understanding of the primary psychiatric disorders. Such knowledge includes symptom presentation, age of onset, sex ratio, natural course, family involvement, and likelihood of response to treatment. For example, major depression is more frequent in women, has its onset during the 20s to 40s, runs a recurrent course, has a higher incidence in other members of the family, has few or no residual symptoms between episodes, and has a good likelihood of response to cyclic antidepressants or other antidepressant therapies. Therefore, if a patient presents for the first time in his or her 70s, has no history of emotional problems, other family members have had no difficulty with affective problems, and the symptoms are cluttered with unusual complaints, then causes for the psychiatric presentation other than primary depression should be given greater consideration.

DSM-IV Case Formulation

Refer to, or reread, the case of RH presented at the beginning of this chapter. This case presentation describes a middle-aged man with a lifelong history of alcohol abuse that progressed to the point that he abstained only when sleep, unconsciousness, illness, or the inability to procure more intervened. He was admitted agitated and incoherent with paranoid thoughts and physical signs and symptoms suggesting alcohol withdrawal. Other causes of delirium were possible, because the patient had liver enzyme and electrolyte disturbances, pancreatitis, a gastrointestinal bleed, and cerebral trauma. Nonetheless, because the clinical history from the patient, the police, and the family was most compatible with alcohol withdrawal delirium (delirium tremens), it was considered the most likely Axis I diagnosis (Table 1–9). Despite this working diagnosis, other possible causes of the patient's mental state were being considered or corrected while the patient was treated for alcohol withdrawal.

During the years before admission, he demonstrated dependence and tolerance to alcohol. His education was shortened, marriage broken, job lost, and health impaired because of alcohol consumption. Despite attempts at in- and outpatient treatment, he persisted in nearly continuous intoxication. He showed drinking behavior consistent with that of other first- and second-degree family members. This tight history of mental and emotional problems related to alcohol ingestion supports the Axis I diagnosis of alcohol dependence (see DSM-IV for criteria). Figure 1–1 outlines additional diagnostic issues for RH. RH displayed evidence of delirium, which should trigger a search for specific causes. It is common for multiple causes of delirium to be identified.

Other psychiatric syndromes are seen frequently in men with alcohol dependence. These include depression, other forms of substance abuse, antisocial personality disorder, anxiety, and dementia. RH had a history of antisocial traits, but these were insufficient to make the diagnosis of antisocial personality disorder. Furthermore, the antisocial traits that were present (school expulsion, difficulties with teachers, frequent fights, arrests) always occurred under the influence of alcohol. RH denied abuse of other substances, and this was confirmed, at least at the time of admission, by the absence of other substances of abuse in his urine. The family also confirmed that he didn't use "pills."

RH had a history of depressed affect during intoxication or withdrawal accompanied by suicidal ideation on several occasions. During periods of abstinence, depression had never been a problem. Both during and after treatment of the patient's withdrawal delirium, there was no evidence of depression, despite an apparently dismal life situation. Despite treatment with antianxiety medications, he showed no evidence for current or past anxiety disorder. RH reported significant paranoid delusions. Although these may have occurred as part of a recurrent withdrawal pattern, it appears that paranoid symptoms also occurred independent of withdrawal. DSM-IV would classify this alcoholic paranoia as an alcohol psychotic disorder, with delusions.

It was impossible to assess cognitive function of the patient during the delirious state. After adequate treatment, however, he was able to score 29 of 30 on the MMSE (see screening tests section and Chapter 4). Although this does not exclude the possibility that more subtle evidence for cognitive impairment is present in this high-risk patient, it does suggest that dementia is not a major problem. More specialized cognitive testing was not performed in RH for reasons that will be discussed later. As in many patients with alcohol dependence, the patient exhibits some traits of avoidant, dependent, and schizoid personality disorders. There is insufficient evidence to make the diagnosis of any one of these or to make a diagnosis of mixed personality disorder because the influence that alcohol has on these traits cannot be parceled out, even when the chart is reviewed thoroughly. The Axis II diagnosis is therefore deferred. As previously mentioned, antisocial personality disorder, which has greater validity and reliability than other personality disorders, has been excluded.

The Axis III diagnoses for RH are listed in Table 1–9 and are primarily related to complications of alcohol abuse. The patient, however, had a seizure 3 weeks into his hospital stay. Although alcohol withdrawal seizure is a logical choice in the differential, it occurred outside the expected period (3 to 14 days) for this complication to happen. The EEG and CT, documenting a subdural hematoma, were done not only because the presentation was atypical (although this would have been enough) but also because RH was at high risk for an alternative cause of new seizure onset because of his history of alcohol abuse and thrombocytopenia. In addition, it may be recalled that the patient had a head bruise on physical examination, and the fundoscopic examination had not been performed because of poor patient compliance.

The subdural hematoma could have been identified earlier had a more aggressive central nervous system workup for delirium been done at the outset. This is where systematic and thorough examination and informed clinical judgment become so important. The patient is at a high risk for other causes of central nervous system pathology because of the unreliable alcoholic state and a fundoscopic examination was not initially possible during the delirium. Delirium alone should be sufficient to warrant further evaluation in such a case. Decisions such as these have important implications regarding patient care.

Before the onset of this admission, the patient experienced no acute stressors (Axis IV) that would have predisposed him to admission. Although not receiving his disability check could have been considered an acute stressor, it is more likely that the lack of alcohol was a major factor in his presentation. However, he was unemployed, had no social support system, and suffered from intermittent medical problems related to his alcohol abuse, which qualify as severe, enduring stressful circumstances. The patient's global assessment of function during the delirious state suggests that he wouldn't have been able to maintain his personal care on his own (Axis V).

RH responded well to high-dose benzodiazepines for withdrawal within a few days of initial hospitalization. Other medical factors were evaluated and treated during the initial hospital stay. As the patient's delirium resolved, further information was obtained from the patient, and his behavior was observed to confirm the initial impression and determine whether other psychiatric conditions might be present, especially those with a high frequency in alcohol dependence. Particular emphasis was placed on observing the patient's ability to identify familiar personnel, locate his room, and perform activities of daily living. He did these without trouble after the delirium cleared, suggesting that he would be able to function satisfactorily outside a structured environment. Furthermore, documenting these behaviors obviated the need to perform more formalized and expensive neuropsychological testing.

RH had participated in several alcohol treatment programs without lasting benefit. For this reason, legal commitment to an inpatient treatment center was deemed unlikely to benefit him. This particular admission was occasioned by a serious threat to the patient's life. It is at times like these that some alcoholics become sufficiently frightened that they enter and follow through on their resolve to stay sober. He expressed an interest in reinitiating contact with Alcoholics Anonymous, which was encouraged during his hospital stay. Such a program, if adhered to, effectively uses group support, confrontation, religious motivation, and behavior modification to modify the long-term behavior of alcoholics. Because it is run by former alcoholics, rationalizations and ploys are much more difficult to get away with than when mental health professionals administer treatment.

Social factors also often play a role in when and how much alcoholics drink. One thing that has not been done is to have the patient live in a more structured environment such as a nursing home in the hope that opportunities to imbibe would not be as frequent. The patient would have to agree to this and be willing to cooperate with the personnel in abiding by rules at the facility.

When the clinical situation warrants, a systematic psychiatric assessment is important for appropriate patient care, regardless of the setting. It requires an understanding of current psychiatric nomenclature (DSM-IV) and predictive value of the disorders being diagnosed. Because psychiatric conditions are no longer diagnosed merely by excluding other illnesses that can cause similar complaints, it is important to know what questions to ask and how to ask them, as well as to accurately observe the behaviors that lead to making a psychiatric diagnosis. The skilled use of the mental status examination, psychological and neuropsychological tests, and laboratory evaluations will help differentiate medical from psychiatric problems or identify the relationship between the two. DSM-IV provides a framework, albeit not perfect, for considering psychiatric diagnosis in the differential diagnosis of many patient problems. Chapter 2 discusses basic aspects of the psychosocial and psychodynamic assessment, and other chapters will discuss the major psychiatric diagnostic categories in more detail, including specific issues relevant to clinical diagnosis and treatment.

CLINICAL PEARLS

- The principles of psychiatric assessment are identical to physical disorder assessment. Symptoms are elicited and signs are reviewed. Differential diagnosis is carried out using all available evidence including laboratory and X-ray findings.
- Medical patients will usually accept psychiatric assessment when it is explained as part of a comprehensive assessment of the role of physical and stress factors influencing their symptoms.
- Because psychiatric symptoms are many times colored by subjective factors, the extra effort to interview the patient's family and friends often pays off in more accurate assessment.
- Thyroid function abnormalities are a common medical cause of psychiatric symptoms.
- The setting of a patient encounter will influence the types of common psychopathology. However, mood disorders, anxiety disorders, and alcohol/drug disorders are commonly found in all settings.
- All mental status examination reports should indicate whether homicidal or suicidal ideation present.
- When a patient is unable to relate an understandable history, consider cognitive impairment disorder and psychiatric disorders associated with thought disorder such as schizophrenia or bipolar disorder.
- An EEG may be helpful when there is a question of whether a patient's symptoms are due to brain dysfunction or a functional psychiatric disorder.
- Presenting an extensive five-axis formulation will provide the major aspects of a biopsychosocial assessment.
- New psychiatric symptoms in a geriatric patient should trigger a vigorous search for mental disorders due to medical, neurologic, toxic, or medication-related factors.

ANNOTATED BIBLIOGRAPHY

American Psychiatric Association: Diagnostic and Statistical Manual of Mental Disorders, 4th ed. Washington, DC, American Psychiatric Association, in press [1994]

American Psychiatric Association: DSM-IV Draft Criteria 3/1/93. Washington DC, American Psychiatric Association, 1993

> Contains diagnostic criteria for over 200 defined psychiatric diagnoses. Also includes information about age of onset, predisposing factors, prevalence, sex ratios, and differential diagnosis for each disorder.

Berg R, Franzen M, Wedding D: Screening for Brain Impairment. New York, Springer-Verlag, 1987

> Excellent summary of neuropsychological tests that have relevance for evaluation of psychiatric patients. Gives historical information about individual tests and reviews briefer neuropsychological screening batteries.

Frances AJ, First MB, Widiger TA et al: An A to Z guide to DSM-IV conundrums. J Abnormal Psychol 100:407–412, 1991

> This article outlines the changes for DSM-IV which is scheduled for publication in 1994.

Goodwin DW, Guze SB: Psychiatric Diagnosis. New York, Oxford University Press, 1984

> Reviews essentials of diagnosis for major psychiatric disorders and provides summary of clinical validation for each disorder, including epidemiology, natural history, and family studies.

Kaufman D: Clinical Neurology for Psychiatrists. New York, Grune & Stratton, 1987

> For students interested in details of the neurological exam as applied to psychiatric patients, this is a practical and lucid guide.

MacKinnon RA, Yudofsky SC (eds): The Psychiatric Evaluation in Clinical Practice. Philadelphia, JB Lippincott, 1986

> This book provides an authoritative and well-written discussion of the psychiatric interview and history from a psychodynamic perspective. It also provides excellent discussions of the mental status examination and other aspects of the neuropsychiatric evaluation.

Mesulam M (ed): Principles of Behavioral Neurology. Philadelphia, FA Davis, 1985

> This is a splendid presentation of the basic science and clinical application of behavioral neurology with a strong emphasis on neuropsychiatric assessment.

van Riezan H, Segal M: Comparative Evaluation of Rating Scales for Clinical Psychopharmacology. Amsterdam, Elsevier, 1988

> Extensive review of psychiatric rating scales used for research and clinical purposes. Includes information on how to obtain scales and copyright considerations.

REFERENCES

American Psychiatric Association: DSM-IV Draft Criteria 3/1/93. Washington DC, American Psychiatric Association, 1993

American Psychiatric Association: Diagnostic and Statistical Manual of Mental Disorders, 4th ed. Washington, DC, American Psychiatric Association, in press [1994]

Baron M: Behavioral genetics. In Stoudemire A. (ed): Human Behavior: An Introduction for Medical Students, 2nd ed. Philadelphia, J. B. Lippincott Company, 1994

Bates B, Hoekelman RA: Interviewing and the health history. In Bates B (ed): A Guide to Physical Examination. Philadelphia, JB Lippincott, 1983

Berg R, Franzen M, Wedding D: Screening for Brain Impairment. New York, Springer-Verlag, 1987

Chandler JD, Gerndt JE: The role of medical evaluation in psychiatric inpatients. Psychosomatics 29:410–416, 1988

Colligan RC, Osborne D, Swenson WM, Offord KP: The MMPI: A Contemporary Normative Study. New York, Praeger, 1983

Elstein AS, Shulman LS, Sprafka SA: Medical Problem Solving: An Analysis of Clinical Reasoning. Cambridge, MA, Harvard University Press, 1978

Feighner JP, Robins E, Guze SB et al: Diagnostic criteria for use in psychiatric research. Arch Gen Psychiatry 26:57–63, 1972

Fink PJ: Response to the presidential address: Is "biopsychosocial" the psychiatric shibboleth? Arch Gen Psychiatry 145:1061–1067, 1988

Hall RCW, Gardiner ER, Stickney SK et al: Physical illness manifesting as psychiatric disease: II. Analysis of a state hospital inpatient population. Arch Gen Psychiatry 35:989–995, 1980

Hampton JR, Harrison MJG, Mitchell JRA et al: Relative contributions of history-taking, physical examination, and laboratory investigation to diagnosis and management of medical outpatients. Br Med J 2:486–489, 1975

Hoffman RS: Diagnostic errors in the evaluation of behavioral disorders. JAMA 248:964–967, 1982

Kathol RG, Mutgi A, Williams J, Clamon G, Noyes R: Diagnosis of major depression in cancer patients according to four sets of criteria. Am J Psychiatry 147:1021–1024, 1990

Koranyi EK: Somatic illness in psychiatric patients. Psychosomatics 21:887–891, 1980

Krummel S, Kathol RG: What you should know about physical evaluations in psychiatric patients: Results of a survey. Gen Hosp Psychiatry 9:275–279, 1987

LaBruzza AL: Physical illness presenting as psychiatric disorder: Guidelines for differential diagnosis. J Operational Psychiatry 12:24–31, 1981

Osborne D: The MMPI in medical practice. Psychiatr Ann 15(9):534–541, 1985

Olfson M: Utilization of neuropsychotic diagnostic tests for general hospital psychiatry patients with mental disorders. Am J Psychiatry 149:1711–1717, 1992

Regier DA, Goldberg ID, Taube CA: The de facto U.S. mental health system. Arch Gen Psychiatry 35:685–693, 1978

Reich J: Personality disorders in primary care. In: Yates WR (ed): Primary Care Clinics—Psychiatry Issue Volume 14, Philadelphia, WB Saunders, 1987

Robins E, Guze SB: Establishment of diagnostic validity in psychiatric illness: Its application to schizophrenia. Am J Psychiatry 126:983–987, 1970

Rosenhan DL: On being sane in insane places. Science 179:250–258, 1979

Spitzer RL, Endicott J, Robins E: Research diagnostic criteria. Rationale and reliability. Arch Gen Psychiatry 35:773–782, 1978

Stoudemire A: Somatothymia: Part I. Psychosomatics 32:365–370, 1991a

Stoudemire A: Somatothymia: Part II. Psychosomatics 32:371–381, 1991b

Stoudemire A (ed): Human Behavior: An Introduction for Medical Students, 2nd ed. Philadelphia, J. B. Lippincott Company, 1994

Taylor MA, Sierles FS, Abrams R: The neuropsychiatric evaluation. In Hales RE, Yudofsky SC: Textbook of Neuropsychiatry. Washington, DC, American Psychiatric Press, Inc, 1987

van Riezen H, Segal M: Comparative Evaluation of Rating Scales for Clinical Psychopharmacology. Amsterdam, Elsevier, 1988

Appendix to Chapter One

STRUCTURE OF DSM-IV DIAGNOSTIC CATEGORIES

(Adapted from: DSM-IV Draft Criteria [3/1/93 version], Task Force on DSM-IV, American Psychiatric Association) Readers should check the final published version of DSM-IV as last-minute changes may be made both in the nomenclature as well as specific diagnostic criteria.

MULTIAXIAL SYSTEM

Axis I   Clinical Syndromes
              V Codes

Axis II   Personality Disorders

Axis III   General Medical Conditions

Axis IV   Psychosocial and Environmental Problems

Axis V   Global Assessment of Functioning

Disorders Usually First Diagnosed in Infancy, Childhood, or Adolescence

Mental Retardation

      Mild Mental Retardation
      Moderate Retardation

Severe Mental Retardation
Profound Mental Retardation
Mental Retardation, Severity Unspecified

Learning Disorders (Academic Skills Disorder)

Reading Disorder (Developmental Reading Disorder)
Mathematics Disorder (Developmental Arithmetic Disorder)
Disorder of Written Expression (Developmental Expressive Writing Disorder)
Learning Disorder NOS

Motor Skills Disorder

Developmental Coordination Disorder

Pervasive Developmental Disorders

Autistic Disorder
Rett's Disorder
Childhood Disintegrative Disorder
Asperger's Disorder
Pervasive Developmental Disorder NOS (including Atypical Autism)

Disruptive Behavior and Attention-deficit Disorders

Attention-deficit/Hyperactivity Disorders
    predominantly inattentive type
    predominantly hyperactive-impulsive type
    combined type
Attention-deficit/Hyperactivity Disorder NOS
Oppositional Defiant Disorder
Conduct Disorder
Disruptive Behavior Disorder NOS

Feeding and Eating Disorders of Infancy or Early Childhood

Pica
Rumination Disorder
Feeding Disorder of Infancy or Early Childhood

Tic Disorders

Tourette's Disorder
Chronic Motor or Vocal Tic Disorder
Transient Tic Disorder
Tic Disorder NOS

Communication Disorders

Expressive Language Disorder (Developmental Expressive Language Disorder)

Mixed Receptive/Expressive Language Disorder (Developmental Receptive Language Disorder)
Phonological Disorder (Developmental Articulation Disorder)
Stuttering
Communication Disorder NOS

Elimination Disorders
Encopresis
Enuresis

Other Disorders of Infancy, Childhood, or Adolescence
Separation Anxiety Disorder
Selective Mutism (Elective Mutism)
Reactive Attachment Disorder of Infancy or Early Childhood
Stereotypic Movement Disorder (Stereotypy/Habit Disorder)
Disorder of Infancy, Childhood, or Adolescence NOS

Delirium, Dementia, Amnestic and Other Cognitive Disorders

Deliria
Delirium Due to a General Medical Condition
Substance-induced Delirium
(refer to specific substance for code)
Delirium Due to Multiple Etiologies
(use multiple codes based on specific etiologies)
Delirium NOS

Dementias
Dementia of the Alzheimer's Type With Early Onset:
if onset at age 65 or below
   uncomplicated
   with delirium
   with delusions
   with depressed mood
   with hallucinations
   with perceptual disturbance
   with behavioral disturbance
   with communication disturbance
With Late Onset: if onset after age 65
   uncomplicated
   with delirium
   with delusions
   with depressed mood
   with hallucinations
   with perceptual disturbance

with behavioral disturbance
with communication disturbance
Vascular Dementia
uncomplicated
with delirium
with delusions
with depressed mood
with hallucinations
with perceptual disturbance
with behavioral disturbance
with communication disturbance

Dementias Due to Other General Medical Conditions

Dementia Due to HIV Disease *(Code 043.1 on Axis III)*
Dementia Due to Head Trauma *(Code 905.0 on Axis III)*
Dementia Due to Parkinson's Disease *(Code 332.0 on Axis III)*
Dementia Due to Huntington's Disease *(Code 333.4 on Axis III)*
Dementia Due to Pick's Disease *(Code 331.1 on Axis III)*
Dementia Due to Creutzfeldt-Jakob Disease *(Code 046.1 on Axis III)*
Dementia Due to Other General Medical Disease
Substance-induced Persisting Dementia
(refer to specific substance for code)
Dementia Due to Multiple Etiologies
(use multiple codes based on specific etiologies)
Dementia NOS

Amnestic Disorders

Amnestic Disorder Due to a General Medical Condition
Substance-induced Persisting Amnestic Disorder
(refer to specific substance for code)
Amnestic Disorder NOS

Cognitive Disorder NOS

Mental Disorders Due to a General Medical Condition Not Elsewhere Classified

Catatonic Disorder Due to a General Medical Condition
Personality Change Due to a General Medical Condition
Mental Disorder NOS Due to a General Medical Condition

Substance Related Disorders

Alcohol Use Disorders
Alcohol Dependence
Alcohol Abuse
Alcohol Intoxication

Alcohol Withdrawal
Alcohol Delirium
Alcohol Persisting Dementia
Alcohol Persisting Amnestic Disorder
Alcohol Psychotic Disorder
  with delusions
  with hallucinations
Alcohol Mood Disorder
Alcohol Anxiety Disorder
Alcohol Sexual Dysfunction
Alcohol Sleep Disorder
Alcohol Use Disorder NOS
Amphetamine (or Related Substance) Use Disorders
Amphetamine (or Related Substance) Dependence
Amphetamine (or Related Substance) Abuse
Amphetamine (or Related Substance) Intoxication
Amphetamine (or Related Substance) Withdrawal
Amphetamine (or Related Substance) Delirium
Amphetamine (or Related Substance) Psychotic Disorder
  with delusions
  with hallucinations
Amphetamine (or Related Substance) Mood Disorder
Amphetamine (or Related Substance) Anxiety Disorder
Amphetamine (or Related Substance) Sexual Dysfunction
Amphetamine (or Related Substance) Sleep Disorder
Amphetamine (or Related Substance) Use Disorder NOS
Caffeine Use Disorders
Caffeine Intoxication
Caffeine Anxiety Disorder
Caffeine Sleep Disorder
Caffeine Use Disorder NOS
Cannabis Use Disorders
Cannabis Dependence
Cannabis Abuse
Cannabis Intoxication
Cannabis Delirium
Cannabis Psychotic Disorder
  with delusions
  with hallucinations
Cannabis Anxiety Disorder
Cannabis Use Disorder NOS
Cocaine Use Disorders
Cocaine Dependence
Cocaine Abuse
Cocaine Intoxication
Cocaine Withdrawal

Cocaine Delirium
Cocaine Psychotic Disorder
  with delusions
  with hallucinations
Cocaine Mood Disorder
Cocaine Anxiety Disorder
Cocaine Sexual Dysfunction
Cocaine Sleep Disorder
Cocaine Use Disorder NOS
Hallucinogen Use Disorders
  Hallucinogen Dependence
  Hallucinogen Abuse
  Hallucinogen Intoxication
  Hallucinogen Persisting Perception Disorder
  Hallucinogen Delirium
  Hallucinogen Psychotic Disorder
    with delusions
    with hallucinations
  Hallucinogen Mood Disorder
  Hallucinogen Anxiety Disorder
  Hallucinogen Use Disorder NOS
Inhalant Use Disorders
  Inhalant Dependence
  Inhalant Abuse
  Inhalant Intoxication
  Inhalant Delirium
  Inhalant Persisting Dementia
  Inhalant Psychotic Disorder
    with delusions
    with hallucinations
  Inhalant Mood Disorder
  Inhalant Anxiety Disorder
  Inhalant Use Disorder NOS
Nicotine Use Disorders
  Nicotine Dependence
  Nicotine Withdrawal
  Nicotine Use Disorder NOS
Opioid Use Disorder
  Opioid Dependence
  Opioid Abuse
  Opioid Intoxication
  Opioid Withdrawal
  Opioid Delirium
  Opioid Psychotic Disorder
    with delusions
    with hallucinations

Opioid Mood Disorder
Opioid Sleep Disorder
Opioid Sexual Dysfunction
Opioid Use Disorder NOS
Phencyclidine (or Related Substance) Use Disorders
Phencyclidine (or Related Substance) Dependence
Phencyclidine (or Related Substance) Abuse
Phencyclidine (or Related Substance) Intoxication
Phencyclidine (or Related Substance) Delirium
Phencyclidine (or Related Substance) Psychotic Disorder
  with delusions
  with hallucinations
Phencyclidine (or Related Substance) Mood Disorder
Phencyclidine (or Related Substance) Anxiety Disorder
Phencyclidine (or Related Substance) Use Disorder NOS
Sedative, Hypnotic, or Anxiolytic Substance Use Disorders
Sedative, Hypnotic, or Anxiolytic Dependence
Sedative, Hypnotic, or Anxiolytic Abuse
Sedative, Hypnotic, or Anxiolytic Intoxication
Sedative, Hypnotic, or Anxiolytic Withdrawal
Sedative, Hypnotic, or Anxiolytic Delirium
Sedative, Hypnotic, or Anxiolytic Persisting Dementia
Sedative, Hypnotic, or Anxiolytic Persisting Amnestic Disorder
Sedative, Hypnotic, or Anxiolytic Psychotic Disorder
  with delusions
  with hallucinations
Sedative, Hypnotic, or Anxiolytic Mood Disorder
Sedative, Hypnotic, or Anxiolytic Anxiety Disorder
Sedative, Hypnotic, or Anxiolytic Sleep Disorder
Sedative, Hypnotic, or Anxiolytic Sexual Dysfunction
Sedative, Hypnotic, or Anxiolytic Use Disorder NOS
Polysubstance Use Disorder
Polysubstance Dependence
Other (or Unknown) Substance Use Disorders
Other (or Unknown) Substance Dependence
Other (or Unknown) Substance Abuse
Other (or Unknown) Substance Intoxication
Other (or Unknown) Substance Withdrawal
Other (or Unknown) Substance Delirium
Other (or Unknown) Substance Persisting Dementia
Other (or Unknown) Substance Persisting Amnestic
Disorder
Other (or Substance Substance Psychotic Disorder
  with delusions
  with hallucinations
Other (or Unknown) Substance Mood Disorder

Other (or Unknown) Substance Anxiety Disorder
Other (or Unknown) Substance Sexual Dysfunction
Other (or Unknown) Substance Sleep Disorder
Other (or Unknown) Substance Use Disorder NOS

Schizophrenia and Other Psychotic Disorders

Schizophrenia–paranoid type
Schizophrenia–disorganized type
Schizophrenia–catatonic type
Schizophrenia–undifferentiated type
Schizophrenia–residual type
Schizophreniform Disorder
Schizoaffective Disorder
Delusional Disorder
Brief Psychotic Disorder
Shared Psychotic Disorder (Folie a Deux)
Psychotic Disorder Due to a General Medical Condition
    with delusions
    with hallucinations
Substance-Induced Psychotic Disorder
(refer to specific substance for codes)
Psychotic Disorder NOS

Mood Disorders

Code current state of Major Depressive Disorder or Bipolar Disorder in fifth digit:

0 unspecified
1 mild
2 moderate
3 severe, without psychotic features
4 severe, with psychotic features
5 in partial remission
6 in full remission

Depressive Disorders
    Major Depressive Disorder, single episode
    Major Depressive Disorder, recurrent
    Dysthymic Disorder
    Depressive Disorder NOS
Bipolar Disorders
    Bipolar I Disorder, single manic episode
    Bipolar I Disorder, most recent episode hypomanic
    Bipolar I Disorder, most recent episode manic
    Bipolar I Disorder, most recent episode mixed
    Bipolar I Disorder, most recent episode depressed
    Bipolar I Disorder, most recent episode unspecified

Bipolar II Disorder (recurrent major depressive episodes with hypomania)
Cyclothymic Disorder
Bipolar Disorder NOS

Mood Disorder Due to a General Medical Condition
Substance-Induced Mood Disorder
(refer to specific substances for codes)
Mood Disorder NOS

Anxiety Disorders

Panic Disorder Without Agoraphobia
Panic Disorder With Agoraphobia
Agoraphobia Without History of Panic Disorder
Specific Phobia (Simple Phobia)
Social Phobia (Social Anxiety Disorder)
Obsessive–Compulsive Disorder
Posttraumatic Stress Disorder
Acute Stress Disorder
Generalized Anxiety Disorder (includes Overanxious Disorder of Childhood)
Anxiety Disorder Due to a General Medical Condition
Substance-Induced Anxiety Disorder
(refer to specific substances for codes)
Anxiety Disorder NOS

Somatoform Disorders

Somatization Disorder
Conversion Disorder
Hypochondriasis
Body Dysmorphic Disorder
Pain Disorder Associated with Psychological Factors
Pain Disorder Associated with Psychological Factors and a General Medical Condition
Undifferentiated Somatoform Disorder
Somatoform Disorder NOS

Factitious Disorders

Factitious Disorder with Predominantly Psychological Signs and Symptoms
Factitious Disorder with Predominantly Physical Signs and Symptoms
Factitious Disorder with Combined Psychological and Physical Signs and Symptoms
Factitious Disorder NOS

Dissociative Disorders

Dissociative Amnesia
Dissociative Fugue

Dissociative Identity Disorder (Multiple Personality Disorder)
Depersonalization Disorder
Dissociative Disorder NOS

Sexual and Gender Identity Disorders
Sexual Dysfunctions
       Sexual Desire Disorders
         Hypoactive Sexual Desire Disorder
         Sexual Aversion Disorder
       Sexual Arousal Disorders
         Female Sexual Arousal Disorder
         Male Erectile Disorder
       Orgasm Disorders
         Female Orgasmic Disorder (Inhibited Female Orgasm)
         Male Orgasmic Disorder (Inhibited Male Orgasm)
         Premature Ejaculation
       Sexual Pain Disorders
         Dyspareunia
         Vaginismus
       Sexual Dysfunctions Due to a General Medical Condition
         Male Erectile Disorder Due to a General Medical Condition
         Male Dyspareunia Due to a General Medical Condition
         Female Dyspareunia Due to a General Medical Condition
         Male Hypoactive Sexual Desire Disorder
         Due to a General Medical Condition
         Female Hypoactive Sexual Desire Disorder
         Due to a General Medical Condition
         Other Male Sexual Dysfunction Due to a General Medical Condition
         Other Female Sexual Dysfunction Due to a General Medical Condition
         Substance-induced Sexual Dysfunction
         (refer to specific substances for codes)
         Sexual Dysfunction NOS
Paraphilias
         Exhibitionism
         Fetishism
         Frotteurism
         Pedophilia
         Sexual Masochism
         Sexual Sadism
         Voyeurism
         Transvestic Fetishism
         Paraphilia NOS
         Sexual Disorder NOS
Gender Identity Disorders
         Gender Identity Disorder
           in Children
           in Adolescents and Adults
         Gender Identity Disorder NOS

Eating Disorders
Anorexia Nervosa
Bulimia Nervosa
Eating Disorder NOS

Sleep Disorders
Primary Sleep Disorders
Dyssomnias
Primary Insomnia
Primary Hypersomnia
Narcolepsy
Breathing-Related Sleep Disorder
Circadian Rhythm Sleep Disorder (Sleep-Wake Schedule Disorder)
Dyssomnia NOS
Parasomnias
Nightmare Disorder (Dream Anxiety Disorder)
Sleep Terror Disorder
Sleepwalking Disorder
Parasomnia NOS
Sleep Disorders Related to Another Mental Disorder
Insomnia Related to [Axis I or Axis II Disorder]
Insomnia Related to [Axis I or Axis II Disorder]
Other Sleep Disorders
Sleep Disorder Due to a General Medical Condition
insomnia type
hypersomnia type
parasomnia type
mixed type
Substance-Induced Sleep Disorder
(refer to specific substances for codes)

Impulse Control Disorders Not Elsewhere Classified
Intermittent Explosive Disorder
Kleptomania
Pyromania
Pathological Gambling
Trichotillomania
Impulse Control NOS

Adjustment Disorders
Adjustment Disorder with Anxiety
Adjustment Disorder with Depressed Mood
Adjustment Disorder with Disturbance of Conduct
Adjustment Disorder with Mixed Disturbance of Emotions and Conduct
Adjustment Disorders with Mixed Anxiety and Depressed Mood
Adjustment Disorder Unspecified

Personality Disorders
Paranoid Personality Disorder

Schizoid Personality Disorder
Schizotypal Personality Disorder
Antisocial Personality Disorder
Borderline Personality Disorder
Histrionic Personality Disorder
Narcissistic Personality Disorder
Avoidant Personality Disorder
Dependent Personality Disorder
Obsessive–Compulsive Personality Disorder
Personality Disorder NOS

Other Conditions That May Be a Focus of Clinical Attention

(Psychological Factors) Affecting Medical Condition
Choose name based on nature of factors:
  Mental Disorder Affecting Medical Condition
  Psychological Symptoms Affecting Medical Condition
  Personality Traits or Coping Style Affecting Medical Condition
  Maladaptive Health Behaviors Affecting Medical Condition
  Unspecified Psychological Factors Affecting Medical Condition

Medication-Induced Movement Disorders

Neuroleptic-Induced Parkinsonism
Neuroleptic Malignant Syndrome
Neuroleptic-Induced Acute Dystonia
Neuroleptic-Induced Acute Akathisia
Neuroleptic-Induced Tardive Dyskinesia
Neuroleptic-Induced Postural Tremor
Medication-Induced Movement Disorder NOS

Adverse Effects of Medication NOS

Relational Problems

Relational Problem Related to a Mental Disorder
or a General Medical Condition
Parent–Child Relational Problem
Partner Relational Problem
Sibling Relational Problem
Relational Problem NOS

Problems Related to Abuse or Neglect

Physical Abuse of Child
Sexual Abuse of Child
Neglect of a Child
Physical Abuse of Adult
Sexual Abuse of Adult

Additional Conditions That May Be a Focus of Clinical Attention

Bereavement
Borderline Intellectual Function
Academic Problem
Occupational Problem
Childhood or Adolescent Antisocial Behavior
Adult Antisocial Behavior
Malingering
Phase of Life Problem
Noncompliance with treatment for a mental disorder
Identity Problem
Religious or Spiritual Problem
Acculturation Problem
Age-Associated Memory Decline

Additional Codes

Unspecified Mental Disorder
No Diagnosis or Condition on Axis I
Diagnosis or Condition Deferred on Axis I
No Diagnosis on Axis II
Diagnosis Deferred on Axis II

Axis IV: Psychosocial and Environmental Problems

Check:
____ Problems with primary support group (Childhood [V61.9], Adult [V61.9], Parent-Child [V61.2]). Specify: _____
____ Problems related to the social environment (V62.4). Specify: _____
____ Educational problem (V62.3). Specify: _____
____ Occupational problem (V62.2). Specify: _____
____ Housing problem (V60.9). Specify: _____
____ Economic problem (V60.9). Specify: _____
____ Problems with access to health care services (V63.9). Specify: _____
____ Problems related to interaction with the legal system/crime (V62.5). Specify: _____
____ Other psychosocial problem (V62.9). Specify: _____

Global Assessment of Functioning Scale (GAF) Scale[1]

Consider psychological, social, and occupational functioning on a hypothetical continuum of mental health-illness. Do not include impairment in functioning due to physical (or environmental) limitations.

Code (Note: Use intermediate codes when appropriate, e.g., 45, 68, 72.)

100   **Superior functioning in a wide range of activities, life's problems never seem to get out of hand, is sought out by others because of his many positive qualities. No symptoms.**
|
91

90   **Absent or minimal symptoms** (e.g., mild anxiety before an exam), **good functioning in all areas, interested and involved in a wide range of activities, socially effective, generally satisfied with life, no more than everyday problems or concerns** (e.g., an occasional argument with
|
81   family members).

80   **If symptoms are present, they are transient and expectable reactions to psychosocial stressors** (e.g., difficulty concentrating after family argument); **no more than slight impairment in social, occupational, or**
|
71   **school functioning** (e.g., temporarily falling behind in school work).

70   **Some mild symptoms** (e.g., depressed mood and mild insomnia) **OR some difficulty in social, occupational, or school functioning** (e.g., occasional truancy, or theft within the household), **but generally functioning**
|
61   **pretty well, has some meaningful interpersonal relationships.**

60   **Moderate symptoms** (e.g., flat affect and circumstantial speech, occasional panic attacks) **OR moderate difficulty in social, occupational, or**
|
51   **school functioning** (e.g., friends, conflicts with co-workers).

50   **Serious symptoms** (e.g., suicidal ideation, severe obsessional rituals, frequent shoplifting) **OR any serious impairment in social, occupational,**
|
41   **or school functioning** (e.g., no friends, unable to keep a job).

40   **Some impairment in reality testing or communication** (e.g., speech is at times illogical, obscure, or irrelevant) **OR major impairment in several areas, such as work or school, family relations, judgment, thinking, or mood** (e.g., depressed man avoids friends, neglects family, and is unable to work; child frequently beats up younger children, is defiant at home, and is
|
31   failing at school).

30   **Behavior is considerably influenced by delusions or hallucinations OR serious impairment in communication or judgment** (e.g., sometimes incoherent, acts grossly inappropriately, suicidal preoccupation) **OR inability to function in almost all areas** (e.g., stays in bed all day; no job,
|
21   home, or friends).

20   **Some danger of hurting self or others** (e.g., suicide attempts without clear expectation of death, frequently violent, manic excitement) **OR occasionally fails to maintain minimal personal hygiene** (e.g., smears feces) **OR gross impairment in communication** (e.g., largely incoherent or
|
11   mute).

10   **Persistent danger of severely hurting self or others** (e.g., recurrent violence) **OR persistent inability to maintain minimal personal hygiene OR serious suicidal act with clear expectation of death.**
|
1

0   **Inadequate information.**

1 The GAF Scale is a revision of the GAS (Endicott J, Spitzer RL, Fleiss, et al: The Global Assessment Scale: A procedure for measuring overall severity of psychiatric disturbance. *Archives of General Psychiatry* 33:766–771, 1976) and the CGAS (Shaffer D, Gould MS, Brasic J, et al: Children's Global Assessment Scale (CGAS). *Archives of General Psychiatry* 40:1228–1231, 1983). These are revisions of the Global Scale of the Health-Sickness Rating Scale (Luborsky L: Clinicians' judgments of mental health. *Archives of General Psychiatry* 7:407–417, 1962).

2

Biopsychosocial Assessment and Case Formulation

Alan Stoudemire

The preceding chapter focused on the basics of the psychiatric history, mental status examination, physical and laboratory assessment, and DSM-IV as a descriptive psychiatric classification system. Based on the information gathered in this type of initial assessment, a preliminary diagnosis and treatment plan can then be made. A more in-depth psychological evaluation, however, is then required. Examples of patients in whom an in-depth psychosocial assessment is called for include the following:

1. Patients who appear to have complex or problematic family, marital, or interpersonal problems.
2. Patients who appear to have *repetitive* patterns of conflicts or difficulties in their interpersonal relationships.
3. Individuals who appear to have psychiatric disorders and symptoms that are apparently precipitated or exacerbated by social, occupational, family, or interpersonal factors.
4. Patients who have unexplained somatic symptoms that cannot be explained on the basis of physical or laboratory findings.
5. Children and adolescents with psychiatric symptoms.

By emphasizing the importance of psychosocial assessment, one should not necessarily assume that such factors are the direct *cause* of the patient's psychiatric disorder—this may or may not be the case. The relative contribution of psychosocial factors in precipitating the onset or exacerbation of psychiatric disorders and symptoms varies depending on the disorder being evaluated. Moreover, the relative contribution of psychosocial factors to the cause of many psychiatric disorders remains highly controversial in the psychiatric literature. To take the position that psychosocial factors are important in the assessment of a patient who has a psychiatric disorder such as schizophrenia, however, is not the same as saying that schizophrenia is *caused by* psychosocial factors, because schizophrenia is now considered to derive primarily from predisposing genetic and biological factors. Nevertheless, few psychiatrists would argue against the position that psychosocial and environmental factors may be involved in relapses of schizophrenia or that schizophrenia has profound effects on the patient's social and interpersonal functioning. Likewise, vulnerability to panic disorder and the major mood disorders appears to be strongly determined by biological factors, yet certain patients may have their symptoms precipitated or exacerbated under certain types of emotionally stressful conditions. *Hence, even though certain disorders may have a primarily genetic and biological basis in respect to their underlying pathophysiology, the disorder's onset and relapse may be affected by social or environmental factors in the biologically predisposed individual.* Even in physical disorders, acute and chronic illness always poses a form of stress for the individual that may potentially affect every aspect of their family, social, and occupational life. For example, cancer and chronic renal disease may have devastating effects on the patient's emotional and social functioning (Green, 1994). Psychological reactions to physical illness are further discussed in Chapters 9 and 20.

GOALS OF PSYCHOSOCIAL ASSESSMENT

The primary goals of a comprehensive psychosocial evaluation are to: (1) assess if psychological or social factors are important in contributing to the patient's vulnerability to psychiatric illness, (2) assess if psychosocial factors are significant in causing relapse or exacerbation of symptoms, and (3) identify areas in the psychological or social realm where treatment efforts might be focused. In addition, such an assessment also will identify areas in the patient's support system that may be a resource. In patients who suffer primarily from repetitive problems in their interpersonal relationships or who have dysfunction within the family system, the psychosocial assessment may be the only means of fully understanding their condition and planning an effective course of treatment.

PSYCHODYNAMIC ASSESSMENT

A *psychodynamic* assessment is a more specialized form of psychological evaluation that is usually performed by a psychiatrist who endorses and is trained in this method of evaluation. An in-depth psychodynamic assessment may be needed as part of the psychosocial assessment in some situations and involves examining the key developmental life experiences that may have affected the patient's personality formation, the nature of the patient's past and current family relationships, the patient's psychological strengths and vulnerabilities, and the patient's characteristic defense mechanisms. A psychodynamic assessment also evaluates current interpersonal stresses that may be affecting the patient and therefore overlaps with the general psychosocial evaluation. Individuals and important environmental and family events that have influenced the patient in either a positive or negative manner are identified, and the effect they currently have or have had on the patient is evaluated. Psychodynamic assessment is often critical not only in developing a comprehensive understanding of the patient's personality and current difficulties but also in determining whether or not psychotherapy is required, and, if so, what type of psychotherapy would be most appropriate.

Psychodynamic assessment is a form of evaluation somewhat more specialized than a general psychosocial assessment and is largely based on a psychoanalytic frame of reference. Psychodynamic assessment imparts major significance to developmental influences on the patient within the family system and potential unconscious factors that may be affecting the patient's behavior, motivations, and interpersonal relationships. Psychodynamic assessment thus focuses on the influence of early relationships on the patient's personality formation, the patient's ego defense mechanisms, and the effects that these early relationships have on their interpersonal relationships.

Some psychoanalytic and psychodynamic theorists have attempted to explain all psychiatric illness—including major disorders such as schizophrenia, major depression, and anxiety disorders—in their most doctrinaire form as deriving from intrapsychic and unconscious mental processes. Personality disorders and other disturbances in behavior also were explained primarily on a psychodynamic basis as deriving from abnormal or otherwise conflicted childhood developmental experiences and dysfunction within the family system.

Recent advances in biological psychiatry and psychopharmacology in some instances have almost completely usurped primarily psychoanalytic and psychodynamic viewpoints with respect to *etiological* explanations for the major mental disorders such as schizophrenia, major depression, and bipolar disorder. In addition, psychoanalytically oriented therapies for these disorders based on these types of purist etiological explanations have been under serious criticism. Although considerable polarization and strain exist within the field of psychiatry regarding the relative contribution of psychodynamic factors in the cause of the major psychiatric disorders, there has been a recent trend to attempt to integrate biological and psychological viewpoints regarding the etiology and treatment of psychiatric illness (Cooper, 1985; Kandel, 1979, 1983; Reiser, 1984; van der Kolk, 1994). In addition, it is recognized that the relative contribution of psychological and biological factors varies with the psychiatric disorder being studied and that even within a given disorder (such as major depression) considerable heterogeneity exists among patients who may carry the same primary diagnosis.

Further discussion of this area is beyond the scope of this text, and the philosophy of this text that, given our limited knowledge of the precise cause of most psychiatric disorders, a balanced approach should be taken in patient evaluation so as to always consider the possible contributions of biological, psychological, and sociological factors relevant to the patient's condition. In every case, however, a psychosocial assessment should be part of the patient's evaluation. If a detailed assessment of the patient's personality structure is indicated, this is often best performed by a psychoanalyst or psychodynamically oriented psychotherapist. The theoretical basis for such assessments are primarily based on psychoanalytic theory that is discussed in depth in a chapter in the companion text to this volume on human behavior (Inderbitzen and James, 1994).

THE PRIMARY PHYSICIAN'S ROLE IN PSYCHOSOCIAL ASSESSMENT

It should be emphasized that a complete psychosocial assessment may be a complex and time-consuming process. In many cases, performing such an evaluation will exceed the skills and time of even the most psychologically minded physician. In such situations it may be necessary to refer the patient to a psychiatrist for a more in-depth assessment. Nevertheless, it is still the responsibility of the primary physician to gather certain basic information to assess and identify patients who may need referral.

The responsibility of the primary physician to elicit basic psychosocial data in this situation has analogies in general medical practice. For example, a general internist will assess the signs and symptoms of a patient with chest pain and, after this initial assessment, might then refer the patient to a cardiologist for possible cardiac catheterization and definitive cardiologic diagnosis and treatment. The internist would hardly consider initiating such a referral without gathering the basic medical history and performing a physical examination. Similarly, gathering basic psychosocial information about the patient will assure that patients in need of more specialized evaluation will be identified appropriately.

PSYCHOSOCIAL ASSESSMENT: BASIC APPROACHES

When the psychosocial assessment is conducted, there are several fundamental questions that should be posed to the patient, and if adequate time is allowed for exploration of the patient's responses, an excellent initial data base can be assimilated by the primary physician regarding the patient's general developmental history and current psychosocial status.

For example, the physician may ask questions directed toward determining the key events and important people in the patient's childhood, adolescence, and adulthood that appear to have had or continue to have an effect on the patient. Were there past traumas, losses, or problems within the family system, or difficulties in other childhood and adult relationships that had a major impact on the patient? Are there conflicted or unresolved relationships with family, friends, or significant other individuals that are a source of distress for the patient? Have there been particularly difficult times in the patient's life? What have been the patient's sources of happiness and satisfaction or unhappiness and frustration? Answers to open-ended questions of this sort will usually yield information that will form the rubric of a preliminary psychosocial and psychodynamic understanding of the patient. Patients who are guarded or who deny the significance or importance of psychological matters will require more extended psychiatric evaluations, or the physician will need to gather information from other sources such as family members.

PSYCHOSOCIAL STRESSES AND SOMATIC SYMPTOMS

Many patients under psychosocial stress in the general medical setting will present to their primary care physicians with somatic symptoms (insomnia, headaches, gastrointestinal distress). Somatic symptoms are also extremely common and may develop as a response to even minor stresses (e.g., tension headaches). Patients will also seek help in the medical sector for somatic symptoms that are part of a major depressive disorder long before the symptoms are recognized or considered as part of a primary psychiatric syndrome.

Somatothymia

Some patients have a limited capacity to describe their feelings verbally. This limitation in the ability to articulate and communicate feeling states in verbal language has been termed *somatothymia*, a term derived from Greek terms to mean "a bodily state of feeling." Research in child development has shown that the fundamental "language" children use to communicate physical or emotional distress is in somatic or physical terms. It is only later in development that children begin to learn "feeling" words to label and verbally communicate internal emotional distress, fear, or—alternately—their affectionate feelings. In some individuals, because of cultural, educational, intellectual, familial, and psychological factors, the ability to articulate and communicate emotional states is never developed or is developed to a very limited degree. The multiple determinants of the capacity for affective language have been discussed in detail elsewhere (Stoudemire, 1991a, b).

In some cultures the *primary* means of communicating emotional distress remains based on the use of somatic language. The tendency to describe strong emotional reactions persists in our own culture ("the news just made me *sick*"; "he died of a *broken heart*"; "the news gave me great *pain*"; etc.). Hence, the capacity for directly communicating emotional distress in abstract "psychological" language varies from individual to individual and is subject to strong cultural and subcultural influences. The task of the physician is to learn the "emotional language" of the patient and to interpret it appropriately. For many patients, the language of emotion will continue to be predominantly based on somatic or physical words. The concept of somatothymia will also be mentioned in respect to the somatoform disorders in Chapter 9 as well as in the somatic presentations of depression in Chapter 7. Particularly in respect to depression, it should be noted that somatic symptoms are the principle way that disturbances in mood present in the medical setting.

Two Caveats

It should not, however, be assumed that all physical symptoms with a negative medical workup are "psychosomatic" or "stress related" in nature. Two caveats should always be kept in mind: first, symptoms of medical illness and stress/psychiatrically related symptoms may coexist and be enmeshed; hence, even if stress-related symptoms are identified as such, this does not rule out the possibility of concurrent medical illness. Second, stress and the presence of a concurrent psychiatric illness (such as depression) may greatly magnify the symptoms of clearly documented underlying physical illnesses.

BIOPSYCHOSOCIAL ASSESSMENT

The DSM-IV system discussed in Chapter 1 (see Chapter 1 Appendix) is used primarily for purposes of description and classification and is based on data that can be documented objectively. Integrating the descriptive approach of DSM-IV with a psychosocial and psychodynamic understanding of the patient, however, is useful in determining what types of psychiatric treatment would be most helpful for the patient, especially in determining the need for psychotherapy.

As mentioned in Chapter 1, the biopsychosocial model uses a systems approach in attempting to integrate biological, psychological, and social aspects of the patient's condition (Alexander, 1950; Bertalanffy, 1968; Cohen-Cole & Levinson 1994; Engel, 1977; Fink, 1988; Meyer, 1957; Reiser, 1988). This approach inherently validates the potential importance of biogenetic, psychological, social, and environmental factors in the diagnosis and treatment of the patient.

The basic clinical principles of the type of biopsychosocially oriented case assessment of patients in medical *or* psychiatric settings presented in this text would take the following into consideration:

1. Genetic and biological factors are deemed to be of major importance in the pathogenesis and treatment of certain psychiatric disorders (such as schizophrenia and mood disorders) and also may play a part in determining the patient's resilience or vulnerability to stress.

2. Certain problematic developmental experiences and conflicted relationships within the family and social system may confer vulnerabilities to certain types of psychiatric illness; alternatively, positive developmental experiences and relationships and good social support may provide a buffering effect.

3. Current life stresses may precipitate the onset of certain psychiatric disorders and symptoms or contribute to relapses of preexisting conditions.

This chapter focuses on the practical clinical applications of these principles, and space does not permit a critical review of the overwhelming scientific evidence to support the biopsychosocial model. In the companion volume on human behavior for medical students, the scientific basis for the biopsychosocial model is discussed in depth, particularly by Cohen-Cole and Levinson. Students are referred to selected articles in the annotated bibliography and reference list and other chapters in the text on human behavior that precedes this volume for substantiating information (Aneshensel, Stone, 1982; Bifulco, Brown, Harris, 1987; Birley, Brown, 1970; Bolton, Oatley, 1987; Breier, Kelsoe, Kirwin et al, 1988; Bryer, Nelson, Miller et al, 1987; Cadoret, O'Gorman, Troughton et al, 1985; Coyne, 1991; Dew, Bromet & Penkower, 1992; Doane, West, Goldstein et al, 1981; Galanter, 1988; Goldberg, Bridges, Cook et al, 1990; Greenblatt, Becerra, Serafetinides, 1982; Harris, Brown, Bifulco, 1986, 1987; Kendler, 1988; MacMillan, Gold, Crow et al, 1986; Miklowitz, Goldstein, Neuchterlein et al, 1987; Miklowitz, Goldstein, Neuchterlein et al, 1988; Miller, Ingham, Davidson, 1976; Parry, Shapiro, 1986; Pellegrini, 1990; Penkower, Bromet, Dew, 1988; Romans, Walton, Herbison et al, 1992; Roy, 1980; Rutter, 1985; Schwartz, Myers, 1977a & b; Stansfeld, Gallacher, Sharp et al, 1991; Tennant, 1983, 1988; Tennant, Bebbington, Hurry, 1982; Tennant, Hurry, Bebbington, 1982a & b; Tennant, Smith, Bebbington et al, 1981; Uhlenhuth, Paykel, 1973; van der Kolk, 1986, 1994; Weissman, Gammon, John, et al, 1987).

CLINICAL APPLICATIONS

Diagnosis and treatment using the biopsychosocial model are multimodal and are directed toward stabilizing each sphere of the patient's life that appears to be under stress—biological, psychological, and/or social. To reiterate, in this conceptual framework it is essential to (1) accurately assess the pertinent biological and physical factors associated with the patient's condition, (2) evaluate the effects of past and present environmental, social, and family stressors, and (3) appraise the psychological significance of the illness for the patient (e.g., how the patient experiences the illness in light of significant current and past life experiences).

The following prototypical case describes how the biopsychosocial model, the DSM-IV descriptive approach, and a psychosocial/psychodynamic formulation can be integrated into patient evaluation and comprehensive treatment planning.

CASE STUDY: MR. A

Mr. A, a 50-year-old married attorney, presented to his internist 4 weeks after successful coronary artery bypass surgery. He appeared to have deteriorated after his successful surgery, was chronically fatigued, had severe insomnia, had lost his appetite, and had lost interest in doing almost everything, including returning to work. Because of his inability to return to work, he was sinking into financial debt, and his position in his law firm was in jeopardy. Although he had little interest in sex, he did attempt intercourse with his wife several times but was impotent.

The internist performed a complete medical evaluation and checked his laboratory profile. He was slightly hypokalemic because of the use of a thiazide diuretic. He was also taking the beta-adrenergic blocking agent propranolol for hypertension. Other than being overweight and continuing to smoke two packs of cigarettes a day, his examination was unremarkable, including a screening thyroid profile.

The internist assessed that the patient was primarily depressed, so he tapered and discontinued his propranolol (the physician knew the drug has been associated with inducing depression). He "reassured" the patient and prescribed a low dose of a cyclic antidepressant and a benzodiazepine sleeping medication and scheduled a follow-up appointment for 4 weeks.

Despite these measures, the patient continued to deteriorate. He began to have crying spells, guilty ruminations, and suicidal thoughts. He took his antidepressant inconsistently. He returned to the internist after a week at his wife's insistence. The internist felt a psychiatric consultation was then necessary.

The psychiatrist evaluated the patient and, because the patient had recently had an extensive physical and laboratory evaluation, he decided to begin treatment with a cyclic antidepressant with incremental increases, giving no more than a week's supply at a time because of the possibility of a suicidal overdose. Because the patient's wife could stay with him during the day and the patient denied any suicidal plans, the decision was made to treat him initially as an outpatient with twice-weekly visits.

Before deciding on this treatment plan, however, the psychiatrist first performed a full psychiatric history and mental status examination. The patient was found to be cognitively intact, and his symptoms were all consistent with the diagnosis of major depression. The patient's personality assessment revealed marked obsessive–compulsive traits in that he was a "workaholic," a perfectionist, driven to achieve, and rarely ever "relaxed." He was generally rigid and strict with his children and emotionally aloof. Although he loved and was devoted to his family, he had severe difficulty in directly expressing any affection or personal feelings toward them or other people. Although things had gone well for him professionally, he believed he was never totally happy and had a tendency to be chronically mildly depressed, dysphoric, and dissatisfied with himself and life in general. He never believed he had "done enough" professionally and always thought he had to prove himself to others, and he had doubts about his basic self-worth. He had marked difficulties in expressing not only affectionate feelings but anger as well. When angry, he would generally "bottle it up," become preoccupied with the person or situation he was angry with, and "stew" for days.

Exploration of his developmental history revealed that his mother was generally available to him, but she had periods of apparent depressive episodes that were disabling, and she would emotionally withdraw from the family. She had never sought or received professional treatment for these apparent depressive episodes. His father was emotionally remote, cold, critical, and "pushed him" to do well in school. Because of the pressure and criticism from his father (and the fact that he felt he had to "earn" his father's love and approval), he gradually became more distant from him, silently resenting him, and sometimes "wished he were dead."

His father died suddenly of a myocardial infarction at age 49 when the patient was 15. The patient described his father's death as traumatic, not only because of the loss of his father but because he felt as if the anger and hostility he felt toward his father "had something to do with his death." Although he realized that this was not rationally possible, he nevertheless felt guilty about having been angry at his father and felt that he had to make it up to him "in some way." In addition, he felt that when his father died he had forever lost the chance to be close to him.

The patient ultimately went on to finish high school and college and decided to become an attorney, similar to his father. The patient always had a fear of dying at an early age—of a heart attack, similar to his father—but nevertheless smoked, was overweight, and did not exercise.

Based on the patient's chronic history of depression, the psychiatrist believed that, in addition to his antidepressant treatment, the patient could benefit from psychotherapy. The psychiatrist, who had a psychodynamic orientation, initially formulated the patient's case as follows: Part of the patient's problems with depression and low self-esteem were associated with problematic relationships with his parents. His mother's periodic depressions would, at times, make her unavailable to him when the patient needed support as a child, and he often interpreted her lack of interest and responsiveness as a sign of rejection. Moreover, his father was hypercritical and demanding, leaving the patient with feelings of worthlessness and guilt when he did not perfectly please his father, and he was frustrated by his inability to be close to him. In addition to this frustration, he was also resentful and angry and hated his father at times, although he also loved him and craved his attention and approval. When his father died, the patient was stricken with not only a sense of loss but also remorse and guilt. His guilt centered on his hostility toward his father in that he may have unconsciously related his father's death to his hostile feelings and blamed himself for it.

Because both parents often were unavailable to him emotionally and communication of feelings in the family was poor, he felt trapped with his loneliness and did not know to whom or how he could express his inner feelings. Because of his guilt and pattern of having to "achieve" and produce to maintain his self-esteem, he gradually became more engrossed in school and work. His compulsive work habits also served to help him avoid his inner feelings of mild depression and contributed to his compulsive personality traits. The patient nevertheless channeled his compulsive style and need for achievement into his work and did well academically and professionally. His marriage was generally stable, although his wife felt that he was always emotionally remote from her, neglected the family for his work, and could not express his feelings. He tended to be distant, hypercritical, and demanding of his own children, repeating the pattern of his own father. He had drifted further and further from both his wife and children.

The psychiatrist believed that the patient's own heart attack could have reactivated the memories and feelings associated with the grief surrounding his father's death. The patient may have identified with the father, and his own heart attack fulfilled his lifelong fear that he too would die at an early age. The psychiatrist also believed that the patient was at high risk genetically for depression because of his mother's probable history of depression and the patient's use of the beta-adrenergic blocking agent propranolol. Both of these factors may have contributed to his biological vulnerability to depression, as may have the acute stress of his coronary artery bypass surgery.

In the course of the patient's subsequent psychotherapy, the memories and feelings related to his childhood experiences were explored. The patient gained a new understanding of the impact that his father's death had on him and came to fully realize that his angry feelings toward his father were largely justified and had nothing to do with his father's death; thus, his sense of guilt, which had been largely unconscious, was relieved. He began to realize more fully how he was still trying to "earn" approval by way of work and achievement, a central conflict related to his need to be close to his father and earn his love.

Concurrent with his psychotherapy and antidepressant medication, the patient was referred to a cardiac rehabilitation program, where he was placed on a diet, an exercise regimen, and a smoking cessation program. Brief office counseling with the patient's wife reassured them both about the safety of gradually resuming normal sexual activity.

The patient complied with this multimodal approach and responded well to his antidepressant, psychotherapy, and cardiac rehabilitation program and returned to work. Formal psychotherapy was terminated after 6 months, although he continued on his antidepressant for 1 year, after which it was gradually tapered and discontinued. The patient did well subsequently.

DIAGNOSIS AND BIOPSYCHOSOCIAL ASSESSMENT

In the DSM-IV schemata, the patient would have initially been diagnosed as follows:

Axis I: Major depression, single episode, severe, without psychotic features
Dysthymic disorder, primary type, early onset (provisional diagnosis)
Nicotine dependence
Axis II: Obsessive–compulsive personality traits (premorbid)
Axis III: Coronary artery disease, status post coronary artery bypass surgery. Status post hypokalemia, essential hypertension, overweight

Axis IV: Psychosocial and Environmental Problems: Occupational Problem (threat of job loss)

Axis V: Global Assessment of Functioning (GAF): 45

The biopsychosocial assessment applied to this case provided a structured and systematic way of understanding the patient's condition by attributing significance to each sphere of his life—psychological, biological, and social—as well as understanding key developmental influences that affected the patient's personality development and vulnerability to depression (Fig. 2–1). In this manner, the treatment interventions that were devised (medical/biological, psychotherapeutic, and rehabilitative/social) addressed *each aspect* of the patient's life and sources of stress. Hence, the descriptive approach of DSM-IV, which is based clearly on the biopsychosocial model with its multiaxial system, combined with a basic psychodynamic assessment that attempts to analyze the meaning of an illness for patients from the standpoint of both past and current life experiences, provides a comprehensive method to formulate an integrated plan of treatment. Table 2–1 summarizes a structured treatment approach to psychiatric assessment and treatment planning based on this approach.

Although the relative *weight* attached to biological, psychological, and social aspects of each individual patient varies, it is essential that each area at least be considered to be potentially important. This philosophy and approach to patient care is the essential theme that runs throughout the course of this text.

In the remaining chapters of this text, students will become familiar with major psychopathological syndromes in clinical psychiatry and the management of behavioral and psychiatric disorders that are encountered in medical, surgical, and pediatric

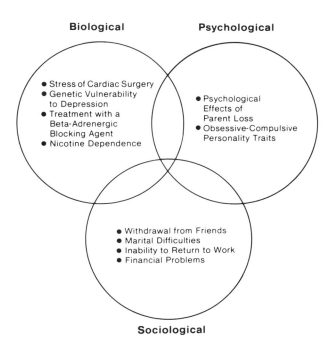

Figure 2–1. *The interaction of biological, psychological, and social factors in the case of Mr. A.*

Table 2–1 **Outline of Psychiatric Assessment and Treatment Planning**

Psychiatric history
Mental status examination
Medical evaluation
Differential diagnosis: psychiatric and medical
DSM-IV diagnoses (definitive or provisional)
   Psychiatric disorders (Axis I)
   Personality diagnosis (Axis II)
   Medical diagnoses (Axis III)
   Identification of major psychosocial stressors (Axis IV)
   Assessment of psychosocial functioning (Axis V)
Psychosocial assessment and case formulation
Treatment plan
   Psychological—need for and choice of psychotherapy; inpatient or outpatient treatment
   Biological—need for further medical/neurological evaluation or treatment; psychopharmacological treatment; rehabilitation programs
   Social—need for intervention in environmental conditions and social conditions; referral to support agencies, occupational counseling, financial or legal assistance

settings. As the student studies these conditions and encounters them in his or her future medical practice, it is hoped that they will take an integrated approach to patient assessment and treatment based on the biopsychosocial model presented in these introductory chapters.

CLINICAL PEARLS

The following ten questions, which should be modified by the interviewer to be asked in an open-ended manner, will facilitate uncovering the source of psychosocial stress connected with the onset or relapse of psychiatric symptoms, assuming the patient is open and cooperative with the interviewer.

- Has there been any recent serious illness or death in your family?
- Have you been having any problems with money or with your job? Are you seriously in debt?
- Have you had any serious problems with your children, your marriage, or other close relationships?
- Have you had any recent illness or surgery, and are you on any medications?
- Have you ever thought you might have a problem with drinking too much alcohol or taking drugs?
- Have you been under any stress or pressure recently that has been difficult for you to manage?

Regarding the patient's past history, the following questions will help identify any significant psychodynamic problems or major stresses in the patient's developmental years. These are "lead" questions that will identify any major developmental traumas, but the development history should not be limited solely to these four questions.

- Tell me about growing up with your family and your relationship with your parents. Did you have any special problems with your parents or within your family when you

were growing up? Was there frequent fighting between your parents when you were a child or teenager?
- Did either one of your parents have a problem with alcohol or drugs?
- Did your parents divorce or separate when you were a child, or did one of your parents die when you were young?
- Were you ever physically or sexually molested when you were a child or teenager?

ANNOTATED BIBLIOGRAPHY

Nemiah JC: Foundations of Clinical Psychopathology. New York, Oxford University Press, 1961
> This is an intriguing and beautifully written text that remains a classic as an introduction to psychodynamic theory.

Balint M: The Doctor, His Patient and the Illness. New York, International University Press, 1957
> Balint was a psychoanalyst who worked extensively with primary care doctors in evaluating and treating the common psychiatric conditions of general medical patients. This text remains a classic for exploring and understanding the psychological aspects of medical practice.

For students interested in excellent resources on psychiatric interviewing, the following books are recommended:

Shea SC: Psychiatric Interviewing. The Art of Understanding. Philadelphia, WB Saunders, 1988

Cohen-Cole SA: The Medical Interview: The Three-Function Approach. Washington DC, C. V. Mosby Company, 1991

REFERENCES

Alexander F: Psychosomatic medicine. Its principles and applications. New York, Norton, 1950

Aneshensel CS, Stone JD: Stress and depression: A test of the buffering model of social support. Arch Gen Psychiatry 39:1392–1396, 1982

Bertalanffy L von: General system theory: A critical review. In Buckley W (ed): Modern Systems Research for the Behavioral Scientist, pp 11–30. Chicago, Aldine, 1968

Bifulco AT, Brown GW, Harris TO: Childhood loss of parent, lack of adequate parental care and adult depression: A replication. J Affective Discord 12:115–128, 1987

Birley JLT, Brown GW: Crises and life changes preceding the onset or relapse of acute schizophrenia: Clinical aspects. Br J Psychiatry 116:327–333, 1970

Bolton W, Oatley K: A longitudinal study of social support and depression in unemployed men. Psychol Med 17:453–460, 1987

Breier A, Kelsoe JR, Kirwin PD et al: Early parental loss and development of adult psychopathology. Arch Gen Psychiatry 45:987–993, 1988

Bryer JB, Nelson BA, Miller JB et al: Childhood sexual and physical abuse as factors in adult psychiatric illness. Am J Psychiatry 144:1426–1430, 1987

Cadoret RJ, O'Gorman TW, Troughton E et al: Alcoholism and antisocial personality: Interrelationships, genetic and environmental factors. Arch Gen Psychiatry 42:161–167, 1985

Cobb S: Social support as a moderator of life stress. Psychosom Med 38:300–314, 1976

Cohen-Cole SA, Levinson R: The biopsychosocial model in medical practice. In Stoudemire A (ed): Human Behavior: An Introduction for Medical Students, 2nd ed. Philadelphia, JB Lippincott, 1994

Cooper AM: Will neurobiology influence psychoanalysis? Am J Psychiatry 142:1395–1402, 1985

Coyne JC: Social factors and psychopathology: stress, social support, and coping processes. Annu Rev Psychol 42:401–425, 1991

Dew MA, Bromet EJ & Penkower L: Mental health effects of job loss in women. Psycho Med 22:751–764, 1992

Doane JA, West KL, Goldstein MJ et al: Parental communication deviance and affective style: Predictors of subsequent schizophrenia spectrum disorders in vulnerable adolescents. Arch Gen Psychiatry 38:679–685, 1981

Engel GL: The need for a new medical model: A challenge for biomedicine. Science 196:129–136, 1977

Fink PJ: Response to the presidential address: Is "Biopsychosocial" the psychiatric shibboleth? Am J Psychiatry 145:1061–1067, 1988

Galanter M: Research on social supports and mental illness. Am J Psychiatry 145:1270–1272, 1988 (editorial)

Goldberg D, Bridges K, Cook D et al: The influence of social factors on common mental disorders. Br J Psychiatry 156:704–713, 1990

Green SA: Supportive psychological care of the medically ill: A Synthesis of the Biopsychosocial Approach in Medical Care. In Stoudemire A (ed): Human Behavior: An Introduction for Medical Students 2nd ed. Philadelphia, JB Lippincott, 1994

Greenblatt M, Becerra R, Serafetinides EA: Social networks and mental health: An overview. Am J Psychiatry 8:977–984, 1982

Harris T, Brown GW, Bifulco A: Loss of parent in childhood and adult psychiatric disorder: The role of lack of adequate parental care. Psychol Med 16:641–659, 1986

Harris T, Brown GW, Bifulco A: Loss of parent in childhood and adult psychiatric disorder: The role of social class position and premarital pregnancy. Psychol Med 17:163–183, 1987

Inderbitzin LB, James ME: Psychoanalytic Psychology. In Stoudemire A (ed): Human Behavior: An Introduction for Medical Students, 2nd ed. Philadelphia, JB Lippincott, 1994

Kandel ER: Psychotherapy and the single synapse. The impact of psychiatric thought on neurobiologic research. N Engl J Med 301:1028–1037, 1979

Kandel ER: From metapsychology to molecular biology: Explorations into the nature of anxiety. Am J Psychiatry 140:1277–1293, 1983

Kendler KS: Indirect vertical cultural transmission: A model for nongenetic parental influences on the liability to psychiatric illness. Am J Psychiatry 145:657–665, 1988

Leavy RL: Social support and psychological disorder: A review. Community Psychology 11:3–21, 1983

Lindberg F, Distad L: Post-traumatic stress disorders in women who experienced childhood incest. Child Abuse Negl 9:329–334, 1985

MacMillan JF, Gold A, Crow TJ et al: The Northwick Park study of first episodes of schizophrenia: IV. Expressed emotion and relapse. Br J Psychiatry 148:133–143, 1986

Meyer A: Psychobiology, A Science of Man. Springfield, IL, Charles C Thomas, 1957

Miklowitz DJ, Goldstein MJ, Neuchterlein KH et al: The family and the course of recent-onset mania. In Hahlweg K, Goldstein MJ (eds): Understanding Major Mental Disorder: The Contribution of Family Interaction Research, pp 195–211. New York, Family Process Press, 1987

Miklowitz DJ, Goldstein MJ, Neuchterlein KH et al: Family factors and the course of bipolar affective disorder. Arch Gen Psychiatry 45:225–231, 1988

Miller PM, Ingham JG, Davidson S: Life events, symptoms and social support. J Psychosom Res 20:515–522, 1976

Parry G, Shapiro DA: Social support and life events in working class women. Arch Gen Psychiatry 43:315–323, 1986

Pellegrini DS: Psychosocial risk and protective factors in childhood. Dev Behav Pediatrics 11:201–209, 1990

Penkower L, Bromet EJ, Dew MA: Husbands' layoff and wives' mental health. Arch Gen Psychiatry 45:994–1000, 1988

Reiser MF: Mind, Brain, Body. New York, Basic Books, 1984

Romans SE, Walton VA, Herbison GP et al: Social networks and psychiatric morbidity in New Zealand women. Aust N Zeal J Psychiatry 26:485–492, 1992

Roy A: Parental loss in childhood and onset of manic-depressive illness. Br J Psychiatry 136:86–88, 1980

Rutter M: Psychopathology and development: Links between childhood and adult life. In Rutter M, Hersov L (eds): Child and Adolescent Psychiatry. London, Blackwell Scientific Publications, 1985

Schwartz CC, Myers JK: Life events and schizophrenia. I: Comparison of schizophrenics with a community sample. Arch Gen Psychiatry 34:1238–1241, 1977a

Schwartz CC, Myers JK: Life events and schizophrenia. II: Impact of life events on symptom configuration. Arch Gen Psychiatry 34:1242–1245, 1977b

Stansfeld SA, Gallacher JEJ, Sharp DS et al: Social factors and minor psychiatric disorder in middle-aged men: a validation study and a population survey. Psychol Med 21:157–167, 1991

Stoudemire A: Somatothymia: Part I. Psychosomatics 32:365–370, 1991a

Stoudemire A: Somatothymia: Part II. Psychosomatics 32:371–381, 1991b

Tennant C: Life events and psychological morbidity: The evidence from prospective studies. Psychol Med 13:483–486, 1983

Tennant C: Parental loss in childhood: Its effect in adult life. Arch Gen Psychiatry 45:1045–1050, 1988

Tennant C, Bebbington P, Hurry J: Social experiences in childhood and adult psychiatric morbidity: A multiple regression analysis. Psychol Med 12:321–327, 1982

Tennant C, Hurry J, Beddington P: The relation of childhood separation experiences to adult depressive and anxiety states. Br J Psychiatry 141:475–482, 1982a

Tennant C, Hurry J, Bebbington P: The relationship of different types of childhood separation experiences to adult psychiatric disorders. Br J Psychiatry 141:475–482, 1982b

Tennant C, Smith A, Bebbington P et al: Parental loss in childhood: Relationship to adult psychiatric impairment and contact with psychiatric services. Arch Gen Psychiatry 38:309–314, 1981

Uhlenhuth EG, Paykel ES: Symptom intensity and life events. Arch Gen Psychiatry 28:473–477, 1973

van der Kolk B: The psychological consequences of overwhelming life experiences. In van der Kolk B (ed): Psychological Trauma. Washington, DC, American Psychiatric Press, 1986

van der Kolk B: Behavioral and psychobiological effects of developmental trauma. In Stoudemire A (ed): Human Behavior: An Introduction for Medical Students, 2nd ed. Philadelphia, JB Lippincott, 1994

Vaughn CE, Snyder KS, Jones S et al: Family factors in schizophrenic relapse: Replication in California of British research on expressed emotion. Arch Gen Psychiatry 41:1169–1177, 1984

Warr P, Jackson P: Factors influencing the psychological impact of prolonged unemployment and of re-employment. Psychol Med 15:795–807, 1985

Weissman MM, Gammon GD, John K et al: Children of depressed parents: Increased psychopathology and early onset of major depression. Arch Gen Psychiatry 44:847–853, 1987

Alan Stoudemire (ed). *Clinical Psychiatry for Medical Students,* Second Edition. Copyright © 1994, 1990 by J. B. Lippincott Company.

3 *Psychological Testing in Medical Practice*

Nadine J. Kaslow and Eugene W. Farber

This chapter focuses on the uses of psychological testing including the types of clinical questions that can be addressed, the nature of psychological testing, and how the information gleaned from testing can be used in formulating and implementing a treatment plan. Special emphasis is placed on the types of problems that may arise in medical or psychiatric practice in which psychological testing would be practically helpful in patient care. Case vignettes will illustrate several major assessment instruments and how findings obtained from these tests are used to assist with the clinical care of patients.

THE USES OF PSYCHOLOGICAL TESTING

Psychological tests assess intellectual, neuropsychological, and personality functioning and are standardized empirical methods of sampling behavior. The results of psychological testing may aid in the diagnosis, case formulation, treatment planning, and prediction of behavior. The results of psychological testing should be integrated with other forms of pertinent clinical data including behavioral observation, clinical presentation, and psychiatric and medical history in providing a comprehensive portrait of the individual's overall psychological functioning. In developing referral questions to the consulting psychologist, physicians should specify what information is needed, how it will be helpful, and for what it will be used. The psychologist will select the most appropriate test or battery of tests (a combination of tests that measure different psychological domains) based upon the specific referral questions that are presented.

Formulating Referral Questions

Psychological testing can be useful in addressing a range of clinical problems. Brief vignettes will be used to illustrate circumstances in which physicians may wish to request formal psychological testing.

1. <u>Intellectual functioning.</u> *Mr. and Mrs. Jones spoke with their pediatrician about concerns regarding their son Adam's school performance. Although Adam was well behaved and popular, he was not learning as quickly as his classmates and was feeling frustrated that "the other kids were smarter." The pediatrician made a referral to a child psychologist for psychological testing to receive information regarding Adam's intellectual abilities.*

   Intellectual assessment provides an estimation of intellectual ability (e.g., IQ score) and a determination of cognitive and intellectual strengths and weaknesses (e.g., learning disabilities). These data may be used to formulate appropriate modes of clinical intervention (i.e., strategies for communicating information in a manner consistent with cognitive functioning level and style) and to help the individual obtain necessary remedial services for intellectual handicaps or learning disabilities. If questions about mental retardation arise, measures of adaptive functioning can also be administered. Examples of specific questions that can be answered by psychological testing include the following: (a) What is the overall level of this person's intellectual functioning, including areas of relative strength and weakness? (b) Is this person able to understand the nature of their physical condition and follow instructions for self-care? (c) For an individual who is currently receiving Workmen's Compensation or disability payments for a physical disability, what are their cognitive strengths that can be used in pursuing occupational alternatives?

2. <u>Neuropsychological functioning.</u> *Dr. Stuart, a neurologist, was consulted by a hematologist who was treating a sickle cell patient who had recently suffered a cerebral vascular accident (CVA). This sickle cell patient had functioned effectively prior to his CVA but was now reporting difficulties with language comprehension and distractibility. As part of the workup, the neurologist requested a neuropsychological evaluation.*

   Neuropsychological testing is useful in efforts to ascertain the neurologic contributions to the symptom picture or assess the impact of brain impairments/lesions on cognitive functioning. In conjunction with neurological data, neuropsychological test findings can answer questions regarding the nature, extent, and impact of the brain impairment and provide directions for cognitive rehabilitation. Specific questions may include: (a) What impact does this middle cerebral vascular accident have on this person's cognitive functioning? (b) What is the impact of this temporal lobe lesion on this individual's memory? (c) What type of cognitive rehabilitation programming would be most efficacious for this patient? (d) Is there evidence for a neurologic component to this person's impulse control problems?

3. Thought disorder and reality testing. *Dr. Costner, a psychiatric resident, was treating an intelligent 26-year-old male in outpatient psychotherapy. As the patient became more self-revealing, Dr. Costner found it difficult to follow the patient's odd line of thinking. Dr. Costner noticed that his patient misinterpreted events and displayed magical thinking. The patient, however, denied hallucinations and delusions. Dr. Costner requested psychological testing to assess for the presence of an underlying thought disorder and for difficulties with reality testing.*

Information regarding the nature and severity of the person's thought disorder and the degree of impaired reality testing may aid in differential diagnosis between a schizophrenia spectrum disorder, a personality disorder with transient psychotic symptoms, a drug-induced psychosis, or a mood disorder with psychotic features. Specific questions might include: (a) Does this person have difficulties with accurate perception of events and stimuli and how pervasive and serious are these impairments? (b) Is there evidence for disorganized thinking? (c) What are the specific conditions under which thought disturbance or reality-testing problems might emerge and/or be exacerbated? (d) What clinical strategies might the treatment team use to help improve this person's thinking and reality testing?

4. Mood disorder. *Dr. Newman, an internist, was following the case of Suzanne, a 31-year-old female with a diagnosis of chronic fatigue syndrome. For the past year, Suzanne complained of fatigue, low energy, and anhedonia. Her symptoms recently had worsened, and she reported such extreme bouts of tiredness and low energy that she was no longer able to maintain her full-time job. Dr. Newman requested psychological testing in order to ascertain whether or not Suzanne was experiencing a depressive disorder in addition to chronic fatigue syndrome.*

Information regarding the nature and severity of the person's affective distress may assist in differential diagnosis where the following diagnoses are being considered: major depression with or without psychotic features, dysthymia, bipolar disorder with or without psychotic features, schizoaffective disorder, or affective instability secondary to the presence of a personality disorder. Examples of specific referral questions regarding the presence and nature of a mood disorder may include: (a) Is this woman with chronic fatigue syndrome also experiencing a major depressive episode or dysthymia? (b) Is this mother's difficulty caring for her newborn consistent with a diagnosis of a major depressive episode in the postpartum period or reflective of an underlying personality disorder? (c) Since this patient evidences both psychotic and depressive symptoms, which symptom complex is primary and what are appropriate treatment recommendations?

5. Ego functioning (coping ability). *Dr. Jennings, a forensic psychiatrist, was asked to evaluate the violence potential of Ms. Terry, a prison inmate who had been incarcerated for her involvement in a cocaine distribution ring. She had provided key evidence enabling law enforcement personnel to make arrests of the leaders of the drug ring. As the trial date approached in which she would be asked to testify against her former bosses, she became increasingly emotionally labile and at one point she made suicide threats. In an effort to gather a more complete picture of Ms. Terry's impulse control, frustration tolerance, and affect regulation, Dr. Jennings requested a psychological evaluation.*

   Data regarding impulse control, frustration tolerance, and affect regulation provide information about the quality of ego functioning and defenses utilized to cope with stress. Questions may include: (a) What is this individual's potential for losing control? Under what circumstances might his or her impulse control be most problematic? Under what conditions is this person likely to become suicidal or violent? (b) What is this person's capacity for delaying gratification? (c) How does this person manage affective stimulation and their own emotional responses? (d) What are prominent defenses or adaptive mechanisms this person employs to cope with stressful circumstances?

6. Psychodynamics and personality functioning. *George, a successful stockbroker, was significantly disfigured by burns suffered in an automobile accident. Upon discharge from the burn unit, he returned home to his family and soon thereafter resumed his work. His physician, Dr. Hawthorne, was concerned that George did not appear to be adjusting to his disfigurement and recommended psychotherapy. During psychotherapy sessions, George was guarded and often silent. While his distress about his disfigurement was understandable, his inability to articulate his thoughts and feelings left his therapist uncertain about how to be most helpful. Thus, psychological testing was requested to assist in more fully understanding the psychodynamic issues contributing to George's adjustment difficulties.*

Psychological testing can be used to provide information regarding self-esteem, identity formation, major areas of conflict, and typical interpersonal modes of relating and interacting. Pertinent questions may include: (a) How has this patient's physical condition affected his or her self-concept? (b) What types of interpersonal difficulties is this person most likely to encounter? (c) How will this individual's personality style influence their interactions in the doctor–patient relationship and treatment compliance?

7. Validity of complaints. *Pete Donaldson, a 23-year-old first-year law student, fractured his pelvic bone in a rock-climbing accident. Although X-rays and CT scans revealed no additional complications, Pete complained that he was unable to walk because his legs did not "feel right." His orthopedist, Dr. Wilkins, found no physical reason to explain Pete's complaints. The physical therapy team also could find no underlying physical reason that Pete could not walk once his pelvic bone had healed. Dr. Wilkins and members of Pete's medical team began to question the validity of his complaints. He was thus referred for psychological testing to ascertain whether or not there was a significant psychogenic basis for his alleged inability to walk.*

Information from psychological testing may be useful in ruling out a primarily psychological etiology of a given complaint and may be helpful in differential diagnosis of a malingering, factitious, or somatoform disorder, as well as other DSM-IV Axis I and Axis II disorders (Schretlen, 1988). Examples of questions are: (a) Is there a significant discrepancy between symptom claims and psychological test findings suggestive of malingering? (b) Are the test results consistent with a conversion or dissociative disorder?

Indications for Testing Children

As Dr. Dulcan articulates in Chapter 16, there are developmental considerations that differentiate clinical approaches in child and adult psychiatry. With regard to such considerations, Racusin and Moss (1991) outline referral questions specific to the psychological assessment of children and adolescents. Such questions may focus on: (a) the child's developmental progress in cognitive, emotional, and interpersonal functioning, as well as adaptive behavior and skill acquisition; (b) provision of a reliable estimate of intellectual functioning; (c) comparison of the child's intellectual functioning and achievement in order to diagnose learning disabilities; (d) differential diagnosis of psychopathological conditions; and (e) obtaining information to make treatment disposition decisions, to predict the course of therapy, and to provide the necessary documentation for the child or adolescent to receive special services (e.g., classes for the intellectually gifted, behaviorally or emotionally disordered, learning disabled, or services for the mentally retarded including residential placement).

Communication of Findings

Providing feedback regarding test results is an interactive process between professions in which all concerned parties discuss the findings, their meanings, and the limitations of the results (Pope, 1992). The format and content of the communication of test findings varies depending upon the referral source, the questions being addressed, and the person(s) to whom the results are being presented. In addition to receiving verbal feedback, test results will be communicated to the physician via a testing report. The testing report involves analysis, synthesis, and integration of the material gathered during the testing (Tallent, 1988). Testing reports typically include the following sections: identifying information, reason for referral, pertinent background information, behavioral observations, intellectual and neuropsychological functioning, achievement and aptitude, personality and/or emotional functioning, and a summary and recommendations.

NATURE OF PSYCHOLOGICAL TESTING

Psychometric Properties

The utility of a given test may be evaluated on the basis of three psychometric properties: standardization, reliability, and validity.

Standardization refers to the use of consistent stimuli to elicit information, uniformity in test administration, and the availability of norms based upon data from demographically and clinically representative samples (Anastasi, 1988).

Reliability refers to the consistency, accuracy, and reproducibility of the test results. If a measure is reliable, scores obtained are relatively consistent within the given test (internal consistency reliability), across administrations (test-retest reliability), and across examiners (interrater reliability) (Anastasi, 1988).

Validity refers to the extent to which the test measures what it is purported to measure. Valid tests include items that accurately represent the psychological domain being assessed (content validity), that are effective in predicting a person's performance in a specific area of functioning (predictive validity), and that adequately measure the theoretical construct or trait for which the test was developed (construct validity) (Anastasi, 1988).

Classification of Psychological Test Instruments

Test instruments may be classified in several ways.

Functional Domains

One classification refers to the *domains* of functioning assessed. Tests commonly used to assess the psychological functioning of psychiatric and medical patients assess domains that include intelligence, educational achievement, aptitude, adaptive behavior functioning, vocational skills and interests, neuropsychological functioning, personality, and psychiatric symptomatology.

Intelligence tests assess an individual's present functioning and capacity to understand and cope with the world (Wechsler, 1991). Rather than emphasizing particular abilities, these tests assess a broad range of intellectual functions, such as verbal and nonverbal reasoning, the capacity for abstraction, the fund of knowledge, attention and concentration, visual-spatial skills, and facility with simultaneous (concurrent processing of many stimuli) and sequential (arrangement of stimuli in sequential or serial order) processing. Based upon an individual's performance on verbal and performance tasks, an overall Intelligence Quotient (IQ) can be determined. IQ scores, a quantitative interpretation of a total test score in relation to appropriate group norms, are derived using the following formula: IQ = MA/CA × 100. Mental age (MA) is the average intellectual level of a particular age, while chronological age (CA) is the individual's chronological age. Individuals with average IQs have equivalent mental and chronological ages; thus, their IQ scores approximate 100. An IQ of 100 is the mean score, with a standard deviation of 15 points on the major intelligence tests. When a psychologist provides feedback regarding the intellectual functioning of a particular individual, the psychologist offers an IQ score and describes the individual's level of functioning according to the classification listed in Table 3–1. Recently, the meaningfulness of IQ scores interpreted in isolation has been questioned. For example, some authors assert that the IQ classification schemas are arbitrary, varying according to test authors, diagnostic and classification manuals, and government criteria (Kaufman, 1990). In this regard, two individuals with comparable IQ scores will not necessarily demonstrate similar intellectual capabilities. Concurrent with the concern about the usefulness of IQ scores is an increased emphasis on qualitative evaluation of the individual's intellectual strengths and weaknesses relative to overall IQ and on the consideration of the individual's IQ score in the context of sociocultural factors and adaptive behavior functioning.

Table 3–1 **IQ Score Classification
of Intellectual Functioning Level**

CLASSIFICATION	CORRESPONDING IQ RANGE
Very Superior	130 and above*
Superior	120 to 129*
High Average	110 to 119*
Average	90 to 109*
Low Average	80 to 89*
Borderline	70 to 79*
Mild Mental Retardation	50–55 to approx. 70**
Moderate Mental Retardation	35–40 to 50–55**
Severe Mental Retardation	20–25 to 35–40**
Profound Mental Retardation	Below 20 or 25**

*Criteria correspond to those described in the WAIS-R Manual.
**Criteria correspond to those described in the DSM-IV.

Educational achievement tests measure the effects of a specific educational program of study on academic achievement (Anastasi, 1988). These tests identify academic skills deficits and are used to develop interventions addressing skill deficits (Sattler, 1988). In combination with intelligence test results, achievement test findings identify specific learning disabilities or DSM-IV academic skills disorders (i.e., developmental arithmetic, expressive writing, or reading disorders).

Aptitude tests measure abilities in specified skill domains and are employed to predict subsequent performance. For example, the MCAT, which measures competencies important for medical practice, is an aptitude test presumed to have predictive validity for medical school performance.

Tests of adaptive behavior measure the capacity to effectively meet the natural and social demands of one's environment in accord with cultural and age expectations. The areas of personal and social sufficiency addressed include: independent functioning, social and communication skills, physical skill capacities, language development, and academic competencies. In the DSM-IV, a diagnosis of mental retardation includes documentation of an IQ of 70 or below *and* adaptive functioning impairments.

Vocational skills and interest tests assess job and career preferences and are used by career counselors, industrial-organizational psychologists, school psychologists, and guidance counselors.

Neuropsychological tests measure brain-behavior relationships in the following domains: orientation, language, memory, perception, perceptual-motor, attention and concentration, concept-formation, and executive functions (planning and problem-solving abilities). Neuropsychological tests help detect the presence of brain pathology and the nature of associated cognitive or behavioral deficits (Lezak, 1983).

Personality tests measure emotional, motivational, interpersonal, and attitudinal characteristics of the individual (Anastasi, 1988).

Semistructured diagnostic interviews permit more precise and standardized psychiatric diagnoses (Widiger and Frances, 1987). These measures assess symptom and personality patterns consistent with DSM-IV Axis I and Axis II diagnoses.

Format of Administration

A second classification refers to the format of test administration, with distinctions made between tests administered to individuals and those given to groups. *Individually administered tests* allow for careful observation and evaluation of psychological functioning in a given individual. *Group tests* offer the advantage of easy administration and scoring and thus are time and cost efficient.

Objective and Projective Tests

Objective tests typically are self-report pencil-and-paper measures utilizing specific questions and a standardized response format that can be mechanically scored and statistically analyzed. Although the format of such tests is objective, the meaning of the results and scores is not and requires interpretation by a skilled clinician. In contrast, *projective tests* are less structured with regard to response format and scoring and require the testee to provide responses based upon his or her perception and interpretation of relatively ambiguous stimuli for which a wide range of responses is possible. It is posited that such perceptions and interpretations are influenced by core aspects of psychological functioning as the individual projects their characteristic modes of organizing experience, needs, motivations, feelings, meanings, and salient intrapsychic and interpersonal conflicts and psychodynamics. This has been referred to as the *projective hypothesis* (Frank, 1939). Proponents of projective techniques, who often utilize a psychodynamic approach to test interpretation, assert that this method of assessment is particularly effective in revealing unconscious aspects of personality functioning.

See Table 3–2 for examples of test instruments according the classification scheme outlined above. Table 3–3 presents a synopsis of clinical questions, types of psychological tests indicated, and pertinent information derived.

Clinical Vignettes

Having reviewed the basic principles of psychological testing, the following vignettes illustrate the usefulness of psychological tests for physicians. These vignettes introduce commonly used psychological tests, information gleaned from the assessment process, and treatment implications of test results.

VIGNETTE 1

Mr. Jordan, a 32-year-old single advertising executive, presented to his primary care physician complaining of chest pain. He jogs four miles three times per week and plays tennis on the weekend. He denies smoking cigarettes and his weight is within the normal range. He denies prior history of cardiac difficulties, although his family history is positive for heart disease. Specifically, his paternal and maternal grandfathers died secondary to myocardial infarctions in their 60s. While he reported that work typically was fast paced, he did not report subjective feelings of anxiety or stress. Additionally, he stated that his personal life was satisfactory. A thorough physical examination was conducted, including an electrocardiogram (EKG), and all findings were negative. His primary care physician recommended that Mr. Jordan recontact her should his symptoms continue or worsen. A few weeks later, the patient was seen for a follow-up appointment, with complaints of continued intermittent chest pains. He was then referred for a full cardiology workup, which was negative. At this point, his primary care physician and cardiologist referred him for psychological evaluation because his pain symptoms defied etiological diagnosis, and they were interested in information regarding a functional component to his physical distress.

Having received a referral with the question, "Does this individual evidence personality characteristics consistent with persons who experience chronic pain with no apparent physical etiology?" the psychologist elected to administer the Minnesota Multiphasic Personality Inventory-2.

Minnesota Multiphasic Personality Inventory-2 (MMPI-2)

The MMPI-2, a 567-item personality inventory, is the most commonly used and thoroughly researched objective self-report personality inventory. It is a psycho-

Table 3–2 **Classification of Commonly Used Psychological Testing Instruments**

TEST TYPE	EXAMPLES
Intelligence	Wechsler Scales (WAIS-R, WISC-III, WPPSI) Stanford-Binet, 4th ed McCarthy Scales of Children's Abilities Kaufman Assessment Battery for Children (K-ABC)
Achievement	Wide Range Achievement Test-Revised (WRAT-R) Woodcock-Johnson Psychoeducational Battery Kaufman Test of Educational Achievement (K-TEA)
Aptitude	Scholastic Aptitude Test (SAT) Differential Aptitude Test (DAT) Medical College Admissions Test (MCAT)
Adaptive Behavior	Vineland Adaptive Behavior Scales Scales of Independent Behavior
Vocational	Strong Vocational Interest Blank (SVIB)
Neuro-psychological	Halstead-Reitan Test Battery (HRB) Luria-Nebraska Neuropsychological Battery (LNNB) Bender Visual-Motor Gestalt Test Wechsler Memory Scales-Revised (WMS-R)
Personality Objective	 Minnesota Multiphasic Personality Inventory (MMPI-2) MMPI-Adolescent Millon Clinical Multiaxial Inventory (MCMI) Beck Depression Inventory (BDI) Symptom Checklist-90 (SCL-90) Myers-Briggs Type Indicator (MBTI)
Projective	Rorschach Inkblot Test Thematic Apperception Test (TAT) Children's Apperception Test (CAT) Sentence Completion Test (SCT) Draw-A-Person Test (DAP)
Interview	Structured Clinical Interview for Diagnosis (SCID) Diagnostic Interview Schedule (DIS) Diagnostic Interview Schedule for Children (DISC)
Individual	Wechsler Adult Intelligence Scale-Revised (WAIS-R) Rorschach Inkblot Test
Group	Medical College Admission Test (MCAT) California Achievement Test (CAT)

Table 3–3 **Examples of the Clinical Uses of Common Psychological Tests**

CLINICAL QUESTION	TEST(S) INDICATED	INFORMATION DERIVED
Intellectual Functioning	WAIS-R, WISC-III, Stanford-Binet	IQ estimate, cognitive strengths/ weaknesses
Academic Achievement	WRAT-R, K-TEA, Woodcock-Johnson	Academic skills and strengths and weaknesses
Skill Aptitude	DAT, SAT, MCAT	Skill level and prediction of performance/competence
Adaptive Behavior	Vineland	Capacity to effectively meet environmental demands
Vocational Skills	SVIB, MBTI	Job and career suitability and interests according to interests/ personality preferences
Brain Impairment	Halstead-Reitan, Luria-Nebraska	Presence and effects of brain lesions
Psychiatric Diagnosis	SCID	DSM diagnostic considerations
Psychosis	Rorschach, MMPI-2	Disordered thinking, impaired reality testing
Mood Disorder	Rorschach, MMPI-2, BDI, SCL-90	Depression, mania, affect regulation
Global Personality Functioning	Rorschach, MMPI-2, TAT, MCMI	Self-esteem, interpersonal style, dynamic conflicts

metrically valid and reliable test that has been well standardized across representative demographic groups (Graham, 1990). The MMPI-2 requires the respondent to answer true or false to statements describing psychological symptoms, preferences, interpersonal relationships, and emotional responses to commonly encountered situations. The MMPI-2 provides indices addressing response style, including measures of guardedness, underreporting or overreporting of psychological difficulties, and random responding. The measure also provides information on ten clinical scales: hypochondriasis, depression, hysteria, psychopathic deviate, masculinity-femininity, paranoia, psychasthenia, schizophrenia, hypomania, and social introversion. A brief description of the three validity scales and the ten clinical scales can be found in Table 3–4.

The MMPI-2 also includes supplementary and content scales measuring a variety of personality characteristics that aid in the interpretation of the results obtained on the main clinical scales. A high score on a given scale does not necessarily indicate that the respondent has that psychiatric disorder. For example, a high score on the hypomania scale does not necessarily imply a diagnosis of bipolar disorder; this elevation may be seen in active, accomplished, and extroverted individuals with no history of a mood disorder.

The MMPI-2 and its predecessor, the MMPI (Hathaway and McKinley, 1943), are often used in medical practice (e.g., Osborne, 1985), as in the psychological evaluation of chronic pain patients (Keller and Butcher, 1991). The MMPI/MMPI-2 have been used with medical patients to screen for serious psychopathology and substance abuse, to ascertain the patient's likely responses to medical interventions and psychosocial adjustment to their medical condition, and to distinguish between psychiatric

Table 3–4 **MMPI-2 Validity and Clinical Scales**

Validity Scales	
L: Lie	Measures frankness in responding to test items, including willingness to admit minor shortcomings. Detects deliberate and unsophisticated efforts to present oneself in a positive light.
F: Infrequency	Detects atypical response sets. Serves as an index of overall degree of psychopathology.
K: Suppressor	Measures subtle forms of defensive responding and, conversely, responding that suggests an unusually frank or self-critical approach. Adjusts clinical scale elevations according to degree of response defensiveness.
Clinical Scales	
1: Hypochondriasis	Measures somatic focus and preoccupation with bodily functioning.
2: Depression	Measures symptomatic depression, including low morale, lack of hope, and general dissatisfaction with one's life situation.
3: Hysteria	Measures tendency to rely on "hysteroid" defenses, including denial, repression, and inhibition, and proneness to conversion or somatoform symptoms in response to stress.
4: Psychopathic Deviate	Measures general social maladjustment, family conflict, authority problems, rebelliousness, and antisocial patterns.
5: Masculinity-Femininity	Measures a range of personality and interest areas, including aesthetic interests, sensitivity, and passivity, as well as sex-role stereotyped behavior patterns.
6: Paranoia	Identifies paranoid symptoms and assesses interpersonal sensitivity, suspiciousness, vigilance, and distrust.
7: Psychasthenia	Measures anxiety, fear, tension and obsessive–compulsive tendencies.
8: Schizophrenia	Measures bizarre thinking, unusual perceptions, social alienation, identity confusion, and feelings of general inadequacy.
9: Hypomania	Measures degree of hypomanic personality features, including elated but unstable mood, psychomotor excitement, flight of ideas, and overactivity.
0: Social Introversion	Assesses level of comfort in social situations, degree of withdrawal or gregariousness, and extent of social anxiety and social inhibition.

and medical illness (Graham, 1990; Osborne, 1985). It is important to underscore, however, that the MMPI/MMPI-2 cannot and should not be used in isolation to diagnose or rule out the presence of a physical condition. Rather, MMPI/MMPI-2 data regarding personality functioning can be used along with other available medical and psychological information to make inferences regarding the compatibility of personality characteristics expressed on the MMPI/MMPI-2 and a functional etiology for physical symptoms (Graham, 1990).

Interpretation of Test Findings

Mr. Jordan provided a valid MMPI-2 protocol according to the validity scales. He showed a mild elevation on scale 7, the psychasthenia scale, and scale 9, the hypomania scale. These elevations typically are indicative of tension, anxiety, obsessive–compulsive traits, and the use of hypomanic defenses (i.e., high activity level as a defense against an underlying depression) that make it difficult for him to relax (Greene, 1991). There were no additional elevations on the main clinical scales.

Mr. Jordan's profile was not consistent with protocols typically obtained from chronic pain sufferers. Such patients most frequently exhibit one of the following profiles: (a) clinically significant elevations on scale 1 (hypochondriasis), scale 2 (depression), and scale 3 (hysteria); (b) clinical scale scores within the normal range, with scales 1, 2, and 3 being the most elevated, though not significantly so; and (c) clinically significant elevations on several clinical scales in addition to scales 1, 2, and 3, namely scale 6 (paranoia), scale 7 (psychasthenia), and scale 8 (schizophrenia) (Strassberg et al, 1992).

While Mr. Jordan's profile is not consistent with that of chronic pain sufferers, his elevation on scale 7 may suggest that he is frightened and worried about the possibility of having cardiac difficulties. Alternatively, his profile might reflect a Type A behavior pattern characterized by high levels of competitiveness and achievement strivings, hard-driving behavior, and high levels of hostility. The Type A behavior pattern has been found by some researchers to be a risk factor for cardiac disease and is discussed in Chapter 24 by Goldstein et al (Friedman and Rosenman, 1974; Williams, 1986; see Thoresen and Powell [1992] for a recent critical review of this literature). An examination of his MMPI-2 content and supplementary scale scores revealed a significant elevation on the Type A subscale (TPA).

Based upon these MMPI-2 findings, the psychologist informed the referring physician that the patient's self-reported personality style was not consistent with that of individuals who somatize. Rather, while the results from psychological testing cannot be used as documentation of cardiac difficulties, they are indicative of an individual whose behavior and personality style may put them at risk for cardiovascular symptoms. Thus, the psychologist and cardiologist spoke together with the patient and recommended psychotherapy to help Mr. Jordan address the dynamics associated with his anxious, obsessive, and hard-driving style, combined with cognitive-behavioral interventions including relaxation training.

VIGNETTE 2

Ms. Foster, a 21-year-old cashier, was brought into the psychiatric emergency room by her co-worker because she had been acting "strange" the past few days. Her co-worker reported that Ms. Foster was "suspicious and became angry a lot." Upon evaluation, she appeared disorganized, her affect was labile and often inappropriate to content, and she reported hearing her dead grandmother's voice calling her name. She acknowledged suicidal ideation and had contemplated using a knife to stab herself. A complete mental status examination revealed that she was alert and fully oriented and that cognitive functions were intact. She acknowledged occasional alcohol use, denied past or current drug abuse, and her toxicology findings were negative. Her family history was significant for maternal depression and a paternal uncle who was hospitalized for "nerve problems." A breakup with her boyfriend of two years precipitated her recent deterioration. According to reports obtained from family members, Ms. Foster had no previous psychiatric history. She was hospitalized and a complete psychiatric and medical evaluation was conducted. Laboratory findings were within normal limits, and head computerized tomography (CT) and electroencephalogram (EEG) were normal. Within three days of being on the inpatient unit, she denied psychotic symptoms and showed evidence of increasing personality reorganization without neuroleptic treatment. She acknowledged mild depressive symptoms but demanded discharge as soon as possible. The psychiatric resident requested a testing consultation to aid in differential diagnosis. The resident queried whether or not the patient's psychological functioning was consistent with that of an individual with a personality disorder manifesting a transient psychotic episode, an underlying thought disorder consistent with a schizophrenia spectrum diagnosis, or a mood disorder with psychotic features.

Due to the complexity and variability of the patient's symptom picture and the importance of a thorough psychological assessment given that this patient presented with her first psychotic episode, the psychologist conducted a relatively standard battery of psychological tests, including the Wechsler Adult Intelligence Scale-Revised (WAIS-R; Wechsler, 1981), the Rorschach Inkblot Test (Rorschach, 1921/1949), the Thematic Apperception Test (TAT; Murray, 1943), and the MMPI-2.

Wechsler Adult Intelligence Scale-Revised (WAIS-R)

The WAIS-R, the most widely used and psychometrically sound intelligence test for adults, is comprised of 11 subtests, including six subtests measuring verbal IQ (information, digit span, vocabulary, arithmetic, comprehension, and similarities) and five subtests measuring predominantly nonverbal perceptual and motor capacities, which are termed performance IQ (picture completion, picture arrangement, block design, object assembly, and digit symbol). The range of functions measured allows the psychologist to determine areas of strength and weakness relative to the individual's overall intellectual functioning and to make comparisons with an age-matched national sample. Additionally, for purposes of interpretation, Kaufman (1990) has suggested three major domains of intellectual functioning assessed by the WAIS-R: verbal comprehension (information, vocabulary, comprehension, and similarities subtests), perceptual organization (picture completion, block design, and object assembly subtests), and freedom from distractibility (arithmetic and digit span subtests). Further, subtest score patterns can be used as a screening device for neuropsychological deficits (Lezak, 1983). Table 3–5 presents descriptions of the WAIS-R subtests.

Rorschach Inkblot Test

The Rorschach, a projective instrument, consists of ten symmetrical inkblot designs of varying complexity and color administered in a standardized order. The examiner records verbatim responses to each card. Although a number of systems have been devised to score the patient's responses, increasingly psychologists rely upon the scoring guidelines delineated by Exner (1991; 1993), a highly structured and psychometrically reliable scoring system. Based upon certain combinations of scores, indices related to key diagnostic questions are computed, assessing schizophrenia,

Table 3–5 **Description of WAIS-R Subtests**

SUBTEST	DESCRIPTION
Verbal Scales	
Information	Measures range of general factual knowledge.
Digit Span	Measures immediate rote recall/reversibility skills and involves short-term auditory memory and sequential and attentional processes.
Vocabulary	Measures word knowledge and provides index of language development.
Arithmetic	Measures computational skill and taps attentional, sequential, and numerical reasoning processes.
Comprehension	Measures social judgment, practical knowledge, and ability to apply past experience in formulating solutions to specific problems.
Similarities	Measures verbal concept formation and verbal reasoning skills.
Performance Scales	
Picture Completion	Measures ability to differentiate essential from nonessential details and taps long-term visual memory skills.
Picture Arrangement	Measures planning ability, capacity to anticipate consequences, and temporal sequencing and time concepts.
Block Design	Measures nonverbal concept formation, spatial visualization skills, and the capacity for analysis and synthesis of abstract visual stimuli.
Object Assembly	Measures anticipation of relationships among parts to form familiar objects, and ability to benefit from sensory-motor feedback.
Digit Symbol	Measures speed and accuracy of visual-motor coordination, psychomotor speed (speed of mental operation), and visual short-term memory.

depression, coping deficits, suicide potential, hypervigilance, and obsessive style. Systematic analysis of Rorschach content material is used to obtain information regarding intrapsychic conflicts, predominant defenses, and interpersonal dynamics.

Thematic Apperception Test (TAT)

The TAT, a projective device, consists of 30 pictures representing a particular scene or interpersonal situation as well as one blank card. Examiners administer approximately ten cards selected based upon common interpersonal situations depicted in the cards and information about interpersonal dynamics relevant to the given patient. In response to each card, the patient is asked to make up a story about what is being depicted in the card and the examiner records these responses verbatim.

The TAT investigates personality dynamics manifested in interpersonal relationships via the patient's meaningful interpretations (apperceptions) of the environment as depicted on the cards. The TAT differs from the Rorschach by providing less ambiguous stimuli, a more clearly specified task structure, and a greater focus on interpersonal dynamics than on perceptual functioning and reality testing. The absence of accepted formal scoring procedures has resulted in a standard practice of qualitative analysis of test data requiring clinical acumen and experience. Typical categories that provide a systematic focus for TAT interpretation include interpersonal relationships, significant intrapsychic and interpersonal conflicts, and adequacy of ego and superego functioning (Bellak, 1992).

Interpretation of Test Findings

Ms. Foster's WAIS-R results placed her in the superior range of overall intellectual functioning, as she obtained a Full Scale IQ of 127. Her Verbal IQ was 119 and her Performance IQ was 127. There was no statistically significant difference between her verbal and performance scores. Her verbal comprehension and perceptual organization scores were comparable, suggesting that these abilities were fairly evenly developed. However, her performance on the Digit Span subtest, which loads on the freedom from distractibility factor, was significantly lower than all other subtest scores, suggesting that psychological factors impaired her attention and concentration. These results were not indicative of any neuropsychiatric condition or learning disability. Additionally, the comparability in verbal and performance subscale scores is not consistent with what might be expected from a depressed person whose depressive symptoms would likely interfere with performance on nonverbal timed tasks. Qualitative and quantitative analyses of the data revealed no evidence of a thought disorder, as might be expected from an individual with a schizophrenia spectrum disorder.

Despite the lack of evidence for a thought disorder on the WAIS-R, Ms. Foster showed signs of a mild thought disorder on the Rorschach, a test sensitive in detecting subtle underlying disturbances in thinking. Although she did not offer responses reflective of a severe thought disorder, on occasion she provided realistically implausible and odd responses, including "two pigs fighting over a baseball bat" and responses reflecting boundary disturbance, such as "two women joined at the hip." Ms. Foster's overall Rorschach protocol also revealed reality-testing difficulties. However, no gross perceptual distortions were noted.

Her Rorschach responses suggested difficulties with impulse control and a tendency to become overwhelmed by her feelings. On the first card in which there is some color present (red blot areas), she commented, "Oh boy, this makes me nervous! Wait a minute. I'm confused. Okay. That looks like blood, like menstrual blood, like when I have my period." The manner in which color is incorporated into percepts indicates the degree of emotional control, with more emphasis on color than form suggesting that affect is likely to be expressed more intensely. Ms. Foster provided a significant number of Rorschach responses depicting aggressive activity and interaction, including "an angel and a devil in a fist fight." This response also suggests the use of splitting as a defense, as she offers a "good" object (angel) fighting with a "bad" object (devil).

Finally, her Rorschach Coping Deficit Index and Suicide Constellation were positive. These findings are indicative of chronic susceptibility to difficulties coping with everyday stressors and interpersonal conflicts and of increased risk for suicidal ideation and/or behavior.

Her TAT responses were consistent with her Rorschach results. Her responses reflected aggressive themes and tumultuous interpersonal relationships marked by impulsivity, difficulty with affect regulation, and a propensity to consider suicidal behavior to cope with stress. For example, on a card in which a woman is touching the shoulders of a man who is turned away from her as if he were trying to pull away, Ms. Foster produced the following story. "They are having an argument over whether he's having an affair. She yells that she has always been faithful and he constantly betrays her. She demands that he stay with her, because if he leaves she will overdose. The fight started because he came home a half hour late from work and wasn't very sociable when he arrived. She was furious and he didn't seem to care. As always, they will probably make up, but fight about the same problem later. Or, he may leave and she may take an overdose."

Her MMPI-2 was valid and interpretively useful. It yielded a 3-point code (the three highest clinical scale elevations) of 8-4-2 (schizophrenia, psychopathic deviate, and depression scales). Individuals with this profile typically present with social alienation and social adjustment difficulties, proneness to frequent relationship conflicts, angry and impulsive behavior, and underlying dysphoria. Additionally, such persons often present with identity confusion and distortions in thinking.

Taken together, Ms. Foster's test findings are consistent with a diagnosis of borderline personality disorder with a propensity to experience transient psychotic episodes and dysphoria (borderline personality disorder is discussed in Chapter 6). At her best, which occurs in relatively structured and affectively neutral circumstances, she is an intelligent woman with a capacity for positive interpersonal interactions. Given the extent of her coping deficits, however, her equilibrium becomes easily disrupted under stressful conditions, particularly those marked by interpersonal conflict. At these times, she may become affectively labile, impulsive, and hostile. Under conditions that she experiences as extremely stressful, namely when confronted with threats of abandonment and actual loss, she may become actively suicidal, and the quality of her thinking and reality testing are likely to deteriorate and give way to psychotic distortions of reality. However, her thinking and reality-testing impairments are not so severe as to be consistent with a diagnosis of schizophrenia or major depression with psychotic features. Based upon these results, long-term psychodynamic psychotherapy was recommended to help the patient develop more effective coping strategies for dealing with interpersonal conflicts and painful affects. Additionally, group therapy was deemed advisable, as this is a particularly effective modality for addressing interpersonal difficulties (Yalom, 1985).

VIGNETTE 3

Mr. Lee, a 40-year-old computer software specialist, was diagnosed as HIV + 4 years prior to being referred by his internist for psychiatric evaluation of his complaints of unmanageable anxiety and insomnia. These difficulties began 4 months earlier, concurrent with his first HIV/ AIDS-related hospitalization for pneumocystis pneumonia (PCP). He had no previous psychiatric history, although he reported a tendency to worry and to be "high strung." During the evaluation, the psychiatrist conducted a Mini-Mental State Examination (Folstein, Folstein, and McHugh, 1975), which suggested possible difficulties with short-term memory. Upon questioning, Mr. Lee acknowledged that he had "not been as sharp as usual at work." As it was unclear whether or not his memory difficulties were secondary to his anxiety problems or indicative of deteriorated cognitive functioning associated with HIV-related neurocognitive impairments, head CT and magnetic resonance imaging (MRI) were ordered. The results were negative. Thus, the psychiatrist referred

Mr. Lee for neuropsychological evaluation to ascertain whether or not there was a physical basis to his short-term memory difficulties not detected on neurological workup.

The psychologist conducted a brief screening evaluation for specific memory deficits, which included the WAIS-R, Trail-Making Test (a subtest of the Halstead-Reitan Battery), Bender Visual-Motor Gestalt Test (Bender-Gestalt), and California Verbal Learning Test (CVLT). The MMPI-2 was administered to assess personality functioning.

Trail-Making Test

The Trail-Making Test, assessing motor speed, visuomotor tracking, and attention, is sensitive to the effects of brain injury (Lezak, 1983). Part A asks the patient to draw lines to connect consecutively numbered circles on a worksheet. For Part B, the patient is asked to connect consecutively numbered and lettered circles by alternating between the two sequences (i.e., 1-A-2-B-3-C, etc.). For both Parts A and B, the respondent is asked to complete the task as quickly as possible without lifting the pencil from the paper.

Bender Visual-Motor Gestalt Test (Bender-Gestalt)

The Bender-Gestalt, a visual motor task widely used as a screen for organic impairment, consists of nine simple designs displayed on separate cards presented to the patient one at a time. The patient is instructed to copy each design exactly as it appears on the card in front of them (Direct Copy Trial). Objective scoring systems provide a means to evaluate whether or not there is likely to be physical impairment. The Bender-Gestalt can also be used to assess visual memory deficits. For these purposes, after the direct copy trial the patient is asked to recall the nine designs from memory by drawing them (Immediate Recall Trial). Then, after working for 20 minutes on an interference task, the respondent is again asked to draw the nine designs from memory (Delayed Recall Trial).

California Verbal Learning Test (CVLT)

The CVLT assesses retention, recognition, and recall in the verbal memory system and results enable the examiner to distinguish deficits in these three areas. The CVLT assesses the capacity to learn new aurally presented material, retain this information in short- and long-term memory, and recall this information in the context of semantic cues. Additionally, it assesses long-term recognition memory.

Interpretation of Test Findings

Results of the brief neuropsychological evaluation suggested that Mr. Lee's memory difficulties may reflect both high levels of anxiety and neurologic difficulties. On the WAIS-R, Mr. Lee obtained a Full Scale IQ of 110, a Verbal IQ of 115, and a Performance IQ of 104, placing him in the average range of intellectual functioning. The 11-point Verbal-Performance IQ difference is statistically significant but not an abnormally large discrepancy, suggesting that his verbal skills are better developed than his nonverbal skills. Intra- and intersubtest scatter on the Performance subtests was minimal, revealing relatively consistent intellectual functioning in the nonverbal area. Although five of the six Verbal subtest scores were above average, on the Digit Span subtest he evidenced moderate impairments on the digits forward portion and considerable difficulty repeating digits backward. This suggests that his anxiety interfered with his capacity to attend (digits forward) and raised the possibility of short-term auditory memory difficulties (significant discrepancy between digits forward and digits backward).

On the Trail-Making Test, Mr. Lee's times for completing Parts A and B were not significantly different. However, his time to completion on both sections was slower than expected for an individual achieving an average Full Scale IQ and fell below the average time to completion for persons without brain impairment.

Mr. Lee's direct copy of the Bender-Gestalt yielded an overall score in the borderline range for the task, raising questions about possible neurologic impairment. His immediate and delayed recall trials were slightly below average, suggesting mild impairment of short- and long-term visual memory.

On the CVLT, he evidenced considerably more difficulty in learning newly presented material than would be expected for an individual with an average IQ. Further, he demonstrated impaired short- and long-term retention, with minimal improvement noted when semantic cues were provided. Further, he demonstrated only slightly improved performance on the delayed recognition portion of the CVLT. This overall pattern of results on the CVLT and Bender-Gestalt suggests the presence of verbal and visual memory deficits. Specifically, the results are indicative of encoding, retention, and recall difficulties inhibiting his capacity to learn and retain new information.

The patient provided a valid MMPI-2, albeit with some indication of guardedness (mild elevation on the K validity scale). All of his clinical scale scores were in the normal range except for scales 2 (depression) and 7 (psychasthenia), which were mildly elevated. This profile typically is seen in individuals who feel nervous, tense, guilty, and dysphoric. Such persons are also prone to excessive worry and obsessional thinking.

Overall, results from this screening battery led the psychologist to conclude that Mr. Lee's overall intellectual functioning is in the average range. The findings showed evidence for mild attentional difficulties and specific memory deficits. Mr. Lee appears to experience significant levels of anxiety that may exacerbate his encoding and retention difficulties, although his anxiety is unlikely to account for the extent of his apparent memory deficits. However, his pattern of results does not suggest impairments significant enough to profoundly interfere with his capacity to function effectively at work. Finally, there were some data suggesting possible diffuse neurologic impairment (e.g., borderline performance on the Bender-Gestalt and Trail-Making tests, Verbal-Performance IQ difference on the WAIS-R).

Based upon these findings, the psychologist recommended further and more complete neuropsychological evaluation to ascertain the presence and extent of diffuse neurologic impairment and its impact on cognitive functioning. The psychologist also recommended that the internist provide written instructions regarding medical management in order to enhance proper compliance. Further, a combination of stress management, cognitive-behavioral interventions, and evaluation for anxiolytic medications were suggested as means to address the patient's anxiety. Finally, the importance of helping him develop strategies for coping with his memory deficit was underscored.

SUMMARY AND CONCLUDING COMMENTS

Psychological assessment is a process that entails collecting, organizing, and interpreting information about a person's cognitive and emotional functioning and situational influences. Psychological tests enable the measurement, description, evaluation, and prediction of some human behaviors. The reliability and validity of the results are influenced by the patient's attitudes toward testing and the degree of compliance, the psychometric properties of the assessment devices used, the manner in which the testing is conducted (i.e., degree of standardization of test administration), and the ways in which the examiner interprets the findings. Choice of assessment devices and interpretation of findings often are guided by the referral questions, theoretical biases of the examiner, and context in which the testing is conducted. Physicians may request psychological testing when further information is needed regarding a patient's intellectual and neuropsychological functioning, the presence of underlying psychotic processes and affective disturbances, the quality of ego functioning, intrapsychic and interpersonal dynamics and personality style, and the veracity of patient's complaints. Psychological testing results, if communicated clearly and in a manner relevant to the referral questions, can be used by the referring physician to aid in diagnosis, case formulation, and treatment planning.

Mental health professionals may request a psychological testing consultation during any phase of psychotherapy. In the evaluation phase, test results may be useful in matching patients to treatment modality, theoretical orientation, and clinician. In the early stages of psychotherapy, testing may provide a comprehensive understanding of the patient's psychological functioning across functional domains. This helps the therapist anticipate potential difficulties that may complicate the therapeutic alliance, sensitizes the therapist to central areas of conflict, suggests areas of focus in treatment, elucidates potentially useful intervention strategies, and assists the therapist in more effectively managing resistances. In the later stages of psychotherapy, testing can be of value when therapeutic impasses emerge requiring outside consultation and may be useful as a barometer of therapeutic progress and future areas of work.

Like all assessment tools, psychological tests are not without their limitations. Interpretation of test findings often varies between psychologists, who may differentially emphasize various pieces of test data. Interpretation is influenced by the interpersonal dynamics of the testing situation (Schafer, 1954), the theoretical orientation of the psychologist, the types and format of the tests utilized, and the interpretive systems employed. These factors influence which psychological themes become the focus of the assessment and treatment process.

Another potential limitation of psychological assessment is the questionable applicability of tests for individuals from various cultural and ethnic groups. Psychological tests vary with regard to the degree of cross-cultural standardization used in their psychometric construction. As such, psychologists must use care in test selection to determine the psychometric appropriateness of a given test for use with persons from a specific cultural group. Further, knowledge of normative differences in performance among different ethnic and cultural groups is essential to the interpretive process.

Some have argued that a potential limitation of the psychological testing process is an excessive emphasis on deficits and pathology to the relative exclusion of the person's strengths and health. These advocate a more balanced approach in test design and the interpretation of test findings. They stress the importance of identifying the individual's adaptive modes of functioning. Finally, research regarding the psychometric soundness (e.g., adequacy of reliability and validity) of various assessment instruments has yielded equivocal results. This in turn leads to questions regarding the usefulness and meaningfulness of test findings. Some researchers and clinicians assert that many of the psychological tests described in this chapter, particularly personality inventories and projective tests, are of minimal value. For example, behavioral psychologists avoid subjective interpretation of the person, as they eschew the notion of internal psychological dynamics or traits in favor of an emphasis on the functional analysis of observable behavior patterns and associated environmental events (Skinner, 1974).

These potential limitations underscore the importance of interpreting psychological test findings in the context of a person's medical status, psychiatric symptom presentation, and sociocultural milieu. Thus, the integration of interdisciplinary sources of assessment data allows for comprehensive patient evaluation and well-informed treatment planning sensitive to the uniqueness of each patient's situation.

CLINICAL PEARLS

- Referral for psychological testing is appropriate when there is a need to assess intellectual, neuropsychological, and personality functioning.
- Psychological testing results should be integrated with other pertinent clinical data when tests are used to aid in diagnosis, case formulation, treatment planning, and prediction of behavior.
- In order to maximize the usefulness of testing results, it is important that the physician clearly articulate specific referral questions to be addressed in the psychological evaluation.
- The utility of a given psychological test instrument should be evaluated on the basis of the psychometric properties of standardization, reliability, and validity.
- Although psychological tests are standardized instruments, individual differences and cultural context must be taken into account in test interpretation.

ANNOTATED BIBLIOGRAPHY

Anastasi A: *Psychological Testing*, 6th ed. New York, Macmillan, 1988

> This classic text provides an introduction to the nature and uses of psychological testing. It includes a review of the history of psychological testing, a discussion of ethical considerations in testing, an overview of basic psychometric issues pertaining to psychological tests, and a description of a wide range of commonly used tests.

Exner JE: The Rorschach: A Comprehensive System. Vol 1, Basic Foundations, 3rd ed. New York, John Wiley and Sons, 1993

> This is an excellent introduction to the Comprehensive System of Rorschach administration, scoring, and basic interpretation. It also includes a brief history of the Rorschach as a clinical assessment tool, as well as a discussion of research findings relevant to Rorschach interpretation.

Exner JE: The Rorschach: A Comprehensive System. Vol 2, Interpretation, 2nd ed. New York, John Wiley and Sons, 1991

> A companion to Exner's first volume, this text offers a detailed focus on methods of Rorschach interpretation, including discussion of issues in diagnosis and treatment planning. It also outlines changes and revisions in scoring and interpretation made subsequent to publication of the first volume.

Greene RL: The MMPI-2/MMPI: An Interpretive Manual. Needham Heights, MA, Allyn and Bacon, 1991

> An excellent introduction to the MMPI-2 is presented in this book. In addition to an overview of basic psychometric properties of the MMPI-2, a comprehensive step-by-step discussion of test interpretation is also provided.

Kaufman AS: Assessing Adolescent and Adult Intelligence. Boston, Allyn and Bacon, 1990

> This book offers a detailed discussion of intellectual testing with an emphasis on the WAIS-R, providing an excellent detailed account of the breadth and depth of interpretive usefulness of intellectual test results. An overview of important issues and debates relevant to intellectual testing is also included.

Lezak MD: Neuropsychological Assessment, 2nd ed. Oxford, Oxford University Press, 1983

> This classic reference offers an overview of the nature and uses of neuropsychological testing. It provides descriptions of a wide range of available test instruments and includes discussion of their interpretive usefulness.

Sattler JM: Assessment of Children, 3rd ed. San Diego, Jerome M. Sattler Publisher, 1988

> This standard reference text offers an overview and introduction to psychological assessment with children. The emphasis is on assessment of abilities (e.g. intellectual functioning, achievement). Such specialized topics as mental retardation, learning disabilities, developmental disorders, attention-deficit hyperactivity disorder, and adaptive behavior are also discussed.

Tallent N: Psychological Report Writing. 3rd ed. Englewood Cliffs, NJ, Prentice-Hall, 1988

> An introduction to considerations in communication of test findings in a report is provided in this text. Even for those who are not likely to need knowledge of how to write a report, this book may offer insights into the types of information that might be derived from psychological testing.

REFERENCES

Anastasi A: Psychological Testing, 6th ed. New York, Macmillan, 1988

Bellak L: The T.A.T., C.A.T. and S.A.T. in clinical use, 5th ed. Needham, MA, Allyn & Bacon, 1992

Exner JE: The Rorschach: A Comprehensive System. Vol 1, Basic Foundations, 3rd ed. New York, John Wiley and Sons, 1993

Exner JE: The Rorschach: A Comprehensive System. Vol 2, Interpretation, 2nd ed. New York, John Wiley and Sons, 1991

Folstein MF, Folstein SE, McHugh PR: Mini-mental state. J Psychiatr Res 12:189–198, 1975

Frank LK: Projective methods for the study of personality. J Psychol 8:389–413, 1939

Friedman M, Rosenman RH: Type A Behavior and Your Heart. New York, Knopf, 1974

Graham JR: MMPI-2: Assessing Personality and Psychopathology. New York, Oxford University Press, 1990

Greene RL: The MMPI-2/MMPI: An Interpretive Manual. Needham Heights, MA, Allyn and Bacon, 1991

Hathaway SR, McKinley JC: The Minnesota Multiphasic Personality Inventory, rev. ed. Minneapolis, University of Minnesota Press, 1943

Kaufman AS: Assessing Adolescent and Adult Intelligence. Boston, Allyn and Bacon, 1990

Keller LS, Butcher JN: Assessment of Chronic Pain Patients with the MMPI-2. Minneapolis, University of Minnesota Press, 1991

Lezak MD: Neuropsychological Assessment, 2nd ed. Oxford, Oxford University Press, 1983

Murray HA: Thematic Apperception Test Manual. Cambridge, Harvard University Press, 1943

Osborne D: The MMPI in medical practice. Psychiatric Annals 15:534–541, 1985

Pope KS: Responsibilities in providing psychological test feedback to clients. Psychol Assessment 4:268–271, 1992

Racusin GR, Moss NE: Psychological Assessment of Children and Adolescents. In Lewis M (ed.): Child and Adolescent Psychiatry: A Comprehensive Textbook, pp 472–485. Baltimore, Williams & Wilkins, 1991

Rorschach H: Psychodiagnostics. New York, Grune & Stratton, 1921/1949.

Sattler JM: Assessment of Children, 3rd ed. San Diego, Jerome M. Sattler Publisher, 1988

Schafer R: Psychoanalytic Interpretation in Rorschach Testing. New York, Grune & Stratton, 1954

Schretlen DJ: The use of psychological tests to identify malingered symptoms of mental disorder. Clin Psychol Rev 8:451–476, 1988

Skinner BF: About Behaviorism. New York, Vintage Books, 1974

Strassberg DS, Tilley D, Bristone S, Oei TPS: The MMPI and chronic pain: A cross-cultural view. Psychol Assessment 4:493–497, 1992

Tallent N: Psychological Report Writing, 3rd ed. Englewood Cliffs, NJ, Prentice-Hall, 1988

Thoresen CE, Powell LH: Type A behavior pattern: New perspectives on theory, assessment, and intervention. J Consult Clin Psychol 60:595–604, 1992

Wechsler D: Manual for the Wechsler Adult Intelligence Scale-Revised. New York, Psychological Corporation, 1981

Wechsler D: Manual for the Wechsler Intelligence Scale for Children, 3rd ed. New York, Psychological Corporation, 1991

Widiger TA, Frances A: Interviews and inventories for the measurement of personality disorders. Clin Psychol Review 7:49–75, 1987

Williams RB: Biobehavioral Factors in Cardiovascular Disease. In Houpt JL, and Brodie HKH (eds.): Psychiatry, Vol 3, pp 391–399. New York, Basic Books, 1986

Yalom IB: The Theory and Practice of Group Psychotherapy, 3rd ed. New York, Basic Books, 1985

Alan Stoudemire (ed). *Clinical Psychiatry for Medical Students*, Second
Edition. Copyright © 1994, 1990 by J. B. Lippincott Company.

Delirium, Dementia, and Other Disorders Associated with Cognitive Impairment

Alan Stoudemire

This chapter will discuss diagnosis and treatment of delirium, dementia, and other psychiatric conditions associated with cognitive impairment. The term "cognitive impairment" has replaced the anachronistic term "organic" in DSM-IV because it is now recognized that *many* of the *major* psychiatric disorders involve some degree of neuropsychological dysfunction and that all behavior has a neurochemical (organic) substrate. Taken as a whole, dementia, delirium, and other cognitive impairment disorders are among the most common psychiatric disorders encountered by general medical and surgical physicians in clinical practice.

Before proceeding in this area, a few basic terms will be defined to guide the discussion (Tucker et al, 1992; Popkin and Tucker, 1992).

1. *Delirium.* Delirium is a disorder, usually acute and fluctuating, characterized by an altered state of consciousness (that is, reduced awareness of and ability to respond to one's environment) (Table 4–1). Cognitive defects in attention, concentration, thinking, memory, and goal-directed behavior are almost always present. Delirium may be accompanied by hallucinations, misperceptions of sensory stimuli (illusions), emotional lability, alterations in the sleep–wake cycle, psychomotor slowing, or hyperactivity. The onset of delirium is often abrupt but may be insidious in nature. The cause is usually traced to a medication

The editor gratefully acknowledges the help of Drs. Marshall Folstein and Paul McHugh who supplied textual material for the original version of the chapter in the first edition of this textbook.

Table 4–1 **Major Signs and Symptoms of Delirium**

Altered state of alertness, awareness, and consciousness (hyperalert or obtunded; patient's level of consciousness may vary from time to time; lucid intervals may occur)
Fluctuating course—as above
Onset may be dramatic but may be subtle and evolve over days or weeks
Disorientation and confusion
Decreased attention, concentration, and memory
Psychotic symptoms—paranoia, hallucinations (often visual), delusions
Behavioral disinhibition, emotional lability, irritability
Psychomotor retardation or agitation—may vary in a 24-hour period
Fragmented sleep/wake cycle; increased agitation at night
Usually reversible with correction of underlying etiology
Apraxia, dysgraphia, dysnomia and tremors, abnormal reflexes (myoclonus or asterixis)

side effect, metabolic abnormalities, toxic agents, acute central nervous system (CNS) abnormalities, or medication/drug intoxication or withdrawal. If the cause of the delirium can be identified and corrected, the condition usually remits relatively promptly. In DSM-IV the subtypes "substance-induced delirium" and "delirium due to multiple etiologies" are listed.

2. *Substance-induced delirium.* Substance-induced delirium is associated with psychoactive agents due to either intoxication or withdrawal. This category of mental disorders is used to designate behavioral abnormalities caused by direct effects of psychoactive agents on the brain. DSM-IV addresses the following drugs associated with intoxication syndromes: alcohol, amphetamines (and similar sympathomimetics), caffeine, cannabis, opioids, cocaine, hallucinogens, inhalants, phencyclidine (and similarly acting arylcyclohexylamines), sedative-hypnotics, and anxiolytics. *Withdrawal* deliria are possible with alcohol, sedative-hypnotics, and anxiolytics. Certain medical drugs (including narcotics) can cause delirium, including histamine (H-2) blocking agents, digitalis, and anticholinergics. In many cases it is difficult to ascertain a precise etiology of the patient's delirium (such as a patient with fever, electrolyte abnormalities, and renal failure who is being treated with multiple medications including narcotics) in which case the delirium is noted to be caused by "multiple etiologies." Table 4–2 is a *partial* listing of drugs that have been reported to cause delirium. They are discussed further in Chapter 10 by Dr. Swift.

3. *Dementia.* Dementia is characterized by (usually) insidious (but sometimes acute) development of generalized brain dysfunction with *multiple* cognitive deficits (Table 4–3). It is essential that the patients' cognitive deficits result in an impairment in their so-

Table 4–2 **Drugs Causing Delirium (Partial Listing)**

Antibiotics

Acyclovir (antiviral)
Amphotericin B (antifungal)
Cephalexin
Chloroquine (antimalarial)
Fluoroquinilones (ciprofloxin)

Anticholinergic

Antihistamines
  Chlorpheniramine
  Diphenhydramine
Anticholinergics
  Benztropine
  Biperiden
Antispasmodics
Atropine/homatropine
Belladonna alkaloids
Phenothiazines (especially
  thioridazine)
Promethazine
Scopolamine
Tricyclic antidepressants
  (especially amitriptyline)
Trihexyphenidyl

Anticonvulsants

Phenobarbital
Phenytoin
Sodium valproate

Antiinflammatory

Adrenocorticotropic hormone
Corticosteroids
Ibuprofen
Indomethacin
Naproxen
Phenylbutazone

Antineoplastic

5-fluorouracil

Antiparkinson

Amantadine
Carbidopa
Levodopa

Antituberculous

Isoniazid
Rifampicin

Analgesics

Opiates
Salicylates
Synthetic narcotics

Cardiac

Beta-blockers
  Propranolol
Clonidine
Digitalis
Disopyramide
Lidocaine
Mexiletine
Methyldopa
Quinidine
Procainamide

Drug intoxication/withdrawal

Alcohol
Barbiturates
Benzodiazepines

Sedative-Hypnotics

Barbiturates
Benzodiazepines
Glutethimide

Sympathomimetics

Amphetamines
Phenylephrine
Phenylpropanolamine

Miscellaneous

Aminophylline
Bromides
Chlorpropamide
Cimetidine
Cyclosporine
Disulfiram
Lithium
Metrizamide
Metronidazole
Ranitidine
Podophyllin by absorption
Propylthiouracil
Quinacrine
Theophylline
Timolol ophthalmic

**Over-the-Counter (most have
anticholinergic effects)**

Compoz
Sleep-Eze
Sominex

(Adapted and used with permission from Wise MG: Delirium. In Hales RE, Yudofsky SC
(eds): Textbook of Neuropsychiatry. Washington, DC, American Psychiatric Press, 1987)

Table 4–3 **Major signs and symptoms of dementia***

ALZHEIMER'S TYPE

Multiple Cognitive Deficits Characterized by
  Memory impairment
  At least one of the following disturbances:
    Aphasia
    Apraxia
    Agnosia
    Executive functioning (planning, organizing, sequencing, abstraction)
Gradual onset and continued decline
Cognitive deficits lead to significant impairment in social and/or occupational
functioning and represents decline from previous level of functioning
Cognitive deficits are *not* due to another identifiable metabolic, or neuro-
logic disorder, or due to another psychiatric disorder (such as depressive
pseudodementia or schizophrenia)
Cognitive deficits not primarily caused by delirium

VASCULAR DEMENTIA

Multiple Cognitive Deficits Characterized by:
  Memory impairment
  At least one of the following disturbances:
    Aphasia
    Apraxia
    Agnosia
    Executive functioning (planning, organizing, sequencing, abstraction)
Focal neurologic signs (see text) or radiographic evidence of cerebral
vascular disease
Cognitive deficits lead to significant impairment in social and/or occupa-
  tional functioning and represents decline from previous level of function-
  ing
Cognitive deficits are not due to a delirium

DEMENTIA DUE TO OTHER CONDITIONS

Multiple Cognitive Deficits Characterized by
  Memory impairment
  At least one of the following disturbances:
    Aphasia
    Apraxia
    Agnosia
    Executive functioning (planning, organizing, sequencing, abstraction)
Cognitive deficits lead to significant impairment in social and/or occupa-
  tional functioning and represents decline from previous level of function-
  ing
Cognitive deficits not primarily caused by delirium
Evidence exists from physical exam, laboratory or radiographic evidence
  that the cognitive dysfunction is caused by one or more of the following:
    HIV
    Head Trauma
    Parkinson's Disease
    Huntington's Disease
    Pick's Disease
    Jakob-Creutzfeldt Disease
    Other causes (hypothyroidism, B_{12} deficiency, normal pressure hydro-
    cephalus, brain tumors, etc., see Table 4–4)

*Adapted from DSM-IV (APA 1993, in press [1994])

cial and/or occupational functioning and a decline from their previous level of functioning. The patients' level of awareness and mental alertness is intact and stable in the early phases of a dementia—in contrast to the unstable alternating level of consciousness seen in delirium. These cognitive deficits are often (but not always) predominately manifested by memory impairment—both the inability to learn new information and to recall previously learned information. Alzheimer's-type dementia *must* also be accompanied by one more of the following signs or symptoms (indicating dementia is more than just a memory disorder): aphasia (language dysfunction), apraxia (difficulty or inability to carry out most activities), agnosia (difficulty or failure to recognize or identify objects), and disturbances in executive functioning (APA [DSM-IV], 1993, in press [1994]). The course is usually chronic and deteriorating unless an identifiable, treatable cause of the brain dysfunction is identified (such as B_{12} deficiency or hypothyroidism). The most common causes of the dementia symptoms are Alzheimer's disease, vascular dementia (multi-infarct or cerebrovascular dementia), Parkinson's disease, Huntington's disease, HIV, head trauma, Pick's disease, Jakob-Creutzfeldt disease, brain tumors, hypothyroidism, normal pressure hydrocephalus, and substance-induced conditions (such as alcohol) (Table 4–4).

Table 4–4 **Causes of Dementia (Partial Listing)**

Alcohol-related dementia
Alzheimer's disease
Amyotrophic lateral sclerosis
Bromide poisoning
Chronic granulomatous meningitis
  (tuberculous, fungal)
Folic acid deficiency
Head trauma
Human immunodeficiency virus (HIV)
Huntington's chorea
Hypothyroidism
Multi-infarct dementia
Multiple sclerosis
Neoplasms
Normal-pressure hydrocephalus
Parkinson-dementia complex
Parkinson's disease
Postanoxic states
Progressive supranuclear palsy
Tertiary neurosyphilis
Transmissible virus dementia
  (Jakob-Creutzfeldt disease)
Vitamin B_{12} deficiency

The most common form of dementia is Alzheimer's disease and can be associated with superimposed delirium, delusions, and symptoms of depressed mood. If the patient's depressive symptoms are of such severe proportion to meet diagnostic criteria for major depression, then major depression should be listed as a separate concurrent diagnosis.

The other major cause of dementia in the elderly is *vascular dementia* (also referred to as multi-infarct dementia or cerebrovascular dementia). In DSM-IV its criteria differ little from those of Alzheimer's disease except that evidence of focal neurologic signs and symptoms should be present (e.g., hyperactive deep tendon reflexes, extensor plantar (Babinski) response, pseudobulbar palsy, gait abnormalities, weakness, etc.) *or* radiographic evidence of cerebral vascular disease such as multiple infarction of the cerebral cortex or white matter. Vascular dementia can be "subtyped" based on the presence or absence of concurrent deliria, delusions, or depressive symptoms (APA, 1993).

Dementia is a disorder of cognitive impairment—*in addition* to impairments in short- and long-term memory, problems exist in abstract thinking, logical judgment, personality changes, orientation, interpersonal relationships, and higher cortical functions such as language and calculations. The onset is usually insidious and slowly progressive. As noted above, unlike in delirium, the patient's *level of awareness and alertness is usually intact* in the early and middle stages of the illness and usually becomes impaired only in the *latter stages* of the illness; the retention and stability of *alertness* is a primary symptom that distinguishes *dementia* from *delirium*. Examples of dementia include Alzheimer's disease, Pick's disease, AIDS-related dementia, vascular (multi-infarct) dementia, dementia of Parkinson's disease, and normal pressure hydrocephalus. Table 4–5 contrasts the clinical differences between delirium and dementia.

4. *Substance-induced dementia*. Dementia syndromes induced by substances are also characterized by multiple cognitive deficits and by memory impairment (usually the inability to learn new information or to recall previously learned information) along with one or more of the following symptoms: aphasia, apraxia, agnosia, or disturbances in executive functioning (planning, organization, and abstract thought). The symptoms should represent a change in the patient's usual level of functioning. The primary substance associated with this form of dementia is *alcohol* but it may occur with certain types of inhalants as well as the chronic use of sedative hypnotics and has been reported with anxiolytics such as benzodiazepines.

5. *Amnestic disorders*. These are disorders characterized by a relatively focal disorder of short-term memory characterized by the

Table 4–5 **Differential Diagnosis of Delirium and Dementia**

FEATURE	DELIRIUM	DEMENTIA
Onset	Acute, often at night	Insidious
Course	Fluctuating, with lucid intervals, during day; worse at night	Stable over course of day
Duration	Hours to weeks	Months or years
Awareness	Reduced	Clear
Alertness	Abnormally low or high	Usually normal
Attention	Lacks direction and selectivity, distractibility, fluctuates over course of day	Relatively unaffected
Orientation	Usually impaired for time, tendency to mistake unfamiliar for familiar place and persons	Often impaired
Memory	Immediate and recent impaired	Recent and remote impaired
Thinking	Disorganized	Impoverished
Perception	Illusions and hallucinations usually visual and common	Often absent
Speech	Incoherent, hesitant, slow or rapid	Difficulty in finding words
Sleep–wake cycle	Always disrupted	Fragmented sleep
Physical illness or drug toxicity	Either or both present	Often absent, especially in Alzheimer's disease

(Used with permission from Lipowski ZJ: Delirium (acute confusional states). JAMA 258:1789–1792, 1987)

inability to learn new information or the inability to recall previously learned information; other cognitive functions are intact. The memory disturbance must be accompanied by impaired social or occupational functions. The memory problem should not occur as part of a primary delirium or dementia syndrome. The most common cause of substance-induced amnestic disorders is alcoholism. The most common neuroanatomic abnormality that has been described with the amnestic syndrome is bilateral sclerosis of the mamillary bodies probably due to hemorrhage. Degenerative changes also have been described in the dorsal medial nucleus of the thalamus, which serves as a relay point between memory centers and the frontal cortex.

Transient global amnesia (TGA) is a form of amnestic disorder that usually occurs in middle-aged or elderly individuals and is characterized by the sudden loss of memory of recent events and the inability to recall new information. In DSM-IV, TGA would be coded as an *amnestic disorder with transient features.* The essential feature of this condition is the transitory inability to learn new information (encoding memory problems) with a variable retrograde amnesia that "shrinks" following recovery such that the amnestic gap is confined to that time period predominantly between the acute onset of the disorder and its resolution (Caine, 1993). The level of consciousness usually is normal during the course of TGA and personal identity remains intact. Patients are aware of their deficits and may ask questions about their circumstances. Such episodes may last from minutes to hours, and attacks usually are episodic. The "spells" often remit within 24 hours. Most experts consider the episodes to be caused by transient vascular insufficiency of the mesial temporal lobe, but other disorders such as tumors, use of short-acting benzodiazepines (such as triazolam), cardiac arrhythmias, cerebral embolism, migraine, polycythemia vera, and mitral valvular disease have been reported to cause episodes of TGA. Most patients with TGA also have associated risk factors for cerebrovascular stroke. Amnestic disorders may be classified based upon whether they are due to medical causes or due to psychoactive substances (Caine, 1993). Amnestic disorders are characterized as being either *transient* or *chronic* based on the time course and persistence of the amnesia.

6. *Anxiety, mood, and psychotic disorders due to general medical conditions and substances.* These diagnoses are made when evidence of brain dysfunction affecting behavior (anxiety, mood, psychosis) exists but a *primary* dementia or delirium has been ruled out; the symptoms should occur in the presence of a relatively clear mental status. These conditions involve abnormalities in *mood, anxiety*, or *the presence of psychotic symptoms, delusions*, and *hallucinations* that can usually be attributed directly to some specific cause or agent. *As noted above, these diagnoses should not be made if the patient primarily meets diagnostic criteria for delirium or a dementia.*

   A patient with a clear mental status who becomes depressed because of *hypothyroidism* would be considered to have a depressive disorder due to a general medical condition. A complete review of these syndromes is beyond the scope of this text, but the most common causes of these mood and psychotic disorders are summarized in Tables 4–6, 4–7, and 4–8.

7. *Personality change due to a general medical condition.* This disorder applies to situations where patients develop personality changes from the usual pattern due to a specific medical or neurological condition (such as temporal lobe epilepsy). The disorder is subtyped into the following categories: *labile, disinhibited, aggressive, apathetic*, and *paranoid*, although mixtures of symptoms are perhaps most common clinically (combined type) (Table 4–9).

8. *Catatonic disorder due to a general medical condition.* Catatonic behavior is characterized by negativism, profound with-

Table 4–6 **Major Reported Causes of Depressive Syndromes Due to General Medical Conditions, Medications and Other Substances**

Medications

Antihypertensives (reserpine, methyldopa, propranolol)
Barbiturates
Corticosteroids
Guanethidine
Indomethacin
Levodopa
Psychostimulants (amphetamine and cocaine in the postwithdrawal phase)

Medical illnesses

Carcinoid syndrome
Carcinomas (pancreatic)
Cerebrovascular disease (stroke)
Collagen-vascular disease (systemic lupus erythematosus)
Endocrinopathies (Cushing's syndrome, Addison's disease, hypo-
  glycemia, hyper- and hypocalcemia, hyper- and hypothyroidism)
Lymphomas
Parkinson's disease
Pernicious anemia (B_{12} deficiency)
Viral illnesses (hepatitis, mononucleosis, influenza)

(Adapted from Stoudemire A: Selected organic mental disorders. In Hales RE, Yudofsky SC (eds): Textbook of Neuropsychiatry. Washington, DC, American Psychiatric Press, 1987)

Table 4–7 **Major Reported Causes of Manic Syndromes Due to General Medical Conditions, Medications and Other Substances**

Medications

Antidepressants
Corticosteroids/ACTH
Decongestants (containing phenylephrine)
Levodopa
Monoamine oxidase inhibitors
Sympathomimetics/bronchodilators (containing theophylline
  and/or ephedrine/isophedrine)

Metabolic abnormalities

Hyperthyroidism

Seizure/neurologic disorders

Multiple sclerosis
Right hemispheric damage
Temporal lobe seizures

Neoplasms

(Adapted from Stoudemire A: Selected organic mental disorders. In Hales RE, Yudofsky SC (eds): Textbook of Neuropsychiatry. Washington, DC, American Psychiatric Press, 1987)

Table 4–8 **Major Reported Causes of Psychotic Disorders Due to General Medical Conditions, Medications and Other Substances (Partial Listing)**

CNS disorders	Endocrinopathies
Cerebrovascular disease	Adrenal insufficiency
Idiopathic basal ganglia calcification	Cushing's disease
Multiple sclerosis	Hyperthyroidism
Neoplasms	Hypothyroidism
Parkinson's disease	Hypo- and hypercalcemia
Spinocerebellar degeneration	Panhypopituitarism
Temporal lobe epilepsy	**Miscellaneous**
Connective tissue disease	Amphetamines
Systemic lupus erythematosus	Bromide
Temporal arteritis	Corticosteroids
Deficiency states	Heavy metal toxicity
B_{12}	Huntington's chorea
Folate	Pentazocine
Niacin	Porphyria
Drug/medications	
Antidepressants	
Antihypertensives	
Antimalarials, anticonvulsants	
Antiparkinsonian agents	
Antituberculosis agents	
Hallucinogens	

(Adapted from Stoudemire A: Selected organic mental disorders. In Hales RE, Yudofsky SC (eds): Textbook of Neuropsychiatry. Washington, DC, American Psychiatric Press, 1987)

drawal, mutism, motor rigidity, and catalepsy ("waxy" flexibility that may alternate with severe agitation). The disorder is most commonly associated with mood disorders but may also occur as a presenting symptom of a variety of medical and neurological disorders such as herpes encephalitis, vascular insults, or as a

Table 4–9 **Major Reported Causes of Personality Changes Due To Medical and Neurological Conditions**

Adrenocortical disease
Head trauma
Heavy metal poisoning
Hypothyroidism
Multiple sclerosis
Neoplasms
Systemic lupus erythematosus
Temporal lobe seizure disorders
Vascular disease

profound parkinsonian-like reaction to neuroleptics (neuroleptic-induced catatonia) (Popkin and Tucker, 1992; Stoudemire, 1982). In DSM-IV, the category is deemed "catatonic disorder due to a general medical condition" where medical and neurologic disorders are the causative factor.

9. *Postconcussional syndrome as proposed for inclusion in DSM-IV.* This syndrome follows a history of head trauma and should involve at least two of the following symptoms: loss of consciousness for at least *five minutes*, posttraumatic amnesia for at least a 12-hour duration, and onset of seizure within 6 months of the injury. Evidence should exist from neuropsychological testing of impairments in attention, concentration, performing simultaneous cognitive tasks, and impairments in learning new memory or recalling information that occurs shortly after the traumatic injury. Other symptoms associated with the postconcussive syndrome include easy fatiguability, vertigo, dizziness, irritability, emotional lability, impulsivity (sometimes involving aggression), anxiety, depression, personality changes, inappropriate sexual or social behaviors, and apathy. Patients should not meet criteria for dementia, including dementia due to head trauma. Hence, the postconcussive syndrome is *not* a form of dementia. This disorder is listed in the Appendix to DSM-IV and will undergo further study before becoming an "official" disorder in this diagnostic manual (APA, 1993).

Arriving at the diagnosis of delirium, dementia, and other cognitive impairment disorders requires a carefully structured cognitive and behavioral assessment of the patient. The following section discusses the clinical assessment of the patient's condition.

CLINICAL EXAMINATION OF THE PATIENT WITH COGNITIVE DYSFUNCTION: USE OF THE MINI-MENTAL STATE EXAMINATION

Perhaps the most serious clinical error made in medicine is underdiagnosis of cognitive disorders in medical and surgical settings. It is common for physicians to label a patient's abnormal behavior caused by a cognitive disorder erroneously as "functional" (that is, due to a "psychiatric" or emotional problem). Although the reasons for underdiagnosis or misdiagnosis of cognitive impairment disorders are not entirely clear, they probably result from a lack of rigor and structure in performing a mental status examination, if one is performed at all. Because of this pervasive problem in clinical medicine, a significant portion of this chapter is devoted to presenting in some detail a structured cognitive mental status examination using the Mini-Mental State Examination (MMSE) (Folstein, Folstein, McHugh, 1975). The MMSE is a practical and efficient instrument for assessing, documenting, and tracking a patient's cognitive functioning over time. This cognitive screening instrument has been extensively validated in both clinical and research settings. Its brevity, accuracy, and efficiency make it immensely practical for routine clinical use (see Appendix at end of chapter).

There are, however, several disadvantages to this approach. Symptoms such as delusions and hallucinations, which could not be quantitated as easily, are not included. A total score does not specifically characterize the patient's cognitive capacity in terms such as amnesia, aphasia, or apraxia. Hence, the MMSE is *not* to be considered a comprehensive behavioral or cognitive mental status examination but a reliable means of screening and monitoring gross changes in cognitive functioning.

Mini-Mental State Examination

The set of items called the Mini-Mental State Examination briefly surveys important cognitive functions, including language function, that are omitted from most other brief screening tests (Chapter 4 Appendix). It is useful in screening patients and also is useful in teaching aspects of the cognitive examination that can be embellished by the examiner asking for such things as the interpretation of proverbs, a listing of the presidents in reverse order, or a drawing of a cube or a clock. It also can be amplified by the addition of more formal neuropsychological testing, including symbol digit and trails test, to delineate in more detail preserved and impaired functions.

The MMSE begins with a set of questions about orientation in time and place. The patient is asked, "Where are you?" and the patient is expected to be able to tell us the place they are in space and time, specific to the day of the week and the month of the year. Thus, orientation to time and place can be graded, and a patient is *more or less* oriented rather than *absolutely* disoriented or oriented. Patients can acquire 10 points out of 30 on the examination for giving a complete answer to the questions concerning *orientation*. Orientation is the first and easiest capacity to assess because it is so frequently disturbed among patients. Although disorientation can be as subtle as a mild sense of bewilderment over the date, it can be so severe that patients may not know whether they are indoors or outdoors, standing or lying, in the hospital or at home.

Because one cause of disorientation might be the inability of patients to learn from an assessment of their surroundings, the disorientation could be the outcome of a memory disorder. The next set of probes tests the ability of the patient to learn and remember.

Questions in this segment of the exam begin with the test of the patient's capacity to register and repeat three simple words that are presented orally. The patient is asked to repeat three words given approximately 1 second apart, such as pony, quarter, and orange, and is given one point for each of the three correctly repeated. This task is also an assessment of the patient's capacity to hear, attend, and repeat words, as well as the capacity to remember three objects mentioned in a very short period of time. To determine their capacity to recall for a longer period of time, the patient is asked to recall the three objects a short while later, after which he or she performs another task that is presented to prevent constant rehearsal of the three objects.

During this interval, another capacity is tested; the patient is asked to attend to a task and carry it through to completion. The best tasks testing attention and concentration are those that demand a continuing focus on and performance of a serial problem. Thus, a subtraction of 7 from 100 for five consecutive subtractions requires patients to be able to attend and at the same time perform an arithmetic function without losing track of the task that they are performing. Another similar, but less difficult, task is the spelling of the word "world" backward. This task is offered to patients only when they refuse to perform the serial 7s, because the serial 7s task is more difficult.

After the assessment of attention and calculation by the serial 7s task, it is determined whether patients can recall three words presented to them previously in the registration task; thus, they are able to tap a longer-term aspect of memory.

This completes the *first section* of the MMSE. Many aspects of the tests of orientation, registration, attention and calculation, and recall depend to some extent on the patient's capacity to comprehend and use language. The second part of the examination is designed explicitly to test the patient's language capacity. It is then determined whether the patient can name a visually presented object; repeat the phrase "No ifs, ands, or buts"; follow a three-stage verbal command—"Take this piece of paper in your right hand, fold it in half, and put it on the floor"; read a simple sentence—"Close your eyes"; write a sentence spontaneously; and copy a design. This aspect of the MMSE can be supplemented with evaluation by the physician of the patient's speech—whether it is fluent, dysarthric, or of normal rate, rhythm, and prosody. Thus, one then makes make a judgment as to whether the patient speaks clearly with normal intonation or whether the speech is monotonic or slurred. In addition, it is noted whether the patient uses appropriate vocabulary or whether mistakes are made in the meaning of particular words, such as when new words are constructed or old words are pronounced incorrectly. It is also noted whether patients use appropriate syntax with complex or simple sentences in their response to questions, and finally whether the patient in the course of the examination addresses the examiner in the expected fashion, with appropriate eye contact and demeanor. In this way, in addition to being able to score the patient's performance on a series of simple tasks, it is possible to appraise the patient's phonology, semantics, syntax, and pragmatics of language function. These last aspects are not scored but should be entered as commentary on the patient's performance on the examination. The language section of the MMSE can be affected by disease processes of several types, including focal brain diseases of the left hemisphere, such as those produced by a stroke, as well as by diffuse brain disease, such as that produced by Alzheimer's disease.

Consciousness

The examination is concluded by an assessment of the patient's level of consciousness, which is rated on an analog scale from comatose to fully alert. This rating can be performed reliably and is a measure of the patient's alertness, responsiveness, and accessibility to the examiner (Anthony, LeResche, Von Korff et al, 1985). Although this aspect of the examination is not taken into the total score, it serves to distinguish those patients who are cognitively impaired in a clear state of consciousness, as in dementia, from those who are cognitively impaired with an altered state of alertness and consciousness, as in delirium.

In a medical setting, the usual procedure is to try to determine whether the impairments as assessed by the MMSE in fact cluster into groups of symptoms, such as the syndromes of dementia and delirium. After that assessment, one then attempts to determine whether an *identifiable* pathological process is present, such as a stroke, Alzheimer's disease, or drug intoxication. In a final step of the overall evaluation, it is determined whether a recognizable risk factor or causal agent is present, such as hypertension or a genetic abnormality. Thus, one reasons from symptoms and signs to syndromes to pathology to etiology.

The Syndromes

One conceptual approach to syndromes of cognitive impairment is to divide them into two main groups, the *developmental syndromes* and the *deteriorations*. The *developmental syndromes* include those aspects of *mental retardation, developmental dyslexia, and attention-deficit hyperactivity disorders*, which are apparently present from *birth or early childhood.* These syndromes are contrasted with the *deteriorations* of cognition, which represent a decline from a previous level of functioning. Examples of deteriorations of cognition include dementia, delirium, aphasic syndromes, and amnestic syndromes. In this chapter, we consider only the *deteriorations* that are called dementia and delirium. Several of the developmental syndromes are discussed in chapter 16 on child psychiatry by Dr. Dulcan.

Dementia

Dementia is a deterioration of multiple cognitive impairments occurring in clear consciousness and alertness and may have multiple causes (Tables 4–3 and 4–4). Dementia should be distinguished from cognitive impairments that are not deteriorating in nature and from more focal deteriorations of the brain, which may affect single functions such as language.

The determination of brain deterioration requires confirming evidence other than what is observed directly or elicited from the patient (e.g., family members or employers who can give examples of functions that the patient could once perform but in which there has been a change). Useful functions that can be evaluated and that may indicate cognitive decline include the ability to manage finances and a checkbook, the capacity to travel without becoming lost, the ability to use the telephone and take messages, and the ability to recall the place of objects, such as the patient's wallet, keys, and eyeglasses. Observations such as these from the patient's family are correlated with impairments in orientation, recall, attention, and sometimes language function, which can be documented with the MMSE. When a decline has been reported and found to be accompanied by multiple cognitive impairments on formal examination, the syndrome of dementia can be diagnosed if the patient is otherwise generally alert.

Contrary to popular clinical lore, the syndrome of dementia can occur *suddenly*, as seen after stroke or hypoxic insults, but more commonly develops *insidiously and progresses gradually*, as seen in association with Alzheimer's disease. The syndrome may at times be totally or partially reversible, such as when it occurs because of hypothyroidism, although the patient may be left with permanent impairments. Most dementia is irreversible, such as that associated with Alzheimer's disease. From an epidemiological point of view, most cases of dementia seen in the community are insidious, gradually progress, and are, at the present time, not reversible (Folstein, Anthony, Parhad et al, 1985). These facts clearly are subject to revision, however, if adequate treatments are discovered. The epidemiology of dementia in elderly patients is discussed in Chapter 11 on geriatric psychiatry.

Some authorities have found it useful to divide dementia into two types, the *cortical* type and the *subcortical* type. This distinction is based on the clinical impression or "gestalt" of the presentation of patients. For example, dementias of the *cortical* type, as in Alzheimer's disease, tend to be characterized by a profound memory deficit and often a semantic aphasia, but the patient is fluent, moderately attentive, normally responsive to questions, and normally active in his environment at home or in the office (Brandt, Folstein, Folstein, 1987).

In contrast, patients with the *subcortical* dementing illness, such as Huntington's disease and occult hydrocephalus, are relatively alert but slowly responsive and inactive and usually are not fluent in their language. They are often dysarthric and have difficulty with forming complex sentences. These patients have little difficulty with semantic processing, however, and usually comprehend language fully, even when severely affected. They may have relatively mild disorders of memory or have marked attentional problems and show difficulty with "executive" functions, such as changing from one cognitive "set" to another, as demonstrated by the Wisconsin Card Sort Task or the Trail-Making Test (Brandt and Butters, 1986). In addition to their cognitive features, patients with subcortical dementia frequently suffer from motor disorders such as involuntary movements, as seen in Parkinson's disease and Huntington's disease. They often are found to have a depressive syndrome in addition to their cognitive syndrome. Thus, the patient with subcortical syndrome is slow in response, apathetic, behaviorally inactive, and has a cognitive disorder associated with disorders of movement and mood. The distinction between cortical and noncortical dementias is not universally accepted by clinicians, and a significant amount of overlap exists between symptoms in the two categories.

Noncognitive Symptoms Accompanying Dementia

Disorders of mood, perception, belief, and behavior are often associated with dementia. Disorders of mood of several types are seen. A sustained depressive syndrome occurs in 30 to 60% of patients with subcortical dementia and 10 to 20% of cortical dementia patients (Rovner, Kafonek, Filipp et al, 1986). Hence, dementia and depressive states can coexist, and the mood disorder component of the patient's condition can be responsive to antidepressants or electroconvulsive therapy.

Pathological laughter or crying occurs when the dementia syndrome is caused by bilateral corticobulbar lesions, such as in multiple strokes and multiple sclerosis. The disruption in mood may be transient, lasting seconds or minutes, and is often prompted by a meaningful psychological stimulus, such as a conversation, music, or a sentimental memory. The laughter or crying observed is often abnormal because it is expressed against the will of the patient, who does not always actually feel sad or happy and in fact is often embarrassed by it.

Irritability and explosiveness is another type of emotional disorder seen with dementia, especially with the dementia of Huntington's disease. Excessive emotional outbursts that occur after task failure have been called "catastrophic reactions" and may occur in the dementia of Alzheimer's disease. Precipitational catastrophic reactions can be modulated by educating family members so as to avoid confrontations of memory deficits.

Delusions and hallucinations occur about 10 to 20% of the time at some phase of the dementia process. Paranoid delusions may arise out of the cognitive impairment, as when misplaced objects are reported by the patient to be stolen; hence, the patient attempts to make "sense" out of the fact that an object is gone by arriving at what he or she believes must be a logical explanation. It's not "there" because someone has apparently stolen it.

Hallucinations of all types occur, but visual hallucinations tend to be the most common. In Parkinson's disease or diencephalic vascular disease, peduncular hallucinosis is seen. In this condition, pleasant or relatively benign simple visions, such as falling handkerchiefs, usually occur. Lilliputian hallucinations of small people often dressed in colorful costumes also occur. In addition to these primary hallucinatory experiences, patients with dementia also experience a variety of misinterpretations of environmental stimuli (illusions). Patients with agnosia often misinterpret their environment and become fearful or aggressive (Cummings, Miller, Hill et al, 1987). A wide variety of abnormal behaviors is encountered, including suicide, aggression, agitation, emotional lability, wandering, and insomnia.

The relationship of dementia to other psychiatric disorders, such as depressive disorders, schizophrenia, and hysterical disorders, requires some clarification. Cognitive dysfunction also may occur in severe depression to the extent that it has been reported to "mimic" dementia in some respects. When cognitive dysfunction occurs in depression or in another psychiatric disorder, it may be referred to as the "dementia syndrome of depression" or "dementia of schizophrenia" (Folstein and McHugh, 1978). Perhaps more accurately, one may refer to it as "depression-related cognitive dysfunction" (DRCD). Clinically, cognitive dysfunction due to depression *rarely*, if ever, resembles the global progressive deficits seen in dementia unless the patient already has a preexisting dementia on which the depressive disorder becomes superimposed. Primary dementia and depression may be superimposed on each other, although depression is frequently overlooked, dismissed, or otherwise not aggressively treated in patients with dementia (Stoudemire, Hill, Kaplan et al, 1988).

Causes of Dementia

Among the 6% of elderly individuals in the general population who are suffering from a dementia syndrome of some sort, approximately one-third to one-half are suffering from Alzheimer's disease, and approximately one-fifth to one-third are suffering from dementia related to stroke, with the remaining 20 to 30% suffering from other causes, including head trauma, alcoholism, Parkinson's disease, HIV, and miscellaneous causes (Table 4–4).

In the general community, dementia related to *reversible* disorders is extremely low; the majority are due to stroke (vascular or multi-infarct dementia) and Alzheimer's disease. In hospital settings, however, individuals with dementia syndromes are often suffering from reversible cognitive dysfunction that requires treatment (Rocca, Amaducci, Schoenberg, 1986). It is also extremely common for delirium to occur concurrently with dementia in the hospitalized elderly because of unstable metabolic problems and medications (see following section on delirium).

The full evaluation of dementia (which consists of history, physical examination, laboratory tests for drug levels and toxins, electrolytes, liver function tests, calcium, phosphorus, thyroid, Venereal Disease Research Laboratory (VDRL) test, serum B_{12} level, sedimentation rate, chest X-ray, EKG, CT scan, and EEG) is usually unrevealing of reversible causes of cognitive dysfunction, although about 5 to 15% of patients may have a reversible or partially reversible condition affecting their cognitive dysfunction (Table 4–10).

Cortical Dementia

The leading example of a cortical dementia syndrome is Alzheimer's disease (Alzheimer, 1907). Approximate estimates of the prevalence of Alzheimer's disease in the community vary from 2 to 10% of the population over age 65 and from 15 to 20% of the population over age 85 (Rocca, Amaducci, Schoenberg, 1986). Patients with Alzheimer's disease constitute more than half of all patients in nursing homes. These patients in the community or in nursing homes seldom have access to adequate psychiatric care and thus present a major public health problem in terms of the prevention of complications that result from the secondary symptoms of the disease.

Alzheimer's disease (AD) is a clinical pathological entity characterized by a dementia syndrome consisting of prominent memory deficits that usually begin with short-term memory and then progress to more pervasive memory deficits and global deficits such as aphasia, apraxia, and agnosia. Alzheimer's disease has an insidious onset and a gradual progression to death on average 7 years after onset, although great variability exists in the course of the illness (Katzman, 1986). The MMSE score in AD is approximately 14 (out of 30) after 4 years of illness.

On postmortem examination, the brain is found to be small and atrophic with a remarkable accumulation of neurofibrillary tangles and neuritic plaques with amyloid core and a deposition of amyloid in blood vessels in most cases. The composition of the neuritic tangle is under active investigation. However, there is some evidence that it consists of an amyloid fibril decorated with a variety of proteins, including ubiquitin and tau. The neuritic plaque consists of a beta pleated sheet of amyloid probably derived from a transmembrane protein. Embedded in the amyloid mass are bits of neurons derived primarily from *cholinergic* and *adrenergic* systems.

Two systems of neurons appear to be primarily involved in AD. One of them is the cholinergic system originating in the basal forebrain, the so-called *nucleus basalis of Meynert*. Reductions in brain acetylcholine and its rate-limiting enzyme

Table 4–10 **Comprehensive Workup of Dementia and Delirium**

Physical exam, including thorough neurologic exam
Vital signs
Mental status examination
Mini-Mental State Exam (MMSE)
Review of medications and drug levels
Blood and urine screens for alcohol, drugs, and heavy metals*
Physiologic workup
   Serum electrolytes/glucose/Ca^{++}, Mg$^+$
   Liver, renal function tests
   SMA-12 or equivalent serum chemistry profile
   Urinalysis
   Complete blood cell count with differential cell type count
   Thyroid function tests (including TSH level)
   RPR (serum screen)
   FTA-ABS (if CNS disease suspected)
   Serum B$_{12}$
   Folate levels
   Urine corticosteroids*
   Erythrocyte sedimentation rate (Westergren)
   Antinuclear antibody* (ANA), C$_3$C$_4$, Anti-DS DNA*
   Arterial blood gases*
   HIV screen*†
   Urine porphobilinogens*
Chest x-ray
Electrocardiogram
Neurologic workup
   CT or MRI scan of head*‡
   SPECT**
   Lumbar puncture*
   EEG*
Neuropsychological testing§

*If indicated by history and physical examination
†Requires special consent and counseling
‡See Table 4-11 for relative discriminating power
**May detect cerebral blood flow perfusion deficits
§May be useful in differentiating dementia from other neuropsychiatric syndromes if this cannot be done clinically
(Adapted with permission from Stoudemire A, Thompson TL: Recognizing and treating dementia. Geriatrics 36:112–120, 1981)

choline acetyltransferase *are* the most consistent neurotransmitter abnormalities observed in the brains of AD patients. The other neurotransmitter system also consistently observed to be abnormal is the *adrenergic* system originating in the *locus ceruleus* (Rosser, Iverson, 1986). There is some evidence that these two systems are affected independently in the disease, because some patients can be found with more or less adrenergic involvement. Involvement of the adrenergic system may be at least partially related to the high degree of disruptions in mood and anxiety regulation seen in AD.

GENETICS OF ALZHEIMER'S DISEASE

The cause of the neuronal death and subsequent deposition of neurofibrillary plaques and tangles is currently unknown. However, some cases have been found to be linked to a restriction fragment length polymorphism (RFLP) marker on chromosome 21, and others have been found to be associated with trisomy 21. Furthermore, the gene for the regulation of the protein that is precipitated in amyloid is also found on chromosome 21. In addition, Down's syndrome appears more likely to occur in families with AD than in families without histories of AD (Heston, Mastri, Anderson et al, 1981). DNA markers on chromosome 21 have been linked to the genetic defect causing familial AD in three of four large pedigrees (St George-Hyslop, Tanzi, Polinsky et al, 1987). The gene that encodes amyloid, which is a major component in neuritic plaques, is located nearby on chromosome 21.

Several family lines have been identified in which the early onset of AD appears to segregate in an autosomal dominant pattern, and in a subset of early-onset familial AD kindreds, mutations of the amyloid precursor protein (APP) gene appear to be responsible for the disease (Schellenberg et al, 1992). The majority of early-onset familial AD families, however, do not show linkage or have mutations on the APP gene. Recent data indicates a familial AD locus on chromosome 14 (Schellenberg et al, 1992). The most current data suggests that AD is a genetically heterogeneous disease caused by two or more genes located on two or more chromosomes (14, 19, and 21 have been most consistently implicated to date). Identifying the gene loci involved is a much more complex process, but one that will eventually unravel the core biochemical defect of the disease as well as resolve the issue as to whether or not abnormalities in beta amyloid metabolism are a primary or secondary element of the disease.

Other theories of causation of AD include the excess deposition of aluminum in the brain and the possibility of a slow viral infection. A review of current theories of Alzheimer's disease is beyond the scope of this discussion, but students should be aware that research is moving so rapidly in this area that "dated" information may be only a few months old.

For many years, Alzheimer's disease was thought to be a disorder with an early age of onset (before age 65) that was distinct from so-called "senile dementia," which occurred much later and was common in the elderly. Because the neuropathology and the clinical presentation of Alzheimer's disease, or "presenile dementia" and "senile dementia," are the same, the early-onset and later-onset types are considered to have the same pathophysiology. In recent years, however, evidence is emerging that the disorder might very well be heterogeneous, with one form having an early age of onset that is associated with more severe neuropathological changes, more rapid progression, dermatoglyphic changes similar to those found in Down's syndrome, and platelet membrane abnormalities (such as increased platelet membrane fluidity).

In the families where there appears to be a genetic component in the development of Alzheimer's disease, several investigators have attempted to estimate the morbid risk among first-degree relatives of patients with Alzheimer's disease. One method involves the life-table method, which estimates the age-specific cumulative incidence of a disease in a manner that adjusts for the fact that individuals die of other causes before the disease's onset (Breitner, Folstein, 1984; Mohs, Breitner, Silverman et al, 1987; Zubenko, Huff, Beyer et al, 1988). Using this technique, the morbid risk among first-degree relatives of patients has been estimated to be as high as 50% by age 90 (Mohs, Breitner, Silverman et al, 1987). These calculations have been used to suggest that there is a dominant mode of inheritance for the Alzheimer's disease gene, although it appears that the genetic predisposition to the illness shows variable penetrance.

During the next several years, the genetic basis of Alzheimer's disease may be defined, along with the factors that may influence its expression. Alzheimer's is probably not a single disease entity but rather a heterogeneous disorder with varying degrees of behavioral, neurochemical, and neuropathological differences (Small, Greenberg, 1988).

BRAIN IMAGING
AND ALZHEIMER'S DISEASE

Abnormalities have also been noted on computed tomography (CT), magnetic resonance imaging (MRI), single photon emission computed tomography (SPECT), and positron emission tomography (PET) scanning (Riege, Metter, 1988). Cerebral atrophy, cortical sulci widening, deep white matter lesions with periventricular distribution, and ventricular enlargement changes have been observed on CT/MRI scanning, but these changes also can be seen in elderly patients without Alzheimer's disease; alternatively, many patients *with* Alzheimer's disease will have normal CT/MRI scans. The primary use of CT/MRI scanning is to *exclude* any potentially treatable causes of cognitive dysfunction, such as a brain tumor or chronic subdural hematoma.

The most consistent observations made to date with PET scanning have been decreases in the regional cerebral metabolic rate of glucose using the marker F-18-deoxyglucose (FDG). These findings also appear to correlate with decreased cerebral blood flow, as measured by SPECT techniques (Bonte et al, 1990). The deficits that have been observed are predominantly in the *temporoparietal area* but are also in *frontal* regions in more severe cases. Decreased glucose use observed by PET scanning, however, is not always uniform or symmetric in the hemispheres. In addition, there is a significant amount of interpatient variability (Riege, Metter, 1988). Metabolic dysfunction revealed by PET is an indication of the first cortical degeneration while the anatomic changes with CT and MRI reflect later manifestations of the disease (Faulstich, 1991; Albert, Lafleche, 1991).

PICK'S DISEASE AND
JAKOB-CREUTZFELDT DISEASE

Two other disorders that are differentiated from Alzheimer's disease and are primarily cortical in their expression are *Pick's disease* and *Jakob-Creutzfeldt disease*. Pick's disease can occur in patients in their 60s and 70s and presents with an insidious and progressive change in behavior and cognition. Usually the patients show marked unpredictable and unexplainable behavioral abnormalities in association with relatively mild cognitive problems early in the illness. Although the patient subsequently develops a clear dementia syndrome, the disease is characterized by a lobar or focal atrophy that often affects the *frontal and temporal lobes* and is clearly detectable with CT or MRI scans.

Jakob-Creutzfeldt disease is a subacute dementia syndrome that affects the same age group as Alzheimer's and Pick's disease and presents with a cortical syndrome that is both insidious and progressive, usually over a period of weeks to months rather than months to years. The patient becomes moderately to severely demented 6 months to a year after the initial symptom. Patients have a typical cortical dementia syndrome with amnesia, aphasia, apraxia, and agnosia, but in addition often have tremor, ataxia of gait, and a *typical burst pattern on the EEG*. It is the rapid course of the illness that suggests the diagnosis. This condition is associated with a spongiform degeneration of the brain that is transmissible to animals and has been found to be caused by a slow virus of the scrapie type. The disease is remarkable in that it has a long latent period between exposure to the virus and subsequent expression of its effects. Although it is caused by an infectious agent, the typical inflammatory changes in the brain, which are usually associated with infection, are absent. This has led to the speculation that perhaps other psychiatric disorders, including Alzheimer's disease and even schizophrenia, could be caused by a similar virus. However, there has been no evidence of transmissibility in any of the other disorders, with the exception of the so-called Gerstmann's syndrome.

Pick's disease and Jakob-Creutzfeldt disease are rare disorders. There are other cerebral degenerations, even more rare, that are occasionally seen presenting as a dementia syndrome. These include Kufs' disease or a late-onset form of Tay-Sachs disorder, cortical striatal degenerations, and a variety of dementia syndromes associated with atypical neuropathological findings, and occasionally a case of dementia syndrome of the cortical type with an apparently normal brain. Although all of these disorders are extremely rare, they are exceptions that might reveal important mechanisms of the disease.

Subcortical Dementia

The subcortical dementias are distinguished from the cortical dementias by symptoms and pathology. An important clinical distinction is that patients with disease entities causing a subcortical dementia often have a gait disorder in the presence of a moderate dementia, whereas with Alzheimer's disease and other cortical dementia, a gait disorder occurs only late in the illness.

The discussion of subcortical disorders will begin with multi-infarct dementia. Although this is clearly a disorder that could have either cortical or subcortical signs depending on the location of the lesions, small lacunar infarctions associated with hypertension are most often found in the basal ganglia and in the subcortical white matter.

Multi-infarct dementia is a term used for a dementia syndrome associated with prominent infarctions of the brain, which can be due to a variety of causes but is usually associated with either hypertension or atrial fibrillation with multiple cerebral emboli. The clinical diagnosis is based on the sudden and episodic appearance of worsening of the patient's mental state, usually associated with asymmetrical motor signs and CT or MRI signs of cerebral infarction. The natural history of the disease is not well described. Claims have been made that its course may be altered by vigorous treatment of hypertension (Hachinski, Lassen, Marshall, 1974).

Occult hydrocephalus or "normal pressure" hydrocephalus is a more typical subcortical disorder characterized by a triad of *dementia, ataxia,* and *urinary incontinence* and associated with a large dilatation of the cerebral ventricles with relatively mild cerebral atrophy. The disorder is caused by the defective drainage of cerebral spinal fluid, which is usually due to a blockage of reabsorption sites secondary to head trauma, previous hemorrhage, or infection. Some of these cases have been reported to respond to surgical drainage of cerebral spinal fluid but the technique remains controversial and response to shunting procedures is unpredictable; thus, diagnosis is important (McHugh, 1964).

Huntington's disease is characterized by hereditary chorea beginning in the 30s and 40s and associated with a prominent subcortical dementia syndrome. The caudate nucleus and eventually other striatal centers atrophy. Cortical atrophy is sometimes seen. The cause of the disease is an abnormal gene on the long arm of chromosome 4 whose product is unknown. However, a marked loss of n-methyl-d-aspartate receptors in the striatum is noted. The abnormality in this receptor could lead to excessive cellular excitation by incoming glutaminergic fibers and then to cell death through calcium influx, kinase activation, and eventually free radical oxygen accumulation (Folstein, Leigh, Parhad et al, 1986).

Another subcortical dementia disorder is *Parkinson's disease*, which is characterized by the triad of akinesia, rigidity, and tremor, associated with degeneration of the dopamine-containing neurons of the substantia nigra. In recent years, Parkinson's disease has been divided into two types—that associated with the neuritic plaques and tangles of Alzheimer's disease and that with a pure nigral degeneration. At this point, the clinical distinction between these types is uncertain.

Parkinson's disease is associated with a clear dementia syndrome. A high proportion of patients with Parkinson's disease also develop depressive disorders, and treatment of the parkinsonian patient often includes L-dopa and an antidepressant or electroconvulsive therapy, which is effective in the motoric, cognitive, and mood features of the disorder. Delusions and hallucinations are also commonly seen in Parkinson's disease and may at times be caused by L-dopa itself.

HIV (AIDS)-RELATED DEMENTIA

AIDS-related cognitive disorders are not fully addressed in this chapter and are dealt with in depth by Moran in Chapter 21. One should note, however, that AIDS involvement in the central nervous system has been well documented to occur as a *primary symptom of the illness with clinical signs and symptoms that may appear well before any systemic signs of immunosuppression.* In the later, more advanced stages of AIDS, behavioral observations of both delirium and dementia may be seen as a direct result of HIV infection or secondary fungal, parasitic, or viral disease (Grant, Atkinson, Hesselink et al, 1987; Ostrow, Grant, Atkinson, 1988).

CNS involvement with HIV pervades the course of the illness from beginning to end. The initial infection of HIV likely involves the brain in almost all cases, and this initial viral infection may be neurologically asymptomatic or be accompanied by aseptic meningitis or meningoencephalitis. The most common symptom of acute infection involves flulike symptoms and headache (Robertson and Hall, 1992). Bell's palsy and other cranial nerve abnormalities may occur soon after acute exposure as well as peripheral neuropathy. Seizures may occur at any time during the course of infection and demand a search for the cause (infections, tumors) but in about 50% of cases no specific etiology is identified (Wong, Suite, Labar, 1990).

Some reports demonstrate signs of neuropsychologic dysfunction early in the course of HIV infection, but others do not. There is support for early CNS dysfunction in HIV infection as evidenced by declines in evoked potentials and abnormalities detected by MRI and SPECT brain scanning (Masde et al, 1991). As has been emphasized by others (Robertson and Hall, 1992), despite evidence that the CNS is affected early in the course of HIV, general intellectual functioning remains relatively intact until the latter stages of AIDS.

In latter phases of the illness, patients with AIDS Dementia Complex (ADC) show a variety of intellectual and motor impairments. One of the more common findings are delays in response time and shortening of the attention span. Functional areas of impairment include not only attention, concentration, and speed of processing but also memory, visuospatial skills, and mental flexibility (Robertson and Hall, 1992).

Motor decline tends to parallel intellectual decline and may include impairments in fine motor skills, gait difficulties, incoordination, a fine or course tremor, and general "clumsiness." Bradykinesia, apraxia, and abnormalities of saccadic and pursuit eye movements are common. Muscle stretch (deep tendon) reflexes may be hyperactive, or possibly decreased, indicating a concomitant peripheral neuropathy. Plantar (Babinski) responses may be extensor. Primitive reflexes may be observed including grasp, suck, snout, and palmomental responses. Diffuse muscle weakness is also typical. More details regarding neuropsychiatric aspects of HIV/AIDS are in Chapter 21.

OTHER TYPES OF DEMENTIA

Multiple Sclerosis

Multiple sclerosis (MS) is characterized by multifocal lesions in the white matter of the central nervous system. Neuropsychiatric symptoms in patients with multiple sclerosis are, therefore, relatively common, particularly as the disease progresses. Because of the shifting and transient nature of both the neurological and neuropsychiatric symptoms associated with multiple sclerosis, many of these patients may be diagnosed as "hysterical" or as having conversion disorders early in the course of their illness. In the advanced stages of this illness, global dysfunction may occur in cognitive and behavioral functioning and a dementia syndrome. In addition, depression is relatively common in MS. Mood disorders such as depression in multiple sclerosis and mania may be caused by treatment with exogenous steroids and adrenocorticotropic hormone (ACTH) treatment.

Vitamin B$_{12}$ Deficiency

Failure of the gastric mucosa to secrete intrinsic factor results in abnormal absorption of vitamin B$_{12}$ from the ileum. B$_{12}$ deficiency can result in peripheral neuropathy and a variety of neuropsychiatric disturbances. The megaloblastic anemia (pernicious anemia) is the most obvious hematologic manifestation of the illness. Nevertheless, *neurological changes, including CNS degeneration, may appear before megaloblastic changes.* Behavioral changes associated with vitamin B$_{12}$ deficiency include depression, emotional lability, irritability, and the spectrum of signs and symptoms associated with dementia. Screening for serum B$_{12}$ level is a standard component of a dementia evaluation.

Hypothyroidism (Myxedema)

Hypothyroidism may cause a form of dementia in addition to a classic depressive disorder. The onset may be insidious and be overlooked for months or years. The psychiatric picture is usually characterized by lethargy, mental sluggishness, and slowing of cognition. These symptoms occur in concert with the typical physical signs of the illness, which include dry skin, decreased ear canal cerumen, nonpitting edema over the face and limbs, hair loss, menstrual changes, and a "froglike" voice due to laryngeal edema. A variety of metabolic findings may be seen, including hyponatremia and hypokalemia. With progression of disease there is increased cognitive dysfunction. Gross psychosis (myxedema madness) in addition to the cognitive and depressive features may be seen. In screening patients for possible hypothyroidism, it is essential to obtain a serum thyroid-stimulating hormone level (TSH) to detect subclinical levels of the illness.

Wilson's Disease

A degenerative form of dementia is caused by Wilson's disease, which is an inherited defect in copper metabolism that affects the putamen of the lenticular nucleus and the liver (hepatolenticular degeneration). Neuropsychiatric symptoms often precede overt manifestations of the dementia syndrome. This is a disorder that usually presents in the second decade of life and is associated with cirrhosis, golden brown pigmentation on the posterior corneal surface (Kayser-Fleischer rings), tremor, and rigidity. The diagnosis can be made by presence of decreased serum ceruloplasmin in association with aminoaciduria.

DIAGNOSTIC EVALUATION OF DEMENTIA

The screening diagnostic evaluation for dementia is relatively straightforward and parallels the evaluation for a delirium, although usually without the same dramatic urgency that accompanies a patient with delirium. The basic diagnostic workup is listed in Table 4–10 but a few special points might be considered:

1. If AIDS-related dementia is suspected, special consent and counseling will be required for HIV antibody testing.
2. As noted above, the serum B_{12} level should be ascertained.
3. The serum VDRL may be negative in older patients with tertiary syphilis, and a serum FTA is usually recommended for a definitive answer. If the serum FTA is positive, the same test should be performed on the CSF to assess for tertiary CNS syphilis.
4. CT and MRI scanning have differential powers in assessing for dementia and other CNS lesions. While Table 4–11 (AMA Council Report, 1988) offers a guide to their relative sensitivities, consultation with a neuroradiologist may be a measure that will save both money and patient duress (the isolation involved in MRI scanning may be stressful for older patients with cognitive impairment) (see also Chapter 1 by Drs. Yates, Kathol, and Carter).
5. The EEG is not sensitive for detecting dementia (high rate of false-negatives) and is often normal in both the early and middle phases of AD. However, the EEG is quite sensitive for detecting delirium.

PHYSICIAN'S ROLE IN THE MANAGEMENT OF DEMENTIA

Beyond the diagnostic evaluation, the role of the general medical physician in the care of dementia patients is as follows:

1. Provide long-term supportive medical care for the patient.
2. Provide emotional support for the patient and family as a triage point for medical and community resources.
3. Provide assistance with management of disruptive behavior.

In respect to the latter items, major behavioral difficulties often arise in patients with dementia, particularly dementia of the Alzheimer's type. The most problematic are agitation, insomnia, emotional lability, personality changes, and psychotic symptoms—most commonly paranoia. There are, however, a surprisingly small number of systematic studies of the psychopharmacologic treatment of the behavioral disorders of dementia. Low doses of neuroleptic agents, such as haloperidol or loxapine, will help control agitation, emotional lability, and paranoia, but often symptoms are only suppressed rather than eliminated. Disturbed sleep is an extremely common component of dementia and is probably the problematic symptom that most exhausts caregivers. Again, low-dose neuroleptic agents near bedtime may help, but other sedative-hypnotics such as chloral hydrate may be needed. Low doses of shorter acting benzodiazepines such as temazepam, which has a short half-life (13–16 hours) and whose metabolism is not affected by aging, can help on an "as needed" basis. More recently, some clinicians have reported the efficacy of trazodone (50–200 mg), a sedating antidepressant also effective for nocturnal agitation. The anxiolytic agent buspirone may also have some efficacy in the control of agitation in dementia. This

Table 4–11 **CT Versus MRI as a Neurodiagnostic Probe**

DISEASE	MRI	CT	METRIZAMIDE-ENHANCED CT
Cerebrovascular disease			
TIA-RIND	+ +	±	—
Emboli	+ + +	+	—
Ischemic infarction	+ + + +	+ + +	—
Vasculitis	+ + +	±	—
Intracerebral hemorrhage	+ + +	+ + + +	—
Trauma			
Craniocerebral	+ +	+ + +	—
Spinal	+ + +!	+ + +	+ + +
Tumors			
Glioma			
Low-grade (1–2)			
Supratentorial	+ + +	+ +	—
Infratentorial	+ + + +	+ +	—
High-grade (3–4)			
Supretentorial	+ + + +	+ + + +	—
Infratentorial	+ + + +	+ +	—
Metastases			
Supretentorial	+ + +	+ +	—
Infratentorial	+ + +	+	—
Meningioma			
Supratentorial	+ +	+ + + +	—
Infratentorial	+ +	+ +	—
Pituitary	+ +	+ + + +	—
Sinuses and orbits	+ + + +	+ + +	—
Demyelinating disease	+ + + +	+ +	—
Dementia			
SAE	+ + + +	+ +	—
Alzheimer's, Huntington's, and PSP	±	±	—
NPH	+	+	+ + +

(continued)

drug has no habit-forming or sedating properties and takes 2 to 4 weeks to reach its full therapeutic effect.

If possible, psychotropic drugs should be used on an "as needed" basis rather than given automatically for long periods of time, until the necessity of their ongoing use becomes absolutely necessary. Caution should be used, especially with the high-potency neuroleptic agents (e.g., haloperidol), because elderly patients may be quite prone to extrapyramidal reactions (see Chapter 18 by Drs. Silver, Hales, and Yudofsky). Psychotropic agents are often used excessively and inappropriately in nursing home patients because they are frequently used as "chemical restraints" by overextended staffs (Beers, Avorn, Soumerai, 1988). Physicians should carefully reassess the need for psychotropic agents in this population on a regular basis.

Table 4–11 **(continued)**

DISEASE	MRI	CT	METRIZAMIDE-ENHANCED CT
Cervicomedullary junction and cervical spinal cord			
Syrinx (and congenital anomalies)	+ + + +	+	+ +
Tumors (intra-axial)			
Brain stem	+ + + +	+	+ +
Cerebellopontine angle	+ + +	+ +	+ + +
Cervical spine	+ + + +	±	+ +
Tumors (extra-axial)			
Brain stem	+ + + +	+	+ +
Cervical spine	+ + + +	±	+ + +
Cervical disk disease	+ + +	+ + +	+ + + +
Lumbar disk disease	+ + +	+ + +	+ + + +
Regional cerebral blood flow	***	+ + +#	—

±, of questionable value;
+, of some value, but other technologies are definitely superior;
+ +, of moderate value at present and frequently competitive with other technologies, but should not be considered as the initial diagnostic approach;
+ + +, of definite value;
+ + + +, of definite value and the preferred initial approach;
***, research phase—of great potential importance for the future as a first-line diagnostic tool;
MRI, magnetic resonance imaging;
CT, computed tomography;
TIA-RIND, transient ischemic attacks and reversible ischemic neurological deficits;
SAE, subcortical arteriosclerotic encephalopathy;
PSP, progressive supranuclear palsy;
NPH, normal-pressure hydrocephalus;
!, roentgenographic CT is superior in visualizing bone abnormalities, while MRI may be superior in demonstrating blood and spinal cord injury;
#, roentgenographic CT combined with inhalation of stable xenon or intravenous administration of contrast medium.
(Used with permission from American Medical Association Council on Scientific Affairs, Report of the panel on Magnetic Resonance Imaging: Magnetic resonance imaging of the central nervous system. JAMA 259:1211–1222, 1988)

Perhaps one of the most valuable things a physician can do for a patient's family is to refer them to a community social worker or other geriatric specialist who has an interest in geriatrics to assist in resource planning. In addition, a referral to a support organization, such as the Alzheimer's Association, will assist the family in receiving help through support groups and education as to the patient's care and management. Referral to an attorney for legal planning, in addition to getting a durable power of attorney for the family to be made when the diagnosis becomes evident, will save the family enormous amounts of time, trouble, and money (Overman, Stoudemire, 1988).

Finally, physicians should be careful to follow the patient periodically for concurrent medical problems and to continue as a source of support and information for the family. Many families often feel abandoned by their physicians if no regular plans for follow-up appointments are made. Dementia is a *chronic* illness with a duration of years, during which the family will often be under enormous emotional stress. The primary physician's role in the ongoing support of the patient and family is crucial. (Students are referred to Chapter 11 for more information regarding the overall management of psychiatric illness in the elderly.)

DELIRIA

As noted in the introductory comments, delirium (previously known as acute organic brain syndrome) is characterized by an alteration in the level of consciousness that often fluctuates. Patients may have either a clouding or fogging of consciousness, or they may be hyperalert and agitated at times, such as in alcohol withdrawal delirium. Multiple signs and symptoms may accompany delirium and include gross psychotic symptoms such as paranoia, delusions, and hallucinations (tactile, auditory, visual, and olfactory). Patients also may exhibit evidence of thought disorganization and incoherent language that may resemble a schizophrenic psychosis.

The sleep–wake cycle may be grossly disrupted, with agitation often exacerbated during the evening hours (the same observation may be seen in relatively stable dementias)—the "sundowning" syndrome. Cognitive signs usually receive the most attention, but they may be subtle and undetected in patients who are "quietly delirious" and are not exhibiting any overt behavioral disturbances or who are overmedicated with sedatives and tranquilizers. Cognitive dysfunction may be exhibited in defects in memory, attention, concentration, and orientation. Behaviorally, the patients may be agitated, combative, and hostile. Many times the uncooperative, irritable, and aggressive nature of the delirious patient—combined with his paranoia—is assumed to be a "functional psychosis," and the underlying metabolic component driving the patient's abnormal behavior overlooked.

As noted earlier, the primary feature of a delirium is a diminution in the level of consciousness that fluctuates in a sine wave fashion over time. Consistent with this sine wave pattern, patients may actually experience *periods of relative lucidity*. As noted above, "clouding" of consciousness and decreased alertness are the most common symptoms, but some patients can also show hyperalert activity. Sleep is usually fragmented and poor, with the patients being anxious, irritable, and restless. Disturbances in psychomotor functioning vary from hyperactivity to lethargy, stupor, obtundation, and catatonia. Neurological signs and symptoms may be seen, such as tremor, asterixis (particularly in deliria caused by metabolic and hepatic encephalopathies), or drug intoxications or withdrawal.

Deliria by definition are usually "acute" in onset, but some, particularly those due to subtle or insidious metabolic deficits, may develop and persist over days, weeks, or months with mild forms of fluctuating cognitive dysfunction. Most cases of delirium should improve or resolve within a week to 10 days if sufficient attention is given to correcting and stabilizing the underlying condition causing cerebral dysfunction.

Delirium is an extremely common disorder within the general hospital population—particularly the elderly. One study found that as many as 35% of patients over 65 years of age will have signs and symptoms of delirium on admission, or they will develop it sometime during the course of their hospitalization (Hodkinson, 1973). Other surveys have shown prevalence rates of delirium for the hospitalized elderly to range from 16 to 25% in general medical wards (Bergmann, Eastham, 1974; Seymour, Henschke, Cape et al, 1980) and from 10 to 15% in surgical wards (Millar, 1981). In addition, the presence of delirium is often a grave prognostic sign for survival. One study reported that one-third of over 4000 patients admitted with a primary diagnosis of delirium died within a month (Bedford, 1959). Other studies have found general mortality associated with delirium and its affiliated causes to be 25% (Hodkinson, 1973; Simon, Cahan, 1963).

Diagnosis

The diagnosis of delirium is made by a combination of clinical observations and formal changes in the patient's mental status. Of paramount importance is checking on the observations of the nursing staff either verbally or by reviewing the chart. This is especially helpful in assessing for fluctuations in the patient's mental status over a 24-hour period. Documenting the patient's baseline mental status before the hospitalization or onset of the cognitive dysfunction from information provided by the family is essential. The family will also be helpful in documenting the use of drugs or alcohol.

Factors Associated with Delirium and High-Risk Groups

Lipowski (1983) has documented the most common physical illnesses associated with delirium (in the elderly), and these include congestive heart failure, pneumonia, urinary tract infections, cancer, uremia, malnutrition, hypokalemia, dehydration, hyponatremia, and cerebrovascular accidents (Flint, Richards, 1956; Hodkinson, 1973; Kay, Roth, 1955; Roth, 1955; Seymour, Henschke, Cape et al, 1980; Simon, Cahan, 1963). Systemic illnesses that result in brain dysfunction are more common causes of delirium than are primary CNS disorders. Intoxication with medical drugs and psychotropic agents is probably the most common causes of delirium in the elderly patient, particularly iatrogenic drugs that have sedative and anticholinergic side effects such as amitriptyline (Lipowski, 1983).

Alcoholics, particularly those with a history of recent heavy drinking where there is a possibility of a withdrawal syndrome, should be watched very closely. A history of other drugs that involve significant potential for withdrawal, such as barbiturates, sedative-hypnotics, and benzodiazepines, should also be monitored carefully and treated with the appropriate detoxification regimen (see Chapters 10 and 19).

Patients with a history of trauma, especially head trauma, are at extremely high risk medically for complications. Patients with sensory impairment (blindness, deafness, history of cataract surgery, or those facing extensive bandaging or casting) are prone to become delirious because of sensory deprivation and may need special care to promote orientation to the environment. Patients with preexisting cognitive dysfunction, mental retardation, or dementia have less of an ability to organize and adjust to the strangeness of the hospital and also are prone to delirium.

The differentiation between dementia and delirium is important, and Table 4–5 lists key differentiating factors (Lipowski, 1987). It is essential to note, however, that dementia and delirium may coexist and be superimposed on one another.

Etiology

Delirium can derive from failure or dysfunction in any organ system (pulmonary, cardiac, hepatic, renal, endocrine, gastrointestinal) because of either direct or secondary metabolic abnormalities of the central nervous system (electrolyte imbalances, hypoglycemia, adrenal insufficiency, hyperosmolarity or hypoosmolarity, uremia, hypoxemia, hypercarbia, hypercalcemia or hypocalcemia, or severe hypertension). Decreases in cardiac output from congestive heart failure can lead to decreased perfusion of the CNS and confusion. Peripheral as well as central nervous infections can cause fever and sepsis, leading to altered mental status. Infiltration of the meninges from certain forms of leukemia can also cause delirium.

Direct insults to the CNS from bacterial meningitis, viral encephalitis, cerebrovascular hemorrhage, subdural hematoma, strokes, and vasculitis from connective tissue diseases, such as systemic lupus erythematosus, may cause delirium with or without psychotic symptoms. Gliomas and meningiomas may cause delirium or resemble dementia, and their onset may be insidious if the tumor is growing slowly and may not be associated with focal neurological findings in their early stages.

Patients who suffer from intermittent delirium (often with psychotic features) in addition to having a history of chronic abdominal pain and a peripheral neuropathy should be suspected of having acute intermittent porphyria. The family history, if it can be reconstructed, is usually positive. Although the diagnosis is confirmed by special urine tests (porphobilinogen levels), the diagnosis has occasionally been made by exposing the patient's urine to sunlight, in which it turns beet red.

Medication side effects, particularly in the elderly and even in "therapeutic" doses, may cause delirium, especially when there are coexisting medical problems that may alter the pharmacokinetics of the drug. Common offenders include narcotic analgesics, barbiturates, benzodiazepines, and other sedative-hypnotics. Antidepressant drugs, particularly cyclic antidepressants with strong anticholinergic and sedating side effects, such as amitriptyline, are notorious for causing delirium in the elderly (anticholinergic delirium).

A variety of nonpsychiatric medications cause symptoms of delirium. These include antihistamines (some of which also have relatively potent anticholinergic effects), atropine-like drugs, H-2 (histamine receptor) blockers (cimetidine, ranitidine), phenytoin, phenobarbital, digitalis (even at "therapeutic levels"), procainamide, lidocaine, L-dopa, and antihypertensive agents if they are sedating (such as clonidine). Steroids, particularly when administered rapidly in high doses, can cause a delirium usually known as "steroid psychosis." Table 4–2 presents a partial listing of drugs reported to potentially cause delirium.

DELIRIUM AND
INTENSIVE CARE UNIT SYNDROMES

Special note should be made of the so-called "intensive care unit syndrome," "intensive care unit psychosis," and "postcardiotomy syndrome." Although the abnormalities that have been described in intensive care unit patients often have been called "postoperative psychosis," the majority of these patients suffer from what is best characterized as a delirium with psychotic components. Delirious states in the ICU are usually multifactorially determined and may arise from the inherent stresses of the ICU itself, particularly its sleep-depriving effects. The environmental stresses of the ICU may include being placed in a strange, technologically oriented environment; incapacitation; noisy monitors; restriction in movement by intravenous lines and catheters; and the lack of privacy. Most patients in the intensive care unit are gravely ill and compromised medically and receive multiple medications. In addition, sleep deprivation and loss of the normal diurnal light–dark rhythm in units without windows may be biologically disrupting.

Delirium after cardiothoracic surgery also has been described and has been termed "postcardiotomy delirium." This condition classically occurs 3 or 4 days after surgery. The patient may be lucid but then suffers from progressive deterioration, confusion, and other features of delirium such as psychosis. Factors that may contribute to the development of postcardiotomy delirium include increasing age, total time spent on cardiopulmonary bypass, intraoperative hypotension, severity of illness, sleep deprivation, and sensory monotony. Postcardiotomy delirium may be related to decreased postoperative cardiac index, leading to a greater likelihood of impaired cerebral perfusion and oxygenation (Heller, Kornfeld, Frank et al, 1979).

Diagnosis

The cardinal rule in evaluating patients with delirium is to detect and correct the underlying disorder contributing to the patient's cerebral dysfunction. Appropriate treatment must be anteceded by an extensive and thorough search for the cause of the patient's cognitive dysfunction. Although the differential diagnosis of potential causes of delirium is extensive, the actual diagnostic workup is straightforward.

First, a review of all factors leading up to the patient's hospitalization is essential. If the patient is postsurgical, a review of the operative record also is important. In terms of premorbid factors, the presence of alcoholism, medication use, or coexisting dementia is also important. Because medications are almost always high on the list in the hospitalized elderly, the cumulative dose of medications received over the past week should be checked in the patient's chart, along with serum levels for drugs when possible (anticonvulsants, digoxin, theophylline, and so forth). Any psychotropics that the patient has been taking should be scrutinized, particularly the relationship between the onset of cognitive dysfunction and any new drugs or changes in doses. Anticholinergic agents are particularly worrisome in the elderly.

Once the patient has been examined medically and neurologically, the history has been reviewed, and the events leading up to the hospitalization or surgery have been documented, the patient should undergo an evaluation of vital signs. The assessment is based on an organ system-by-organ system search, looking for evidence of metabolic dysfunction, such as cardiovascular (arterial blood gasses, chest X-ray), pulmonary, renal (electrolyte imbalances, uremia), endocrine (thyroid panel, hypoglycemia, calcium), liver (hepatic encephalopathy), and gastrointestinal (impaction, obstruction, ileus, hemorrhage, volvulus) disease. A search for infection (sepsis, occult abscess, meningitis, urinary tract infection, pneumonia) is crucial. *The fundamental clinical principle remains that of detecting and correcting to whatever extent possible the underlying abnormality causing the patient's altered mental status.*

Special note should be made regarding the use of the EEG in the evaluation of delirium. Although the EEG may be normal in dementia, it is almost always abnormal in delirium, making it a very sensitive test in this clinical situation. The EEG abnormalities, however, are not always characterized by slowing, and the patterns can be low amplitude–fast activity, as may be found in alcohol withdrawal and sedative-hypnotic withdrawal. EEG abnormalities, which almost always accompany delirium, may persist after the clinical manifestations of the brain syndrome remit.

Treatment

The treatment of patients with delirium primarily involves treating the underlying cause of the cerebral dysfunction as noted above. Until that can be identified and corrected, however, some environmental and psychopharmacologic strategies can facilitate keeping patients safe and stabilizing their behavior. Environmental strategies include having a window from which the patient can observe normal light–dark cycles to help correct his diurnal rhythm (windows should be secured to prevent jumping or sitters should be provided). A familiar family member or 24-hour sitters should be allowed at the bedside if at all possible to facilitate orientation. Large calendars on which days can be marked off, clocks, familiar photographs, and having a radio or television playing during waking hours can also help the patient stay connected to the outside world and provide sensory stimulation. Providing night-lights and other types of additional sensory input for heavily bandaged or casted patients can be helpful. Elderly patients with cataracts are at risk for delirium, leading to the practice of performing such procedures "one eye at a time" to prevent "black patch delirium." Patients who are on ventilators or are unable to speak because of tube placement or mechanical problems should nevertheless be communicated with by handwriting, hand signals, or lap-computer keyboards.

Pharmacologic Strategies

The psychopharmacologic management of agitated and psychotic behavior will be described in other sections of this text, particularly Chapters 10, 18, and 19. In general, however, the "higher potency" antipsychotic agents such as haloperidol are the drugs of choice in this setting because they have minimal effects on blood pressure. These drugs tend to be slightly less sedating and also have very few anticholinergic side effects. "Lower potency" antipsychotic agents such as chlorpromazine and thioridazine tend to cause hypotension.

The prototypical drug used for stabilization of delirium is haloperidol, which can be given in tablet or liquid form orally or through the intramuscular and intravenous routes (see Chapter 18). A typical starting dose of haloperidol would be 2 mg p.o. or i.m. q.1h. or until the patient is sedated. Some clinicians advocate the use of parenteral benzodiazepines such as lorazepam for this purpose as well. For example, lorazepam may be used by giving the patient 1–2 mg orally, sublingually, or intramuscularly every hour until the patient is calm and slightly drowsy. Lorazepam, however, can cause anterograde amnesia when given in this manner, and benzodiazepines may exacerbate disinhibited behavior.

If a patient is suffering from a severe anticholinergic delirium, physostigmine salicylate 1–2 mg can be given slowly intravenously or intramuscularly and repeated after 15 minutes. Contraindications to using this potent cholinergic agonist include a history of heart disease, asthma, diabetes, peptic ulcer disease, or the possibility of bladder or bowel obstruction (Lipowski, 1987).

After the patient is stabilized, haloperidol may then be given in supplemental doses every 3 to 4 hours as needed. The need for continuous medication should then be reevaluated every 24 hours and the doses decreased and discontinued as rapidly as possible commensurate with stabilization of the patient medically and the patient's overall mental status. In most instances, resolution of the delirium should be accompanied by discontinuation of the antipsychotic agent as soon as possible.

Patients also should be carefully monitored for the presence of extrapyramidal side effects, neuroleptic-induced catatonia, and neuroleptic-induced malignant syndrome. Diagnosis and management of these particular side effects of the neuroleptic are discussed in Chapters 5 and 18. Chapter 11 on geriatric psychiatry discusses special considerations in using psychotropic drugs in the elderly in more detail.

CLINICAL PEARLS

- Several of the most frequently underdiagnosed disorders in medicine are delirium and early dementia.
- The most common causes of delirium in hospitalized patients are medication side effects.
- Delirious patients are not always either obtunded or agitated; some may by hyperaroused and excitable or quietly delirious.
- The EEG is very sensitive for delirium but relatively nonsensitive in dementia.
- A mild dementia may be one of the earliest signs of HIV infection occurring before signs of systemic immunosuppression.
- Intravenous haloperidol may be given for rapid control of severely agitated delirious patients, but the necessity of its use should be carefully documented.
- Neurological signs and symptoms of B_{12} deficiency have been reported before hematologic changes and in the presence of a normal serum B_{12} level.
- Depression and dementia may coexist, and the mood disturbance may exacerbate the cognitive and psychosocial dysfunction of the demented patient. Major depression rarely mimics the pervasive and progressive picture of dementia unless the patient already has some degree of underlying dementing illness.

ANNOTATED BIBLIOGRAPHY

Lishman WA: Organic Psychiatry, 2nd ed. Oxford, Blackwell Scientific Publication, 1987

> This is a classic textbook that reviews in detail neuropsychiatric disorders.

Lipowski ZJ: Delirium (acute confusional states). JAMA 258:1789–1792, 1987

> An excellent and practical review of the clinical assessment of delirium.

Slaby AE, Erle SR: Dementia and Delirium. In Stoudemire A, Fogel BS (eds): Psychiatric Care of the Medical Patient, pp 415–453. New York, Oxford University Press, 1993

> This is an excellent and in-depth overview of the diagnosis and management of delirium and dementia.

Yudofsky SC, Hales RD (eds): Textbook of Neuropsychiatry, 2nd ed. Washington, DC, American Psychiatric Press, 1992.

> This is an eminently readable textbook that provides practical reviews of the major disorders in clinical neuropsychiatry.

REFERENCES

Albert MS, Lafleche G: Neuroimaging in Alzheimer's disease. Psychiatric Clinics N Am 14:443–459, 1991

Alzheimer A: About a peculiar disease of the cerebral cortex. Jarvik L, Greenson H (trans): Alzheimer Disease and Associated Disorders 1:7–8, 1987

Alzheimer A: Uber eine eigenartige Erkrankund der Hirnrinde. Allg Z Psychiatry Psychisch-Gerichtlich Med 64:146–148, 1907

American Medical Association Council on Scientific Affairs, Report of the Panel on Magnetic Resonance Imaging Magnetic resonance imaging of the central nervous system. JAMA 259:1211–1222, 1988.

American Psychiatric Association: DSM-IV Draft Criteria 3/1/93. Washington DC, American Psychiatric Association, 1993

American Psychiatric Association: Diagnostic and Statistical Manual of Mental Disorders, 4th ed. Washington DC, American Psychiatric Association, in press [1994]

Anthony JC, LeResche LA, Von Korff MR et al: Screening for delirium on a general medical ward: The tachistoscope and a global accessibility rating. Gen Hosp Psychiatry 7:36–42, 1985

Bedford PD: General medical aspects of confusional states in elderly people. Br Med J 2:185–188, 1959

Beers M, Avorn J, Soumerai SB et al: Psychoactive medication use in intermediate-care facility residents. JAMA 260:3016–3020, 1988

Bergmann K, Eastham EJ: Psychogeriatric ascertainment and assessment for treatment in an acute medical ward setting. Age Ageing 3:174–188, 1974

Bonte FJ, Hom J, Tintner R et al: Single photon tomography in Alzheimer's disease and the dementias. Seminars in Nuclear Med 20:342–352, 1990

Brandt J, Butters N: The neuropsychology of Huntington's disease. Trends Neurosci 93:118–120, 1986

Brandt J, Folstein S, Folstein M: Differential cognitive impairment in Alzheimer's disease and Huntington's disease. Ann Neurol 9:21, 1987

Breitner JCS, Folstein MF: Familial Alzheimer's dementia: A prevalent disorder with specific clinical features. Psychol Med 14:63–80, 1984

Caine ED: Amnesic disorders. J Neuropsychiatry Clin Neurosciences 5:6–8, 1993

Cummings JL, Miller B, Hill MA et al: Neuropsychiatric aspects of multiinfarct dementia & dementia of the Alzheimer type. Arch Neurol 44:389–393, 1987

Engel GL, Romano J: Delirium, a syndrome of cerebral insufficiency. J Chronic Dis 9:260, 1959

Faulstich ME: Brain imaging in the dementia of the Alzheimer type. Intern J Neuroscience 57:39–49, 1991

Flint FJ, Richards SM: Organic basis of confusional states in the elderly. Br Med J 2:1537–1539, 1956

Folstein MF, Anthony JC, Parhad I et al: The meaning of cognitive impairment in the elderly. J Am Geriatr Soc 33:228–235, 1985.

Folstein MF, Folstein SE, McHugh PR: Mini-Mental State. A practical method for grading the cognitive state of patients for the clinician. J Psychiatr Res 12:189–198, 1975

Folstein S, Leigh RJ, Parhad I et al: Diagnosis of Huntington's disease. Neurology 36:1279–1283, 1986

Folstein MF, McHugh PR: Dementia syndrome of depression. In Katzman R, Terry RD, Rick KL (eds): Alzheimer's Disease: Senile Dementia and Related Disorders, Vol 7, pp 87–96. New York, Raven Press, 1978

Grant I, Atkinson JH, Hesselink JR et al: Evidence for early nervous system involvement in the acquired immunodeficiency syndrome (AIDS) and other human immunodeficiency virus (HIV) infections. Ann Intern Med 107:828–836, 1987

Hachinski VC, Lassen NA, Marshall J: Multi-infarct dementia: A cause of mental deterioration in the elderly. Lancet 2:207–210, 1974

Heller SS, Kornfeld DS, Frank KA et al: Postcardiotomy delirium and cardiac output. Am J Psychiatry 136:337–339, 1979

Heston LL, Mastri AR, Anderson E et al: Dementia of the Alzheimer type: Clinical genetics, natural history, and associated conditions. Arch Gen Psychiatry 38:1085–1090, 1981

Hodkinson HM: Mental impairment in the elderly. J R Coll Physicians Lond 7:305–317, 1973

Katzman R: Alzheimer's disease. Trends Neurosci 9:522–525, 1986

Kay DWK, Roth M: Physical accompaniments of mental disorder in old age. Lancet 2:740–745, 1955

Lindenbaum J, Healton EB, Savage DG et al: Neuropsychiatric disorders caused by cobalamin deficiency in the absence of anemia or macrocytosis. N Engl J Med 318:1720–1728, 1988

Lipowski ZJ: Transient cognitive disorders (delirium, acute confusional states) in the elderly. Am J Psychiatry 140:1426–1436, 1983

Lipowski ZJ: Delirium (acute confusional state). JAMA 258:1789–1792, 1987

McHugh PR: Occult hydrocephalus. Q J Med 33:297–308, 1964

Masde JC, Yudd A, Van Heertum RI et al: Single-photon emission computed tomography in human immunodeficiency virus encephalopathy: A preliminary report. J Nucl Med 32:1471–1475, 1991

Millar HR: Psychiatric morbidity in elderly surgical patients. Br J Psychiatry 138:17–20, 1981

Mohs RC, Breitner JCS, Silverman JM et al: Alzheimer's disease: Morbid risk among first-degree relatives approximates 50% by 90 years of age. Arch Gen Psychiatry 44:405–408, 1987

Ostrow D, Grant I, Atkinson H: Assessment and management of the AIDS patient with neuropsychiatric disturbances. J Clin Psychiatry 49:14–22, 1988

Overman W, Stoudemire A: Guidelines for legal and financial counseling of Alzheimer's disease patients and their families. Am J Psychiatry 145:1495–1500, 1988

Popkin MK, Tucker GJ: "Secondary" and drug-induced mood, anxiety, psychotic, catatonic, and personality disorders: A review of the literature. J Neuropsychiatry Clin Neurosciences 4:369–385, 1992

Riege WH, Metter EJ: Cognitive and brain imaging measures of Alzheimer's disease. Neurobiol Aging 9:69–86, 1988

Robertson KR, Hall CD: Human immnodeficiency virus-related cognitive impairment and the acquired immunodeficiency syndrome dementia complex. Seminars Neurology 12:18–27, 1992

Rocca WA, Amaducci LA, Schoenberg BS: Epidemiology of clinically diagnosed AD. Ann Neurol 19:415–424, 1986

Rosser M, Iverson LL: Non-cholinergic neurotransmitter abnormalities in Alzheimer's disease. Br Med Bull 42:70–74, 1986

Roth M: The natural history of medical disorder in old age. J Ment Sci 101:281–301, 1955

Rovner BW, Kafonek S, Flipp L et al: The prevalence of mental illness in a community nursing home Am J Psychiatry 143:1446–1449 1986

Schellenberg GD, Bird TD, Wijsman EJ et al: Genetic linkage evidence for a familial Alzheimer's disease locus on chromosome 14. Science 258:668–671, 1992

Seymour DG, Henschke PJ, Cape RDT et al: Acute confusional states and dementia in the elderly: The role of dehydration/volume depletion, physical illness and age. Age Ageing 9:137–146, 1980

Simon A, Cahan RB: The acute brain syndrome in geriatric patients. Psychiatr Res Rep 16:8–21, 1963

Small GW, Greenberg DA: Biologic markers, genetics, and Alzheimer's disease. Arch Gen Psychiatry 45:945–947, 1988

St George-Hyslop PH, Tanzi RE, Polinsky RJ et al: The genetic defect causing familial Alzheimer's disease maps on chromosome 21. Science 235:885–890, 1987

Stoudemire A: Selected organic mental disorders. In Hales R, Yudofsky S: Textbook of Neuropsychiatry. Washington, DC, American Psychiatric Press, 1987

Stoudemire A: The differential diagnosis of catatonic states. Psychosomatics 23:245–252, 1982

Stoudemire A, Hill C, Kaplan W et al: Clinical issues in the assessment of dementia and depression in the elderly. Psychiatr Med 6:40–52, 1988

Stoudemire A, Thompson TL: Recognizing and treating dementia. Geriatrics 36:112–120, 1981

Tucker GJ, Caine ED, Folstein MF et al: Introduction to background papers for the suggested changes to DSM-IV: Cognitive Disorders. J Neuropsychiatry Clin Neurosciences 4:360–368, 1992

Wong MC, Suite ND, Labar DR: Seizures in human immunodeficiency virus infection. Arch Neurol 47:640–642, 1990

Zubenko GS, Huff FJ, Beyer J et al: Familial risk of dementia associated with a biologic subtype of Alzheimer's disease. Arch Gen Psychiatry 45:889–893, 1988

Appendix to Chapter 4: Mini-Mental State Examination and Instructions

Patient _____

Examiner _____

Date _____

MINI-MENTAL STATE EXAMINATION

Maximum

Score	Score	
		Orientation
5	( )	What is the (year) (season) (date) (day) (month)?
5	( )	Where are we: (state) (county) (town) (hospital) (floor)
		Registration
3	( )	Name three objects: 1 second to say each. Then ask the patient all three after you have said them. Give 1 point for each correct answer. Then repeat them until he learns all three. Count trials and record.

Trials _____

Used with permission from Folstein MF, Folstein SE, McHugh PR: Mini-Mental State: A practical method for grading the cognitive state of patients for the clinician. J Psychiat Res 12:189–198, 1975

Attention and Calculation

5   ( )   Serial 7s. 1 point for each correct. Stop after five answers. Alternatively, spell "world" backwards.

Recall

3   ( )   Ask for the three objects repeated above. Give 1 point for each correct.

Language

9   ( )   Name a pencil, and watch. (2 points).
Repeat the following: "No ifs, ands, or buts." (1 point)
Follow a three-stage command:
   "Take a paper in your right hand, fold it in half, and put it on the floor." (3 points)
Read and obey the following:
   Close your eyes. (1 point)
   Write a sentence. (1 point)
   Copy design. (1 point)

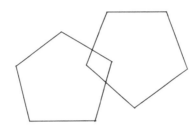

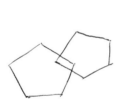

Total Score

Perfect score = 30
Any score below 25 indicates the presence of significant cognitive dysfunction.

Assess the level of consciousness along a continuum:

    Alert   Drowsy   Stupor   Coma

INSTRUCTIONS FOR ADMINISTRATION OF MINI-MENTAL STATE EXAMINATION

Orientation

(1) Ask for the date. Then ask specifically for parts omitted, e.g., "Can you also tell me what season it is?" One point for each correct.

(2) Ask in turn "Can you tell me the name of this hospital?" (town, county, etc.). One point for each correct.

Registration

Ask the patient if you may test his memory. Then say the names of three unrelated objects, clearly and slowly, about 1 second for each. After you have said all three, ask him to repeat them. This first repetition determines his score (0–3) but keep saying them until he can repeat all three, up to six trials. If he does not eventually learn all three, recall cannot be meaningfully tested.

Attention and Calculation

Ask the patient to begin with 100 and subtract backwards by 7. Stop after 5 subtractions (93, 86, 79, 72, 65). Score the total number of correct answers.

If the patient cannot or will not perform this task, ask him to spell the word "world" backwards. The score is the number of letters in correct order, e.g., dlrow = 5, dlorw = 3.

Recall

Ask the patient if he can recall the three words you previously asked him to remember. Score 0–3.

Language

Naming: Show the patient a wrist watch and ask him what it is. Repeat for pencil. Score 0–2.

Repetition: Ask the patient to repeat the sentence after you. Allow only one trial. Score 0 or 1.

Three-stage command: Give the patient a piece of plain blank paper and repeat the command. Score 1 point for each part correctly executed.

Reading: On a blank piece of paper print the sentence "Close your eyes," in letters large enough for the patient to see clearly. Ask him to read it and do what it says. Score 1 point only if he actually closes his eyes.

Writing: Give the patient a blank piece of paper and ask him to write a sentence for you. Do not dictate a sentence, it is to be written spontaneously. It must contain a subject and verb and be sensible. Correct grammar and punctuation are not necessary.

Copying: On a clean piece of paper, draw intersecting pentagons, each side about 1 in., and ask him to copy it exactly as is. All 10 angles must be present and 2 must intersect to score 1 point. Tremor and rotation are ignored.

Estimate the patient's level of sensorium along a continuum, from alert on the left to coma on the right.

Alan Stoudemire (ed). *Clinical Psychiatry for Medical Students*, Second
Edition. Copyright © 1994, 1990 by J. B. Lippincott Company.

5

Schizophrenia and Other Psychotic Disorders

Philip T. Ninan and Rosalind Mance

Traditionally, psychoses have been historically divided into "organic" (caused by underlying neurologic or metabolic abnormalities) and "functional." This differentiation is now obsolete because even "functional" psychotic disorders have an underlying biochemical substrate in the brain. DSM-IV labels psychotic disorders resulting from neurologic and metabolic conditions as "Psychotic Disorder due to a General Medical Condition." This chapter will discuss schizophrenia, schizophreniform disorder, brief psychotic disorder, schizoaffective disorder, and delusional disorder. Mood disorders with psychotic features (psychotic depression) will be dealt with in Chapter 7.

"Psychosis" is a generic descriptive term applied to behavior marked by a *break from reality*. This often presents as disorganization of mental processes, emotional aberrations, difficulty in interpersonal relationships, and a decrease in functional capacity. Mundane daily responsibilities can become burdensome or impossible to manage. Schizophrenia is the prototypical psychotic disorder and hence will be the primary focus of this chapter.

It should be emphasized before proceeding any further that psychotic symptoms may occur in multiple medical, neurological, and substance-abuse disorders, and a vigorous search should be made for a medical or neurologic cause of the patient's symptoms before a primary psychiatric diagnosis is made (Table 5–1). In addition, psychotic symptoms may occur in a *variety* of psychiatric disorders and are *not* by any means specific for schizophrenia (Table 5–2). For

This work was supported in part by U.S. Public Health Service (NIMH) grants MH 40597 and MH 42298.

Table 5–1 **Brief Differential Diagnosis of Psychosis**

MEDICAL, NEUROLOGIC
AND SUBSTANCE-INDUCED DISORDERS

Psychotic disorders due to general medical conditions
Dementia
Delirium (includes side effects of medications)
Substance-induced (e.g., amphetamine, phencyclidine, etc.) psychotic
disorder

MOOD DISORDERS

Bipolar disorder (mania)
Major depression with psychotic features

PSYCHOTIC DISORDERS

Brief psychotic disorder
Schizophreniform disorder
Schizophrenia
Schizoaffective disorder
Delusional disorder

PERSONALITY DISORDERS*

Schizotypal
Schizoid
Paranoid
Borderline

*Usually have brief psychotic disorders. See Chapter 6

Table 5–2 **Schizophrenia and Other Psychotic Disorders***

Schizophrenia
  Catatonic
  Disorganized
  Paranoid
  Undifferentiated
  Residual
Schizophreniform Disorder
Schizoaffective Disorder
Delusional Disorder
Brief Psychotic Disorder
Shared Psychotic Disorder
Psychotic Disorder due to a general medical condition
Substance-Induced Psychotic Disorder
Psychotic Disorder not otherwise specified

*Derived from DSM-IV Draft Criteria 3/1/93. See DSM-IV (APA 1993, in press [1994]) for
details.

example, psychotic symptoms may be seen in mood disorders (psychotic depression and mania), in personality disorders (often during brief psychotic breaks), and in "encapsulated" form as part of a delusional (paranoid) disorder. Psychotic symptoms found in psychotic depression and mania are discussed in the appropriate chapters found elsewhere in this text (Chapter 7). The differential diagnosis for psychosis in dementia, delirium, and neurologic disorders may be found in Chapters 4 (Dr. Stoudemire) and 19 (Dr. Dubin).

SCHIZOPHRENIA

Schizophrenia is an illness that is present in all cultures. Early writings indicating the presence of schizophrenia go back to the twelfth century B.C. In more modern times, epidemiological studies suggest that there is a 1–2% chance that an individual will develop an episode of schizophrenia during his or her lifetime (Robins, Helzer, Weissman et al 1984). The cost to society is huge—over 100,000 psychiatric beds are occupied by patients suffering from schizophrenia in the U.S., and their treatment costs are estimated at $7 billion annually. What cannot be quantified is the enormous emotional cost to the patient and loved ones.

Phenomenology and Diagnosis

Schizophrenia is a *brain disorder* that is characterized by abnormalities in thinking, emotions, and behavior. Because we have no laboratory test yet that can confirm the diagnosis of schizophrenia, we are dependent on a descriptive or phenomenological definition of the disorder. Unfortunately, *there is no symptom that is pathognomonic of the illness or a symptom that is present in every patient with the illness*. Thus, no one symptom is necessary or sufficient for the diagnosis. The criterion for diagnosis is a particular *constellation of symptoms* rather than a single symptom.

Such a diagnostic system does not define a homogenous group of patients with a single etiology, pathophysiology, treatment response, and outcome but a *heterogenous* group of disorders. This *heterogeneity* of schizophrenia has been a significant hurdle to the advancement of our understanding of schizophrenia, because findings relevant to one subgroup of schizophrenic patients are obscured by the heterogeneity of the population studied.

As our knowledge has advanced, various attempts have been made to describe the constellation of symptoms that would best make the diagnosis of schizophrenia. Different diagnostic criteria can either define the illness broadly, which results in a large number of patients meeting the criteria for the illness, or provide a narrow definition of the illness, which would result in just a small (presumably core) group of patients being diagnosed. If the illness lies along a spectrum of severity, then casting a wide net would include those patients with milder, nonpsychotic versions of the illness (schizophrenia spectrum disorders) but would also risk some nonschizophrenics being given the label (i.e., a false–positive diagnosis).

The most reliably recognized symptoms of the illness are its more dramatic ones, such as hallucinations, delusions, and bizarre behavior. These are called "positive" symptoms because they are symptoms that are added to the premorbid state. However, there is a long tradition in *not* considering these the *central* elements of schizophrenia. "Negative" symptoms, such as *emotional blunting, apathy,* and *avolition,* are symptoms marked by the absence of functions. These negative symptoms are less dramatic in presentation. Some have postulated the negative symptoms to be the core elements of schizophrenia, but negative symptoms are agreed on less reliably. Thus, an illness defined purely by its more dramatic presentations could correctly label one group of patients as having schizophrenia, but it also could potentially exclude a number of patients who suffer predominantly from the core negative expressions that result from the pathophysiology of the illness, but without its more dramatic manifestations.

Historical Development

Emil Kraepelin (1907) coined the term "dementia praecox," which he differentiated from manic-depressive (bipolar) illness. Dementia praecox, or the precocious development of intellectual impairment, was based on acute symptomatology marked by hallucinations, delusions, withdrawal, loss of interest, and poor attention associated with a dissociation of thought content and affect. Kraepelin believed that the illness usually began early in life and tended to result in an end state of dementia. The cause was postulated to be a disease process that affected cortical neurons. Inherent in Kraepelin's definition of dementia praecox was a cross-sectional description of psychotic symptoms that included both positive and negative symptoms, an early onset, and a deteriorating course over time.

Eugen Bleuler (1911) coined the term "schizophrenia" and described it as a group of illnesses. *He shifted the focus from the course of illness to a purely cross-sectional approach* in making the diagnosis of schizophrenia. He thus described schizophrenia as being marked by problems with (thought) association, affect, autistic thinking, and psychotic ambivalence ("Bleuler's four A's") and called these the fundamental symptoms of the illness. He did *not* include a deteriorating course as inherent in the illness. Bleuler believed that the delusions and hallucinations often associated with schizophrenia were really secondary and derived from the fundamental symptoms. Bleuler also postulated a basic neurologic or metabolic defect as the cause of schizophrenia. He believed that the illness of schizophrenia could present itself with the fundamental symptoms without the secondary manifestations of delusions and hallucinations and called it "simple schizophrenia." Bleuler also thought that the basic defect causing schizophrenia also could exist without expressing itself in either the fundamental symptoms or the secondary manifestations and called this "latent schizophrenia."

The inherent problem with the approach taken by Bleuler in diagnosing schizophrenia was the lack of a well-defined threshold of how prominent a symptom (e.g., autistic thinking) had to be before the diagnosis of schizophrenia could be made. Thus, nonpsychotic individuals with personality aberrations (for example, the current concept of schizotypal personality disorder) were diagnosed as having schizophrenia.

The concepts of latent and simple schizophrenia blurred the distinction between patients who had schizophrenia and those who had nonpsychotic pathology.

Subsequent authors tried various methods to address the basic conflict of diagnosing an illness that required *both* cross-sectional symptomatology *and* longitudinal course of illness in its diagnostic criteria. Thus, Langfeldt (1956) developed the term *schizophreniform* to define a group of patients who had psychotic symptoms but did not have a deteriorating course. Kurt Schneider (1959) defined the list of symptoms that he thought were pathognomonic of schizophrenia. However, these have been shown subsequently to be present in functional psychotic illnesses other than schizophrenia so that the diagnostic value of these symptoms was diluted.

Current Nomenclature

The DSM-IV has a relatively stringent approach to the diagnosis of schizophrenia that requires specific psychotic symptoms to be present for at least a month (Table 5–3). To prevent many false–positive diagnoses, *the course of illness* also is included in the diagnostic requirements. Thus, a *deteriorating course* is part of the diagnostic criteria. This combination of a cross-sectional and longitudinal approach provides for improved reliability in the diagnosis. Patients who might have an illness that is related to schizophrenia in some ways but is atypical in others are given other diagnostic labels. For example, patients who have the symptoms of schizophrenia but recover without residual symptoms within a 6-month period of time are classified as having *schizophreniform disorder.* Patients with schizophreniform disorder also may be subclassified into those with or without good prognostic features. Good prognostic features include an acute onset, good premorbid functioning, and absence of flat affect. In patients who meet the criteria for schizophreniform disorder but have not recovered yet, the diagnosis is provisional.

If a patient has symptoms of depression or mania with psychotic symptoms, then the diagnoses of either *schizoaffective disorder* or a primary *mood disorder* with

Table 5–3 **Key Features of Schizophrenia***

Psychotic Symptoms, *at least two*, present for at least a month
   Hallucinations
   Delusions
   Disorganized Speech (Incoherence, Evidence of a Thought Disorder)
   Disorganized or Catatonic Behavior
   Negative Symptoms (Affective flattening, Lack of motivation)
Impairment in Social or Occupational Functioning
Duration of the illness for at least six months
Symptoms are not primarily due to a Mood Disorder or Schizoaffective
   Disorder
Symptoms are not due to a Medical, Neurologic or Substance-Induced
   Disorder

*Summarized from DSM-IV Draft Criteria 3/1/93. See DSM-IV (APA 1993, in press [1994]) for specific diagnostic criteria.

psychotic features should be considered. *Schizoaffective disorder* is usually diagnosed when depressive or manic symptoms are a prominent and consistent feature of a patient's longterm psychotic illness. The diagnosis of schizoaffective disorder is supported if the longitudinal course of the patient's condition is consistent with schizophrenia and where residual schizophrenic-like symptoms persist when the patient is not depressed or manic. If the psychotic symptoms are present *only* when the patient is depressed or manic, and the patient has relatively good interim functioning between episodes, then the patient should be considered to have a primary *mood disorder* (major depression or bipolar disorder) with psychotic features.

Schizophrenia has been subclassified into *catatonic* (dominated by motoric abnormalities such as rigidity and posturing), *disorganized* (marked by flat affect and disorganized speech and behavior), *paranoid* (paranoid symptoms in the absence of catatonic and disorganized features), and *undifferentiated* types. The *prodromal phase* of the illness refers to the period of time when the patient's functioning changes before the onset of frank psychotic symptoms. Because it is difficult to prospectively "predict" when a schizophrenic break will occur, the prodromal phase is most safely labeled retrospectively. Residual symptoms exist when the frank psychotic features, such as prominent delusions, hallucinations, incoherence, and bizarre behavior, are controlled but other symptoms (e.g., negative symptoms) remain. The course of the illness is classified into continuous or episodic with complete or incomplete remissions.

DELUSIONAL DISORDER AND
BRIEF PSYCHOTIC DISORDER

Delusional disorder is a condition in which the patient has a delusion lasting for at least 1 month in the absence of prominent hallucinations or bizarre behavior. The delusion is usually confined to a single area or person (i.e., it is encapsulated or relatively confined to a specific idea). Other gross psychotic symptoms evident in schizophrenia are absent in delusional disorder. Patients with delusional disorder are subclassified into erotomania, grandiose, jealous, persecutory, somatic, and mixed types based on their symptomatic presentation.

Brief psychotic disorder is characterized by a relatively sudden onset of psychosis that lasts for a few hours to a month with a return to premorbid functioning afterwards. The psychotic symptoms could be in response to a significant stressor, though not necessarily so, or during 4 weeks postpartum. The patient should recover and return to premorbid levels of functioning within approximately a period of a month to receive this diagnosis.

DIFFERENTIAL DIAGNOSIS

The psychotic disorders described above should be differentiated from psychotic disorders due to substances such as hallucinogens as well as those caused by primary medical and neurologic conditions. This can be done by gathering historical information that would provide clues as to the presence of a specific diagnosis that could be etiologically related to the psychosis. Principal among these would be a history of alcohol or substance abuse, especially of the stimulant (e.g., amphetamine) type. Amphetamine-induced psychosis is clinically indistinguishable in presentation from paranoid schizophrenia. A sudden, unexplained development of a psychotic illness in an otherwise well-functioning individual without a family history of a psychiatric illness is a justifiable reason for exploring possible secondary conditions. A complete physical examination, with particular emphasis on the neurological examination, also should be completed. In the mental status examination, clouding of consciousness or fluctuating levels of consciousness, memory difficulties, disorientation, and confusion should raise the possibility of a neurologic or metabolic process underlying the psychotic presentation (see Chapter 4).

The diagnostic criteria for *psychotic disorders implies that medical including neurological and toxic causes should be ruled out as part of the diagnostic evaluation* . . .

CASE STUDY
Clinical Case Vignette of Schizophrenia
Jim was 20 years old when his family and friends started to see a change in his behavior. During the previous months he had begun to withdraw from those around him, preferring to spend more and more time by himself. He lost interest in his scholastic work and his extracurricular activities. He seemed less interested in his personal appearance. He developed a sudden interest in philosophy and spent hours reading philosophical texts.

He had difficulty sleeping for a few nights, and his mother discovered him mumbling to himself. She noticed that he would talk to himself and pause as though he were listening, and then start talking again. When questioned about this, he would stop, turn, and walk away. He began getting suspicious, telling his mother that his friends had turned against him and were plotting to kill him. He subsequently began to read special meanings into the everyday events in his life. Thus, a blue car parked on the road meant that somebody was trying to contact him.

When taken for an evaluation, he told the psychiatrist that a voice was suggesting to him that he jump in front of traffic. He was hospitalized. After a 2-day observation period and a full medical and neurological workup, he was started on a neuroleptic agent. Within a couple of days his sleep pattern seemed to improve considerably, and he became more interested in his hygiene. Within a week he was able to follow the routine on the ward and take part in the structured activities. He seemed much less focused on the internal concerns that had preoccupied him before admission and was able to talk about current affairs without interjecting his pathological symptoms into the conversation. Although he did not think there was anything seriously wrong with him, he was willing to take medications and was discharged to outpatient treatment.

Within a few months of his hospitalization he was doing relatively well, and he attempted to return to college. He became more paranoid, however, and refused to take his medication. Over a period of a week he became more symptomatic and developed gross psychotic symptoms, resulting in a repeat hospitalization.

The next 5 years were marked by periodic hospitalizations, lasting a few weeks at a time, and outpatient treatment, which included medications and individual and family sessions. The family sessions were aimed at educating the family about the illness and helping them accept Jim's limitations. Interpersonal problems in the family were dealt with by improving communication skills. Stress-management and problem-solving skills were also addressed.

Jim finally began to accept the fact that he had an illness and that he needed long-term treatment. He attended day treatment for a while and then was able to use vocational rehabilitation to begin to look for a job within his limitations. He moved out of his parents' home into a semi-structured group home. He was compliant with his medication and was able to tell his therapist when he felt an impending relapse.

Symptoms of Schizophrenia

Psychotic symptoms are marked by abnormalities in the form of thought (called *formal thought disorder*), content of thought, perceptual disturbances, and alterations in emotions and behavior (Andreasen, 1987).

Formal thought disorder is an abnormality in the form of thought. It is differentiated from lack of speech, which is called *poverty of speech*. The extreme form of poverty of speech can present itself as muteness. Examples of formal thought disorders are as follows:

a) *Derailment* or *loose associations* is a condition in which the sequential connection between ideas is difficult or impossible to follow because the patient wanders to relatively or totally unrelated subjects. This can be present in a single sentence or in a series of sentences.

b) *Tangentiality* is the tendency to wander to points that are distantly connected, but be unable to return spontaneously to the original point. Returning to the original line of thought through a circuitous route is called *circumstantiality*.

c) *Incoherence* is a condition in which even sentences are impossible to follow. It is different from derailment and loose associations, in which the connections between clauses or sentences are problematic. Lack of understanding because of incomprehensible verbalization of speech is excluded from this description.

Delusions are the result of an abnormality in the *content* of thought. Delusions are false beliefs that are often fixed and cannot be explained based on the cultural background of the individual. If the intensity of the delusions is minor, patients may have some insight into their nonsensical nature and therefore may doubt them. Beliefs that can be possibly explained within the realm of reality (e.g., the patient has paranoid delusions that someone is trying to kill him) are differentiated from bizarre delusions that can have no basis in reality (e.g., the television is controlling the patient's behavior against his or her will). A systematized delusion (compared with an encapsulated one) is one that is complex with elaborate connections and multiple implications.

The concept of *mood congruence and incongruence* essentially assesses whether the delusions are consistent with the overall affective state of the patient. Thus, delusions of grandeur are often associated with manic states, and nihilistic delusions can be seen in major depression with psychotic features. Mood-*incongruent* delusions are more likely to be associated with schizophrenic states.

The intensity of a delusion is based on how firmly the belief is held, lack of insight, whether the delusion preoccupies the individual to the exclusion of other concerns, and whether the individual bases his actions on the delusion. The different types of delusions are as follows:

a) *Paranoid* delusions are convincing feelings that one is being persecuted, in the absence of such a reality. Paranoid patients may believe that they are being followed, their personal belongings are being tampered with, their telephone is tapped, and they are being harassed. The persecution can come from individuals or organizations (such as the FBI or CIA). The delusion can be a simple, isolated one or an intricate one that pervades all aspects of the individual's life such that all experiences are explained by the delusion.

b) *Ideas and delusions of reference* occur when the patient believes that some event, often of no consequence, is related to them specifically (i.e., a baby in a stroller signifies that the patient should cross the street). Often the delusions can have a paranoid flavor, whereby someone talking in the distance is misinterpreted as talking about and having designs on the patient; or a statement made on the radio or television has special reference to the patient. The questioning of these beliefs by the patient would make them ideas of reference, while their acceptance as reality would make them delusions.

c) *Delusion of being controlled* is the belief that one's actions are under the control of someone or some external force with malicious intent. The patient feels powerless in the face of such a force and will often relinquish responsibility for their actions or thoughts. The voluntary release of control over one's beliefs and actions, which is seen in cult situations, is not delusional because control is real and given voluntarily.

d) *Thought broadcasting* is the delusion that one's thoughts are broadcast so that they can be heard by others or transmitted to others even in the absence of vocalizations. Some patients might feel that their thoughts are heard audibly by themselves, or that their mind can be read by someone, even in the absence of verbalization.

e) *Thought insertion and withdrawal* are delusions that the patient's mind is having alien thoughts inserted or thoughts withdrawn outside of their control.

f) Delusions of *jealousy* are ones in which the individual believes that a loved one is being unfaithful, in the absence of such a reality. The love might be real or imagined (where the recipient of the love does not know that he or she is the object of such admiration by the patient).

g) Delusions of *guilt* are ones in which patients feel that, by acts of omission or commission, they are guilty of some deed for which they blame themselves excessively. Often the delusion is based on an insignificant detail in the patient's past that he or she is unable to forget. At times the patient will confess to being the cause of major catastrophes and will focus attention on confessing a deed that is obviously not of their doing. Delusions of guilt are often in the context of overzealous religious beliefs. Delusions of guilt are not specific for schizophrenia and are also common in psychotic depressions.

h) *Grandiose* delusions are delusions in which the patient believes they have special powers that are beyond those of the normal individual. The patient may think that he or she is someone special, such as Jesus or the president, or believe that they have a special mission or significance to society and the world (e.g., developing a theory that would finally explain all of nature). A paranoid flavor is at times associated with grandiose delusions. Grandiose delusions are often associated with manic states and frequently are accompanied by excess irritability. Because paranoid delusions can be present in mania, they provide little help in differentiating schizophrenia from manic psychosis.

i) *Religious* delusions also are a frequent phenomenon and include exaggerations of conventional religious beliefs. The beliefs have to be taken within a sociocultural context before they are labeled as delusional. These can be seen in schizophrenic and affective psychoses.

j) *Somatic* delusions are false beliefs related to the body. These frequently take the form that the body or a part of it is rotting or does not exist. Similar delusions may occur in major depression with psychotic features.

Hallucinations are the experiencing of stimuli in any of the senses in the absence of external stimulation. Based on the particular sense involved, the hallucination is called auditory, visual, tactile, olfactory, or gustatory. In functional psychotic conditions, auditory hallucinations are frequent, visual hallucinations are relatively uncommon, and hallucinations in the other senses are rare. The presence of visual hallucinations should raise the possibility of primary neurologic disorders or the presence of metabolic or toxin/drug/medication-induced delirium, whereas the presence of olfactory hallucinations should raise the likelihood of seizure disorders, especially complex partial seizures.

Auditory hallucinations are the most frequently reported hallucination in schizophrenic patients. These include one or more voices talking to or about the patient. Infrequently calling the patient by name is not by itself evidence that the patient is schizophrenic, but continuous hallucinations lasting all day or on and off for a couple of weeks are indicative of a schizophrenic psychosis. Typically, the patient experiences them as unpleasant, although he or she can get used to them and miss them in their absence. The voices can keep a running commentary of the patient's actions as they happen or can predict actions. The auditory hallucinations can be heard either inside the patient's head or coming from outside. At times, patients responding to treatment will report the progression of voices from outside to inside the head, to audible thoughts that may initially be alien but may later be their own before they go away. Auditory hallucinations of a self-critical or damning nature also may appear in major depression with psychotic features.

Visual hallucinations that occur with the use of hallucinogenic drugs or transiently just as the patient is about to fall asleep (hypnagogic) or wake up (hypnopompic) should not be considered schizophrenic in nature.

Bizarre behaviors include socially inappropriate behaviors such as dressing totally out of context (e.g., wearing a heavy woolen coat in the middle of summer) or disinhibition of behavior that would not be socially accepted, such as masturbating in public. The sociocultural contexts of the behavior should be taken into consideration before they are labeled as bizarre. Stereotyped behaviors are repetitive part actions, often symbolic, that have some contextual meaning to the patient.

Catatonic behavior is the presence of a marked reduction of psychomotor activity. This may present as rigidity, causing passive resistance to movement, or waxy flexibility, in which the patient maintains postures induced by the examiner. Lesser forms of catatonic behavior include mutism and negativism (passive resistance to any attempt to move).

Psychotic depression also may present with catatonic states, and catatonia is more frequently associated with affective states than schizophrenia. Catatonia also may be caused by a variety of medical and neurological disorders or may be a side effect of neuroleptic treatment.

Affect is the outward expression of emotion and is observed in facial features that routinely accompany the experience of emotions during communication. In schizophrenic patients there is a paucity of emotional expression or affect, and terms such as emotional blunting or flat affect are used to describe this situation. A dissociation between affect and behavior or cognition is described as incongruent affect.

Positive–Negative Symptoms Dichotomy

The symptoms of schizophrenia can be labeled positive or negative. Positive symptoms are symptoms that are added on to the premorbid state and include symptoms such as delusions, hallucinations, and bizarre behaviors. Negative symptoms are symptoms marked by the absence of functioning that were or should have been present in the premorbid state. Andreasen (1982) has defined the negative symptoms as *affective flattening, alogia, avolition, anhedonia,* and *attentional impairment.* There is some difficulty in differentiating negative symptoms from the "defect state" (which is the end state of chronic schizophrenia), depression, and (neuroleptic) medication-induced side effects such as bradykinesia.

On the basis of the positive–negative symptom dichotomy, Crow (1985) postulated a two-syndrome concept of schizophrenia in which *Type I schizophrenia* was marked by a predominance of *positive symptoms,* reversible outcome, good response to neuroleptic medications, and lack of intellectual impairment, and Type II schizophrenia was characterized by *negative symptoms,* possible irreversible outcome, poor responsiveness to neuroleptics, and intellectual impairment.

Although such a division is potentially useful, it is difficult to divide patients into such syndromes because the vast majority of them seem to have a clinically mixed picture symptomatically and be partially responsive to treatment. However, a theory that attempts to explain the clinical manifestations of the illness, its cognitive aspects, morphological abnormalities, and response to treatment is a significant advance because it allows the proposal of testable hypotheses.

Factors in the Expression of Schizophrenia

Environmental Factors

Historical Overview. At the turn of the century, emphasis by late contemporary European researchers in schizophrenia such as Kraepelin focused on the phenomenology and definition of psychotic disorders. Adolf Meyer (1866–1950) introduced the first empirical approach to investigating the role of environmental factors in the development of psychiatric disorders. Meyer's "psychobiologic" approach advocated the use of a life chart to map life events, the relationship of which to the development of psychotic behavior and symptomatology could then be examined.

The subsequent development of psychoanalytic theory led to interest in the childhood experiences that might be responsible for the development of schizophrenia. The focus was on the child's interpersonal experience within the family, which might lead to faulty ego development and intrapsychic conflict, which in turn put the child at risk for psychotic regression in adult life. The role of the mother was the first to be cited in the search for a cause. Freida Fromm-Reichmann coined the term *schizophrenogenic mother* to describe the emotionally withholding, domineering, and rejecting attitudes she believed to be present in an excessive number of mothers whose children developed schizophrenia. This, she theorized, led to the child growing up feeling in conflict to, distrustful of, and angry toward others, which later is expressed as a psychotic illness. Other theorists noted evidence of overprotection or rejection in the mothers of schizophrenic individuals.

In the 1950s, interest shifted toward patterns of family or parental interaction that could be responsible for schizophrenia developing in a child. Three major groups of theorists emerged with different hypotheses. Bateson, Jackson, Haley et al (1956) described the concept of the *double-bind* type of communication, which, they argued, could cause schizophrenia in a child who was repeatedly exposed to it. In a double-bind message, meaning is conveyed by communication on different levels or in different modes—for example, literal or metaphorical meaning, verbal expression, and body language. Conflicting messages may thus be given simultaneously, and Bateson suggested that this type of communication could lead to deficits in interpreting meaning, which progress to a disorder of cognition and metacommunication that is seen in schizophrenia.

Theodore Lidz (1958) looked more specifically at two types of dysfunctional parental interaction that, he hypothesized, interfere with personality maturation in the offspring and lead to the development of schizophrenia. In the *schismatic* marriage, parental conflict and lack of trust and communication are seen, whereas in *skewed* marriages, the serious psychopathology of one parent is supported by the masochistic and submissive attitude of the other.

Lyman Wynne and Margaret Singer (1963) at the National Institute of Mental Health (NIMH) developed the concept of *communication deviance*. They argued that parents of schizophrenics show idiosyncratic, disconnected, and confused patterns of speech analogous to the thought disorder seen in schizophrenic patients.

In spite of significant methodologic problems associated with these studies, these theorists postulated that serious disturbances are found in a majority of families with a schizophrenic offspring. Later studies have revealed that these original studies, on which these psychological theories were based, had seriously flawed methodologies and did not confirm their findings. Dysfunction in families in which a member had already developed schizophrenia *may be due to the effects of living with a disturbed person.* Retrospective reports of early life experience are unreliable, especially in someone who has become ill; the reported abnormal interaction patterns also are found in families of alcoholic and affectively disordered patients, making the findings nonspecific.

The etiological significance of communication deviance is continuing to be explored. It could be a subclinical manifestation of schizophrenia present in family members, a reflection of the social isolation resulting from the stigma of mental illness, or an environmental inducer of schizophrenia (a vulnerability or a causative factor) (Doane, West, Goldstein et al, 1981). Recent controlled studies using a prospective follow-up design should shed additional light on these complex issues. For example, preliminary data suggest that disturbed adolescents in families showing communication deviance are more likely to develop one of the schizophrenia spectrum disorders later.

The possibility remains that types of psychological stresses at critical developmental stages could lead to an increased likelihood of a genetically vulnerable individual developing schizophrenia.

Expressed Emotion

Once established, schizophrenia and the major psychoses have considerable variability in their course and outcome. Only part of this variance is related to response to medication. Thus, environmental influences on the course of illness have become a fertile area of investigation.

The course of the illness may be measured by the frequency and severity of relapse and the level of functioning between acute episodes. Follow-up studies of schizophrenic patients returning home have identified certain styles of communication in families that are positively correlated with earlier relapse (Leff, Vaughn, 1981). The critical factors as measured during a standardized family interview are criticism, hostility, and overinvolvement, known as "expressed emotion" (EE). Based on specific criteria, when families were divided into "high and low" degrees of EE there were large differences in relapse rates. These relapse rates were not correlated with severity of illness in the patient. Similar findings were made for families of depressed patients. In high EE families, fewer hours of face-to-face contact between patients and adult relatives significantly reduced the relapse rate in the schizophrenic but not the depressed group of patients. Use of prophylactic medications reduced the relapse rate in schizophrenics returning to high EE homes.

Life Events

Stressful life events seem to relate to the onset of relapse in major psychotic illnesses. Stressors can be divided into those that are acute and independent of the person's behavior and influence (such as an acute illness or death of a relative) and those that are chronic (such as poverty or difficulties at work or in the family environment), which also may be dependent on illness factors in the patient. In the three weeks before a psychotic relapse (in both schizophrenia and depression), it has been shown that there is a high frequency of independent social stressors (Brown, Birley, 1968). Moreover, the use of prophylactic medication in schizophrenics seems to protect against relapse under circumstances of acute stress, unless this is superimposed on a situation of chronic life stress.

When discussing the role of stress in the precipitation or maintenance of psychotic symptoms, one must also take into account each individual's variable response to that stress, his or her resources for dealing with it, and the degree to which he or she had control over its occurrence (Dohrenwend, Dohrenwend, 1978).

Social Class

The role of chronic life stress may be relevant to the finding that schizophrenia clusters in the lower socioeconomic classes (especially in urban environments), something that is not found in other psychotic conditions such as bipolar disorder. A second factor contributing to this clustering is the phenomenon of *social drift*. The higher representation of schizophrenia in lower socioeconomic classes has been shown to relate in part to the downward mobility experienced by schizophrenic individuals secondary to their disability. Studies of the occupations of both biological and adopted fathers of schizophrenics show that patients frequently fail to reach the occupational level of their parents, thus confirming that social drift occurs.

Social Network

The interaction between the effects of the environment on schizophrenia and the effects of schizophrenia on social experience is illustrated again in studies of social network. Social network refers to the circle of family members, friends, and associates with whom support and social activity is shared. Schizophrenics tend to have networks that are smaller, more family oriented, and less intimate than those of controls. This tendency becomes more prominent after repeated hospitalizations, and in many cases family members will eventually disengage and be replaced by more formal professional contacts, such as mental health staff. This finding can be explained by the difficulties schizophrenic patients have in initiating and sustaining social relationships. Because an individual's social network serves as a major buffer against the stresses of life, the patient's shrinking social network also tends to influence the progression of the illness.

Genetic Factors

There is considerable evidence that schizophrenia is an illness that runs in some families, although the majority of patients evaluated do not have a first-degree relative (i.e., sibling, parent, or child, each of whom probably shares half of the patient's genes) with schizophrenia. The morbid risk of a schizophrenic patient's first-degree relative developing schizophrenia is approximately between 4 and 9%, based on different studies. Family members more distantly related to a schizophrenic patient have a lesser risk for the development of schizophrenia. What exactly is transmitted is not clear. Twin studies report that monozygotic twins are more likely to be concordant for schizophrenia (range in different studies 31–78%) than dizygotic twins (range in different studies 0–28%). However, the concordance for monozygotic twins is not absolute, suggesting that the illness is transmitted only in a subset of the twins or that environmental influences can have either a triggering or protective influence in individuals. Twinning might cause vulnerability to the development of a number of conditions, including schizophrenia.

Various studies have shown that the likelihood of monozygotic twins being concordant for schizophrenia is over *four times* greater than that for dizygotic twins. It is important to note that approximately 50% of monozygotic twin pairs are discordant for schizophrenia, suggesting that what is transmitted is not the illness per se but the *vulnerability* for the development of it. Adoption studies of offspring of schizophrenic patients show that they have a greater likelihood of developing schizophrenia than do the adopted offspring of healthy individuals. The estimated heritability of a diathesis for schizophrenia based on such studies is between 60 and 90%.

Advances in molecular biology allow chromosomal analysis in which a search for linkage with known genetic markers can be done in families in which schizophrenia is prevalent. The gene that transmits schizophrenia is reported to sit in close proximity to a known DNA marker on the *fifth chromosome* in one study of a large extended family, though a number of attempts to replicate this finding have failed. Questions about the statistical assumptions used in studies like this have been raised. Failure to replicate the original report could also be the result of the heterogeneity of schizophrenia. Another approach is to explore candidate genes, i.e., D_2 receptor gene, as possibly involved in the transmission of schizophrenia. Attempts to link candidate genes to schizophrenia have failed so far.

Schizophrenic mothers are more likely to have pregnancy problems and perinatal problems with their children; thus, patients might have not only the genetic diathesis but also environmental insults both intrauterine and perinatally. Furthermore, children of schizophrenic mothers are more likely to have disruptive early life experiences that make developmental aberrations, including psychological ones, more likely.

There is a complex interaction between the genetic influences and environmental variables leading to the phenotypic expression of schizophrenia. These variables are interactive, not just additive. This complex interaction of nature and nurture affects not only the development of schizophrenia but also its course. In different individuals, differing genetic and environmental factors may thus play lesser or greater roles in cause and pathogenesis, thus contributing, particularly in schizophrenia, to the heterogeneity of the disorder. The most widely accepted view of the pathogenesis of schizophrenia is the *stress diathesis* model, in which constitutional factors determined by heredity (the diathesis) interact with environmental influences (stress) that precipitate overt expression of the clinical symptoms.

Anatomical Factors

Neuropathological studies of postmortem schizophrenic brains have attempted to find lesions that would explain the symptoms of schizophrenia. The search for pathological lesions in schizophrenia has focused on the frontal and medial temporal lobes, particularly the hippocampus and adjacent entorhinal cortex. The pathological findings include nonspecific gliosis and cellular loss and disordered orientation of the pyramidal cells in the hippocampus suggesting a developmental rather than a degenerative disturbance. However, there is still insufficient evidence to clearly indicate a specific site for a pathological lesion in all schizophrenic patients.

Although a resurgence of interest exists in postmortem neuropathological studies of schizophrenic brains, there are a number of potential pitfalls in this methodology. These include the difficulty in dissociating the etiological factors from effects that might be the result of long-term chronic illness and effects of treatment. Other difficulties include changing ideas about diagnosis, the question of appropriate controls, the cause of death, delays in obtaining and fixing the brain after death, and so forth.

Neurochemistry also has been used in postmortem studies to unravel the mysteries of schizophrenia. A number of studies have documented increases in the number of type 2 dopamine (D_2) receptors in areas such as the basal ganglia and nucleus accumbens, although such an increase could be the result of neuroleptic treatment (an issue yet to be resolved).

Imaging techniques, as they have become available, have been used to better understand the morphology and pathophysiology of schizophrenia. Computed tomography (CT) allows a noninvasive technique to be used to obtain X-rays of the brain in transverse slices. Numerous studies have documented *enlargement of the lateral ventricles, increased width of the third ventricle*, and *sulcal enlargement suggestive of cortical atrophy.*

Lateral ventricular enlargement is reported in schizophrenic patients in the vast majority of controlled studies (Fig. 5–1). Enlargement of the lateral ventricles is not necessarily sufficient to be read as clinically abnormal in the majority of schizophrenic patients. However, planimetric and automated measurements clearly show that statistically significant enlargement of the lateral ventricle exists in the majority of schizophrenic patients. Not all schizophrenic patients have enlarged lateral ventricles, so that enlargement of the lateral ventricles is neither sufficient nor necessary for

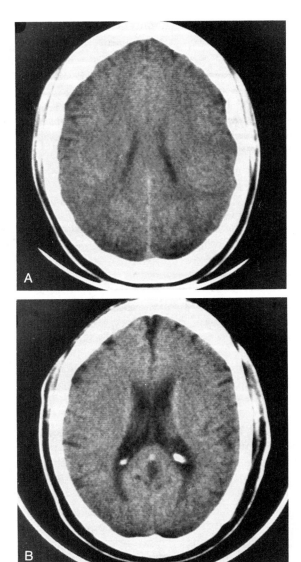

Figure 5–1. *(A) CT scan of patient with schizophrenia with normal lateral ventricles. (B) CT scan of patient with schizophrenia taken at level of bodies of lateral ventricles with enlarged lateral ventricles.*

the diagnosis of schizophrenia. Lateral ventricular enlargement is *not specific* to schizophrenia—it is found in a number of neurological conditions and also in non-schizophrenic psychiatric conditions such as bipolar disorder.

In monozygotic twins discordant for schizophrenia, the lateral ventricles of the schizophrenic twin are enlarged compared with those of the healthy twin.

The lateral ventricular enlargement is seen very early in the onset of the illness, suggesting that it precedes the psychosis. Preliminary data suggest that the finding is not progressive. Lateral ventricular enlargement has been correlated with cognitive disturbances, negative symptoms, poor premorbid psychosocial functioning, poor response to treatment, and poor outcome.

The third ventricle is situated close to anatomical areas of particular interest in schizophrenia. It has been measured in a number of studies, and the majority report its enlargement. Sulcal enlargement also has been reported in a significant number of schizophrenic patients, suggesting diffuse cortical atrophy.

Magnetic resonance imaging (MRI) techniques provide significant advantages over CT scan studies, including better resolution; lack of exposure to radiation; the capacity to have transverse, sagittal, and coronal cuts; and the capacity to do three-dimensional reconstruction of the brain. MRI studies generally confirm the CT findings of enlarged lateral ventricles (Fig. 5–2). In addition, some (but not all) studies report a 3–5% reduction in total brain area and/or volume in schizophrenia. An MRI study also supported the CT study of the affected co-twin with schizophrenia having larger lateral ventricles. MRI studies focusing on the temporal lobe and limbic structures report a reduction in temporal lobe, hippocampal, and amygdala volumes in schizophrenia. The abnormalities are found more often on the left side.

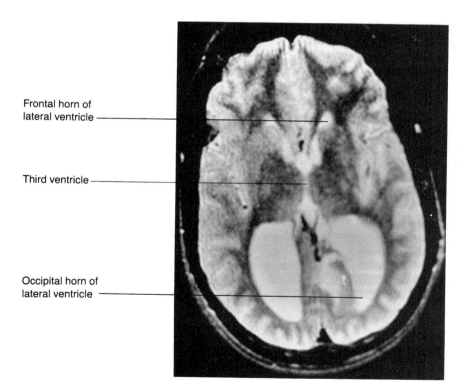

Frontal horn of lateral ventricle

Third ventricle

Occipital horn of lateral ventricle

Figure 5–2. *Axial MRI scan (T₂-weighted image) of a patient with schizophrenia showing enlarged lateral ventricles.*

Morphological studies can provide only a limited understanding of an illness that has some functional basis to it. Hence, static measures of structure are one step removed from physiological processes that need to be studied.

Physiological Factors

Physiological studies connect mental function to underlying physiological processes that are measurable and thus provide insights into normal and pathological psychic functioning. Physiological studies of cerebral blood flow in schizophrenia have been done with xenon 133 inhalation, positron emission tomography (PET), and single photon emission computed tomography (SPECT). Xenon is an inert gas that does not affect physiological or biochemical processes. Thus, measurement of radioactivity using gamma detectors, after inhalation of radiolabeled xenon, is a measure of regional blood flow in the brain. As neuronal activity is directly correlated with blood flow, regional cerebral blood flow is a measure of local neuronal activity. Physiological studies with xenon have the advantage of repetition in individuals because of the limited radioactivity involved, but they give us only information about surface activity. To get an idea about deeper parts of the brain, we turn to techniques such as PET studies. PET allows three-dimensional quantification of physiological activity of the brain—either of blood flow or of receptor activity.

There does not seem to be a difference in the total cerebral blood flow between schizophrenic patients and normal controls. Attempts to study differences in the resting state have resulted in inconsistent results. A number of studies have suggested a *"hypofrontal pattern"* to the regional distribution of cerebral blood flow with a *relative decrease* of blood flow to *the frontal lobes.*

Under activation paradigms, the functional responsivity of the various cerebral areas can be assessed. The most elegant series of studies using this methodology have involved the use of a cognitive task (the Wisconsin Card Sort [WCS]) that activates the dorsolateral prefrontal cortex (DLPFC) in comparison with the use of a nonspecific mental task. Schizophrenic patients failed to activate the DLPFC, and the lack of activation was directly correlated with the number of errors made on the WCS (Fig. 5–3). Similar results have been obtained using a paradigm that activates the left medial frontal cortex with schizophrenic patients failing to activate compared to controls. The interpretation of this series of studies is that schizophrenic patients have a specific abnormality in activating the prefrontal cortex—a part of the brain that is physiologically important in planning, altering strategies in problem solving, and coping with change.

Using a ligand for the dopamine type 2 (D_2) receptor, a preliminary study suggested a functional increase in dopamine receptor activity in the caudate nucleus of schizophrenics, including patients who have never been exposed to neuroleptic medications (suggesting that the alterations in the D_2 receptors were not necessarily an effect of treatment with neuroleptics). However, attempts to replicate this finding have failed, though there were considerable differences in the methodology used in the different studies.

Biochemical Factors

The search for a biochemical understanding of schizophrenia has been plagued by numerous discoveries that have failed to be replicated. The dopamine system has

rCBF % CHANGE ACTIVATION (WCS/NUM) MED FREE

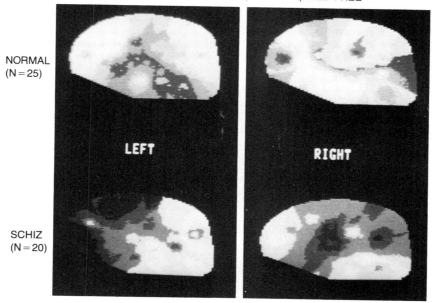

Figure 5–3. *Regional cerebral blood flow using xenon inhalation. Pictures show degree of blood flow changes on color scale with Wisconsin Card Sort test (with the control test being a number matching task). Controls are able to activate the prefrontal cortex bilaterally while schizophrenic patients fail to do so. (Reprinted with permission from Weinberger, Berman & Zec, 1986)*

been a primary focus as a mediator of pathology that could explain the illness of schizophrenia. There is mostly indirect evidence to support a causal role of dopamine in schizophrenia. Thus, all typical antipsychotic medications have the common capacity to block D_2 (non-adenylate cyclase) dopamine receptors. Furthermore, indirect dopamine agonists have the capacity to induce a condition that is clinically indistinguishable from schizophrenia (as in amphetamine psychosis) or exacerbate a psychotic condition, although neither of these effects is consistent in all patients. The affinity that various neuroleptic agents had for the D_2 receptor correlated highly with the average therapeutic dose used for the control of psychotic symptoms. Such data strongly suggest that the neuroleptic action at the D_2 receptor is pharmacologically relevant for the clinical benefits (Table 5–4).

With the cloning of several dopamine receptors, multiple types are now recognized that could not be delineated using previous methodologies (Table 5–5). Of particular interest, the D_4 receptor has a higher affinity for the atypical neuroleptic clozapine and could mediate its greater antipsychotic potency. A number of dopamine systems exist in the mammalian brain. The ones of particular relevance to schizophrenia include the mesolimbic and mesocortical systems, which are thought to be

Table 5–4 Side-Effect Profiles and Dose Equivalents of Commonly Used Neuroleptics

DRUG	EQUIVALENT DOSE (MG)	DOSAGE FORMS	SEDATIVE	SIDE EFFECTS		
				Extra-pyramidal	Hypo-tensive	ANTI-CHOLINERGIC
Phenothiazines						
Chlorpromazine	100	t,i,c,s,r	+++	++	IM +++ oral ++	+++
Thioridazine	95	t,c,s	+++	+	+	++++
Mesoridazine	50	t,i,c	+++	+	++	+++
Fluphenazine	2	t,i,d,s,c	+	+++	+	+
Perphenazine	10	t,i,c	++	++	+	+
Trifluoperazine	5	t,i,c	+	+++	+	+
Butyrophenones						
Haloperidol	2	t,i,c,d	+	+++	+	+
Thioxanthenes						
Thiothixene	5	t,i,c	+ to ++	++	+	+
Dihydroindolone						
Molindone	10	t,c	++	+	0	+
Dibenzoxazepine						
Loxapine	15	t,i,c	+	++	+	++
Diphenylbutylpiperidine						
Pimozide*	2	t	+	+	+	+
Clozapine	50	t	+++	+	+++	++++

0 = none, + = slight, ++ = moderate, +++ = marked, ++++ = pronounced
t = tablet or capsule, i = injectable, c = concentrate, s = suspension, r = rectal suppository, d = depot injection
*Pimozide may have a greater propensity for prolonging the QT interval than other neuroleptics
Information in table extracted in part from:
Mason A & Granacher RP (1980). *Clinical handbook of antipsychotic drug therapy*. New York: Brunner/Mazel, pp. 19–108, and Baldessarini RJ (1978). Chemotherapy. In Nicholi AM (Ed.): *The Harvard Guide to Modern Psychiatry*. Cambridge: Harvard University Press, p. 390. (Used with permission from Stoudemire A, Fogel BS: Psychopharmacology in the medically ill. In Stoudemire A, Fogel BS (eds): Principles of Medical Psychiatry, p 89. Orlando, Grune and Stratton, 1987)

Table 5-5 **Cloned Dopamine Receptors**

TYPE	EFFECT ON ADENYLATE CYCLASE	Anatomic Localization
D_1	stimulates	cerebral cortex
D_2	inhibits	striatum and limbic cortex
D_3	? inhibits	limbic areas
D_4	? inhibits	frontal cortex, midbrain, amygdala, medulla
D_5	? stimulates	limbic system (including hippocampus & amygdala)

integrally related to schizophrenia, and the nigrostriatal and tuberoinfundibular, which are thought to be related more to the side effects of neuroleptics (Table 5-6).

Crow's typology of schizophrenia suggests two different pathological processes in the development of schizophrenia. The first involves the negative symptoms of schizophrenia, which could be reflections of pathological processes in the prefrontal cortex. Damage to the prefrontal cortex results in an amotivated withdrawn state with lack of initiative, thought, and emotion (Fuster, 1980). The positive symptoms, such as hallucinations and delusions, seem to be the result of pathology in the limbic system (Schmajuk, 1987).

Because both the limbic and prefrontal cortex have dopamine projections from the midbrain, it is interesting to look at these systems and their relation to pathology in schizophrenia. There are some differences between the mesocortical and mesolimbic dopamine pathways. The mesocortical dopamine pathway, like the tuberoinfundibular one, does not seem to have autoreceptors on the cell bodies and nerve terminals (Bannon, Roth, 1983). It is believed that as a result of this lack of autoreceptors, the mesocortical dopamine neurons have a higher rate of physiological activity, are less responsive to dopamine agonists and antagonists, and do not develop tolerance to chronic neuroleptic treatment. Thus, it is possible that neuroleptics are used at therapeutic doses that have their predominant effect on the nigrostriatal and the mesolimbic dopamine systems, which result in control of the positive psychotic symptoms and the development of extrapyramidal side effects. At higher doses, neuroleptics may also have an effect on the mesocortical system whereby they can exacerbate negative symptoms.

Table 5-6 **Dopamine Systems Relevant to Schizophrenia**

SYSTEM	CELL BODIES	PROJECTIONS
Nigrostriatal	Substantia nigra (A9)	Neostriatum (putamen + caudate)
Mesolimbic	Ventral tegmental area (A10) Substantia nigra (A9)	Accumbens, olfactory tubercle, amygdala
Mesocortical	Ventral tegmental area (A10)	Prefrontal cortex

Lesion studies of the mesocortical dopamine system (Pycock, Kerwin, Carter et al, 1980) in rats result in disinhibition of the mesolimbic dopamine system with the resulting functional overactivity and up-regulation of the dopamine receptors. Such a finding is congruent with postmortem studies of schizophrenic brains (Weinberger, Kleinman, 1986). These data can suggest a model for explaining the symptomatology in schizophrenia whereby underactivity of the mesocortical dopamine system results in an overactivity of the mesolimbic system, which results in the positive symptoms of schizophrenia (Davis, 1991).

Weinberger (1987) has suggested that insult to the prefrontal cortex early in life would be silent through prepubertal development. However, when the prefrontal cortical functions come on-line with normal brain development associated with sexual maturity and the attainment of early adulthood, such a "lesion" could express itself (possibly triggered by stress) in the form of a psychotic episode. The pathophysiology of this abnormality would be in the form of decreased inhibition of subcortical dopamine systems, which are expressed as psychotic symptoms. Such a model would potentially explain the age of onset of schizophrenia.

There is a growing body of evidence suggesting that cell migration, synapse formations, and programmed cell death might be abnormal in the frontal and temporal cortex and the hippocampus and surrounding areas in schizophrenia. Cell migration is most intense in the early and middle second trimester. Such a period of development might be particularly vulnerable to specific viral infections, failure of gene expression, or other etiological mechanisms that can leave the individual vulnerable to the development of schizophrenic symptoms during adulthood. The influenza epidemic in 1957 has been associated with an increased incidence of schizophrenia in children whose mothers were in the second trimester of pregnancy.

Acute treatment with neuroleptic agents results in an increase in the firing rate of the dopamine cells and an increasing turnover of dopamine at the synaptic sites. However, chronic treatment results in a decrease in the firing rate related to depolarization block of the dopamine cells and the down-regulation of the receptor sensitivity. This is reflected in the reduction of both plasma and cerebrospinal fluid (CSF) homovanillic acid (HVA), a metabolite of dopamine. This reduction in HVA is temporally associated with clinical improvement.

Thus, a number of different lines of information from the clinical, anatomical, physiological, biochemical, and pharmacological areas are coming together to aid in understanding the complex enigma of schizophrenia.

Other Biological Findings in Schizophrenia

Numerous attempts have been made to find biological markers for schizophrenia. Abnormalities in how smoothly the eyes move when tracking a moving object have been reported in about 65% of schizophrenic patients and in a lesser number of other psychiatrically ill patients. At this point it seems to be a *trait* marker, only partially affected by the psychotic state and unrelated to the medication status of the patient. Interestingly, some healthy family members of schizophrenic patients also have this abnormality, suggesting that it could be an abnormality that is genetically transmitted closely with schizophrenia or a vulnerability for the development of schizophrenia.

Treatment of Schizophrenia

Pharmacological Management

The pharmacology of neuroleptic (antipsychotic) medications is covered in Chapter 18. This section will focus on clinical issues in the use of neuroleptics in the treatment of schizophrenia.

Neuroleptic agents are significantly more powerful in controlling the symptoms of psychosis than are antianxiety, antidepressant, and antimanic agents, none of which is any better than placebo. There are two indications for neuroleptic agents in the treatment of schizophrenia. The first is to control the active symptoms of the illness, and the second is to provide a prophylactic effect in preventing relapse. The first is aimed at controlling the acute episode, whereas the second is aimed at maintenance management. In a significant number of patients, however, the control of symptoms is only partial, and therefore the palliative and prophylactic indications for the neuroleptics are often combined.

The typical neuroleptic agents in general use today are all equally effective in the treatment of psychosis (Table 5–4). Thus, in choosing a particular neuroleptic for the treatment of a patient, therapeutic effectiveness is not a factor that guides the physician in the choice of a particular neuroleptic. Even neuroleptics that have a greater sedating effect (e.g., chlorpromazine, thioridazine) seem to improve psychomotor retardation associated with psychosis, whereas less-sedating neuroleptic agents (e.g., haloperidol) have a calming effect in agitated patients.

Side effects can be used when choosing which neuroleptic should be used in a particular individual. Major side effects include anticholinergic ones, postural hypertension, and extrapyramidal ones (acute dystonic reactions, pseudoparkinsonism, akathisia, and tardive dyskinesia). Less common, but with considerable morbidity and mortality, is neuroleptic malignant syndrome. (See Chapter 18)

For the acute episode of schizophrenia, doses in the range of 400–600 mg of chlorpromazine or its equivalent are necessary for successful treatment (Kane, 1987). Megadoses of neuroleptics (over 2000 mg of chlorpromazine or its equivalent) do not seem to result in any greater or faster improvement of schizophrenia. Combining benzodiazepines with neuroleptic agents in the early part of the treatment of an acute schizophrenic episode can be an appropriate strategy to induce sedation and control agitated behavior while using lower doses of neuroleptic agents. Use of benzodiazepines for such an indication should not be for more than a few days at a time because of the potential development of dependence.

The maintenance strategy is to find the lowest useful dose of neuroleptic that will continue to provide protection against psychotic relapse while not interfering with the psychosocial functioning of the individual and reducing the risk for tardive dyskinesia. If high doses of neuroleptics are required for control of an acute episode of schizophrenia, one should consider a slow and gradual reduction in dose once the patient has stabilized and is relatively free of stressful situations. One approach would be to reduce the dosage of chlorpromazine or its equivalent at the rate of 100 mg per month. Such a decrease in dosage should be coupled with education of the patient and significant others and attempts to monitor the development of early warning signs indicative of impending relapse. An unstable environment around the patient and emotional hostility and intrusiveness (high EE) that the patient might have to endure from close relationships are much more likely to be associated with a psychotic relapse. Hence, patients with these situations should have their medications reduced in a more conservative manner.

Neuroleptic Side Effects

Neuroleptics have numerous side effects; this chapter focuses exclusively on the extrapyramidal side effects. These are important because they have a major impact on the patient's compliance with neuroleptic medications.

The extrapyramidal systems are involved in the nonconscious control of all voluntary musculature. Neuroleptics have complex effects on the extrapyramidal systems that are exacerbated by anxiety, disappear during sleep, and can be consciously controlled for a limited time with effort. Extrapyramidal side effects can be classified into those that happen early or late in treatment.

Among the early extrapyramidal side effects are *acute dystonic reactions.* These are involuntary spasms of voluntary muscle groups that are often painful and frightening to patients. Frequently they involve the orofacial and head and neck areas, although any part of the body may be involved. Young men on high-potency neuroleptics (e.g., haloperidol) are at the greatest risk for the development of acute dystonic reactions. Low-potency neuroleptics, especially ones that have significant anticholinergic effects (e.g., thioridazine), have less likelihood of inducing acute dystonic reactions. Acute dystonic reactions tend to happen relatively early in treatment, and there is some tolerance that develops to them. The presumed mechanism of action is an imbalance induced by neuroleptic agents blocking dopamine receptors that are in balance with the cholinergic system. The use of neuroleptics with anticholinergic agents or dopamine agonists results in reestablishment of this dopamine–cholinergic balance and the control of the acute dystonic reaction. Considering the impact of such reactions on compliance of the patient, it is worthwhile to consider using antiparkinsonian agents in a prophylactic manner in patients who are started on neuroleptics, especially the high-potency ones such as haloperidol.

Parkinsonian side effects also associated with the use of neuroleptics include tremor, rigidity, and bradykinesia. These symptoms are indistinguishable from the symptoms of Parkinson's disease, which is caused by degeneration of the dopamine cells in the substantia nigra. Neuroleptic-induced parkinsonian side effects are responsive to anticholinergic and dopamine agonist agents.

Bradykinesia is a state associated with diminished spontaneous motor movements associated with a reduction in spontaneous speech, general apathy, and difficulty initiating activities. Bradykinesia can be difficult to differentiate from depression and negative symptoms. Because anticholinergic agents are effective in treating bradykinesia, such symptoms should be aggressively treated with these agents.

Akathisia is a subjective sense of motor restlessness and is often mistaken for agitation. It is not as responsive as other extrapyramidal side effects to anticholinergic agents. Some patients with akathisia respond to the use of beta-blockers such as propranolol. The most effective treatment for akathisia is a reduction in neuroleptic dose.

Tardive dyskinesia (TD) is a late complication of neuroleptic treatment and has been described as "a syndrome consisting of abnormal stereotyped involuntary movements usually of choreoathetoid type principally affecting the mouth, face, limbs and trunk, which occurs relatively late in the course of drug treatment and the etiology of which the drug treatment is a necessary factor" (Jeste, 1982). There is roughly a 3% annual risk for the development of TD, which is cumulative annually. About one-third of patients treated with neuroleptics seem to be at risk for the development of TD. If detected early, and the neuroleptic is discontinued, the TD is most often reversible. Continued treatment with neuroleptics results in potential worsening of the symptoms of TD and makes them more likely to be irreversible. Risk factors for the development of TD include total lifetime exposure to the dose of neuroleptic medications, older age, female sex, a history of extrapyramidal side effects, and mood disorders.

The presumed pathogenesis of TD is the development of supersensitive dopamine receptors in response to chronic blockade by neuroleptics. However, such supersensitivity probably develops in all patients treated chronically with neuroleptics, but only some go on to develop TD. Hence, supersensitive dopamine receptors might be necessary but not sufficient for the development of TD. Currently, there is no clinically successful strategy for the treatment of TD. Thus, the best approach for avoiding the risk of TD is the use of neuroleptics at the lowest possible dose necessary, regular evaluation for development of the symptoms of TD, and periodic voluntary informed consent for the continued use of neuroleptics.

Clozapine. Clozapine is an atypical antipsychotic agent recently available in the U.S. Clinical studies have shown superior efficacy of clozapine over typical neuroleptics in the treatment of refractory schizophrenic patients. Clozapine is not associated with significant extrapyramidal side effects including the development of TD. However, there is a 1–2% risk for the development of agranulocytosis requiring the weekly monitoring of white cell count (Lieberman, 1989). Other common side effects include sedation, sialorrhea (excessive salivation), hyperthermia, hypotension, grand mal seizures, sexual dysfunction, and enuresis. Clozapine is the first qualitative improvement in antipsychotic pharmacology since chlorpromazine and raises the promise of even further advances in the future. (See also Chapter 18)

Psychosocial Treatment

Psychosocial treatment of the major psychoses must be part of an integrated plan involving the use of a range of therapies appropriate to the phase of illness and the individual characteristics of each patient. Underlying goals are the treatment of symptoms, reduction of stress, mobilization of social supports, assistance with deficits in daily living skills caused by the illness, and gradual rehabilitation to the most autonomous level of functioning possible for the individual patient. Psychosocial treatment modalities include the use of hospitalization, partial hospitalization or day treatment programs, crisis intervention, individual therapy, and family treatment including psychoeducational approaches, social skills and behavioral training, and case management.

Individuals with all major psychotic disorders are likely to need long-term, often lifetime treatment. A consistent relationship with a primary clinician is of key importance to provide support and guidance through different phases of the illness and to coordinate the different treatment modalities that may be needed. Careful attention to maintaining continuity of care between hospital and outpatient clinic, day treatment, vocational rehabilitation, and family treatment programs is of particular importance for patients whose illness may make it difficult for them to make transitions and new relationships or to negotiate complex institutional barriers. Integration of medication and psychosocial programs is essential. Psychosocial treatments are used to target problems not responsive to medications, such as negative symptoms and social and occupational deficits, and to support medication strategies that will be most therapeutic and produce the least possible side effects. Studies indicate that the combination of medication and psychosocial programs is significantly more effective than either used alone (Falloon, Lieberman, 1983).

Acute Phase. In the acute phase of a psychotic illness, hospitalization is often necessary to contain disruptive and dangerous behavior and remove the individual from everyday stresses and responsibilities. Patients should always be medically reevaluated for the presence of medical, neurological, or substance disorders that may be etiologically related to the psychotic break or may have precipitated a relapse.

The push toward deinstitutionalization and community care (founded on the advent of neuroleptics), concern over the iatrogenic effects of long-term institutionalization, and the shifting of public money from state hospitals to community mental health centers has dramatically reduced the length of stay for most psychotic patients. Studies show short-term hospitalization to be at least as effective as longer stays. Interest in partial hospitalization, in which the patient lives at home but attends a structured daily program, has grown. Several studies show that this is feasible and works as well as inpatient treatment for patients who do not present a risk of violence or suicide (Weiss, Dubin, 1982).

The goals of psychosocial intervention in the acute phase of a psychotic experience are to reduce stimulation and provide a safe and structured environment where clear communication, little demand for performance, and firm limit-setting by tolerant and supportive staff can complement the use of medication in achieving a rapid resolution of symptomatic behavior. Immediate contact with the family is important in developing an alliance, providing crisis intervention to resolve stress that may have caused or been caused by the patient's relapse, and planning for future treatment. Connecting the patient with appropriate aftercare treatment is an essential part of the treatment of the acute phase of illness. This requires careful attention because in many public care systems inpatient and outpatient staff are segregated into different institutions and agencies, under different funding and administration, resulting in a high failure rate in keeping first outpatient appointments.

Follow-up Treatment. After an acute psychotic episode, little should be expected of the patient for several months. The principal goals of treatment at this stage are to prevent relapse while adjusting medication to a maintenance level and to help the patient reintegrate into the community. The home environment is now often the major treatment milieu, and it is important for the clinician to attend to the major impact that an acute psychotic episode has on the family system. Emotional turmoil, disruption of family routine and coping strategies, stigma, and restriction of social network are all dimensions that need to be addressed while the family is taught to provide the most therapeutic milieu. Attempts to change specific aspects of family interaction that correlate with higher relapse rates, such as high EE or communication deviance, may be warranted. Family treatment programs involving crisis intervention, education about the illness, stress reduction, and communication skills training have been shown to reduce the risk of relapse in the first year after hospitalization. Day hospital programs can play a useful role in assisting the patient's gradual readjustment to community living and also have been shown to reduce the risk of relapse. They may be particularly helpful for many chronic patients who have little family support and return to boarding homes, halfway houses, or cooperative living arrangements, which provide little in the way of treatment. Psychosocial programs that are too demanding or stimulating are not appropriate for this phase of treatment. Major role therapy (MRT), an intensive problem-solving approach used with schizophrenic outpatients, has been shown to improve social functioning after 18 months of treatment, but if it is offered without the use of prophylactic medication, it is associated with a lower level of adjustment, indicating that too much pressure can be detrimental to patients in the recovery process.

Individual psychotherapy alone has not been shown to improve the outcome for schizophrenic patients over the use of medication alone. This does not preclude its use for a few high-functioning schizophrenic patients. For many patients recovering from an acute psychotic episode, help with living accommodations, food, clothing, income, child care, and medical care is needed immediately. Case management is the term used to describe the social work function of helping the patient access the services that will meet these needs. This model of care is now part of many aftercare systems for psychotic patients. Case management functions may be provided by the primary clinician or may be allocated to separate case managers who work with a specific target population.

For the many patients who do not return to a premorbid level of adjustment following reentry into the community, other types of psychosocial intervention may be indicated. Social skills training programs using behavioral techniques focus on teaching patients verbal and nonverbal behaviors necessary for independent living and everyday social interaction. Assessment of strengths and weaknesses is followed by instruction, modeling, rehearsal (often in role play), and positive reinforcement of behavior that is correctly carried out. This approach has been shown to be helpful for chronic patients left with marked negative symptoms.

Group psychotherapy is useful in developing social skills as well as in encouraging supportive interpersonal relationships, reality testing, giving and receiving advice with practical problems of living, and exploring fears and feelings in a safe environment. With patients who have been psychotic, the group should have a structured, task-oriented focus rather than an exploratory focus. Many mental health centers use a biweekly or monthly medication group to provide an opportunity for patient evaluation, education, and socialization as well as an extension of each patient's social network.

Patients who recover sufficiently from the acute psychotic episode may need assistance in returning to work. Vocational rehabilitation programs such as workshops, job training programs, and transitional employment are offered by state and private agencies, which usually provide a structured and sheltered work environment in which patients may rehearse general job-related skills (such as being on time, completing tasks, and responding to supervision) as well as acquire new skills in preparation for a specific job. Little research has been done to measure the effectiveness of such programs, but they nevertheless address an area of recovery that is sorely in need of help, considering that less than 30% of schizophrenic patients return to work postdischarge.

CONCLUSION

Schizophrenia is an illness that is heterogenous in its cause, pathophysiology, response to treatment, and long-term outcome. Thus, generalizations about the illness and predictability in treatment response and outcome are important factors to consider, but their predictive capacity is small.

CLINICAL PEARLS

- Psychotic symptoms are nonspecific and occur in a variety of medical, psychiatric, neurological, and substance-induced disorders.
- Always rule out a medical, neurologic or substance-induced disorder first before assuming that any patient with psychotic symptoms has a "functional" psychiatric disorder.
- First-onset psychosis after age 45 generally indicates a neurologic, medical or substance-induced disorder or a psychotic depression; the onset of schizophrenia after age 45 is relatively rare.
- It is now believed that schizophrenia is primarily a neurological disorder with a strong genetic component; it is possible, however, that certain types of environmental or developmental stresses in individuals who are genetically vulnerable may contribute to the onset of the illness.
- It has been well demonstrated that the most effective treatment for schizophrenia involves a combination of neuroleptic medication and psychosocial treatment modalities.
- After years of research, abnormalities in the dopaminergic system of the brain remain the most consistent theory for the biological basis of schizophrenia.
- In treating schizophrenia, neuroleptics should be used at the lowest possible dose, and the patient should be monitored closely for tardive dyskinesia. Informed consent regarding tardive dyskinesia should be given at least every six months.

ANNOTATED BIBLIOGRAPHY

Andreasen NC: The diagnosis of schizophrenia. Schizophr Bull 13:9–22, 1987

An overview of the development of the criteria for diagnosing schizophrenia. Assesses both the strengths and limitations of nomenclature in psychiatry.

Arieti S: The Interpretation of Schizophrenia, 2nd ed. New York, Basic Books, 1974

For students interested in an eloquent, psychoanalytically oriented view of the inner world of the schizophrenic, this text is a classic. Its fundamental flaw is that it considers psychological factors as being primary in the etiology of the illness, but it nevertheless enables one to understand the evolution of schizophrenia from the internal world of the patient.

Bloom FE: Advancing a neurodevelopmental origin for schizophrenia. Arch Gen Psychiatry 50:224–227, 1993

> Detailed discussion of neurodevelopment theories on schizophrenia.

Davis KL, Kahn RS, Ko G et al: Dopamine and schizophrenia: Review and reconceptualization. Am J Psychiatry 148:1474–1486, 1991

> Excellent review of dopamine and schizophrenia.

Kendler KS: The genetics of schizophrenia: A current perspective. In Meltzer HY (ed): Psychopharmacology: The Third Generation of Progress, pp 705–713. New York, Raven Press, 1987

> A brilliant review of a confusing area. Frames the right questions and reviews the literature to delineate the answers that are known, and discusses the areas in which knowledge is lacking.

Kane JM: Treatment of schizophrenia. Schizophr Bull 13:133–156, 1987

> A detailed overview of the state-of-the-art knowledge on pharmacological treatment of schizophrenia. Includes strategies on how to address patients who are nonresponders.

Lieberman JA, Kane JM, Johns CA: Clozapine: Guidelines for clinical management. J Clin Psychiatry 50:329–338, 1989

> Everything you wanted to know about clozapine clinically.

Weinberger DR: Implications of normal brain development for the pathogens of schizophrenia. Arch Gen Psychiatry 44:660–669, 1987

> An interesting hypothesis that potentially explains the disparate aspects of schizophrenia, including its symptomatology, age of onset, biochemistry, and pharmacological response. The hypothesis connects morphological abnormality, brain development, and pathogenesis of schizophrenia.

REFERENCES

Akbarian S, Bunney WE, Potkin SG et al: Altered distribution of nicotinamide-adenine dinucleotide phosphate-diaphorase cells in frontal lobe of schizophrenics implies disturbances of cortical development. Arch Gen Psychiatry 50:169–177, 1993

American Psychiatric Association: DSM-IV Draft Criteria 3/1/93. Washington DC, American Psychiatric Association, 1993

American Psychiatric Association: Diagnostic and Statistical Manual of Mental Disorders, 4th ed., Washington, DC, American Psychiatric Association, in press [1994]

Anderson CM: Family intervention with severely disturbed patients. Arch Gen Psychiatry 34:697–702, 1977

Andreasen NC: Negative symptoms in schizophrenia: Definition and reliability. Arch Gen Psychiatry 39:784–788, 1982

Andreason NC: Comprehensive Assessment of Symptoms and History. Department of Psychiatry, University of Iowa College of Medicine, 1987

Andreason NC, Rezai K, Alliger R et al: Hypofrontality in neuroleptic-naive patients and in patients with chronic schizophrenia. Arch Gen Psychiatry 49:943–958, 1992

Baldessarini RJ, Cohen BM, Teicher MM: Significance of neuroleptic dose and plasma level in the pharmacological treatment of psychosis. Arch Gen Psychiatry 45:79–91, 1988

Bannon MJ, Roth RH: Pharmacology of mesocortical dopamine neurons. Pharmacol Rev 35:53–68, 1983

Bateson G, Jackson DD, Haley J et al: Toward a theory of schizophrenia. Behav Sci 1:251–264, 1956

Bleuler E: Dementia Praecox or the Group of Schizophrenias. Zinkin J (trans): New York, Int University Press, 1960 (German ed, 1911)

Brier A, Buchanan RW, Elkashef A et al: Brain morphology and schizophrenia: A magnetic resonance imaging study of limbic prefrontal cortex and caudate structures. Arch of Gen Psychiatry 49:921–926, 1992

Brown GW, Birley JLT: Crises and life changes and the onset of schizophrenia. J Health Soc Behav 9:203–214, 1968

Crow TJ: The two-syndrome concept: Origins and current status. Schizophr Bull 11:471–485, 1985

Crowe RR, Black DW, Wisner R et al: Lack of linkage to Chromosome 5q11–q13 Markers in Six Schizophrenia Pedigrees. Arch Gen Psychiatry 48:357–361, 1991

Davis KL, Kahn RS, Ko G, et al: Dopamine and schizophrenia: Review and reconceptualization. Am J Psychiatry 148:1474–1486, 1991

Doane J, West KL, Goldstein MJ et al: Parental communication deviance and affective style. Arch Gen Psychiatry 38:679–685, 1981

Dohrenwend BS, Dohrenwend BP: Some issues in research on stressful life events. J Nerv Ment Dis 166:7–15, 1978

Falloon IRH, Lieberman RP: Interactions between drug and psychosocial therapy in schizophrenia. Schizophr Bull 9:543–544, 1983

Farde L, Weisel FA, Stone-Elander S et al: D2 dopamine receptor in neuroleptic-naive schizophrenic patients; a position emission tomography study with [11C] raclopride. Arch Gen Psychiatry 47:213–219, 1990

Fromm-Reichmann F: Notes on the development of treatment of schizophrenics by psychoanalytic psychotherapy. Psychiatry 11:263–273, 1948

Fuster J: The Prefrontal Cortex. New York, Raven Press, 1980

Garmezy N, Neuchterlein K: Invulnerable children: Fact and fiction of competence and disadvantage. Presented at the annual meeting of the American Orthopsychiatric Association, Detroit, Michigan, 1972

Gibbons R, Lewine R, Davis J et al: An empirical test of a Kraepelinian vs a Bleulerian view of negative symptoms. Schizophr Bull 11:390–396, 1985

Gottesman II, Shields J: Schizophrenia: The Epigenetic Puzzle. New York, Cambridge University Press, 1982

Herz M: Prodromal symptoms and prevention of relapse in schizophrenia. J Clin Psychiatry 46:22–25, 1985

Hogarty GE, Anderson CM, Reiss DJ et al: Family psychoeducation, social skills training and maintenance chemotherapy in the aftercare treatment of schizophrenia. Arch Gen Psychiatry 43(7):633–642, 1986

Hollingshead AB, Redlich FC: Social Class and Mental Illness: A Community Study. New York, John Wiley & Sons, 1958

Holzman PS: Eye movement dysfunction and psychosis. Int Rev Neurobiol 27:179–205, 1985

Jeste DV, Wyatt RJ: Understanding and Treating Tardive Dyskinesia, p 84. New York, Guilford Press, 1982

Kendler KS: The genetics of schizophrenia: a current perspective. In Mettzer HY (ed): Psychopharmacology: The Third Generation of Progress. New York, Rowen Press, 705–713, 1987

Kraepelin E: Textbook of Psychiatry (abstr). Diefendorf AR (trans): London, Macmillan, 1907

Langfeldt G: The prognosis in schizophrenia. Acta Psychiatr Neurol Scand 110:7–66, 1956

Leff JP: Schizophrenia and sensitivity to the family environment. Schizophr Bull 2:566–574, 1976

Leff J, Vaughn C: The role of maintenance therapy and relatives' expressed emotion in relapse of schizophrenia: A two-year follow-up. Br J Psychiatry 139:102–104, 1981

Lidz T: Schizophrenia and the family. Psychiatry 21:21–27, 1958

Maser JD, Keith SJ: CT scans and schizophrenia—Report on a workshop. Schizophr Bull 9:265–283, 1983

Meyer A: The dynamic interpretation of dementia praecox. Am J Psychol 21:385–403, 1910

Moises HW, Gelernter J, Giuffra LA et al: No linkage between D_2 Dopamine Receptor Gene Region and Schizophrenia. Arch Gen Psychiatry 47:643–647, 1990

O'Callaghan E, Shaw P, Takei N et al: Schizophrenia after prenatal exposure to 1957 AZ influenza epidemic. Lancet 337:1248–1250, 1991.

Pycock CJ, Kerwin RW, Carter CJ: Effect of lesion of cortical dopamine terminals on subcortical dopamine receptors in rats. Nature 286:74–76, 1980

Robins LN, Helzer JE, Weissman MM et al: Lifetime prevalence of specific psychiatric disorders in three sites. Arch Gen Psychiatry 41:949–958, 1984

Scheibel AB, Conrad AS: Hippocampal dysgenesis in mutant mouse and schizophrenic man: Is there a relationship? Schiz Bulletin 19(1) 21–33, 1993

Schmajuk NA: Animal models for schizophrenia. The hippocampally lesioned animal. Schizophr Bull 13(2):317–327, 1987

Schneider K: Clinical Psychopathology. Hamilton MW (trans): New York, Grune & Stratton, 1959

Sherrington R, Brynjolfsson J, Petursson H et al: Localization of a susceptibility locus for schizophrenia on chromosome 5, Nature, 336:164–167, 1988

Tienari P, Sorri A, Lahti I et al: The Finnish adoptive family study of schizophrenia. Yale J Biol Med 58:227–237, 1985

Vaughn CE, Leff JP: The influence of family and social factors on the course of psychiatric illness. Br J Psychiatry 129:125–137, 1976

Weinberger DR: Implication of normal brain development for the pathogens of schizophrenia. Arch Gen Psychiatry 44:660–669, 1987

Weinberger DR, Berman KF, Zec RF: Physiological dysfunction of the dorsolateral prefrontal cortex in schizophrenia. Arch Gen Psychiatry 43:114–124, 1986

Weinberger DR, Kleinman JE: Observations on the brain in schizophrenia. In Hales RE, Frances JA: Psychiatry Update, American Psychiatric Association Annual Review, Vol 5, pp 42–67. Washington, DC, American Psychiatric Press, 1986

Weiss KJ, Dubin WR: Partial hospitalization: State of the art. Hosp Community Psychiatry 33:923–928, 1982

Wong DF, Wagner HN, Tune LE et al: Positron emission tomography reveals elevated D2 dopamine receptors in drug-naive schizophrenics. Science 234:1558–1563, 1986

Wynne L, Singer M: Thought disorder and family relations of schizophrenia. I: Research strategies. Arch Gen Psychiatry 9:191–198, 1963

Alan Stoudemire (ed). *Clinical Psychiatry for Medical Students,* Second
Edition. Copyright © 1994, 1990 by J. B. Lippincott Company.

6 *Personality Disorders*

Deborah B. Marin,
Allen J. Frances, and
Thomas Widiger

Ever since Hippocrates suggested a neuroendocrine model of behavior in which
the relative balance of four bodily humors (blood, black bile, yellow bile, and phlegm)
caused the different personality types (Allport, 1937), physicians have sought to
understand how and why individual personalities differ. Behavioral regression often
accompanies physical illness, and one of the features that separates a great doctor
from a technician is the ability to understand how a patient's personality interacts
with the stress of illness. Physicians who can accurately assess patients' personality
traits and manage their idiosyncrasies in the context of illness will improve their
relationships with patients, enhance compliance, and reduce patient stress (Kahana
and Bibring, 1964). Open and comfortable two-way communication coupled with an
understanding on the part of the physician of the patient's personality, sensitivities,
vulnerabilities, mechanisms of defense, and ways of coping with stress will help
patients recognize that they are being understood.

*Essential to achieving these goals is an understanding that different per-
sonality styles often entail different, yet predictable, ways of coping with illness
that require specific responses from the physician.* For example, as will be seen,
compulsive patients who have a need to be "in control" can best be managed by being
encouraged to become actively involved in treatment decisions. In contrast, the
dependent person who desperately needs to be cared for and reassured will be most
appropriately served by the doctor's being relatively more directive of the decision
making (Kahana and Bibring, 1964).

Physicians of all specialties can learn the techniques of personality assessment
and supportive treatment to obtain optimal doctor–patient relationships. Wise physicians acknowledge their *own* personality patterns and responses and the responses

that different types of patients are likely to elicit from them. Problematic personality traits are ubiquitous in medically ill patients, and personality disorders occur in 5 to 10% of the general population and in up to 60% of inpatient psychiatry samples (Merikangas and Weissman, 1986; Docherty, Fiester, and Shea, 1986). Thus, assessing and managing personality disorders is a common and extremely important part of both general medical and psychiatric practice.

DEFINITION: PERSONALITY TRAITS VS. PERSONALITY DISORDERS

The fact that everyone has a personality is what makes people more or less predictable in their behaviors and reactions. *An individual's personality style is exemplified by typical behavior patterns and characteristic responses to life events and stresses.* The term *personality trait* describes such typical patterns and responses. In distinction to a "trait," a personality *disorder* occurs when an individual's traits are *inflexible* and *maladaptive*, resulting in significant impairments in social, interpersonal, and occupational functioning. Personality *disorders* are chronic behavior disturbances with an early and insidious onset that crystallize by late adolescence or early adulthood. To varying degrees, personality disorders influence all facets of personality, including cognition, mood, behavior, and the interpersonal style of relating to others (Widiger and Frances, 1988).

CLASSIFICATION

The *Diagnostic and Statistical Manual of Mental Disorders* (DSM-IV) (APA in press [1994]) provides the current system for classification of personality disorders. The provision of a separate axis in the DSM-IV system (Axis II) for personality pathologies draws attention to the importance of these pathologies and emphasizes their coexistence with, and contribution to, other psychiatric disorders (Frances and Widiger, 1986; Siever and Klar, 1986). Axis I conditions include all the mental disorders that are not personality disorders. Depression, schizophrenia, and dementia are examples of such conditions. In addition, it acknowledges the coexistence of personality disorders with Axis I conditions.

The DSM-IV personality disorders are grouped into three major clusters (Table 6–1): Cluster A includes the odd or eccentric (schizotypal, schizoid, and paranoid);

Table 6–1 **The Three Clusters of Personality Disorders**

CLUSTER A (ODD)	CLUSTER B (DRAMATIC)	CLUSTER C (ANXIOUS)
Schizotypal	Histrionic	Avoidant
Schizoid	Narcissistic	Dependent
Paranoid	Antisocial	Obsessive–compulsive
	Borderline	

Cluster B includes the dramatic, emotional, or erratic (histrionic, narcissistic, antisocial, and borderline); and Cluster C represents the anxious or fearful (avoidant, dependent, and obsessive–compulsive).

Multiple diagnoses of personality disorders may be made because over 50% of patients with Axis II pathology meet criteria for two categories (Pfohl, 1986). Because all axes must be included in a patient's diagnosis, it is important to list every disorder observed in all the Axis II categories. If a patient's symptoms are not severe enough to warrant a formal diagnosis, the presence of more subtle, subthreshold personality characteristics may be noted in Axis II using the term *traits* rather than *disorder*.

DIAGNOSIS

Several factors make the diagnosis of a personality disorder difficult and should be considered carefully during the clinical assessment of the patient. *Personality characteristics reflect an enduring disposition to react to situations and relate to others in a particular way*. In contrast, *state* conditions reflect a person's condition at a *given point* in time. As an example, a widowed woman may seem dependent or compulsive because she is depressed. It is extremely common to observe regressive behavior, suggestive of a personality disorder, in the context of acute psychiatric illness such as depression. As the patient improves and emotionally reconstitutes, the problematic behavior will tend to decrease in severity. It is also common to see an exacerbation of symptoms in patients with well-defined personality disorders during acute psychiatric illness—which also decreases in severity as the patient's overall condition stabilizes. Distinguishing *trait* from *state* is particularly pertinent when making Axis I and II diagnoses (Frances and Widiger, 1986). It is crucial to try to ascertain whether or not a patient's behavior represents a change from his or her baseline or an enduring personality style.

When determining if a behavior is maladaptive enough to be consistent with a personality disorder, attention must also be turned to the *situation* in which the behavior occurs (Frances and Widiger, 1986). *The physician must not erroneously assign behaviors to personality traits and overlook the contribution of situational factors*. The young man rebelling against authority in military boot camp should not necessarily be diagnosed as having an antisocial personality unless he consistently behaves similarly in other circumstances.

Traits also must be distinguished from roles (Frances and Widiger, 1986). An observed behavior may be a response to the demands of a social role rather than a personality style. When a pathological behavior is evident only in response to a specific stressor or expected role, an adjustment disorder should be diagnosed (Frances and Widiger, 1986). In contrast, an individual with a personality disorder exhibits a maladaptive behavior that is consistent over time in many situations (Millon, 1981).

The traits that constitute the personality disorders frequently occur in diminished number or intensity in the normal population (Frances and Widiger, 1986). The personality disorders differ quantitatively, not qualitatively, from normality. Attention also must be paid to the culture in which certain behaviors occur. It is expectable that cultural norms in different countries and societies will differ significantly. Furthermore, perceptions of the threshold dividing normality from pathology may vary among those performing the evaluation. Determining this boundary is difficult and requires clinical judgment and experience (Frances and Widiger, 1986).

METHOD OF ASSESSMENT

The most frequently used methods to assess personality disorders are the clinical interview, self-report inventories, and semistructured interviews. Self-report inventories for assessment of personality disorders include the Minnesota Multiphasic Personality Inventory, the Millon Clinical Multiaxial Inventory, and the Personality Diagnostic Questionnaire (Widiger and Frances, 1987). The advantages of self-report instruments include ease of administration and scoring as well as documentation of symptoms without the input of a clinician's possible preconceptions and expectations. Yet, interviewing informants and observing the patient over time may indeed yield a more accurate assessment of the person's personality (Dowson, 1992).

Semistructured interviews have facilitated much research in, and understanding of, personality disorders. Examples of such interviews, which include the Structured Interview for the Diagnosis of Personality Disorders, the Personality Disorder Examination, the Structured Clinical Interview for DSM-III-R (SCID), the Personality Interview Questionnaire, and the Diagnostic Interview for Borderlines, are reviewed by Widiger and Frances (1987). These instruments have proved that good interrater reliability can be obtained for the diagnoses of personality disorders if a set of comprehensive and specific questions is provided.

EPIDEMIOLOGY

When evaluating the prevalence of personality disorders, one must consider the population being sampled. The different rates reported below result from the differing instruments used on varied populations. *Most studies assessing the epidemiology of personality disorders have been done in psychiatric inpatients who have concurrent Axis I conditions*. In part, this is because treatment settings are more likely to facilitate comprehensive interviews and to ensure the presence of the experienced raters necessary for a valid assessment of personality traits (Merikangas and Weissman, 1986). Because instruments for establishing criteria for personality disorders in the community are lacking, there are few studies that examine the rates of personality disorders in the general population. To date, there exists no systematic study using DSM criteria to assess all personality disorders in the general population. Because most test instruments to assess personality disorders are standardized on psychiatric patients, their generalizability to epidemiologic studies in other populations is not clear.

Among patients admitted to psychiatric hospitals for depression, 23 to 67% have a concurrent personality disorder (Merikangas and Weissman, 1986). Psychiatric outpatients with mood disorders have rates of personality disorder ranging from 12 to 100% (Merikangas and Weissman, 1986). In the medical setting, a 10% rate of personality disorders has been reported in patients at risk for HIV infection (Jacobsberg, unpublished data). In random community samples, the overall rates of personality disorder appear to range from 5 to 10% (Merikangas and Weissman, 1986). Overall, personality disorders appear to be distributed equally between the sexes and to be more common in the lower socioeconomic classes. Studies of the prevalence of paranoid, schizoid, and schizotypal traits show ranges of 0.03 to 28.4 per 100 people (Merikangas and Weissman, 1986). These figures reflect people who may only have *traits* of these disorders without meeting full threshold criteria for the disorders.

The prevalence of histrionic and borderline personality disorders ranges from 0.2 to 2.2 per 100 people. Antisocial personality disorder is the only Axis II diagnosis that has been studied in a large number of epidemiologic studies. Antisocial traits have prevalence ranging from 0.2 to 9.4 per 100 people. Antisocial personality disorder has been shown to be more common in young men, in lower socioeconomic classes, mobile populations, and in prisons (Merikangas and Weissman, 1986). There are no epidemiologic studies examining narcissistic personality disorder.

The prevalence of avoidant traits ranges from 7 to 41 per 100. The prevalence of dependent traits ranges from 2.5 to 27.2 per 100. Compulsive personality disorder has been shown to have a prevalence of 0.04 to 1.7 per 100 and passive–aggressive personality traits have rates from 0.9 to 2.5 per 100 (Merikangas and Weissman, 1986; Nestadt et al, 1991).

ETIOLOGY

Personality development depends on the interaction of several variables, including the person's constitution, innate temperament, developmental experiences within the family, quality of family relationships, available role models, and opportunities for acquisition of coping skills (Rutter, 1985). Earlier writings favored *either* environment *or* biology as causative factors. In contrast, more recent literature views personality as resulting from a complex interaction of constitutional *and* developmental influences.

Very young infants already differ from one another in several variables, including biologic functioning, autonomic reactivity, sensory alertness to stimuli, adaptability to change, characteristic moods, distractibility, and persistence. These innate endowments constitute each child's *temperament*, which interacts with the environment and caregivers in ways that accentuate and modify behavior (Millon, 1981).

Twin and adoption studies are the most useful research designs for investigating the effects of environment and heredity. Such studies have examined personality traits that may be associated with schizophrenia in a family member. Schizotypal and paranoid personality disorders have been shown to have a familial and genetic association with schizophrenia (Siever and Klar, 1986). There is evidence suggesting that borderline personality disorder also runs in families (Pfohl, 1986).

The rate of Axis I and Axis II disorders in families of patients with personality disorders is coming under increasing investigation. There are data supporting an association between borderline personality disorder and mood disorder, alcoholism and substance abuse in relatives (Pfohl, 1986). A familial transmission of obsessive–compulsive personality has also been supported (Pfohl, 1986).

According to psychoanalytic theory, the infant is born with instinctual drives that are primarily aggressive and sexual in nature. Personality development, as understood by this theory, is a process in which the child learns to control his or her instinctual impulses in order to adapt and adjust to the family environment. Organization and stabilization of this effort for adaptation result in normal behavioral tendencies. During development, if a child's needs are too intense to be satisfied adequately or if expected needs are not satisfied because of lack of response from the environment, the resulting experience may serve as a trauma that may not be completely overcome. Resultant "fixations," which represent unfulfillment of those needs, can occur during any of the major phases of development (Kahana and Bibring, 1964). Disturbances at particular critical development phases will result in certain characteristic personality formations.

It is not possible within the confines of this text to discuss psychoanalytic and other theories of the development of personality disorders in depth, although it should be reiterated that personality is strongly influenced by early developmental influences, the nature and quality of relationships with the parents and siblings, and the psychological adaptations that the individual makes to both positive and negative aspects of the family experience. It is also assumed that although basic personality traits crystallize by late adolescence, experiences and significant relationships with other people later in life may modify the personality. Readers are referred to comprehensive textbooks of psychiatry and selected references for a more in-depth discussion of theories of personality development in general and for discussions of the pathogenesis of specific types of personality disorders (Meissner, 1985). Psychoanalytic theories, including object relations, ego psychology, and self psychology (Kohutian) regarding personality development, are discussed in the companion volume to this text on human behavior (Inderbitzin and James, 1994).

Supporting the role of biogenetic factors is evidence that patients with personality disorders differ from normal and psychiatric controls in a number of biologic parameters. It has been proposed that central nervous system pathology leading to impaired development could result in personality pathology. For example, patients with borderline personality disorder often have a history of brain trauma (Andrulonis, Glueck, Stroebel et al, 1980). EEG abnormalities—in particular, slow wave activity—have been demonstrated in both antisocial and borderline personality disorders (Pfohl, 1986). Sleep EEG abnormalities, including shortened rapid eye movement (REM) latencies, increased REM intensities, and sleep continuity disturbances have been observed in borderline patients (Bell, Lycaki, Jones et al, 1983; Reynolds, Soloff, Kupfer et al, 1985).

Neuroendocrine tests originally used to study the biology of depression have been extended to studies of borderline personality disorder in part because many borderline patients have mood instability and become depressed (Soloff, Anselm, Nathan, 1982). Abnormal dexamethasone suppression test results in borderline patients range between 16 and 61% (Sternbach, Fleming, Exteen et al, 1983). Neuroendocrine challenge tests, which evaluate the overall functional activity of neurotransmitter systems, have documented abnormal central serotonergic function in borderline personality disorder. Studies using fenfluramine, which produces increases in plasma prolactin by virtue of its enhancement of serotonergic availability at postsynaptic receptor sites, have found that patients with borderline personality disorder have a significantly reduced prolactin response when compared to nonborderline personality disorder patients (Coccaro, Siever, Klar et al, 1989). The frequent occurrence of lifetime and concurrent mood disorders in the borderline patients studied, however, complicates interpretation of these results.

Another approach to study the biology of personality has been to investigate personality features that may have a spectrum relationship with Axis I psychopathology. Schizotypal personality disorder tends to "load" in families of proband schizophrenics. Evidence suggests that the biological abnormalities documented in schizophrenic patients are also present in individuals who meet criteria for schizotypal personality disorder. The model that has been most useful in this regard has investigated abnormal smooth pursuit eye movements (SPEM), which are common in schizophrenia (Holzman, Solomon, Levin et al, 1984). Impaired SPEM has been shown to be associated with schizotypal personality disorder or schizotypal traits in college students (Siever, Coursey, Alterman et al, 1984). Schizotypal and paranoid personality disorder patients have significantly more impaired SPEMs than subjects with other personality disorders and normal controls (Siever, Keefe, Bernstein et al, 1990; Siever, Coursey, Alterman et al, 1989). The clinical characteristics associated with impaired SPEM include interpersonal impairment, affective impoverishment, and disturbances of attention and cognition (Siever, Coursey, Alterman et al, 1989). Since SPEM appears to have a genetic basis, impaired SPEM may reflect a genetic vulnerability common to both schizotypal personality disorder and schizophrenia.

The biological correlates of personality pathology that cut across personality disorder diagnoses have been investigated. For example, both borderline and antisocial personality disorders contain criteria describing impulsive and aggressive behavior. Several lines of evidence document the association between impulsivity, physical aggression, and suicide with abnormalities of the serotonergic system. Several studies have investigated the serotonergic system by measuring levels of serotonin's metabolite 5 hydroxyindoleacetic acid (5-HIAA). A correlation between low cerebrospinal fluid (CSF) 5-HIAA and suicidal behavior has been observed in several diagnoses (Roy, Dejong and Linnoila, 1989).

Impulsive and violent behavior without suicidality has also been associated with serotonergic abnormalities. Aggressive behavior, as evidenced in arson and violent acts, has been correlated with low CSF 5-HIAA levels (Virkunnen, Dejong, Bartko et al, 1989). Follow-up studies have also demonstrated that low CSF 5-HIAA at index is associated with subsequent impulsive behavior. Violent offenders and impulsive fire setters who commit such crimes in the future have been shown to have significantly lower CSF 5-HIAA at index than nonrecidivists.

Twin studies provide a powerful method to determine the genetic and environmental contribution to personality. Twin studies include comparison of the heritability of personality traits in monozygotic and dizygotic twins reared together and apart. Research to date has suggested that certain aspects of personality have moderately strong heritability yet are also influenced by environment. For example, twin studies support a genetic component for antisocial personality disorder (Miller and Prinz,

1990). The concordance for antisocial behavior in monozygotic twins has been reported to be as high as 51%. Thirty-six percent of the offspring of criminals have been
shown to meet criteria for antisocial personality disorder. Although most of these
studies are being used for research purposes at present, similar biologic tests may aid
in personality evaluation in the future and lend credibility to the influence of biologic
substrates on personality characteristics.

TREATMENTS

Among the treatment modalities for personality disorders are psychodynamic
supportive, interpersonal, behavioral, cognitive, and pharmacologic therapies. Unlike
the other psychotherapies, *psychodynamic psychotherapy* specifically focuses on
the personality structure and the major developmental experiences in childhood that
have affected the individual (see Chapter 17 by Drs. Ursano, Silberman, and Diaz).
The other techniques are oriented more toward target symptoms but may have a
beneficial impact on personality functioning.

The precise form that psychodynamic therapy takes may vary from time-limited
therapy for several months to psychoanalysis for several years. Fundamental alteration of personality style is frequently an unrealistic goal. Therefore, this form of
therapy usually strives to improve interpersonal functioning by decreasing the *inflexible* nature of the maladaptive traits and increasing the individual's awareness of their
behavior. The goal of therapy is to increase the patient's insight into the nature of their
personality and how certain aspects of their behavior may complicate interpersonal
relationships. By increasing the patient's knowledge about their own personality
through a development reconstruction, the patient is then able to better understand
how personality characteristics may affect relationships with others. This enhanced self-
knowledge ideally leads to changes in thoughts, feelings, and behavior that in the past
may have been problematic. Enhanced insight coupled with newfound flexibility in
relating to others is a major goal of insight-oriented psycho-dynamic therapy. *The
appropriateness of psychodynamic psychotherapy depends in part on the patient's psychological-mindedness and capability and motivation for insight and
character change.* Patients with schizotypal, schizoid, paranoid, and antisocial traits
are less likely to benefit from such a treatment than are patients with dependent,
compulsive, avoidant, and histrionic personality disorders (Frances and Widiger,
1986).

In contrast, *supportive* psychotherapy attempts to aid patients without challenging their basic defenses or attempting to change their fundamental character
structure. Supportive treatment can help the patient through periods of medical,
interpersonal, occupational, or other stresses by minimizing regression and maximizing compliance. For instance, these goals may be met by admiring and being
empathic with the narcissistic patient, providing detailed information to the obsessive–compulsive patient, or maintaining an appropriate and nonintrusive distance
from the schizoid patient. Although psychoanalytic therapy is used for narcissistic
patients, a supportive and empathic approach may aid the patient in overcoming

current narcissistic injuries. The borderline patient who has difficulty tolerating insight-oriented therapy may also benefit from this supportive approach.

Interpersonally oriented psychotherapies are particularly suitable treatments because personality disorders often represent maladaptive interpersonal styles (Frances and Widiger, 1986). This technique can be practiced in *group, family, marital,* and *system-strategic* therapy. This therapy relies on the fact that personality styles frequently elicit complementary responses in others, including the therapist. In this treatment approach, the therapist assumes an interpersonal style that encourages more adaptive and flexible functioning in the patient in order to halt the usual rigid patterns of relating.

Behavioral therapy can be used to reduce target symptoms in appropriate patients. Behavioral techniques involving assertiveness training and graded exposures for social anxiety may be useful for dependent and avoidant patients, respectively (Liebowitz, Stone, and Turkat, 1986). Schizoid patients may benefit from shaping their social behavior. Behavior therapy for patients with antisocial personality disorder may be useful in structured settings, but the behavioral changes observed in these patients may not be sustained.

Cognitive therapy focuses on central, irrational assumptions underlying patients' beliefs and behaviors. Because personality disorders involve debilitating cognitive styles, such a therapeutic approach may be particularly appropriate in patients with these disorders (Millon, 1981). For example, the masochistic-depressive–prone individual may respond to a cognitive treatment similar to that used in treating depression. The borderline patient may benefit from addressing the exaggerated attitudes in order to develop more realistic perceptions of others. Cognitive techniques that focus on assumptions of threat and inadequacy may also be beneficial for the avoidant and dependent patient. Obsessive–compulsive patients may benefit by addressing their irrationally rigid, severe beliefs and moral standards (Widiger and Frances, 1988). The basic principles of psychoanalytic, psychodynamic, cognitive, group behavorial, and family therapy are discussed in Chapter 17.

Pharmacotherapy may be useful when it focuses on such features as mood dysregulation and impulsivity in borderline personality disorder, perceptual disturbances in schizotypal personality disorder, or anxiety in avoidant personality disorder. Low-dose neuroleptics have been found useful for mood and cognitive disturbances in schizotypal and borderline personality disorders (Liebowitz, Stone, and Turkat, 1986; Stein, 1992). Lithium and carbamazepine may ameliorate symptoms of episodic dyscontrol and aggression, even in the absence of epileptic features (Stein, 1992). Antidepressant regimens, including the monoamine oxidase inhibitors, may also be useful for mood disorders frequently seen in patients with Axis II disorders.

There is growing literature on the treatment of personality disorders (Siever and Klar, 1986). This increased attention to Axis II conditions is appropriate, since most patients do have some maladaptive traits that will influence the course and treatment of Axis I syndromes. A treatment chosen for Axis I conditions that considers the patient's personality traits will optimize treatment course and response (Widiger and Frances, 1988).

The Relationship Between Axis I and Axis II Diagnoses

The development of the multiaxial system in the original DSM-III reflected the recognition that personality disorders often coexist with, and impact on, the treatment of the acute psychiatric syndromes (Axis I). A patient's personality traits affect not only the doctor–patient relationship but also compliance and outcome. Axis II psychopathology has been shown to influence predisposition, presentation, course, and treatment response of Axis I conditions (Docherty, Fiester, and Shea, 1986). The exact nature of the relationship between personality disorders and the major syndromes can be conceptualized in different ways. Certain personality traits may (1) predispose toward, (2) modify, (3) represent a complication of, (4) represent an attenuated form of, or (5) coexist independently with specific Axis I disorders (Docherty, Fiester, and Shea, 1986). Below is a review of how specific personality disorders have been shown to be associated with Axis I conditions.

Mood Disorders

Many investigations of the incidence of personality disorders in patients with mood disorders have focused on depressed patients. Up to 61% of patients with mood disorders have been shown to have borderline pathology (Docherty, Fiester, and Shea, 1986). Dependent and avoidant personality disorders also occur frequently in depressed patients (Pfohl, 1986). The presence of character pathology in depressives has been associated with a different clinical presentation from that seen in patients with major depression only. Specifically, the presence of borderline character disorder has been associated with increased anxiety, anger, substance abuse, and attempts at suicide (Docherty, Fiester, and Shea, 1986). The presence of personality pathology in general has been correlated with earlier onset and poorer treatment outcome of depression (Docherty, Fiester, and Shea, 1986).

By definition, patients with personality disorders are often impaired in their ability to adjust to stress. Their inflexible behavioral patterns may, indeed, provoke problematic situations. Consequently, a person with character pathology will be more likely to develop depressive, anxiety, psychotic, and other Axis I disorders. Major depression, bipolar disorder, dysthymic disorder, and cyclothymic disorder have been shown to occur in 14 to 87% of borderline patients (Docherty, Fiester, and Shea, 1986). These rates are substantially higher than would be expected for the general population. Antisocial, schizotypal, compulsive, histrionic, narcissistic, self-defeating, and dependent patients not uncommonly have mood disturbances as well (Docherty, Fiester, and Shea, 1986).

Schizophrenia

Because of the chronic course of schizophrenia, in which personality alterations frequently occur during and after acute psychotic decompensation, it is often difficult to determine premorbid personality traits. McGlashan noted that the most frequently diagnosed personality disorder in schizophrenics is schizotypal, followed by borderline personality disorder (McGlashan, 1983). Schizotypal and borderline patients were reported to have a 55% and 16 to 24% chance, respectively, of developing schizophrenia (McGlashan, 1983). Other studies have noted much lower rates of overlap between schizophrenia and borderline personality disorder (Docherty, Fiester, and Shea, 1986).

Other Axis I Disorders

Both borderline and antisocial patients have been noted to have an increased incidence of alcoholism (Docherty, Fiester, and Shea, 1986). In the borderline patient, substance abuse may reflect an attempt to alleviate affective instability. For the antisocial patient, alcoholism may either result from or initiate an antisocial lifestyle. Social hypersensitivity and perception of threat predispose schizotypal and paranoid patients to develop anxiety disorders. Subjects with anxious cluster personality disorder have also been shown to be at increased risk for the development of anxiety disorders (Nestadt, Romanoski, and Brown et al, 1991).

THE DISORDERS

Included in each of the descriptions of the disorders presented below is an overview of psychiatric treatment, probable presentation in the medical setting, therapeutic strategies for the nonpsychiatric physician, and indications for psychiatric consultation. When evaluating a patient's psychopathology, attention should first be paid to the differential diagnosis of Axis I disorders. *This permits the clinician to determine whether or not a patient's symptoms represent an acute change or a long-lasting pattern.* When a chronic Axis I condition exists, such as dysthymia or an anxiety disorder, Axis II diagnoses can still coexist. Conversely, the presence of an Axis II disorder makes it more likely that an Axis I disorder also will exist.

Schizotypal Personality Disorder

Schizotypal personality disorder encompasses a combination of odd or peculiar behavior, speech, thought, and perception. Patients with such disorders are usually withdrawn and display idiosyncratic and odd speech patterns, eccentric beliefs, paranoid tendencies, perceptual illusion, unusual appearance, inappropriate affect, and social anxiety. When stressed, such a patient may lapse into brief breaks with reality. *Unlike the patient who has the fully developed syndrome of schizophrenia with frank hallucinations or delusions, the schizotypal patient experiences subtle distortions of the environment.* Schizotypal patients may resemble schizophrenia "in remission" and some authorities consider this form of personality disorder a latent type of schizophrenia that never develops into the fully developed schizophrenic syndrome.

When seen in a psychiatric setting, a supportive, structured, and firm approach will help combat the schizotypal patient's misperceptions and fragile grasp of reality. A supportive therapeutic approach would serve to encourage the patient to become involved in activities that are not socially frightening. Social skills training may diminish eccentric behavior and odd appearance and help the patient to feel more at ease in social settings.

Low-dose neuroleptics may alleviate the social anxiety and cognitive symptoms of schizotypal patients (Liebowitz, Stone, and Turkat, 1986). Medical illness may accentuate underlying misperceptions of physical symptoms and possible treatments. As an example, an intravenous line may be viewed by the patient as a device containing something harmful; similar reactions may occur to other medication or to the physician. Basic trust in others is usually a major problem for these individuals—as it is for schizoid, paranoid, and borderline patients.

A physician who can detect these features, understand their significance for the patient's interpersonal relationships and perception of reality, be supportive, reality test, and respect the patient's *need for privacy* and interpersonal distance will ease the patient's hospital course substantially. The staff may be repelled by the patient's "strangeness" and underestimate the degree of attachment such a patient may have for them. It is important to educate the staff that this patient's peculiar behaviors are not meant to be provocative. Psychiatric consultation may be necessary for management of anxiety and cognitive disturbances.

Schizoid Personality Disorder

A central characteristic of schizoid personality disorder is the inability to form relationships or to respond to others in a meaningful manner, leading to social isolation. Indifference to others and lack of response to praise, criticism, or any feelings experienced by others is typical. Yet, beneath the surface of this indifference often exists a loneliness and a desire for close relationships. Such a patient frequently experiences little pleasure or pain and has an affect that is constricted and apathetic. Unlike a schizotypal patient, this patient does not experience cognitive distortions. As with schizotypical personality disorder, schizoid patients may resemble schizophrenia in remission.

Group therapy with similar individuals may demonstrate to the patient that others are also introverted and socially awkward. Behavior therapy that helps the patient with social integration may also be of value (Liebowitz, Stone, and Turkat, 1986). Because such patients dislike new contacts and intrusion into their privacy, medical illness and hospitalization are particularly troubling and anxiety-provoking. A typical response to disease would therefore be further withdrawal. A physician's goal for management should consist of accepting the patient's desire for privacy, fear of intimacy, closeness, and intrusion while still demonstrating interest and concern. Such a therapeutic approach will help engender a perception of the doctor as being both protective and benign.

Paranoid Personality Disorder

Paranoid personality disorder is exemplified by suspiciousness, mistrust, rigidity, and hypervigilance but not grossly psychotic or delusional beliefs. Such a patient is preoccupied with perceived exploitation and infidelity by others. Paranoid beliefs may result in hostility, irritability, anxiety, and an undercurrent of anger. The paranoid patient may be hard to distinguish from the schizotypal patient, since both display mistrust of others and social anxiety. These patients often present as chronically angry, irritable, querulous individuals with a "chip on their shoulder." They mistrust and resent authority and institutions and tend to view the motivations of others in a cynical manner. They mistrust and are suspicious of almost everyone and fear being exploited and controlled by others. They tend to be extremely self-protective of their own interests and are often extremely jealous, controlling, and possessive in whatever relationships they are able to have. It is not unusual to see such individuals fascinated with weapons, survivalist organizations, or with extremist political groups. A profound negativistic, bitter, and cynical attitude often pervades their perception of life and other individuals.

Supportive therapy may be most efficacious for such a patient. An approach that is open, honest, and nonconfrontational will be most likely to engender trust. If the therapist is perceived as a benign, objective, and friendly helper, the patient may be more inclined to entertain alternative explanations and perceptions (Liebowitz, Stone, and Turkat, 1986).

Optimal management of a paranoid patient in a *medical* setting depends on the doctor's recognizing that the patient may believe his or her illness to be due to the inconsiderateness or malice of others. The patient is likely to respond to familiarity or joviality from the physician with withdrawal and suspicious misinterpretation (Nardo, 1986). This type of behavior may cause a physician to become more guarded with the patient, and such a reaction may only engender more distrust. To foster a trusting relationship with a paranoid patient, management should include clear explanations of procedures, medications, and results. The patient's suspicion and mistrust should be met with consideration, information, and impartial recommendation of procedures rather than with annoyance, exasperation, or defensiveness.

Histrionic Personality Disorder

The patient with histrionic (formerly known as hysterical) personality disorder tends to be attention-seeking, self-dramatizing, excessively gregarious, seductive, manipulative, exhibitionistic, shallow, labile, vain, and demanding. Such a patient may, at times, be difficult to distinguish from the borderline or narcissistic patient, and some degree of overlap exists between them. Psychoanalytic psychotherapy has traditionally been the treatment for such patients. The following is a case vignette typifying a histrionic patient admitted to a general hospital.

A CASE VIGNETTE

A 46-year-old woman was admitted for a mastectomy after a breast bi-opsy revealed a malignant tumor. She refused to be admitted to a four-bedded room, stating that she did not intend to share the facilities or staff with any other patients. Her flamboyant and gregarious manner initially ingratiated her to the staff. Her seductive dress and preoccupa-tion with her appearance seemed to overshadow her concern over the implications of her upcoming surgery. After the procedure, her demands for care became so frequent as to interfere with the staff's ability to care for the other patients on the service. She required repeated reassurance and became excessively angered when the staff did not immediately ful-fill her needs.

Medical illness threatens loss of attractiveness, strength, and achievement for any patient, but these are especially profound threats to histrionic patients, whose self-image, self-esteem, and self-worth usually depend on their ability to attract and hold the attention of others with their attractive appearance and entertaining behavior. Although the disorder has stereotypically been applied to women, careful attention should also be paid to identifying the male histrionic patient, who will have the need to display increased masculinity and sexual prowess as exemplified by a "macho" image and to elicit admiration (Nardo, 1986). The physician can greatly aid these patients by complimenting them in a nonpatronizing manner on their appearance and basically acknowledging their need for special attention, while not allowing himself or herself to become overwhelmed by demands. Partially fulfilling such patients' needs combined with limit setting will ease their acceptance of certain restrictions. It is important to convey to these patients that the limits being set do not reflect the doctor's impatience, but rather pressures with which the patient must comply to get the best possible treatment. This approach will offer these patients the knowledge that people are devoted to their care while recognizing the reality of limits.

Fundamental to understanding and treating the histrionic patient is an appreciation of the fact that these patients are fundamentally insecure particularly regarding their self-worth and sexuality and are extremely sensitive to rejection by others. These individuals should be considered to be fundamentally insecure. Behavior that may be superficially interpreted as manipulative, dependent, or even seductive is usually an effort to obtain love, support, attention, and reassurance, which the patient may have been deprived of in childhood. If rejection actually occurs, or if the patient perceives that his or her needs are not being fully met—which is often difficult to do— explosive, dramatic, and turbulent outbursts of emotion may follow. Awareness of the core personality dynamics in such patients will help the physician to manage their behavior and demands in an objective yet empathic manner. It is common to see histrionic and narcissistic personality traits overlap in the same individual.

Narcissistic Personality Disorder

The narcissistic patient, in the extreme form, is egocentric, grandiose, entitled, shallow, exploitive, arrogant, and preoccupied with fame, wealth, and achievement and generally lacks empathy and consideration for the feelings of others. Such a person is, nevertheless, exquisitely hypersensitive to evaluation or criticism by others. Narcissistic individuals crave admiring attention and praise from others and place excessive emphasis on displaying the accoutrements of beauty, power, fame, and wealth. They are typically exploitive of others and use their relationships to meet their own selfish needs with little consideration or empathy for the needs of the other person. Hence, they usually show a profound lack of empathy for others in their relationships. Regardless of the situation, they feel that they are "entitled" to special rights, attention, privileges, and consideration. Because of their sense of entitlement and demands for special treatment, these individuals are often considered to be arrogant and obnoxiously self-centered.

Medical illness is a blow to self-esteem, particularly if it separates these patients from their admirers and other sources of support. The narcissist may try to escape the possibility of illness either by ignoring the effects of the illness or by totally denying its existence. An example of such a patient would be the person with Crohn's disease who refuses to take steroids for fear of the disfigurement caused by this medication (Nardo, 1986). Such patients will benefit most from a medical setting where they feel admired, accepted, and appreciated. This is obviously difficult to do.

It is critical to realize that behind their grandiosity is often a very poorly developed sense of self and a low self-esteem that the patient attempts to hide and compensate for by building up an image of power, wealth, and attractiveness. Efforts to gain attention, praise, and admiration from others is a way of deriving and maintaining self-esteem from external sources since an internalized stable and positive sense of self-worth is lacking or defective. Patients have varying degrees of insight regarding their low self-esteem and examining this aspect of themselves in therapy can be experienced as extremely painful and humiliating. Hence, treatment of these patients in psychotherapy must be handled with a great deal of sensitivity and empathy despite their outwardly entitled, self-centered, and often arrogant behavior.

Psychiatric treatments ranging from long-term insight-oriented to brief, more supportive therapy are useful. These patients may be difficult to treat psychiatrically because of their tendency to be competitive and to alternately devalue or idealize the therapist. Special psychoanalytic techniques using empathic rather than confrontational approaches, originally devised by Heinz Kohut, have been recommended in the treatment of these patients.

Antisocial Personality Disorder

The antisocial (alternatively known as sociopathic or psychopathic) patient typically lacks empathy, social responsibility, guilt, and a sense of social, moral, and interpersonal responsibility. Such a person displays a consistent pattern of behavior that disregards the conventional limitations imposed by society. A veneer of charm and a smooth and ingratiating seductiveness that is hard to resist may mask disregard for the rights and feelings of others, because these patients are interested only in meeting their own needs.

Impulsivity, as manifested by frequent physical fights and abusive behavior, combined with a lack of appropriate responses to obvious consequences of one's actions are apparent. Encounters with the law and other authorities are frequent, as is repetitive criminal behavior. What is not well recognized is that antisocial personalities may often be quite successful in whatever their chosen professional activity. They may have paradoxically reached their position of success, power, and wealth by ruthless exploitiveness of others and carefully concealed lying and dishonesty. Such individuals have no qualms about lying, cheating, or stealing if it meets their self-determined ends. Although severe antisocial personalities are relatively rare and are usually brought to the attention of society when they are "caught," one should appreciate that antisocial personality traits as characterized by a relative lack of guilt and responsibility, as well as a tendency to conveniently lie and cheat when it is in one's self-interest, are a relatively common phenomenon.

In the psychiatric setting, antisocial personality disorder is viewed as one of the most difficult personality disorders to treat. Behavior therapy within very structured environments like prison may be useful. These patients may benefit from a therapeutic technique that attempts to channel their sensation-seeking behavior into more constructive activities (Liebowitz, Stone, and Turkat, 1986). These patients are at high risk for suicide, depression, alcoholism, and substance abuse. In the medical setting, their manipulative behavior and disregard for the staff make them particularly difficult to tolerate. While avoiding the temptation to be punitive, the physician should set limits and not be manipulated or deceived into prescribing excessive medications.

Borderline Personality Disorder

Borderline personality disorder encompasses a behavioral pattern of intense and chaotic relationships with fluctuating and extreme attitudes toward others. In the extreme form, these patients are affectively unstable and impulsive and engage in self-destructive behaviors and lack a clear sense of personal identity. Suicide attempts may be a frequent response to rejections or disappointments in their interpersonal relationships. They often alternate between viewing themselves—and others—as "all good" (idealizing) or as "all bad" (devaluing). Their personal lives tend to be chaotic, unstable, and marked by frequent disappointments and rejections. An underlying mood of chronic anger and depression is ubiquitous. These patients are prone to alcoholism and substance abuse.

During times of crisis or rejection, or under the influence of alcohol or substance abuse, these patients may experience transient psychotic breaks lasting from hours to days. They may show poor control of emotions and impulses that may result in aggressive and destructive behavior toward themselves and others. Borderline personality disorder frequently overlaps with histrionic, schizotypal, and antisocial personality disorders.

From a more subtle standpoint of interpersonal relationships, however, it should be noted that some individuals may show *traits* of borderline personality. These personality characteristics are best understood from a psychodynamic perspective, and include not only unstable personal relationships and chronic smoldering degrees of anger and depression but a tendency to either idealize or devalue others seeing them as "all good" or "all bad." They tend to rapidly alternate from idealizing others to rapidly devaluing them if their expectations of others are not fulfilled or if they are disappointed by them in some way. Permanent, close, and trusting relationships are difficult for these individuals—and what relationships they do have are often characterized by ambivalence.

When diagnosing a borderline patient, attention should be drawn to the possible coexistence of a mood, substance abuse, or eating disorders (Skodol and Oldham, 1991) that should be treated. Various treatment modalities have been used to treat borderline patients in the psychiatric setting. Although intensive, interpretive techniques may be useful, a more supportive, cognitive, and problem-solving approach may be most appropriate. Borderline patients frequently reenact struggles and traumas from childhood, which were often of a depriving or abusive nature, in their current relationships with their physicians by displays of excessive dependency, unrealistic expectations, anger, hostility, and suicidal depression when their emotional needs are not met.

Self-destructive behavior may be treated by behavioral techniques or medication if it is associated with disturbances of mood, impulse, or cognition. The physician must maintain an empathic attitude while setting fair and consistently enforced limits on disruptive, manipulative, or drug-seeking behaviors. Cognitive techniques may aid the patient in developing more realistic perceptions of self and others.

Pharmacotherapy may be useful to treat particular target symptoms. Antidepressants, lithium, and monoamine oxidase inhibitors may be valuable in the treatment of mood disturbances (Gunderson, 1986). Lithium may attenuate impulsive, self-destructive behavior as well as anger. Neuroleptics may lessen distorted cognition. The use of psychotropics in this population may be risky, however, because of these patients' tendency to impulsively attempt suicide by overdosing during crises.

Medical illness, like other stresses, may be met with reactions ranging from intense anger to overwhelming anxiety and depression. Borderline patients may be unclear as to the cause of their physical discomfort. They may blame the pain on others and may perceive painful procedures as hostile and inappropriately intrusive acts. Because of their increased anxiety, regressive behavior, and enhanced dependency in stressful situations, such patients may expect unrealistic and excessive degrees of attention from the staff. If their expectations are not met immediately, these patients may become increasingly hateful and angry.

Provocative and hostile behaviors, which include the tendency to devalue or feel devalued by caregivers, should be met by a stable and calm reaction rather than by a yielding to demands or a rejection of the patient. The physician can help by recognizing the dependency needs of these patients and by providing hope with a sense of stability. Psychiatric consultation may be useful if the patient's extreme response to illness cannot be adequately treated by the medical staff or is accompanied by psychotic symptoms and suicidal behavior. The staff should be educated to expect the patient's tendency to idealize some caregivers and devalue others. Open and continued communication among physicians and staff who are treating the patient is absolutely critical to prevent "splitting"—that is, playing one caregiver against another—which is a classic manipulative technique employed by these patients. Splitting may be detected when intense disagreements arise between health care providers over a patient in which uncharacteristically polarized positions about the patient's care develop—or where miscommunications and misperceptions occur. The "chaos" created by the borderline patient may lead to physicians and nurses "fighting over" a patient. This tendency of the borderline patient to "split"—or divide people in a controversial manner—can only be overcome by recognizing these patterns and helping the different groups of caretakers to carefully and openly communicate with each other.

Dependent Personality Disorder

Dependent personality encompasses a pattern of excessive reliance on others that is reflected in the affected person's tendency to permit others to make decisions for them, to feel helpless when alone, to subjugate their needs to those of others, to tolerate mistreatment, and to be unable to function when self-assertiveness is required. It is not uncommon for such a patient to be living with a controlling, domineering, overprotective, and infantalizing person. The avoidant and dependent personality disorders share the characteristics of interpersonal insecurity, desire for relationships, and low self-esteem.

These patients may benefit from insight-oriented, cognitive, and group therapy. Assertiveness and social skills training may also be useful for both dependent and avoidant patients. When medically ill, these individuals may complain about their suffering and clearly delineate how the physician is unable to allay it. Such patients may become angry and increasingly frustrated if their treatment fails to produce expected results. The dependent patient will often want the physician to "make all the decisions." When informing the patient about procedures, therefore, the physician should be prepared to be very active in treatment planning. Diagnosis of dependent personality disorder in the medical setting is difficult because physically ill patients often display an increase in dependent traits as part of the general behavioral regression that frequently accompanies physical illness.

Avoidant Personality Disorder

The avoidant patient is inhibited, introverted, shy, anxious, and fearful of closeness to and rejection by others. Additional features include low self-esteem, apprehension, social awkwardness, and a chronic fear of being embarrassed. The criteria for social withdrawal overlap with those for schizoid personality disorder. However, the schizoid patient is indifferent to others, whereas the avoidant person desires relationships yet is too shy and insecure to obtain them.

Both insight-oriented and cognitive techniques may benefit the avoidant patient. Assertiveness training and behavior therapy with exposure to the anxiety-producing stimulus may lessen fearfulness. Group therapy will aid the patient in overcoming social anxiety and in obtaining more interpersonal trust and rapport. Anxiety and depression, which may develop in avoidant patients, may be treated by anxiolytics and antidepressants, respectively, depending on their Axis I diagnosis (Liebowitz, Stone, and Turkat, 1986). Medical illness may be embarrassing to avoidant patients both because they have to discuss symptoms and because they are being forced into a new, contact-filled situation in the hospital. Although the avoidant patient will be more fearful at first, both this patient and the dependent person will soon become quite reliant upon and desiring of contact with the doctor. The physician will make the patient feel more at ease in the medical setting by developing an alliance in a timely manner. Such a patient may benefit from not having new and unfamiliar staff and students frequently in rounds at the bedside. Responding to the patient's anxiety with a calm and reassuring demeanor will significantly help the patient to deal with both illness and hospitalization. Physicians should nevertheless avoid taking on a patronizing or parent-like role in treating these individuals and should expect them to take responsibility for their treatment and to participate in the decision-making process.

Obsessive–Compulsive Personality

The person with obsessive–compulsive personality disorder tends to be perfectionistic, constricted, and excessively disciplined. Behavior is rigid, formal, emotionally cool, distant, intellectualizing, and detailed. These patients may be driven, aggressive, competitive, and impatient, with a chronic sense of time pressure and an inability to relax. They have an excessive tendency to be in control of themselves, others, and life situations. They are often tormented with anxiety over matters of uncertainty and ambiguity. Because of their need for perfection, they often have difficulty making decisions and are prone to procrastinate or "obsess." On the other hand, other types of obsessional patients have a hard-driving urge to do "everything now" and expect the same level of efficiency from others. An undercurrent of anger is often visible in their general demeanor, although open expression of anger—or any other emotion—is difficult for them. Superficially, these patients may appear to be drab and monotonous personalities who drone on about topics in excruciating detail. They are usually preoccupied with, and the withholding of, money. They are often "hoarders" of both money and other items.

Although stereotyping these individuals by occupation should be avoided, these individuals tend to gravitate toward occupations involving highly structured methods and techniques, such as accounting, mathematics, computers, and engineering. Although not proven by research, the legal and medical professions have been anecdotally considered to have more than their share of compulsive individuals.

These individuals are also likely to be overly concerned with productivity and achievement. They usually have rigid moralistic attitudes toward life—especially sexuality—and are prone to criticism and moralistic judgment of others because of their rigid superego. They may also be preoccupied with orderliness, neatness, and cleanliness and expect others to meet their expectations. Inflexibility, stubbornness, rigidity, and a need for control dominate their interpersonal relationships. Obsessive–compulsive personality *traits* are extremely common in the general population—particularly among men—and it is only when the traits occur with sufficient rigidity or severity so as to impair the individual's interpersonal relationships or personal functioning that such traits should be considered pathologic.

These patients can benefit from both insight-oriented and cognitive techniques. Following is a case vignette exemplifying such a patient.

A CASE VIGNETTE

A 50-year-old male lawyer with no prior medical history presented to the emergency room with crushing substernal chest pain, shortness of breath, and nausea. He reluctantly cancelled a business meeting to come for an evaluation. Laboratory studies and an electrocardiogram confirmed an acute myocardial infarction. The patient adamantly refused admission, stating that his work could not go unattended. His wife described him as a perfectionist "workaholic" who worked 7 days a week without vacations. He adhered to this rigid and demanding schedule and faulted those who did not subscribe to his standards and morals. He always prided himself on how he was in control of his business and personal affairs and could not allow his health to interfere with his obligations.

When managing a compulsive patient who has a medical problem, the physician must appreciate how illness might represent a disruption in the patient's work, orderly lifestyle, obligations, and sense of control. The patient's response may be to oscillate between minimizing the illness's importance and being overwhelmed with anxiety, anger, and fear of the unknown.

These patients usually will seek as much knowledge as possible about their condition so that they can plan their hospital stay and know exactly when they will be able to return to work. Unlike dependent patients, compulsive patients will not want the doctor to be the primary decision maker and will argue and bicker until they feel they are in control and can make their own decisions about their care. Physicians may approach these patients' overconcern with work by acknowledging the importance of their work but pointing out that inappropriate actions will have harmful consequences and that taking care of themselves will allow them to go on with their responsibilities—that recuperation is a form of "work" in itself. Recognition of these patients' tendencies should lead the physician to treat them by inviting their active cooperation and by providing them with enough information to facilitate a rational understanding of their disease and its treatment. The physician should deal with power struggles and stubbornness by "backing off" and putting decisions solely in the patient's hands.

Passive–Aggressive Personality Characteristics

Although not a formal and separate type of personality disorder in DSM-IV, passive–aggressive personality traits are reflected in a pattern of passive and indirect resistance to authority, responsibility, and obligations. Associated symptoms include complaining, irritability, whining, discontent, and disillusionment. Anger is usually expressed indirectly through resistance, delays, lack of responsiveness, negativism, procrastination, and undermining their own treatment.

Because these individuals cannot express their anger or resentment directly, they display hostile or resentful feelings by postponing or cancelling appointments, procrastinating over assignments and deadlines, not returning phone calls, withholding information, pouting, not paying bills, and being chronically late. When confronted with their actions or queried about being angry or resentful, the patient will usually deny any anger initially and evade dealing with the situation directly.

Social skills training and assertiveness training may help these patients develop alternative ways to deal with frustration. Insight-oriented therapy may be useful for such patients in helping them understand how they handle their anger and to facilitate them in developing a more direct and assertive manner. Direct assertiveness and expression of feelings would theoretically decrease the need for passive–aggressive behaviors in dealing with conflictual situations.

The passive–aggressive patient may undermine procedures and treatment plans suggested by the physician as noted above. It is important to avoid both the power struggles and the withdrawal from the patient that may arise in these circumstances. If the patient is allowed to have a say in treatment, he or she will likely become a more facilitating and active participant in the care.

SUMMARY

It should be emphasized again that while fully developed personality disorders perfectly matching DSM-IV criteria are relatively rare, it is nevertheless extremely common to see *traits* of the personality disorders described in this section in the general population. It is equally common to see various mixtures of the problematic personality traits described rather than seeing them in isolated or pure form. The clinical prototypes described in this chapter represent extremes, but even these disorders appear to overlap in the clinical setting leading to the diagnosis of "mixed personality disorder traits." Readers interested in more detailed descriptions of the personality disorders, including theories regarding their development and psychotherapeutic treatment, are referred to selected references in the Annotated Bibliography.

CLINICAL PEARLS

- A personality disorder is a constellation of intense chronic behavioral traits that result in enduring maladaptive behaviors across many situations.
- These disorders are not uncommon and will influence how a person reacts to the stress of medical illness; elements of a personality disorder are almost always exacerbated by stress and may subside when the crisis is over.
- Physicians who recognize their patients' personality styles and coping mechanisms will be in a better position to understand and appropriately respond to their characteristic responses to illness.
- Axis I and Axis II conditions frequently coexist, necessitating an evaluation for mood, anxiety, psychotic, and alcohol- and substance-abuse disorders.
- The hallmark of a personality disorder is repetitive patterns of problematic interpersonal relationships. Persons with severe personality disorders usually tend to deny their contribution to this pattern and externalize blame for their problems. They tend to *repeat* their mistakes because they fail to learn from them especially in regards to their own contribution to their interpersonal problems.
- A classic sign of when a physician is dealing with a personality disorder is when the doctor feels angry, frustrated, defeated, manipulated, or irritated by the patient. Patients with some types of personality disorders may be flirtatious and seductive yet "turn" on the physician suddenly.
- An objective analysis of the problematic aspects of the patient's behavior can usually only be achieved when the physician "backs off," gains some distance, and reviews the situation formally or informally with a colleague or psychiatric consultant.
- Effective management of patients with personality disorder traits depends, first, on assessing the problematic aspects of the personality and of how these are affecting compliance and the doctor–patient relationship, and second, on developing a plan adapted to accommodate the patient's personality style and characteristic ways of dealing with others.
- Adjunctive psychopharmacology agents may be helpful in treating concurrent Axis I disorders, but the patient's potential to overdose should be carefully assessed.

ANNOTATED BIBLIOGRAPHY

Charney DS, Nelson, CJ, Quinlan DM: Personality traits and disorder in depression. Am J Psychiatry 138:1601–1604, 1981

> A good description of the occurrence of Axis II pathology in depression.

Epstein S, O'Brien E: The person-situational debate in historical and current perceptive. Psychol Bull 988:513–537, 1985

> Highlights issues to be considered in diagnosing a personality disorder.

Fogel BS: Personality disorders in the medical setting. In Stoudemire A, Fogel BS (eds): Psychiatric Care of the Medical Patient. Oxford University Press, New York, 1993, pp 289–305

> Reviews in detail specific strategies for assessing and monitoring personality disorders in the medical setting.

Phohl B, Stangl D, Zimmerman M: The implication of DSM-III personality disorders for patients with major depression. J Affect Disord 7:309–319, 1984

> Emphasizes the effects of personality disorders on the outcome of depression.

Meissner WW: Theories of personality and psychopathology: Classical psychoanalysis. In Kaplan HI, Sadock BJ (eds): Comprehensive Textbook of Psychiatry, 4th ed., vol 1. Baltimore, Williams & Wilkins, 1985

> An in-depth overview of psychoanalytic perspectives on personality development and personality disorders.

Soloff PH, George A, Nathan RS et al: Progress in pharmacotherapy of borderline disorders. Arch Gen Psychiatry 43:691–697, 1986

> A comprehensive review of treatment options for borderline patients.

Stangl P, Pfohl B, Zimmerman M et al: A structured interview for the DSM-III personality disorders: A preliminary report. Arch Gen Psych 42:591–596, 1985

> Reviews the use of a structured instrument that is used to diagnose personality pathology.

Stoudemire A, Thompson TL: The borderline personality in the medical setting. Annals of Internal Medicine 96:76–79, 1982.

> Practical management of the borderline personality in the medical setting.

Weissman MM, Prusoff BA, Lkerman GL: Personality and the prediction of long-term outcome of depression. Am J Psychiatry 135:798–800, 1978

> Emphasizes the impact of personality pathology on outcome of depression.

Widiger T, Frances A, Spitzer R, Williams J: The DSM-IIIR Personality Disorders. An Overview. Am J Psychiatry 145:786–795, 1988.

> Offers an overview of the formulation of Axis II disorders.

REFERENCES

Allport G: Personality: A psychological interpretation. New York, Holt & Company, 1937 American Psychiatric Association: Diagnostic and statistical manual of mental disorder, 3rd edn., revised. Washington, DC, American Psychiatric Association, 1987

American Psychiatric Association: Diagnostic and Statistical Manual of Mental Disorders, 4th ed. Washington, DC, American Psychiatric Association, in press [1994]

Andrulonis PA, Glueck BC, Stroebel CF et al: Organic brain dysfunction and the borderline syndrome. Psychiatr Clin N Am 4:47–66, 1980

Bell J, Lycaki H, Jones P et al: Effect of preexisting borderline personality disorder on clinical and EEG sleep correlates of depression. Psychiatry Res 9:115–123, 1983

Coccaro EF, Siever LJ, Klar HM et al: Serotonergic studies in patients with affective and personality disorders. Arch Gen Psychiatry 46:587–599, 1989

Docherty JP, Fiester SJ, Shea T: Syndrome diagnosis and personality disorder. In Frances AJ, Hales RE (eds): American Psychiatric Association Annual Review, vol 5. Washington, DC, American Psychiatric Press, 1986

Dowson JH: Assessment of DSM III-R personality disorders by self report questionnaire: the role of informants and a screening test for comorbid personality disorders (STCPD). Br J Psychiatry 161:344–52, 1992

Frances AJ, Widiger T: The classification of personality disorders: An overview of problems and solutions. In Frances AJ, Hales RE (eds): American Psychiatric Association Annual Review, vol 5. Washington, DC, American Psychiatric Press, 1986

Gunderson J: Pharmacotherapy for patients with borderline personality disorder. Arch Gen Psychiatry 43:698–700, 1986

Holzman PS, Solomon C, Levin S et al: Pursuit eye movement dysfunction in schizophrenia. Arch Gen Psychiatry 41:136–140, 1984

Inderbitzin LB, James ME: Psychoanalytic Psychology. In Stoudemire A (ed) Human Behavior: An Introduction for Medical Students, 2nd ed. Philadelphia, Lippincott, 1994.

Kahana RL, Bibring GL: Personality types in medical management. In Zinberg NE (ed): Psychiatry and Medical Practice in a General Hospital. New York, International Universities Press, 1964

Kaplan H: History of psychosomatic medicine. In Kaplan H, Sadock J (eds): Comprehensive Textbook of Psychiatry/IV. London, Williams & Wilkins, 1983

Liebowitz MR, Stone MH, Turkat ID: Treatment of personality disorders. In Frances AJ, Hale RE (eds): American Psychiatric Association Annual Review, vol 5. Washington, DC, American Psychiatric Press, 1986

Meissner WW: Theories of personality and psychopathology: Classical psychoanalysis. In Kaplan HI, Sadock BJ (eds): Comprehensive Textbook of Psychiatry, 4th ed., vol 1. Baltimore, Williams & Wilkins, 1985

Merikangas KR, Weissman MM: Epidemiology of DSM-III Axis II Personality Disorders. In Frances AJ, Hales RE (eds): American Psychiatric Association Annual Review, vol 5, pp 258–278. Washington, DC, American Psychiatric Press, 1986

Miller GE, Prinz RJ: Enhancement of social learning family interventions for childhood conduct disorder. Psych Bull 108:291–307, 1990

Millon T: Disorders of personality: DSM-III Axis II. New York, Wiley, 1981

McGlashan TH: The borderline syndrome: II. Is it a variant of schizophrenia or affective disorder? Arch Gen Psychiatry 40:1319–1323, 1983

Nardo JM: The personality in the medical setting: A psychodynamic understanding. In Michels R, Cavenar JO, Brodie HKH et al (eds): Psychiatry. Philadelphia, JB Lippincott, 1986

Nestadt G, Romanoski AJ, Brown CH, Chahal R, Merchant A, Folstein MF, Gruenberg EM, McHugh PR: DSM III Compulsive personality disorder: an epidemiological survey. Psychol Med 21:461–71, 1991

Reynolds CF, Soloff PH, Kupfer DJ et al: Depression in borderline patients: A prospective EEG sleep study. Psychiatry Res 14:1–15, 1985

Roy A, Dejong J, Linnoila M: Cerebrospinal fluid monoanine metabolites and suicidal behavior in depressed patients. A five-year follow-up study. Arch Gen Psychiatry 46:609–612, 1989

Rutter M: Resilience in the face of adversity: Protective factors and resistance to psychiatric disorder. Br J Psychiatry 147:598–611, 1985

Siever LF, Klar H: A Review of DSM-III criteria for the personality disorders. In Frances AJ, Hales RE (eds): American Psychiatric Association Annual Review, vol 5. Washington, DC, American Psychiatric Press, 1986

Siever LJ, Coursey RD, Alterman IS et al: Clinical, psychophysiological, and neurological characteristics of volunteers with impaired smooth pursuit eye movements. Biol Psychiatry 26:35–51, 1989

Siever LJ, Coursey RD, Alterman IS et al: Smooth pursuit eye impairment: A vulnerability marker for schizotypal personality disorder in a volunteer population. Am J Psychiatry 141:1560–1566, 1984

Siever LJ, Keefe R, Bernstein DP et al: Eye tracking impairment in clinically identified patients with schizotypal personality disorder. Am J Psychiatry 142:740–745, 1990

Skodol AE, Oldham JM: Assessment and diagnosis of borderline personality disorder. Hosp Community Psychiatry 42:1021–8, 1991

Soloff PH, Anselm GWA, Nathan S: The dexamethasone suppression test in patients with borderline personality disorders. Am J Psychiatry 139:1621–1623, 1982

Stein JG: Drug treatment of the personality disorders. Br J Psychiatry 161:167–184, 1992

Sternbach HA, Fleming J, Exteen I et al: The dexamethasone suppression and thryrotropin-releasing hormone tests in depressed borderline patients. Psychoneuroendocrinology 8:459–462, 1983

Virkunnen M, DeJong J, Bartko J et al: Relationship of psychobiological variables to recidivism in violent offenders and impulsive fire setters. A follow-up study. Arch Gen Psychiatry 46:600–603, 1989

Widiger T, Frances A: Interviews and inventories for the measurement of personality disorders. Clin Psychol Rev 7:49–75, 1987

Widiger TA, Frances A: Personality disorders. In Talbott JA, Hales RE, Yudofsky S. (eds): Textbook of Psychiatry, pp 621–648. Washington, DC, American Psychiatric Press, 1988

Alan Stoudemire (ed). *Clinical Psychiatry for Medical Students,* Second Edition. Copyright © 1994, 1990 by J. B. Lippincott Company.

7 *Mood Disorders*

Emile D. Risby, S. Craig Risch, and Alan Stoudemire

The "mood disorders" are a heterogeneous group of clinical conditions. A mood disorder generally involves varying degrees of depression, elation, or irritability. Yet the presence of an altered mood in itself is not sufficient to warrant a diagnosis of a mood disorder. A formal psychiatric diagnosis of a mood disorder can be made only when a defined constellation of signs and symptoms occurs for a specified period of time and produces a certain degree of disability. Currently, the *Diagnostic and Statistical Manual of Mental Disorders* (DSM-IV) (APA 1993a, in press [1994]) provides the most widely used criteria for diagnosing psychiatric illnesses in the United States (see Chapter 1 by Drs. Yates, Kathol, and Carter). The DSM-IV identifies the following mood disorders: (1) adjustment disorder with depressed mood, (2) depressive disorders (which include major depressive disorder, depressive disorder unspecified, and dysthymic disorder), (3) bipolar disorders (which include bipolar I disorder, bipolar II disorder, bipolar disorder not otherwise specified, and cyclothymic disorder), (4) mood disorders due to general medical conditions, and (5) substance-induced mood disorders. Although not technically classified as a mood disorder in DSM-IV, premenstrual dysphoric disorder frequently presents with disturbances in the individual's mood. A diagram of the major mood disorders is depicted in Fig. 7–1.

The word "depression" is often used to describe an array of conditions, such as feelings of demoralization, disappointment, or transient psychological reactions to an injury or loss. In addition, the complaint of depression can be seen in almost every psychiatric disorder. The diagnosis of a depressive mood disorder, however, requires more than just the presence of depressive symptoms. Clinically, depression is a

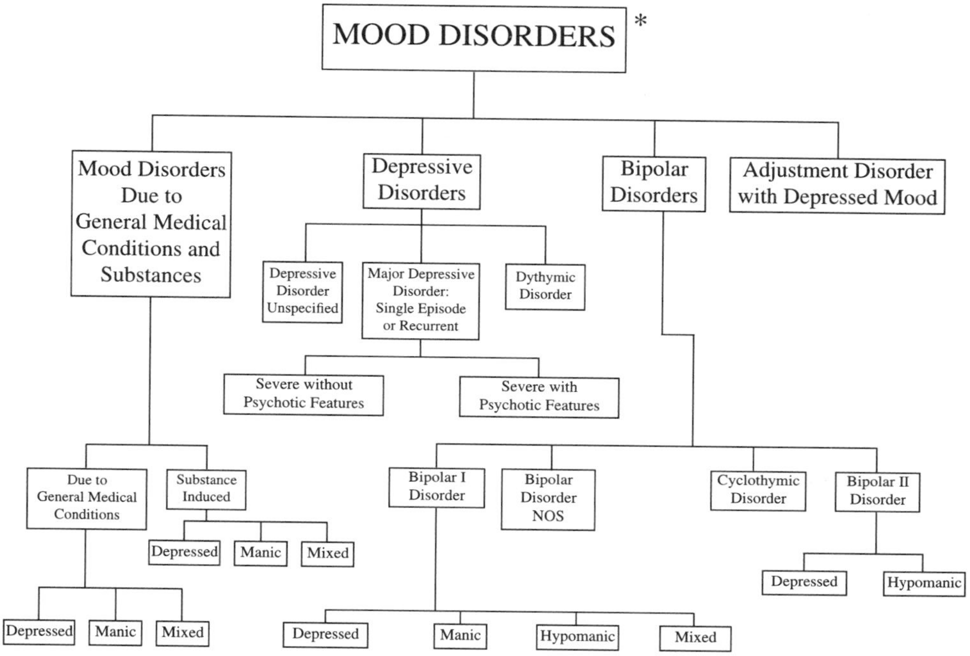

* Derived from DSM-IV (American Psychiatric Association 1993a; in press [1994])

Figure 7–1. *Major mood disorders.*

syndrome that is characterized by a mood disturbance, plus a variety of cognitive, psychological, somatic, and "vegetative" disturbances, which causes *significant impairments* in the individual's ability to function. And while there are numerous symptoms associated with the syndrome of depression, none (not even the complaint of "feeling depressed") is essential for the diagnosis!

The mood disturbance that is the opposite of depression is *mania*. Although a heightened sense of euphoria is typical, anger and irritability may be the predominant feature in some cases. The manic patient may be hyperverbal, hyperactive, overconfident, adventuresome, and irrational. And like some severely depressed individuals, manic patients may become delusional and psychotic.

EPIDEMIOLOGY OF MOOD DISORDERS

In 1980, the Epidemiologic Catchment Area Study (ECA) was initiated by the National Institutes of Mental Health. This study, which involved over 18,000 persons living in five communities, forms the basis of our current understanding of the epidemiology of the major psychiatric disorders in the United States. The ECA data reveals the following American community-based lifetime prevalence rates for the major mood disorders: major depression, 3.5 to 5.8%, with a higher prevalence in women than men; bipolar disorders, 0.7 to 1.6%, with the rates being similar in men and women; and dysthymia, 2.1 to 4.7%, with the rate being twice as high for women than for men (Robins and Regier, 1991). In general medical settings, which selects for patients with emotional distress and physical illness, the prevalence rates for depression have been reported to be as high as 15%. Some studies have estimated that at any given time 13 to 20% of the population has some symptoms of depression (Weissman, Boyd, 1984), and approximately 2 to 3% of the population is hospitalized or seriously impaired because of major mood disorders (Goodwin and Jamison, 1984). Thus, collectively, mood disorders constitute a major public health problem.

Adjustment Disorder with Depressed Mood

An adjustment disorder is a psychiatric disorder that occurs following an identifiable psychosocial stressor (such as a divorce, job loss, physical illness, or natural disaster). The individual's response to that stressor is considered to be extreme or in excess of what would normally be expected or results in significant impairments in the individual's social, occupational, or interpersonal functioning (Table 7–1). It is assumed that the symptoms will remit in time, either when the stressor(s) resolves or when a new level of coping (or adaptation) is reached. Strictly defined, the symptoms should not persist for more than 6 months after termination of the precipitating stressor(s) (APA, 1993a, in press [1994]). If the stressor persists for greater than 6 months, the adjustment disorder is specified as chronic rather than acute. In adjustment disorders with depressed mood, the typical symptoms are sadness, social isolation, difficulty concentrating, and preoccupation with the stressful events, as well as sleep and appetite disturbances. Although it is expected to resolve in time, an adjustment disorder with depressed mood is not necessarily an inconsequential mood disorder. Adjustment disorders may cause major disruptions in the patient's life and

Table 7–1 **Key Features of Adjustment Disorder***

The development of a psychological reaction to identifiable stressors or events.

The reaction reflects a change in the individual's normal personality and is different from the person's usual style of functioning.

The psychological reaction is "maladaptive" in that normal functioning (including social and occupational functioning) is markedly impaired or the reaction is greater than what would normally be expected of others in similar circumstances.

The psychological reaction does not represent an exacerbation of some other mental disorder.

The reaction begins within three months of the onset of the stressor(s) and resolves within six months after termination of the stressful precipitant.

* May present primarily as anxiety, depression, or mixed features. Summarized from DSM-IV Draft Criteria 3/1/93. See DSM-IV (APA 1993a, in press [1994]) for specific diagnostic criteria.

may be associated with severe dysphoria, despondency, suicidal ideations and suicide attempts.

There is no way to predict who will develop an adjustment disorder in the wake of adverse circumstances. The severity of the adjustment disorder does not always parallel the intensity of the precipitating event. The important factors appear to be the relevance or meaning of the event (stressor) to the individual and the ability of the individual to "cope" or manage the stress. Individuals with poor coping skills and inadequate social supports may be more prone to develop adjustment disorders than those with good coping skills and strong social supports.

In general, adjustment disorders with depressed mood are relatively transient and are not accompanied by the major cognitive symptoms seen in major depressions (see below). For example, patients with adjustment disorders feel bad about their situation but do not necessarily feel bad about themselves. And although adjustment disorders can generally be managed by the primary care provider, clergy, a friend, or a family member, the development of extreme withdrawal, hopelessness, suicidal ideations, or failure to improve as circumstances improve are clear indications for psychiatric referral. Treatment of adjustment disorders includes supportive psychotherapy, crisis-orientated psychosocial interventions, and occasionally time-limited pharmacotherapy to alleviate specific target symptoms (e.g., insomnia). Note that depressed mood is only one of the six types of maladaptive adjustment responses that may occur in response to a psychosocial stressor as defined by the DSM-IV.

Dysthymic Disorder

The essential feature of a dysthymic disorder is a *chronically* depressed mood (or possibly an irritable mood in children or adolescents), present for most of the day and occurring on more days than not for at least 2 years (or 1 year for children or adolescents). However, the severity of the mood disturbance does not meet the criteria for major depression (see below). Brief periods of normal mood may be present within the 2-year diagnostic period for adults but should not have lasted more than 2 months. In addition to a depressed mood, there must be some associated symptoms such as low self-esteem, feelings of inadequacy, hopelessness, pessimism, guilt, social withdrawal, decreased productivity, low energy, and difficulty with concentration and memory (Table 7–2). The diagnosis is not made if there is clear evidence of a major depressive episode during the first 2 years of the disturbance, if the disturbance is superimposed on another psychiatric disorder, or if it is judged to be induced by a concurrent medical problem or medication. Dysthymia is designated as either early or late onset, based on the development of the illness before or after age 21 (APA 1993a, in press [1994]).

The differentiation of dysthymia from major depression can be difficult (Table 7–3). Remember, the depressed mood of dysthymia is chronic (at least two years), often without a clear onset, is relatively persistent (patient has only brief periods of relief from depression), and is not associated with psychotic symptoms. The mood disturbance in patients with major depression (as will be discussed in detail later) generally has a period of identifiable onset, is often episodic in nature (with periods of normal functioning between episodes), and may reach psychotic proportions. Al-

Table 7–2 **Key Features of Dysthymic Disorder***

A chronic, mildly depressed mood state that is generally present most of the day, on more days than not, for a period of at least two years (one year in children and adolescents).

There is never a two-month period where there are no depressive symptoms.

The depression is associated with at least three of the following symptoms:
- low self-esteem or feelings of inadequacy
- feeling of pessimism or hopelessness
- generalized loss of interest or pleasure
- social withdrawal
- chronic fatigue or tiredness
- feelings of guilt or brooding about the past
- irritability or excessive anger
- decreased activity or productivity
- poor concentration or difficulty making decisions

There is no evidence of a major depressive episode during the first two years of the disturbance. No history of bipolar disorder and no other major mental disorder is responsible for the patient's symptoms.

There is no physical cause of the patient's depressive symptoms.

*   Adapted from DSM-IV Draft Criteria 3/1/93 (APA 1993a, in press [1994]).

though patients with dysthymia may be socially and occupationally impaired, they are often able to function (e.g., work) and the severity of their symptoms rarely warrant hospitalization. In contrast, patients with major depression are often severely incapacitated by their depression. It is possible, however, for patients with dysthymia to develop a major depressive episode. This combination of dysthymia and major depression is often referred to as a "double depression" (Keller, Lavori, and Endicott, 1983).

There is no universally accepted conceptual framework for the etiology of dysthymia. From a psychological and behavioral perspective, dysthymia may be secondary to poor self-esteem that could have been caused by a lack of nurturing, love, or acceptance during early childhood. Other developmental experiences thought to lead to dysthymia include early parental loss through death or divorce, neglect, sexual

Table 7–3 **Depressive Disorders**

	ADJUSTMENT DISORDER	DYSTHYMIA	MAJOR DEPRESSIVE EPISODE
onset	sudden	no identifiable onset (no history of sustained normal mood during adulthood)	gradual onset (but period of normal functioning during adulthood can be identified)
precipitating event	always	none	occasionally
duration	less than 6 months	at least 2 years	2 weeks to 2 years
response to treatment	good	poor	good

and/or physical abuse, and alcoholism in the home. (Many of these same developmental factors have been identified in patients with major depression as well.) Excessive criticism from parents could be incorporated into the child's own conscience (superego) and cause the development of a personality marked by harsh self-criticism and low self-esteem. These individuals often feel inadequate, unlovable, insecure, and lack the ability to appreciate their value to others. In addition, dysthymics often experience problems in their interpersonal relationships. The combination of dysphoria, low self-esteem, and poor interpersonal relationships often places the dysthymic at an increased risk for substance abuse and suicide.

There are some patients with dysthymia whose depressive symptoms may respond to antidepressant medications, thereby suggesting a biological etiology for at least some of the symptoms in some patients (Akiskal, 1983). Therefore, treatment of the dysthymic patient may include insight-oriented psychotherapy, cognitive therapy, behavioral therapy, and pharmacotherapy. Psychopharmacology may be particularly helpful in those patients with a positive family history of mood disorders and evidence of abnormal neuroendocrine functioning (see below).

Major Depressive Episodes (Unipolar and Bipolar)

Major depression is a serious and often disabling psychiatric disorder. The hallmarks of depression are a subjective sense of dysphoria (sadness) and a loss of interest or pleasure in all activities and pastimes that were previously enjoyed (anhedonia). Depressed individuals often feel discouraged, defeated, helpless, hopeless, and unable to cope with the stresses of everyday life. Severely depressed individuals may find it impossible to motivate themselves to carry out even the most common day-to-day tasks. And while these symptoms of a depressed mood are usually the most prominent feature in many patients with major depression, the essence of the diagnosis is the recognition that major depression is a *syndrome*. The syndrome includes not only a disturbance in mood, but other associated symptoms such as an appetite disturbance; sleep disturbance; psychomotor disturbance; decreased energy; decreased libido; feelings of worthlessness or guilt; difficulty with concentration, memory, or thinking; and thoughts of death or suicide (Weissman and Klerman, 1992; Preskorn, Burke, 1992). Depressed patients may begin to think of themselves in negative terms, to feel like failures, or to believe that their families would be better off without them. The thought processes of some severely depressed people may become so distorted that their thinking becomes delusional and psychotic. Physical activity may be either decreased (psychomotor retardation) or purposefully increased (psychomotor agitation).

Although a depressed mood is frequently the most common complaint in depressed patients, a *subjective* sense of a depressed mood may not be present in every patient who has a major depression. Elderly patients in particular may complain of anxiety, irritability, weakness, or multiple somatic complaints, rather than verbalize complaints of depression per se. Somatic symptoms of depression can involve practically every organ system and include pain (headaches, backaches), gastrointestinal complaints, neurologic complaints (dizziness, numbness), and general fatigue and lethargy. It is important to remember that major depression may present with somatic symptoms as the predominant complaint (see Diagnosis and Treatment of Mood Disorders in the Medical Setting, below). The diagnostic criteria for a major depressive episode are listed in Table 7–4.

The course or natural history of major depression is quite variable. While some people will have only a single episode of depression with full recovery to premorbid levels of functioning, many depressed patients will eventually have another episode. Some people have episodes separated by many years of normal functioning; others have clusters of episodes followed by periods of remission; still others have increasingly frequent episodes as they grow older (APA 1993a, in press [1994]).

During the past decade, researchers and clinicians have become increasingly aware that some major depressions, which were once thought to consist of discrete episodes followed by full recovery, may become chronic in some patients. In the ECA Study, 20% of subjects diagnosed with depression on initial assessment were still depressed one year later. Significantly higher rates of persistent depression were found in women, in subjects who were 30 years old or older, who had more than ten prior episodes, and who had a high co-morbidity index (Katon and Schulberg, 1992). Data from another major study, the Clinical Studies of the National Institute of Mental Health Collaborative Program on the Psychobiology of Depression (the Collaborative Depression Study or CDS), revealed that only 50% of the patients recovered from their major depressive episode in one year, and in the remaining patients, the probability of

Table 7–4 **Key Features of Major Depressive Episodes***

At least two-week period of maladaptive functioning that is a clear change from previous levels of functioning. At least five of the following symptoms must be present during that two-week period, one of which must be (a) or (b).
a) depressed mood
b) inability to experience pleasure or markedly diminished interest in pleasurable activities
c) appetite disturbance with weight change (change > 5% of body weight within one month)
d) sleep disturbance
e) psychomotor disturbance
f) fatigue or loss of energy
g) feelings of worthlessness or excessive or inappropriate guilt
h) diminished ability to concentrate or indecisiveness
i) recurrent thoughts of death or suicidal ideations

The mood disturbance causes marked distress and or significant impairment in social or occupational functioning.

There is no evidence of a physical or substance-included etiology for the patient's symptoms or presence of another major mental disorder that accounts for the patient's depressive symptoms.

* Summarized from DSM-IV Draft Criteria 3/1/93. See DSM-IV (APA 1993a, in press [1994]) for specific diagnostic criteria.

recovery declined with each subsequent year, such that the probability of recovery by the fourth year, after not recovering for three years, was only 18%. Thus, almost one-fifth of the subjects in the CDS cohort remained chronically ill for up to four years (Keller and Baker, 1992).

As previously mentioned, even in patients who recover from a major depressive episode, there is a high probability of recurrence, and each new episode carries renewed risks of chronicity, psychosocial impairment, and suicide (Thase, 1992). In the CDS project, one-quarter of the patients who recovered during the first year of follow-up had relapses within 12 weeks of recovery. The one very strong factor that predicted relapse was a history of three or more previous episodes of major depression (Keller and Baker, 1992). Corollary clinical observations indicate that psychosocial stressors are often (but not always) identifiable before the first affective episodes but become increasingly less apparent with later episodes. Hence, as the illness evolves, relapses appear to occur independently of life events (reviewed by Gold, Goodwin, and Chrousos, 1988a).

Recognition of depression in geriatric populations may be more difficult than in nongeriatric populations. According to the ECA Study, depressive symptoms occur in approximately 15% of community residents over 65 years of age (NIH Consensus Development Panel on Depression in Late Life, 1992). In the elderly, both clinicians and patients may incorrectly assume that some depressive symptoms are expected with aging. For example, because of declining physical abilities, medical illnesses, and social and economic difficulties, it is easy to conclude that depression is a normal consequence of these problems. Remember that many of these problems may be a consequence of depression (or at least made worse by depression) rather than being the cause of depression per se. Also remember that depressed elderly persons are more apt to report somatic symptoms rather than to complain of a depressed mood. Depression in the elderly is discussed in detail in Chapter 11 by Drs. Bienenfeld and Welton.

After a diagnosis of depression has been made the clinician should further characterize the syndrome if possible, into a specific subtype of depression such as unipolar or bipolar; melancholic or nonmelancholic; psychotic or nonpsychotic; or as a predominance of "atypical" features. Some of these subtypes tend to respond to different forms of treatment. Thus, identification of these subtypes can aid the clinician in determining the most appropriate treatment plan for the patient. The presence of mania or hypomania defines bipolar disorder (see below). Melancholic depression, which crosses the boundaries of unipolar and bipolar illnesses, accounts for 40 to 60% of all hospitalizations for depression (Klerman, 1984) and is characterized by anhedonia, excessive or inappropriate guilt, early morning awakening, anorexia, psychomotor disturbance, and diurnal variation in mood. The depressed melancholic patient may appear frantic, fearful, agitated, or withdrawn. Psychotic depressions are characterized by the presence of delusions and/or hallucinations and can also be seen in both unipolar and bipolar patients. Psychotic depressions are not rare and studies suggest that approximately 10 to 25% of patients hospitalized for major depression, especially geriatric patients, have psychotic symptoms (Schatzberg, 1992). Atypical depressions denote neurovegetative symptoms that are generally the opposite of what is seen in melancholia, such as hypersomnia rather than insomnia, hyperphagia (sometimes with carbohydrate craving) rather than anorexia, and reactivity (mood changes with environmental circumstances) and a long-standing pattern of interpersonal rejection sensitivity. Patients with atypical depressions are also frequently reported to have an anxious or irritable mood rather than dysphoria (reviewed by Preskorn and Burke, 1992).

BIOLOGICAL ABNORMALITIES SEEN IN DEPRESSION

Sleep Abnormalities in Depression

The abnormal sleep of depressed patients was one of the earliest findings in biological psychiatry. Sleep may be monitored electroencephalographically and is divided into rapid eye movement (REM) and nonREM sleep (stages 1 to 4). The first REM period usually begins after a period of 70 to 100 minutes of nonREM sleep, which is followed by another 3 to 5 REM periods that usually occur in the latter part of the night. The REM periods generally increase in length as the night progresses (Gold, Goodwin, and Chrousos, 1988b; see also Chapter 22 by Dr. Doghramji).

There are a number of sleep abnormalities that distinguish endogenous ("biologic") depressives from nonendogenous (reactive, situational, or characterological) depressives and normal subjects. Endogenous depressives tend to have prolonged sleep latency (the period of time between going to bed and falling asleep), shortened REM latency (the period of time from the onset of sleep to the first REM period), increased wakefulness, decreased arousal threshold, early morning awakening, and reduced stages 3 and 4 sleep (Coble et al, 1976; Gillin et al, 1979). With respect to REM sleep, in addition to a shorter REM latency (i.e., 30 to 60 minutes instead of 90 minutes), depressed patients may have a redistribution of REM sleep with most of the REM occurring in the first half of the night rather than the second half (Reynolds and Kupfer, 1987) (Table 7–5). These abnormal REM latencies tend to normalize with clinical recovery from depression (Kupfer et al, 1983).

Neuroendocrine Abnormalities in Depression

One of the most frequently reported biologic abnormalities in patients with major depression (particularly those with melancholia) is hyperactivity of the hypothalamic-pituitary-adrenal (HPA) axis, resulting in elevated plasma cortisol levels and loss of normal feedback mechanisms that inhibit adrenocorticotropic hormone (ACTH) (Carroll, 1977; Gold, Goodwin, and Chrousos, 1988b; Nemeroff et al, 1984). The dexamethasone suppression test (DST) is frequently used to access HPA feedback mechanisms (Arano et al, 1985). Dexamethasone is a synthetic corticosteroid that, when given orally, usually suppresses plasma ACTH and cortisol levels for at least 24 hours. In the evaluation of depression, the DST is performed by giving 1 mg dexamethasone at 2300 hours and then drawing plasma cortisol levels at 1600 and 2300 hours the next day. Depressed patients may initially show a normal suppression of blood cortisol (below 5 μg/dl) following dexamethasone, but often escape from suppression signifi-

Table 7–5 **Sleep Abnormalities in Depression**

NON-REM CHANGES IN DEPRESSION

1. Prolonged sleep latency (the period of time between going to bed and falling asleep)
2. Shortened REM latency (the period of time from the onset of sleep to the first REM period)
3. Increased wakefulness
4. Decreased arousal threshold
5. Early morning awakening
6. Reduced stages 3 and 4 sleep

REM SLEEP CHANGES IN DEPRESSION

1. Shorter REM latency (i.e., 30 to 60 minutes instead of 90 minutes)
2. A redistribution of REM sleep to the first half of the night, rather than the second half

cantly earlier than normal. Therefore they may not show suppression when tested 17 to 24 hours later. This nonsuppression 24 hours following administration appears to be more common in the melancholic subgroup (Carroll, 1982). A number of studies have demonstrated that normalization of the dexamethasone suppression test may accompany or precede clinical recovery from depression (Holsboer et al, 1982; Targum, 1983). It has also been observed that a patient who appears to have recovered from depression but fails to suppress cortisol after dexamethasone administration may be at higher risk for relapse. Unfortunately, nonsuppression is not specific for depression, and there may be many false–positive as well as false–negative results. Nonetheless, nonsuppression of the DST may be a helpful variable to consider when faced with difficult diagnostic and/or treatment decisions.

Abnormalities in the thyroid axis have also been reported in depressed patients. Several studies have demonstrated that the normally expected increase in plasma concentrations of thyroid-stimulating hormone (TSH) following an infusion of thyrotropin-releasing hormone (TRH) is blunted in approximately 25% of patients with major depression and tends to normalize with clinical recovery (Loosen and Prange, 1982).

Other neuroendocrine abnormalities often reported in depressed patients are a blunting of the increase in plasma growth hormone induced by alpha-2 adrenergic receptor agonist (reviewed by Willner, 1985) and a blunting in the serotonin-mediated increase in plasma prolactin (reviewed by Lichtenberg et al, 1992; Shapira et al, 1992) (Table 7–6). It should be emphasized that none of these neuroendocrine abnormalities are true "biologic markers" for depression as many patients with a diagnosis of depression will have normal neuroendocrine functioning.

THEORIES OF DEPRESSION

Most studies agree that the likelihood of having an episode of depression is increased five- or sixfold in the six months following stressful "life events." Although reliable, the relationship between life events and depression is not particularly strong.

Table 7–6 **Neuroendocrine Abnormalities in Depression**

1. Hyperactivity of the hypothalamic-pituitary-adrenal (HPA) axis, resulting in elevated plasma cortisol levels and nonsuppression of cortisol following dexamethasone (DST).
2. *Blunting** of the normally expected increase in plasma concentrations of thyroid stimulating hormone (TSH) following an infusion of thyrotropin-releasing hormone (TRH).
3. *Blunting* of the normally expected increase in plasma growth hormone induced by alpha-2 adrenergic receptor agonist.
4. *Blunting* of serotonin-mediated increases in plasma prolactin.

* The term "blunting" refers to decreased physiologic responsiveness

In fact, life events appear to account for at most 10% of the variance in the incidence of depression (Lloyd, 1980). Thus, while many episodes of depression occur during times of stress, only a minority of persons encountering such difficulties develop major depressive episodes, suggesting that there are underlying biological vulnerability factors in those that do (Belsher and Costello, 1987).

A number of factors have been identified that appear to put a person "at increased risk" for developing depression. These variables include the individual's social support system, a history of early parental loss, gender, and a family history of depression. The absence of a positive social support system may predispose an individual to depression (Aneshensel and Stone, 1982; Williams, Ware, and Donald, 1981), and the belief that social reinforcement contributes to psychological well-being is generally well accepted. Although there does not appear to be any single personality trait that is common among all depressives, one psychological attribute that does appear to predispose to depression is introversion, a personality trait that is associated with a decrease in social contacts and support (Akiskal, Hirschfeld, and Yerevanian, 1983). The status of childhood loss as a factor predisposing to depression is controversial. A review by Lloyd (1980), which considered specifically the effects of childhood bereavement, concluded that parental loss in childhood, particularly maternal loss, was associated with a two- to threefold increase in the likelihood of developing an adult depression. More recent research, however, has indicated that the quality of home life in which the parent loss occurred is the most critical variable in determining vulnerability to psychiatric illness in later life (Breier et al, 1988). In regard to gender and depression, women are generally reported to have a two- to threefold higher rate of depression than men (Boyd, Weissman, 1981; Hirschfeld, Cross, 1982). The reasons for this sex difference are not entirely clear. Some investigators have suggested that social or hormonal factors may contribute to the higher incidence of depression in women.

In regard to stressful life events producing "biochemical" depressions, animal studies suggest that exposure to stressful events may sensitize neurotransmitter systems to subsequent stressors (Anisman and Zacharako, 1982). Thus, individuals whose neurologic system has already been sensitized (e.g., because of early parental loss or previous stress) or who have a genetic propensity to develop depression (see Heritability, below), may be more sensitive to a multiplicity of unspecified stressors throughout life that may initiate the cascade of neurophysiological and psychological events characteristic of depression. Therefore, depressions appear to result from the accumulation of psychological, biological, and environmental factors.

A model that attempts to account for many of the longitudinal features of mood disorders is the neurophysiologic "kindling-sensitization" hypothesis advanced by Post and colleagues (Post et al, 1981). In this model, repeated exposures to stress and/ or repeated neurochemical and neuroendocrine changes that accompany an episode of depression may "sensitize" key limbic substrates that integrate affective experiences (e.g., the induction of tearful affect). The potential neurobiologic ravages of each new episode of severe depression, coupled with stress-induced or age-related changes, may permanently alter limbic and various central neurotransmitter systems. The resultant progressive sensitization of limbic substrates may account for many of the trends seen in mood disorders, including the predisposition to develop depression as a result of early stressful experiences, the gradual worsening of affective episodes over time, the progressively shorter latency between an episode's onset and its peak severity, the tendency for the frequency of bipolar mood swings to increase, and the gradual attainment of autonomy and spontaneity (lack of obvious stressors). The prophylactic efficacy of the anticonvulsants carbamazepine and valproic acid (which inhibit certain kindled seizures) in bipolar illness lends support to this hypothesis (Post, 1992; Thase, 1992).

Cognitive Theory of Depression

According to cognitive learning theories, depressed patients have a cognitive style that focuses on what is wrong or negative rather than on what is right or positive. Beck (1974) described a cognitive triad in depression consisting of a person's (1) negative view of self, (2) negative interpretation of experiences, and (3) negative expectation of the future. Thus, in Beck's cognitive model, people are depressed because of their negative view of themselves, the world, and the future. In this model, depressions are viewed as a form of thought disorder of which dysphoric mood is a secondary manifestation, in contrast to the traditional view of depression as a primary mood disorder (Willner, 1985). According to Beck's theory, once a state of depression is established, information processing is biased in such a negative way that the negative mood is reinforced and maintained. Low self-esteem may lead the depressed individual to see himself or herself as being unworthy of pleasure, praise, or reward. Depressed patients do tend to underestimate positives, overestimate negatives, recall more unpleasant memories, have a decreased ability to experience pleasure, and have an increased sensitivity to adverse events. Beck's model may explain the etiology of depressive symptoms in many patients with dysthymia or mild depressions, although it does not seem to account for many of the genetic or biological features seen in many patients with major depressive episodes. (Cognitive psychotherapy is discussed in Chapter 17.)

NEUROTRANSMITTER HYPOTHESIS

Much of the biological literature on depression focuses on the monoamine neurotransmitters norepinephrine (NE), dopamine (DA), and serotonin (5-hydroxytryptamine, 5-HT). Norepinephrine and dopamine are catecholamines, while serotonin is an indoleamine. The catecholamines are degraded by two enzymes, monoamine oxidase (MAO) and catechol-O-methyltransferase (COMT), which produce a variety of breakdown products. However, the degradation of 5-HT is much simpler with MAO producing 5-hydroxyindoleacetic acid (5-HIAA) as the sole breakdown product. The catecholamines and 5-HT are stored in synaptic vesicles and are released when a nerve impulse invades the terminal. The major mechanism for clearing the released neurotransmitter from the synapse is via presynaptic neuronal reuptake, not enzymatic degradation. Following reuptake, much of the neurotransmitter is recycled into the "functional pool" to be reused by the neuron (Willner, 1985).

Norepinephrine and the Catecholamine Hypothesis

The first major hypothesis to address the biologic basis of depression emerged from the observation that approximately 15% of the patients who were treated for hypertension with the biogenic amine-depleting agent reserpine developed depression (Bunney, Davis, 1965; Schildkraut, 1978). Subsequently, drugs that were known to enhance noradrenergic functioning, such as the MAO inhibitors, amphetamines, and the cyclic antidepressants (Hertting et al, 1961), were all found to have antidepressant properties. These observations gave rise to the original catecholamine hypothesis of major depression, which stated that depression resulted from a functional deficit of norepinephrine at critical effector sites in the central nervous system (Schildkraut, 1978).

Although this theory seemed highly plausible given the above observations, there are some additional observations that do not fully support the hypothesis. For example, drugs that interfere with noradrenergic transmission or block catecholamine synthesis do not regularly produce depression in most subjects (note that only 15% of reserpine-treated patients got depressed) (Willner, 1985). Another issue is the time course for antidepressant effects. Blockade of monoamine reuptake or MAO inhibition occurs within hours or days after administration of the antidepressant, but the clinical effects do not usually appear until after 2 to 4 weeks of treatment. To further complicate matters, attempts to demonstrate abnormalities in norepinephrine activity by measuring plasma, urine, and cerebrospinal fluid concentrations of norepinephrine and its major metabolite 3-methoxy-4-hydroxy-phenylglycol (MHPG) have produced conflicting data. Decreases, a lack of change, and even increases in noradrenergic parameters have been reported in depressed subjects compared to normal controls (Davis, Bresnahan, 1987; Jimerson et al, 1983; Mass et al, 1987; Redmond et al, 1986; Roy et al, 1985). Furthermore, chronic treatment (two to three weeks) with most antidepressants reduces the physiologic sensitivity (Vetulani et al, 1976) and number of central beta-adrenergic receptors in the brain of rodents (Banerjee et al, 1977; Smith et al,

1981). This reproducible finding suggests that the efficacy of antidepressants is related to or coincident with downregulation of beta-adrenergic receptor function in the CNS (Maggi et al, 1980; Sulser et al, 1978; Vetulani et al, 1976). In short, these findings do not support the belief that depression is secondary to a generalized decrease in noradrenergic function (Table 7–7). Interestingly, many of the symptoms and physiological changes characteristic of melancholia are strikingly similar to what is seen in acute stress responses. Hence, it has been proposed that the intense arousal, psychomotor agitation, lack of reactivity of mood, decreased sleep, and decreased appetite seen in many melancholic patients might represent a pathological activation of noradrenergic and neurobiological systems (Kling et al, 1989). Nonetheless, the catecholamine hypothesis has had a significant impact on the field of psychiatry and has fostered a cascade of biological investigations into the etiology and treatment of psychiatric illnesses.

Indoleamine Hypothesis of Depression

A burgeoning literature has accumulated over the past three decades implicating the importance of central serotonergic neurotransmission in both the pathophysiology of depression and in the mechanism of action of antidepressant drugs (Table 7–8). The serotonin system is thought to be functionally deficient in depressed patients based on numerous studies revealing: (1) decreases in brain concentrations of serotonin and decreases in CSF concentrations of 5-HIAA in a sizable subgroup of depressed patients; (2) alterations in both presynaptic and postsynaptic central serotonergic receptors in depressed patients; and (3) most antidepressant agents increase the efficacy of CNS serotonin neurotransmission (Risch and Nemeroff, 1992).

Table 7–7 **Noradrenergic Theory of Depression**

DATA SUPPORTING THE THEORY
1. Approximately 15% of patients treated for hypertension with reserpine develop depression.
2. Drugs that enhance noradrenergic functioning (such as stimulants) are often found to have some antidepressant properties.

DATA AGAINST THE THEORY
1. Drugs that interfere with noradrenergic transmission, or block catecholamine synthesis, do not regularly produce depression in most subjects.
2. Blockade of norepinephrine reuptake or MAO inhibition by antidepressant drugs occur within hours or a few days after administration of the antidepressant, but the clinical effects do not usually appear until after 2 to 4 weeks of treatment.
3. Attempts to demonstrate abnormalities in norepinephrine activity by measuring plasma, urine, and cerebrospinal fluid concentrations of norepinephrine and its major metabolite 3-methoxy-4-hydroxy-phenylglycol (MHPG) have produced conflicting data.
4. Chronic treatment with most antidepressants reduces the physiologic sensitivity and number of central beta-adrenergic receptors.

Table 7–8 Data Supporting Serotonin Dysfunction in Major Depression

1. Decreased concentrations of brain serotonin and CSF 5-HIAA in many depressed patients.
2. Most antidepressant agents have been shown to increase the efficacy of central serotonin neurotransmission.
3. Reduction in both central and peripheral 5-HT reuptake sites has been found in depressed subjects.
4. Neuroendocrine challenges have demonstrated that the postsynaptic serotonin-mediated stimulation of prolactin is blunted in depressed patients.

A subgroup of approximately 40% of depressed patients exhibit low concentrations of brain serotonin and its metabolite 5-HIAA (Gibbons and Davis, 1986); and depressed patients with low CSF concentrations of 5-HIAA are more likely to have attempted suicide than depressives with normal 5-HIAA levels (Asberg and Traskman, 1981; Banki and Arato, 1983). Yet low 5-HT turnover may not be specific for depression per se. Low levels of CSF 5-HIAA have also been noted in prison populations and in military personnel with a history of aggressive thinking and behavior. Thus, rather than being associated with depression specifically, it appears that low CSF 5-HIAA may be related to aggression or poor impulse control, which is frequently known to present clinically as suicidal or sociopathic behavior (Willner, 1985; Golden et al, 1991).

Another finding is that low 5-HT turnover (low 5-HIAA) does not appear to be a phenomenon that accompanies an episode of depression, but rather is a state-independent marker that confers a predisposition to becoming depressed. Bipolar patients have been shown to have low CSF 5-HIAA levels while in their manic phase (Banki, 1977; Copper et al, 1972; Mendels et al, 1972). When low CSF levels of 5-HIAA are observed in depressed patients, they usually remain low during periods of remission (Goodwin, Post, and Murphy, 1973; Mendels et al, 1972; van Praag and DeHaan, 1979). In addition, low CSF levels of 5-HIAA may also correlate with a family history of depression in healthy volunteers (Sedvall et al, 1980).

Further support for the role of 5-HT in the pathophysiology of depression is the finding that in many depressed patients there appears to be a reduction in both central and peripheral 5-HT reuptake sites (Risch and Nemeroff, 1992). Because reuptake of the transmitter is the primary method for replenishing the "functional pool," a decrease in reuptake may lead to an eventual decrease in the total amount of available transmitter. Furthermore, as already noted above, neuroendocrine challenges have demonstrated that the postsynaptic serotonin-mediated stimulation of prolactin is blunted in depressed patients.

In summary, multidisciplinary approaches have provided data that support the hypothesis that reductions in serotonergic neurotransmission are associated with a state of depression and successful pharmacologic treatment of depression is associated with enhanced CNS serotonergic neurotransmission (Blier et al, 1987; Risch and Nemeroff, 1992).

BIPOLAR DISORDERS

The presence of mania or hypomania defines bipolar disorder. Mania is a distinct period during which the predominant mood is either elevated, expansive, or irritable, with several associated symptoms such as hyperactivity, pressured speech, racing thoughts, inflated self-esteem, decreased need for sleep, distractibility, and excessive involvement in potentially dangerous activity. In addition, psychotic symptoms such as delusions or perceptual disturbances (hallucinations) may be seen in the acutely manic patient. In mania, the mood disturbance is severe and causes marked impairment in social or occupational functioning (APA 1993a, in press [1994]; Weissman and Klerman, 1992) (Table 7–9). In hypomania, many of the features of mania may be present but the mood disturbance is less severe. At times it may be difficult to differentiate severe hypomania from mania (Table 7–10). Remember, if there are psychotic symptoms or if there is *marked impairment* in normal functioning such that hospitalization is necessary, then the condition has crossed the line into full-blown mania (Table 7–10).

There are two major subtypes of bipolar patients: bipolar I and bipolar II disorders. Bipolar I disorder identifies a patient who has had at least one true manic episode. A history of depression or hypomania may also be present in the bipolar I patient, but neither of these conditions is essential for the diagnosis. Remember, documentation of a bona fide manic episode is all that is needed to make the diagnosis of bipolar I disorder.

In bipolar II disorder, there is a history of hypomania and major depressive episodes but no history of mania. The category "bipolar disorder not otherwise

---

Table 7–9 **Key Features of Bipolar Disorder: Manic Episode***

A distinct period of abnormally and persistently elevated, expansive, or irritable mood, lasting at least one week, and is of sufficient severity to cause marked impairment in social or occupational functioning.

During the period of the mood disturbance, at least three of the following symptoms are also present:

a) grandiosity
b) decreased need for sleep
c) hyperverbal or pressured speech
d) flight of ideas or racing thoughts
e) distractibility
f) increase in goal-directed activity or psychomotor agitation
g) excessive involvement in pleasurable activities that have a high potential for painful consequences

There is no evidence of a physical or substance-induced etiology or the presence of another major mental disorder to account for the patient's symptoms.

---

* Summarized from DSM-IV Draft Criteria 3/1/93. See DSM-IV (APA 1993a, in press [1994]) for specific, diagnostic criteria.

Table 7–10 **Key Features of Hypomanic Episodes***

A distinct period of substained elevated, expansive, or irritable mood, lasting for at least four days, that is clearly different from the individual's nondepressed mood, yet does not cause marked impairment in social or occupational functioning such as in acute mania.
During the mood disturbance, at least three of the following symptoms are also present to a significant degree:
  a) inflated self-esteem or grandiosity
  b) decreased need for sleep
  c) more talkative than usual
  d) flight of ideas or racing thoughts
  e) distractibility
  f) increase in goal-directed activity or psychomotor agitation
  g) excessive involvement in pleasurable activities that have a high potential for painful consequences
The episode is not due to a physical or substance-induced etiology.

* Summarized from DSM-IV Draft Criteria 3/1/93. See DSM-IV (APA 1993a, in press [1994]) for specific diagnostic criteria.

specified" is reserved for an array of bipolar spectrum illnesses that do not meet strict criteria for bipolar I, bipolar II, or cyclothymic disorder (see below). There are some bipolar patients who will present acutely with both manic and depressed symptoms at the same time (yes, this may happen). If the patient meets diagnostic criteria for both mania and depression every day for at least a one-week period, the patient is diagnosed as being in a mixed manic state, sometimes called dysphoric mania. These dysphoric and mixed manic states tend to be more difficult to diagnose and treat than classic mania. Patients with mixed or dysphoric mania tend to be female, have a higher lithium nonresponse rate, and tend to respond best when anticonvulsants such as valproic acid are added to their medication regimen (McElroy et al, 1992).

In general, the clinical presentations of unipolar and bipolar depressions do not appear to differ markedly in the quality or characteristics of their depressions. Antidepressants and electroconvulsive therapy (ECT) effectively treat both unipolar and bipolar depressions, and the prophylactic efficacy of lithium has been consistently demonstrated to be superior to placebo in both conditions. Thus, from a diagnostic standpoint, the major difference between unipolar and bipolar depressed patients is defined by what happens to them when they are not depressed. Remember the distinction between unipolar and bipolar depression is based on the presence or absence of a past history of mania or hypomania. Given the genetic predisposition for bipolar illnesses (see below), a depression in a patient with a family history of bipolar illness is a strong indication that the patient has a bipolar disorder. Recognition that the patient has a bipolar disorder has important treatment implications for the depressed patient (see Treatment of Bipolar Disorders, below).

Cyclothymia

Cyclothymia can be conceptualized as a relatively less-severe form of bipolar illness. The data indicate that approximately 30% of cyclothymics have a positive family history for bipolar illness; that the prevalence of cyclothymia in the relatives of bipolar patients is much higher than the prevalence of cyclothymia in patients with other psychiatric disorders; and that half of the cyclothymics report improvement while on lithium. These data support the conceptualization of cyclothymia as a mild form of bipolar illness (Kaplan and Sadock, 1988). Cyclothymia has an insidious onset usually beginning in the late teens or early 20s. By definition, it is a chronic mood disturbance of at least two years' duration and involving numerous hypomanic and mild depressive episodes (that do not meet the criteria for mania or major depression), with no periods of euthymia greater than two months. The mood disturbance is not severe enough to markedly impair social or occupational functioning (APA 1993a, in press [1994]).

Theories of Mania

Drug-induced behaviors have suggested some possible pathologic mechanisms that may occur during manic episodes. The most striking pharmacologic data is the consistent finding that direct or indirect norepinephrine and dopamine agonists (those drugs that stimulate the noradrenergic and dopaminergic receptors or increase concentrations of these neurotransmitters in the brain) can precipitate mania or hypomania in patients with underlying bipolar illness. Some stimulants (amphetamines, cocaine) can induce manic-like syndromes in humans who do not appear to have an underlying vulnerability to develop a bipolar disorder. Thus, the association of mania or hypomania with hyperadrenergic and/or hyperdopaminergic states is firmly established (Potter, Rudarfer, and Goodwin, 1987).

The diagnosis of bipolar disorder includes patients with a history of both major depressive and manic or hypomanic episodes. Yet how can one illness present itself as two opposite mood states where the explanation for the pathophysiology of one mood state would seem to preclude the existence of the other? Although the answer to this question is unclear, the paradox of having these two opposite pathologic mood states within the same individual may highlight the importance of neurotransmitter balance for normal functioning, and that neurotransmitter imbalances (frequently explained to the patient as a "chemical imbalance") resulting from dysfunction of normal regulatory mechanisms may lead to a dysregulation of normal mood reactivity.

Heritability and Mood Disorders

Genetic factors are undoubtedly important in the etiology of the major mood disorders. The relative risk of major depression is two to five times greater in the relatives of depressed patients than in the relatives of controls. The genetic evidence is even stronger for bipolar illness than for unipolar depression. First-degree relatives (parents, siblings, and offspring) of patients with bipolar illness are reported to be at least 24 times more likely to develop bipolar illness than relatives of control subjects.

The incidence of both bipolar illness and unipolar depression is much higher in first-degree relatives of patients with bipolar illness than in the general population. First-degree relatives of patients with unipolar illness, on the other hand, have an increase only in the incidence of unipolar depression (Gold, Goodwin, and Chrousos, 1988; Willner, 1985).

Since familial aggregation may reflect a shared environmental precipitant, the increased incidence of mood disorders within families does not in itself establish that these illnesses are hereditary. Twin and adoption studies have attempted to address this issue. Twin studies compare the concordance rate for an illness in pairs of monozygotic twins with the rate of the illness in dizygotic twins, and assume that both sets of twins are exposed to the same environment. Due to identical genes, one would expect monozygotic twins to show a greater concordance for hereditary conditions than dizygotic twins. Twin studies have reported the concordance rate for bipolar illness to be approximately 79% in monozygotic twins but only 19% in dizygotic twins. Adoption studies attempt to separate the contributions of nature and nurture by studying children raised away from their biological parents. Adoption studies have shown a greater prevalence of mood disorders among biological relatives of patients with bipolar illness but not in adoptive relatives. Thus, there appears to be a strong genetic predisposition to the development of mood disorders, especially bipolar disorders. Advances in molecular genetic strategies are expected to reveal much more about the inheritance of mood disorders. Nonetheless, the most likely etiology of most mood disorders is multifactorial, with expression of the illness being secondary to a combination of various heredity traits and environmental factors (Pardes et al, 1989) (Table 7–11).

Diagnosis and Treatment of Mood Disorders in the Medical Setting

Depressive symptoms are common in medical-surgical patients. Factors that appear to be involved in the pathogenesis of depressive symptomatology in medically ill patients are multiple, but some common core issues include loss of health, helpless-

Table 7–11 **Genetics in Mood Disorders**

1. The relative risk of major depression is two to five times greater in the relatives of depressed patients than in the relatives of controls.
2. First-degree relatives of patients with bipolar illness are reported to be at least 24 times more likely to develop bipolar illness than relatives of control subjects.
3. The incidence of both bipolar illness and unipolar depression is much higher in first-degree relatives of patients with bipolar illness than in the general population.
4. The concordance rate for bipolar illness is approximately 19% in dizygotic twins but 79% in monozygotic twins
5. Adoption studies have shown a greater prevalence of mood disorders among biological relatives of patients with bipolar illness but not in their adoptive relatives.

ness, chronic disability and pain, injuries to self-esteem, and financial and interpersonal strain secondary to the illness. In some instances the depressive symptoms can be a consequence of the underlying medical illness, or they can be induced by medications.

The issues of loss and stress (either acute or chronic) tend to be recurrent themes in many medically ill depressed patients. The "loss" that the patient experiences may be of body parts (amputation, mastectomy), sexual functioning (spinal cord injury, radical prostatectomy), bodily functions (ostomy placement), or body image (burns). If the physical illness is chronic and debilitating, progressive loss of health, independence, control over one's life, and self-esteem may induce depressive reactions. The financial stress induced by the illness (medical bills, inability to work) may also lead to a certain degree of depression, especially if the patient begins to feel that he is now a burden to the family. Thus, in searching for the psychological precipitances of depression, the physician must look beyond the immediate circumstances of the patient's illness and evaluate the patient's general ability to "cope," the amount of family support available, the degree of financial and occupational strain present, and other conflicts, pressures, or losses that the patient may be struggling with (Stoudemire, in press).

Many depressive reactions in medical-surgical patients do not meet the diagnostic criteria for a mood disorder. These reactions are characterized by sadness over their current circumstances and tend to resolve with stabilization of the medical condition. If major disturbances in social, occupational, interpersonal, or psychological functioning occurs, a diagnosis of an adjustment disorder can be made. However, if the depressive symptoms do not resolve with improvement in the medical condition, this should be considered a *red flag* and the diagnosis of a major depressive episode should be considered.

One of the difficulties in making a diagnosis of major depression in medical-surgical settings is that physical illnesses may produce many of the symptoms that are often associated with depression (fatigue, anorexia, insomnia, etc.). In addition, the patient's "sadness" is often felt to be "normal" or "understandable" given their medical circumstances (Cohen-Cole and Stoudemire, 1987). Although a decrease in mood is expected when one has to deal with unpleasant circumstances, cognitive expressions of decreased self-esteem, worthlessness, excessive guilt, "giving up," or thoughts of death or suicide are not normal reactions to even extreme stressors (i.e., dealing with terminal cancer). When such cognitive symptoms are present, the physician should immediately suspect the development of a depressive disorder and request psychiatric consultation. Although it is "normal" to be sad in view of serious medical illness, it is not "normal" to be depressed. Depression is a serious medical condition.

The relationship between pain, particularly chronic pain, and depression is a frequent question that arises in medical-surgical patients. Chronic pain patients have a high frequency of depressive complaints (sleep disturbance, appetite changes, irritability, decreased libido, social withdrawal, and somatic preoccupation). Whether or not this symptom constellation constitutes true clinical depression remains a matter of controversy. Arguments in this area soon become circular: chronic pain can cause significant reactive depressions, or masked depressions can present as chronic pain. At any rate, the net result is the development of a patient who exhibits chronic pain behavior (the focus of life is on pain complaints and obtaining relief from pain). Invariably, however, if a mood disorder is the basis for the patient's pain complaints, or if depression produces an amplification of legitimate painful symptoms, both an improvement in mood and diminished pain complaints will respond to antidepressant therapy. In these circumstances, it is not known if antidepressants work as a primary mood elevator or have some indirect analgesic effect.

In addition to pain complaints, somatic complaints attributable to almost every organ system have been reported by depressed patients in medical settings (such as weakness, dizziness, nausea, nervousness, and tremor). Depressions presenting with somatic complaints (including pain) in the absence of an obviously depressed mood have been described as "masked depressions" or "somatizing depressions," and the symptoms considered "depressive equivalents." Indeed, a significant percentage of depressed patients in medical settings will present with these "masked depressions"! Thus, a caveat to bear in mind in evaluating depression is that some depressions may be "masked" by the patient being unaware of, in denial of, or having a limited ability to verbalize feelings. Medically ill, elderly, and patients with little education or from low socioeconomic backgrounds may present with a greater percentage of "somatizing" or "masked" depressions and have a host of nonspecific somatic complaints. The physician should not accept denial of depression by the patient as excluding the diagnosis. Often, after a thorough medical workup has completely ruled out a medical basis for the patient's complaints, a therapeutic trial of an antidepressant medication should be considered along with further evaluation of the patient's psychosocial circumstances.

Assessment of Suicide Risk

One of the myths surrounding the assessment of suicidal risk in depressed patients is that asking about suicidal ideation will bring the idea to the patient's mind or serve to "plant" the idea, increasing the chances that suicide will occur. In actuality, the opposite is true: bringing up the subject of suicide and allowing patients to ventilate their possible motives, ideas, and even plans is often a good way to "diffuse" a suicidal situation. Therefore, thorough questioning for suicidal ideation should be conducted in every depressed patient. Questioning the family is also important since the most lethal patient is one who may have already "made up their mind" and are determined that no one will be allowed to intervene. Patients who suddenly begin to "get their affairs in order," make out a will, or who suddenly "get better" inexplicably (due to the idea that they now feel they have a way out of their intractable situation) should be evaluated carefully.

Studies indicate that the rates of suicide in major depression are between 15 and 30% (reviewed by Gold, Goodwin, and Chrousos, 1988). In general, while women tend to attempt suicide more often, men complete the act at a greater rate. A number of factors may help identify patients at higher risk for suicide, such as increasing age, living alone, a recent major loss, chronic illness, and a previous history of depression and/or suicide attempts. Obviously, depressed patients with low self-esteem, excessive guilt, and feelings of helplessness and hopelessness may be extremely suicidal. Patients who have schizophrenia, alcoholism or drug addictions, and cognitive impairment syndromes are more likely to commit suicide because of impaired judgment and impulsivity.

If the patient is a significant suicidal risk, then psychiatric consultation should occur before the patient is allowed to go home. The broad grounds of psychiatric "commitment" usually require that the patient must have a mental illness and be immediately dangerous to themselves, to others, or to be so gravely incapacitated as to be unable to care for themselves. Commitment codes and procedures vary from state to state and psychiatric consultation is advised before pursuing this avenue. Management of suicidal patients is further discussed in Chapters 19 and 20.

Mood Disorders Due to General Medical Conditions

The essential feature of these mood disorders is evidence of a medical or drug-induced etiology for the symptoms. Numerous medical conditions, medications, or illicit drugs may induce mood disturbances (Cohen-Cole and Harpe, 1987). The possibility of a medical or substance-related etiology should always be considered and ruled out in patients presenting with mood disorders. Drugs that have been implicated in inducing mood disorders include steroids, reserpine, alpha-methyldopa, propranolol, carbonic anhydrase inhibitors, stimulants, hallucinogens, alcohol, sedative-hypnotics, benzodiazepines, and narcotics. Medical conditions that may present as mood disorders include endocrinopathies (Cushing's syndrome, Addison's disease, hypothyroidism, hypo- or hypercalcemia), malignancies (occult cancers, lymphomas, pancreatic carcinoma, gliomas), and infections (hepatitis, encephalitis, mononucleosis, HIV). A basic history and physical exam along with a medication review and/or appropriate laboratory screening tests will rule out the majority of these mood disorders. General medical conditions that cause mood disorders are discussed in Chapter 20 by Dr. Levenson.

Indications for Psychopharmacologic Treatment of Depression

Undoubtedly, depressions are an etiologically heterogeneous group of disorders with overlapping symptoms. Thus, there is no one single treatment of choice for all cases of depression. In formulating a treatment plan for the depressed patient, first assess whether the patient meets the DSM-IV criteria for major depressive episode as the primary disorder. Rule out the presence of coexisting substance-abuse disorders and/or general medical conditions. Assess the psychosocial circumstances, the degree of impairment, the chronicity of the disturbance, and the presence of suicidal ideations. Patients with mild depressions or depressions secondary to environmental "stress" or interpersonal conflicts are best treated with counseling or psychotherapy (see below). Moderate to severe depressions will frequently benefit from antidepressant medication.

The pharmaceutical armamentarium of antidepressants includes the cyclic antidepressants, selective serotonin reuptake inhibitors (SSRIs), buproprion, monoamine oxidase inhibitors, and lithium. All of these agents are discussed here as well as in the overview chapter on psychopharmacology in this text (see Chapter 18 by Drs. Silver, Hales, and Yudofsky). No one medication can be recommended as optimal for all patients because of the substantial heterogeneity among patients and among the various antidepressants. There are some general consensus statements that can be made, however. Nonpsychotic melancholia responds well to most antidepressant medications; atypical depressions have a preferential response to monoamine oxidase inhibitors; patients with bipolar depression should be treated with an antidepressant and a mood stabilizer; and psychotically depressed individuals require a combination of an antidepressant and an antipsychotic, or ECT (Schatzberg, 1992). Thus, if it is determined that somatic treatment is warranted, the next step is to define the subtype of depression you will be treating. In general, there is no convincing data to suggest that one antidepressant is superior to any of the other antidepressants in regard to its ability to treat major depressions. The choice of antidepressant in most cases is often predicated on factors such as the patient's age and general health status, the side effect profile of the antidepressant, the cost of the medication, and the patient's past personal or family history of antidepressant treatments. A personal history of prior response to an antidepressant or a favorable response by a family member is a good predictor of a favorable response to that same antidepressant again. The somatic or "vegetative" symptoms (i.e., sleep, appetite, and psychomotor disturbances) are relatively clear target symptoms for antidepressant medication and are usually the first symptoms to improve. The "cognitive" symptoms of depression (low self-esteem, guilt, uncertainty, pessimism, suicidal thoughts) tend to improve more slowly.

In general, a lag time of three to four weeks may be seen before a true mood-elevating effect is seen with the antidepressants, and patients should be warned not to expect results overnight. Significant antidepressant responses in elderly patients often occur later than in younger patients and require at least six to 12 weeks of therapy (NIH Consensus Development Panel on Depression in Late Life, 1992). Improvement in sleep disturbance, agitation, and anxiety may be seen early in the treatment and precede the onset of true antidepressant activity.

Traditionally, the cyclic antidepressants have been the first-line drugs in the treatment of depression, followed by the monoamine oxidase inhibitors if the patient failed to respond. However, more and more clinicians are using the newer generation of antidepressants, such as the selective serotonin reuptake inhibitors, as their first-line drugs.

Tricyclic Antidepressants

A listing of the drugs used to treat major depression and their dose ranges are shown in Table 7–12. In general, the average dose range for most tricyclics is 100 up to a maximum of 300 mg/day. The most prominent exceptions are nortriptyline (50 to 150 mg/day), protriptyline (10 to 60 mg/day), and trazodone (150 to 600 mg/day). In general the tricyclics should be started at low bedtime doses (25 to 50 mg/day) and gradually increased by 25 mg/day every third or fourth night over a 10- to 14-day period of time (with the exceptions as already noted). Elderly patients generally

Table 7–12 **Properties of the CyADs**

	EFFECT ON SEROTONIN REUPTAKE	EFFECT ON NOREPINEPHRINE REUPTAKE	SEDATING EFFECT	ANTICHOLINERGIC EFFECT	ORTHOSTATIC EFFECT	DOSE RANGE (MG)[d]
Amitriptyline[a]	+ + + +	+ +	+ + + +	+ + + +	+ + + +	75–300
Imipramine[a]	+ + + +	+ +	+ + +	+ + +	+ + + +	75–300
Nortriptyline	+ + +	+ + +	+ +	+ +	+	50–150
Protriptyline	+ + +	+ + + +	+	+ + +	+	10–60
Trazodone	+ + +	±	+ + +	±[b]	+ +	200–600
Desipramine	+ + +	+ + + +	+	+	+ +	75–300
Amoxapine[c]	+ +	+ + +	+ +	+ +	+ +	75–400
Maprotiline	+	+ +	+ +	+	+ +	75–400
Doxepin	+ + +	+ +	+ + +	+ +	+ +	150–200
Trimipramine[c]	+	+	+ +	+ +	+ +	75–300
Fluoxetine	+ + + +	−	−	−	−	50–200
Paroxetine	+ + + +	−	−	−	−	20–40
Sertraline	+ + + +	−	−	−	−	10–40
Bupropion	−	−	−	±	−	50–200

Relative potencies (some ratings are approximated) based partly on affinities of these agents for brain receptors in competitive binding studies (Richelson E: Pharmacology of antidepressants in use in the United States. *J Clin Psychiatry* 43:4–11, 1982)

− = none, + = slight, + + = moderate, + + + = marked, + + + + = pronounced, ± = indeterminant.
[a] = Available in injectable form.
There have been case reports, however, of apparent anticholinergic effects.
[b] = Most in vivo and clinical studies report the absence of anticholinergic effects (or no difference from placebo).
[c] = Amoxapine and trimipramine have dopamine receptor blocking activity.
[d] = Dose ranges are for treatment of major depression. Lower doses may be appropriate for other therapeutic uses.
Used with permission from Stoudemire A, Fogel BS, Gulley LR, Moran MG: Psychopharmacology in the Medically Ill. In Stoudemire A, Fogel BS (eds): Psychiatric Care of the Medical Patient, p 160. New York, Oxford University Press, 1993

require lower doses than younger adults (start with 10 or 25 mg/day and build up the dosage gradually, monitoring for side effects). The half-life of most antidepressants is such that they can be administered once daily in the evening. This approach may facilitate both sleep induction and compliance.

Among the most bothersome side effects of the tricyclic antidepressants are their anticholinergic effects, such as dry mouth, blurred vision, urinary retention, constipation, palpitations, and tachycardia. In addition, orthostatic hypotension, which is secondary to alpha-adrenergic blockade, is often a major concern, particularly in the elderly, who are most prone to develop orthostatic hypotension and who are at most risk if it occurs. The orthostatic changes tend to occur before the therapeutic plasma levels are obtained, and frequently there is no tendency for the body to accommodate to this difficult-to-manage side effect. Orthostatic hypotension may precipitate falls as well as cerebrovascular or cardiac events. The demethylated or secondary tricyclics (i.e., desipramine, nortriptyline) are generally better tolerated and less likely to produce anticholinergic and orthostatic side effects.

The use of tricyclics in patients with cardiovascular disease warrants some special concerns. In addition to orthostasis, the tricyclics tend to slow cardiac conduction and, as a group, tend to increase the P-R interval, QRS duration, QTc time, and flatten T-waves on the EKG in patients with cardiac conduction disease (Stoudemire et al, 1993). Thus, patients with either bundle branch blocks or intraventricular conduction defects should be treated very carefully with TCAs. Interestingly, since the tricyclics have properties that are characteristic of type 1A antiarrhythmic compounds (such as quinidine and procainamide), premature ventricular contractions may decrease when tricyclics are administered (Glassman and Bigger, 1981; Veith et al, 1982). Therefore, the combination of tricyclics and type 1A antiarrhythmics should be avoided because of their additive effects on cardiac conduction. One advantage of the newer antidepressant agents (SSRIs and bupropion) is that they have few, if any, effects on cardiac function in healthy adults. Although there are very few controlled studies assessing the effects of these newer agents in diseased hearts, it is widespread clinical practice to use these newer agents in patients with cardiac conditions.

Because of their anticholinergic effects, tricyclic antidepressants may induce a narrow-angle glaucoma crisis, delay gastric emptying, and exacerbate symptoms in patients with dysphagia. Tricyclic antidepressants may lower the seizure threshold in patients with seizure disorders, but the exacerbation of seizures is usually not a problem if seizures are under good control and therapeutic levels of anticonvulsants are maintained.

Monitoring of tricyclic plasma drug levels may be helpful in selected patients, particularly in patients who are unresponsive to usual therapeutic doses. Cigarette smoking, oral contraceptives, alcohol, and barbiturates tend to lower plasma levels of antidepressants through hepatic enzyme induction; disulfiram (Antabuse), antipsychotics, and amphetamine derivatives tend to raise levels, as does the acute administration of other medications competing for the same hepatic enzymes. In evaluating drug levels, the clinician should strive to obtain levels under uniform conditions. A standard procedure is to draw levels in the morning, approximately 12 hours after the last dose of medication (Glenn and Taska, 1984).

Bupropion

Bupropion is a unicyclic antidepressant that differs chemically and pharmacologically from other currently available antidepressants. It does not appreciably inhibit reuptake of norepinephrine or serotonin and is only a weak inhibitor of dopamine reuptake. A number of controlled trials have shown bupropion to be as effective as tricyclics in the treatment of depression. Its side effect profile, however, is much more favorable than the tricyclics. It is essentially devoid of anticholinergic, antihistaminic, and adrenergic side effects. In clinical trials using the recommended dose of 300 mg/day, the most common side effects were dizziness, agitation, insomnia, headache, and nausea. Unfortunately, the risk of drug-induced seizures is greater for bupropion than with any other antidepressant. The increased risk appears to be dose and titration related and can be minimized by gradually increasing the dose, not exceeding 150 mg for any one dose, and not exceeding 450 mg total daily dose. Bupropion is usually started at 150 or 200 mg/day and increased to 300 mg/day over several days (reviewed by Weisler, 1991).

Selective Serotonin Reuptake Inhibitors

The selective serotonin reuptake inhibitors (SSRIs) are rapidly becoming the most commonly prescribed antidepressants in the United States. The combination of clinical efficacy, safety, ease of administration, and favorable side effect profile is responsible for their rapid acceptance and widespread use. They are as effective as the cyclic antidepressants in the treatment of depression but have some distinct tolerability and dosing advantages. Their therapeutic dose and starting dose are generally the same so, unlike other classes of antidepressants, there is no "delay" between initiation of therapy and titration to a therapeutic dose. The SSRIs are not associated with any significant anticholinergic side effects, cardiotoxicity, sedation, or weight gain. Gastrointestinal symptoms, anxiety, headache, and insomnia are the most commonly reported side effects (Leonard, 1992). Sexual complaints may include inhibited orgasm in both men and women. Although the SSRIs share similar pharmacodynamic profiles (they all inhibit serotonin reuptake), structurally they are a heterogeneous group, resulting in different pharmacokinetic properties. Yet there are no differences in their clinical efficacy. Currently there are four SSRIs available in the United States—fluoxetine, sertraline, paroxetine and fluvoxamine, the last of which is indicated for obsessive–compulsive disorder (Rickels and Schweizer, 1990).

Monoamine Oxidase Inhibitors

Monoamine oxidase inhibitors (MAOIs) are not widely prescribed because of their potential to produce a hypertensive crisis if the patient ingests a food source high in tyramine or a sympathomimetic drug. They are generally prescribed for those patients who are unresponsive to cyclic antidepressants, who develop intolerable side effects with cyclic antidepressants, or who give a history of previous response to MAOIs. However, MAOIs may be the drug of choice in patients with "atypical" depression whose mood disorder is characterized by hypersomnia, carbohydrate craving, somatic complaints, phobias, anxiety, or histrionic features (Robinson et al, 1973; Quitkin et al, 1979).

Foods rich in tyramine—aged cheese, yogurt, Chianti wine, foreign beer, liver, snails, pickled herring, chocolate, broad beans, soy sauce, and avocados—should be avoided during treatment with MAOIs. Patients should avoid medications containing sympathomimetic compounds such as amphetamines, diet pills, and over-the-counter common cold preparations. MAOIs should not be used in patients on guanethedine, sympathomimetics of any kind, or in combination with narcotics or the SSRIs. The MAOIs may cause orthostatic hypertension but do not increase cardiac conduction time or have many significant anticholinergic side effects (Snyder and Yamamura, 1977). Patients with congestive heart failure, liver disease, or pheochromocytoma should not receive MAOIs. There are two major types of MAOIs, the hydrazine and the nonhydrazine compounds. Phenelizine (hydrazine) and tranylcypromine (non-hydrazine) are the most frequently used MAOIs. The usual dosage range is 15 to 60 mg for phenelzine and 20 to 30 mg for tranylcypromine, given in divided doses.

Psychostimulants

Stimulants such as methylphenidate, amphetamine, and pemoline have occasionally been used to treat depressed medical patients who cannot tolerate other antidepressant drugs or who refuse electroconvulsive therapy (Katon and Raskind, 1980). However, these drugs may produce rebound depression, insomnia, restlessness, agitation, and even paranoid reactions. Their antidepressant action may be short-lived and they are not approved by the Food and Drug Administration for use as antidepressants. In addition, they have some abuse potential. However, these agents have been reported to be effective in patients with AIDS (see Chapter 21 by Dr. Moran).

Electroconvulsive Therapy

Although there is a large armamentarium of clinically effective antidepressants that are available to the clinician, both psychotic and melancholic depressions tend to respond most predictably to electroconvulsive therapy (ECT). In fact, ECT is clearly the most effective treatment for all major depressions and should be considered in depressed patients who cannot tolerate the side effects of antidepressant medications. Other indications for ECT include: refractory depressions (usually defined as failure to respond to at least two different antidepressants given for 4–6 weeks at therapeutic doses); depressions in frail elderly patients; and in some cases of acute mania, schizoaffective disorders, or acute-onset psychotic episodes (including schizophrenia) presenting with a predominance of affective or catatonic symptoms. The only contraindications to ECT are the presence of CNS mass lesions, recent myocardial infarction, or a history of malignant ventricular arrhythmia (see also Chapter 18).

Duration of Treatment

There are no clear indications as to how long antidepressant drugs should be continued once an antidepressant effect is achieved. In general, antidepressant medications should be continued for an average of nine to 12 months when a gradual taper can be attempted while watching for signs of relapse. If the patient has had multiple episodes of depression in the past or has a strong family history of depression, he or she may well need to be maintained on antidepressants indefinitely. In conjunction with medication treatment, supportive psychotherapy or some form of counseling to deal with conflicts, stressors, or other precipitances that may contribute to depression is usually recommended (even if the therapy is relatively brief and confined to the early stages of treatment).

TREATMENT OF BIPOLAR DISORDERS

Clinically, unipolar depressions cannot be distinguished from bipolar depressions. Yet this differentiation may be critically important since antidepressants may precipitate a manic episode or increase the "cycling" of the mood disorder in bipolar patients. Hence, if the patient has a personal or family history of bipolar disorder, antidepressants (particularly tricyclic antidepressants) should be used cautiously. If a decision is made to give an antidepressant to a depressed bipolar patient, lithium should be started along with the antidepressant to help prevent the induction of mania. Lithium itself has antidepressant properties, especially in bipolar patients, and should be considered as the sole maintenance agent (Glenn and Taska, 1984). In acute mania, although the onset of its therapeutic action is somewhat slow (5 to 10 days), 60 to 70% of manic patients will respond to therapeutic blood levels of this monovalent cation. The efficacy of lithium in preventing or attenuating the recurrence of depression and mania in bipolar illness is well established.

Renal function, electrolytes, EKG, and thyroid function should be evaluated prior to initiating lithium. Lithium has no metabolites and is excreted almost entirely by the kidney. The rates of renal excretion are affected by advancing age, medical conditions that impair renal blood flow, and sodium intake (because the two cations compete with each other for the same ion transport sites in the kidney). The possibility that lithium can produce clinically significant renal damage is controversial. Tubular atrophy, interstitial fibrosis, glomerulosclerosis, and full renal failure secondary to lithium-induced interstitial nephritis have all been reported after long-term use (Hestbach et al, 1977). Yet the risk of clinically significant renal damage in patients treated with therapeutic concentrations of lithium appears to be small (Scully, Galdabini, and McNely, 1981). More commonly, lithium may suppress thyroid functioning and induce thyroid goiters and/or clinical hypothyroidism. The inhibition of thyroid function appears to be dose dependent and is readily reversible with cessation of lithium therapy. Lithium very rarely causes cardiac abnormalities such as inversion and flattening of T-waves on the EKG, sinus node dysfunction, SA block, and ventricular irritability, even at therapeutic blood levels (Glenn and Taska, 1984).

To begin inpatient treatment for acute mania, lithium carbonate can usually be started at 1200 or 1500 mg/day in divided doses, adjusting the dose every several days until a therapeutic blood level is achieved. Lower doses will be needed in patients who are elderly, have renal insufficiency, or who are otherwise medically compromised. The optimal serum blood level during an acute manic episode should be at the upper spectrum of the therapeutic range (between 1.0 and 1.5 mEq/L). Serum levels should be drawn in the morning before the morning lithium dose (approximately 12 hours after the last dose). Serum levels above 1.5 mEq/L often produce signs of toxicity and levels of 5 mEq/L can be fatal. Since clinical response usually takes several days, antipsychotic or sedative medications are frequently needed during the initial treatment. Following the acute episode, maintenance lithium levels between 0.6 and 1.2 are usually sufficient to prevent relapses of both bipolar and recurrent unipolar depressive illnesses (Glenn and Taska, 1984).

It should be emphasized that close monitoring of side effects, not serum lithium concentrations, is the ultimate criterion for lithium toxicity. Signs and symptoms of lithium toxicity include tremor, weakness, ataxia, drowsiness, dysarthria, blurred vision, tinnitus, nausea, vomiting, hyperactive deep tendon reflexes, nystagmus, confusion, seizures, and coma. Some of these side effects (such as tremor, weakness, and gastrointestinal complaints) are seen with therapeutic levels of lithium. The lithium-induced tremor can be alleviated by the addition of 20 to 60 mg of propranolol. Gastrointestinal disturbances can best be treated by dividing total dosage or switching to a slow-release formulation. Some patients develop marked polyuria and polydipsia that may improve by lowering the lithium dose or by adding low doses of a thiazide diuretic (note: monitor for lithium toxicity if you add the diuretic). If hypothyroidism develops (check TSH to find out), decrease the dose of lithium if possible or treat with thyroid supplements (i.e., levothyroxine).

Women of child-bearing potential should be warned of the reported increase in cardiovascular abnormalities in the offspring of lithium-treated mothers. Lithium should be used with caution in patients with unstable renal or cardiovascular disease, severe dehydration, or patients receiving thiazide diuretics or nonsteroidal anti-inflammatory agents. Although there have been some extremely rare reports of neurotoxicity in patients being treated with a combination of lithium and neuroleptics (Cohen and Cohen, 1974), in general the combination of lithium and neuroleptics is well tolerated and safe.

Over the past decade, a growing body of data has emerged supporting the efficacy of the anticonvulsant drugs carbamazepine and valproic acid in the treatment of patients with bipolar disorders. These agents have been demonstrated to be efficacious in the treatment of acute mania and mixed manic states. The mechanism by which these anticonvulsants and/or lithium works in the treatment of mood disturbances is unclear. It can be assumed that these drugs somehow "stabilize" dysregulated brain functioning, which allows one's mood to progress outside "normal" ranges.

The use of psychopharmacological agents in the treatment of mood disorders is more fully discussed in Chapter 18. Discussions of the use of lithium in medically complicated patients may be found elsewhere (Stoudemire et al, 1993).

PSYCHOTHERAPY

There is a wide range of psychotherapeutic interventions that may be useful in the treatment of mood disorders, particularly depressive mood disorders. The establishment of a supportive therapeutic relationship is often crucial in the treatment of the depressed patient. Supportive psychotherapy generally consists of (1) providing a therapeutic rationale or explanation for the patient's symptoms; (2) providing ongoing education, knowledge, and feedback in regard to the patient's illness, prognosis, and treatment; (3) guiding the patient in reference to interpersonal relationships, work, and major life adjustments; (4) helping to bolster the patient's morale; (5) setting realistic goals; and (6) being available in times of crisis.

Psychodynamic psychotherapies embrace, to various degrees, Freud's original conceptualization of depression in which the relationship to a highly ambivalent lost person is of central importance. The importance of early deprivations of love and affection, guilt secondary to a harsh conscience and repressed fantasies, and frustrations related to having excessively high personal ideals are also common psychodynamic themes. Psychodynamic theory affirms that in order for the individual to improve, the unconscious intrapsychic processes underlying depression must be brought into consciousness. Once these forces are made conscious, future difficulties can be anticipated and mastered or future conflicts can be neutralized through the process of insight (reviewed by APA, 1993b).

Interpersonal therapy seeks to recognize and explore depressive precipitants that involve interpersonal losses, role disputes, social isolation, or deficits in social skills (reviewed by APA, 1993b). Cognitive therapy approaches the patient's symptoms as being secondary to irrational beliefs and distorted attitudes towards self, the environment, and the future (see Cognitive Theory of Depression, above).

In general, research on the efficacy of the various psychotherapies in the acute and maintenance phase of major depressions, either in conjunction with pharmacotherapy or alone, is sparse and inconclusive. It is generally agreed that patients with mild depressions or with dysthymic disorders seem most likely to benefit from a purely psychotherapeutic approach. Psychotherapy alone may be equally sufficient and effective for those with primarily situational forms of depression. However, even in cases of mild depression, if the symptoms do not respond to psychotherapy, somatic treatment should be considered. There is general consensus, even though there is little research data to support it, that the optimal treatment of major depression requires some form of somatic intervention coupled with some form of psychotherapeutic management. Psychotherapy can assist the patient in reversing the negative self-images, the negative feelings about the future, and the poor self-esteem that are ubiquitous features of depression. All psychiatric patients, regardless of their diagnosis, seem to benefit from a positive therapeutic relationship with a therapist (APA, 1993b).

PREMENSTRUAL DYSPHORIC DISORDER

Premenstrual dysphoric disorder (frequently called premenstrual syndrome or PMS) is a syndrome characterized by the repeated occurrence of a number of affective, cognitive, and behavioral symptoms during the luteal phase of the menstrual cycle. (The disorder is not an "official" disorder in DSM-IV but is listed in the appendix of the DSM-IV manual pending further research. To make the diagnosis, at least one of the following symptoms must be present most of the time during the luteal phase: depressed mood, anxiety, or tension; affective lability; and irritability or increased interpersonal conflicts. Other associated symptoms include: decreased interest in usual activities, difficulty concentrating, decreased energy, appetite change, sleep disturbance, sense of being overwhelmed or out of control, and various physical symptoms such as bloating, headaches, and breast tenderness. The patient must have a total of at least five of the aforementioned symptoms and their occurrence in relation to the menstrual cycle must be confirmed by using prospective daily ratings. Additionally, the symptoms must be severe enough to interfere with normal occupational, social, or interpersonal relationships. Studies on the prevalence of premenstrual symptoms in women of reproductive age indicate that as many as 80% have physical discomfort and/or alterations in mood before menses. Despite this high figure, a relatively small number of women have symptoms of sufficient severity to warrant the diagnosis of premenstrual dysphoric disorder (Mortola, 1992).

As you can see, many of the symptoms of premenstrual dysphoric disorder overlap with those of depressive disorders, and there may be a high incidence of psychiatric co-morbidity in patients with premenstrual dysphoria. What is pathognomonic for the disorder is the marked fluctuations of symptoms with the menstrual cycle. Although there is no one universal pattern in which the timing of the severity of the symptoms occurs, in general the mean symptom severity increases gradually throughout the luteal phase, reaches a peak just before the onset of menses, and subsequently declines rapidly after the onset of menses. Thus, the hallmark of the diagnosis rests on the presence of a relatively symptom-free interval between days 12 and 14 of the menstrual cycle (Mortola, 1992).

Treatment of the patient with premenstrual dysphoric disorder should include education on the biology of the disorder, supportive psychotherapy, and in severe cases pharmacotherapy. Pharmacologic strategies that have been reported to be successful includes alprazolam, fluoxetine, and gonadotropin-releasing hormone agonists (reviewed by Mortola, 1992).

CLINICAL PEARLS

- Major depression is a *syndrome*, characterized by a mood disturbance, plus a variety of cognitive, psychological, and somatic symptoms.
- It is important to remember that a *subjective* sense of a "depression" may not be present in every patient who has a major depression. Some depressions may be "masked" by the patient being unaware of, in denial of, or having a limited ability to verbalize feelings.
- Elderly patients may complain of anxiety, irritability, weakness, or multiple somatic complaints rather than verbalize complaints of depression per se.
- Somatic symptoms of depression can include pain, gastrointestinal complaints, neurologic complaints, general fatigue, and lethargy.
- The development of extreme withdrawal, hopelessness, or suicidal ideations in a depressed individual are clear indications for psychiatric referral.
- Major depressions, which were once thought to consist of discrete episodes followed by full recovery, may become chronic in some patients.

- There is a high recurrence rate for major depressive episodes.
- An adjustment disorder may occur following an identifiable psychosocial stressor; it may cause major disruptions in the individual's life; and it may be associated with severe dysphoria, despondency, and suicidal ideations.
- The essential feature of a dysthymic disorder is a chronic history of a mild- to moderate-grade depression, with only brief, if any, periods of euthymia.
- Atypical depressions denote neurovegetative symptoms that are generally the opposite of what is seen in melancholia, such as hypersomnia rather than insomnia, hyperphagia rather than anorexia, and environmental reactivity.
- The presence of a mania or hypomania defines bipolar disorder.
- In bipolar disorder, dysphoric or mixed manic states occur when both manic and depressive symptoms occur at the same time. Patients with mixed or dysphoric mania tend to be female, have a higher lithium nonresponse rate, and tend to respond best when anticonvulsants are added to their medication regimen.
- The pharmaceutical armamentarium of antidepressants includes the cyclic antidepressants, monoamine oxidase inhibitors, selective serotonin reuptake inhibitors (SSRIs), bupropion and lithium. No one medication can be recommended as optimal for all patients because of the substantial heterogeneity among patients and among the various antidepressants.
- Nonpsychotic melancholia responds well to most antidepressant medications; atypical depressions have a preferential response to monoamine oxidase inhibitors; and psychotically depressed individuals require a combination of an antidepressant and an antipsychotic, or ECT.
- The most common cause of "refractory" major depression is noncompliance or inadequate doses of antidepressant.
- If a patient does not respond to an adequate trial of an antidepressant, consider lithium or thyroid augmentation before switching the patient to another class of antidepressant.
- Traditionally, the cyclic antidepressants have been the first-line drugs in the treatment of depression. However, more and more clinicians are using the newer generation of antidepressants, such as the selective serotonin reuptake inhibitors, as their first-line drugs.
- At therapeutic doses, anticholinergic effects, sedation, and weight gain are the most problematic side effects of the traditional cyclic antidepressants. The newer antidepressants have almost none of these problems.
- The half-life of most antidepressants is such that they can be administered once daily. This approach may facilitate both sleep induction and compliance.
- Bupropion is essentially devoid of anticholinergic, antihistaminic, and adrenergic side effects, yet has a higher incidence of seizures.
- In addition to having a low incidence of anticholinergic, antihistaminic, and adrenergic side effects, the selective serotonin reuptake inhibitors (SSRIs) have the dosing advantage of having their starting dose also being their therapeutic dose, thus there is no treatment delay while waiting to get to a therapeutic dose.
- Antidepressant medications should be continued for an average of nine to 12 months then a gradual taper can be attempted while watching for signs of relapse. If the patient has had multiple episodes of depression in the past or has a strong family history of depression, he or she may well need to be maintained on antidepressants indefinitely.
- In conjunction with medication treatment, the establishment of a supportive therapeutic relationship is often crucial in the treatment of the depressed patient.
- When prescribing lithium, have the patient take it on a full stomach or use the slow-release preparations to decrease gastric irritation.

- A growing body of data has emerged supporting the efficacy of the anticonvulsants carbamazepine and valproic acid in the treatment of mania. Consider these anticonvulsants in the lithium-refractory or lithium intolerant patient.
- Elderly patients tolerate lithium poorly; keep serum levels at the lower end of the therapeutic spectrum.
- Acute psychotic mania may be indistinguishable from acute schizophrenic psychosis; consider both possibilities in evaluating the acutely psychotic patient.
- In the patient over 40 who develops psychotic symptoms for the first time, consider a mood disorder in addition to ruling out a neurologic, metabolic, or substance-induced etiology as the new onset of schizophrenia after age 40 is uncommon.

ANNOTATED BIBLIOGRAPHY

American Psychiatric Association: Practice guideline for major depressive disorder in adults. Am J Psychiatry 150 (Suppl 4):1–26, 1993

> This very comprehensive document not only gives the American Psychiatric Association's recommended guidelines for the management of major depression in adults, it also reviews the diagnosis, epidemiology, and natural history of the illness. It addresses both pharmacologic and psychotherapeutic strategies for the treatment of depression.

American Psychiatric Association Commission on Psychiatric Therapies: The Psychiatric Therapies. Washington, DC, American Psychiatric Association, 1984, Chapter 2

> Reviews the use of psychotropic agents in the treatment of emotional disorders.

Gold PW, Goldwin FK, Chrousos GP: Clinical and biochemical manifestations of depression, Part I. N Eng J Med 319(6):348–353, 1988

Gold PW, Goldwin FK, Chrousos GP: Clinical and biochemical manifestations of depression, Part II. N Eng J Med 319 (7):413–420, 1988

> Two-part article that reviews the diagnosis, epidemiology, biological findings, and theories of major depression.

Mortola JF: Issues in the diagnosis and research of premenstrual syndrome. Clin Obste Gyn 35(3):587–598, 1992

> Recent update on the diagnosis of PMS and current research challenges.

Potter WZ, Rudorfer MV, Goodwin FK: Biological Findings in Bipolar Disorders. In Hales RE, Frances AJ (ed): American Psychiatric Association Annual Review, Vol 6. Washington, DC, American Psychiatric Press, 1987

> Reviews biological findings in mood disorders with particular emphasis in comparing bipolar with unipolar depressions.

Willner P: Depression: A Psychobiological Synthesis. New York, A Wiley-Interscience Publication, 1985

> A comprehensive review of the biological and cognitive theories of depression

Shader RI, Greenblatt DJ (eds): Journal of Clinical Psychopharmacology 12(1): February 1992 suppl

> A collection of papers appears in this supplement of the journal that covers the differential diagnosis of bipolar disorders, mechanism of action of anticonvulsants in mood disorders, pharmacokinetics of the anticonvulsants, and an algorithm for patient management of acute mania.

Management of Patients Who Are Nonresponders to or Nontolerators of Initial Antidepressant Therapy. J Clin Psychiatry. Monograph Series, Vol. 10, No. 1, May 1992 (entire issue).

> This monograph contains a series of very practical, clinically oriented articles on the treatment of depressed patients.

REFERENCES

Akiskal HS, Hirschfeld RMA, Yerevanian BI: The relationship of personality to affective disorders: A critical review. Arch Gen Psychiatry 40:801–810, 1983

American Psychiatric Association: Diagnostic and Statistical Manual of Mental Disorders, 4th ed. Washington, DC. American Psychiatric Association, in press [1994]

American Psychiatric Association: DSM-IV Draft Criteria 3/1/93. Washington, DC. American Psychiatric Association, 1993a.

American Psychiatric Association: Practice guideline for major depressive disorder in adults. Am J Psychiatry 150(suppl 4):1–26, 1993b

Aneshensel CS, Stone JD: Stress and depression: A test of the buffering model of social support. Arch Gen Psychiatry 39:1392–1396, 1982

Anisman H, Zacharko RM: Depression: The predisposing influence of stress. Behav Brain Sci 5:89–137, 1982

Arano GW, Baldessarini RJ, Ornsteen M: The dexamethasone suppression test for diagnosis and prognosis in psychiatry. Arch Gen Psychiatry 42:1193–1204, 1985

Asberg M, Traskman L: Studies of CSF 5-HIAA in depression and suicidal behavior. Adv Exp Med Biol 133:739–752, 1981

Banerjee SP, Kung CS, Riggi SJ, Chanda SK: Development of beta-adrenergic subsensitivity by antidepressants. London, Nature, 268:455–456, 1977

Banki CM: Correlation of anxiety and related symptoms with cerebrospinal fluid 5-hydroxyindoleacetic acid in depressed women. J Neural Transm. 41(2-3):135–43, 1977

Banki CM, Arato M: Amine metabolites and neurendocrine responses related to depression and suicide. J Affect Disord 5:223–232, 1983

Beck AT: The Development of Depression: A Cognitive Model. In Friedman, Katz MM (eds): The Psychology of Depression: Contemporary Theory and Research, pp 3–20. New York, John Wiley and Sons, 1974

Belsher G, Costello CG. Relapse after recovery from unipolar depression: A critical review. Psychol Bull 104:84–96, 1988

Blier P, de Montigny C, Chaput Y. Modification of the serotonin system by antidepressant treatments: Implications for the therapeutic response in major depression. J Clin Psychopharmacol 7:24S–35S, 1987

Boyd JH, Weissman M: Epidemiology of affective disorder: A reexamination and future directions. Arch Gen Psychiatry 38:1039–1046, 1981

Breier A, Kelsoe JR, Kirwin PD, Beller SA, Wolkowitz OM, Pickar D: Early parental loss and development of adult psychopathology. Arch Gen Psychiatry 45:987–993, 1988

Bunney WE, Jr., Davis JM: Norepinephrine and depressive reactions: A review. Arch Gen Psychiatry 13:483–494, 1965

Carroll BJ: The Hypothalamus-Pituitary-Adrenal Axis in Depression. In G. Burrows (ed): Handbook on Depression, pp 325–341. Amsterdam, Excerpta Medica, 1977

Carroll BJ: The dexamothesone suppression test for melancholia. Br J Psychiatry 140:292–304, 1982

Chouinard G: Bupropion and amitriptyline in the treatment of depressed patients. J Clin Psychiatry 44(5 sec 2):121–129, 1983

Coble P, Foster FG, Kupfer DJ: Electroencephalographic sleep diagnosis of primary depression. Arch Gen Psychiatry 33:1124–1127, 1976

Cohen NH, Cohen NH: Lithium carbonate, haloperidol, and irreversible brain damage. JAMA 230:1283–1287, 1974

Cohen-Cole S, Harpe C: Diagnostic Assessment of Depression in the Medically Ill. In Stoudemire A, Fogel BS (eds): Principles of Medical Psychiatry. Orlando, FL, Grune and Stratton, 1987

Cohen-Cole S, Stoudemire GA: Major depression and physical illness. In Oken D (ed): The psychiatry clinics of North America. Philadelphia, W.B. Saunders, 1987

Copper A, Prange AJ, Whybrow PC, Noguere R: Abnormalities of indoleamines in affective disorders. Arch Gen Psychiatry 26:474–478, 1972

Davidson J, Miller R, Van Wyck Fleet J et al. A double-blind comparison of bupropion and amitriptyline in depressed inpatients. J Clin Psychiatry 44(5, sec 2):115–117, 1983

Davis JM, Bresnahan DB: Psychopharmacology in Clinical Psychiatry. In Holes R, Franes HJ (ed): Psychiatry Update, Vol 6, 159–187. Washington, DC, American Psychiatric Association, 1987

Gibbons RD, Davis JM. Consistent evidence for a biological subtype of depression characterized by low CSF monoamine levels. Acta Psychiatr Scand 74:8–12, 1986

Gillin JC, Duncan W, Pettigrew KD, Erakel BL, Snyder F: Successful separation of depressed, normal and insomniac subjects by EEG sleep data. Arch Gen Psychiatry 36:85–90, 1979

Glassman AH, Bigger JT: Cardiovascular effects of therapeutic doses of tricyclic antidepressants: A review. Arch Gen Psychiatry 38:815–820, 1981

Glenn M, Taska RJ: Antidepressants and Lithium. In Karasu TB (ed): The Psychiatric Therapies. Washington, DC, American Psychiatric Association, 1984

Gold PW, Goodwin FK, Chrousos GP: Clinical and biochemical manifestations of depression, part I: Relation to the neurobiology of stress. N Eng J Med 319(6):348–535, 1988a

Gold PW, Goodwin FK, Chrousos GP: Clinical and biochemical manifestations of depression, part II. Relation to the neurobiology of stress. N Eng J Med 319(7):413–420, 1988b

Golden RN, Gilmore JH, Corrigan MHN et al: Serotonin, suicide, and aggression: Clinical studies. J Clin Psychiatry 52(suppl 12):61–69, 1991

Goodwin FK, Jamison KR: The Natural Course of Manic-Depressive Illness. In Post RM, Ballenger JC (ed): Neurobiology of Mood Disorders, pp 20–37. Baltimore, Williams & Wilkins, 1984

Goodwin FK, Post RM, Murphy DL: Cerebrospinal fluid amine metabolites and therapies for depression. Sci Proc Am Psychiatr Assoc 126:24–25, 1973

Hertting G, Axelrod J, Whitby LG: Effects of drugs on the uptake and metabolism of 3H-norepinephrine. J Pharmacol Exp Ther 134:146–153, 1961

Hestbach J, Hansen HE, Amdisen A, Olsen S: Chronic renal lesions following long-term treatment with lithium. Kidney Int 12:205–213, 1977

Hirschfeld RM, Cross CC: Epidemiology of affective disorders: Psychosocial risk factors. Arch Gen Psychiatry 39:35–47, 1982

Holsboer F, Liebl R, Hofschuster E: Repeated desmethasone suppression test during depressive illness: Normalization of test result compared with clinical improvement. J Affect Disor 4:93–101, 1982

Janowsky DS, Risch SC: Adrenergic-Cholinergic Balance and Affective Disorders: A Review of Clinical Evidence and Therapeutic Implications. In Rusch AJ, Altschuler KC (eds): New Advances and Treatment of Depression. New York, Guilford Press, 1984

Jimerson DC, Insel TR, Reus VI, Kopin IW: Increased plasma MHPG in dexamethasone-resistant depressed patients. Arch Gen Psychiatry 40:173–176, 1983

Kaplan HI, Sadock BJ: Mood Disorders. In Kaplan HI, Sadock BJ (eds): Synopsis of Psychiatry. Baltimore, Williams & Wilkins, 1988

Karasu TB (Chairman): American Psychiatric Association Commission on Psychiatric Therapies, p 90. Washington, DC, American Psychiatric Association, 1984

Katon W, Raskind M: Treatment of depression in the medically ill elderly with methylphenidate. Am J Psychiatry 137:963–965, 1980

Katon W, Schulberg H. Epidemiology of depression in primary care. Gen Hosp Psychiatry 14(4):237–47, 1992

Keller MB, Baker LA: The Clinical Course of Panic Disorder and Depression. J Clin Psychiatry 53(suppl 3) 5–8, 1992

Keller MD, Lavori PW, Endicott J: "Double Depression" two-year follow-up. Am J Psychiatry 140:689–694, 1983

Klerman GL: History and Developments of Modern Concepts of Affective Illness. In Post RM, Ballenger JC (eds): Neurobiology of Mood Disorders, 1–19. Baltimore, Williams & Wilkins, 1984

Kling MA, Perini GI, Demitrack MA, Geracioti TD, Linnoila M, Chrousos GP, Gold PW. Stress-responsive neurohormonal systems and the symptom complex of affective illness. Psychopharmacol Bull 25:312–318, 1989

Kupfer DJ, Thase ME: The use of the sleep laboratory in the diagnosis of affective disorders. Psychiatr Clin North Am 6:3–25, 1983

Kupfer DJ, Spiker DG, Rossi A, Cable PA, Ulrich R, Shaw D: Recent Diagnostic and Treatment Advances in REM Sleep and Depression. In Calyton PJ, Barrett JE (eds): Treatment of Depression: Old Controversies and New Approaches. New York, Raven, 1983

Lichtenberg P, Shapira B, Gillon D, Kindler S, Cooper TB, Newman ME, Lerer B: Hormone responses to fenfluramine and placebo challenge in endogenous depression. Psychiatry Res 43:137–146, 1992

Lloyd C: Life events and depressive disorders reviewed, Part II: Events as precipitating factors. Arch Gen Psychiatry 37:541–548, 1980a

Lloyd C: Life events and depressive disorder reviewed, Part I: Events as predisposing factors. Arch Gen Psychiatry 37:529–535, 1980b

Loosen PT, Prange AJ: Serum thyroptropin response to thyrotropin-releasing hormone in psychiatric patients: A review. Am J Psychiatry 139:405–416, 1982

Maggi A, U'Prichard DC, Enna SJ: Differential effects of antidepressant treatment on brain monoaminergic receptors. Eur J Pharmac vol 61:91–98, 1980

Mass JW, Koslow SH, David J, Katz M, Fraxer A, Bowden CL, Berman N, Gibbons R, Stokes P, Landis DH: Catecholamine metabolism and disposition in health and depressed subjects. Arch Gen Psychiatry 44:337–344, 1987

McElroy SL, Keck PE, Pope HG, Hudson JI, Faedda GL, Swann AC. Dysphoric or mixed mania: Clinical and research implications. Am J Psychiatry 149:1633–1644, 1992

Mendels J, Frazer A, Fitzgerald RG, Ramsey TA, Stokes KW: Biogenic amine metabolites in cerebrospinal fluid of depressed and manic patients. Science 175:1380–1382, 1972

Mortola JF: Issues in the diagnosis and research of premenstrual syndrome. Clin Obste Gyn 35(3):587–598, 1992

Myers JK, Weisman MM, Tischler GL et al: Six-month prevalence of psychiatric disorders in three communities 1980–82. Arch Gen Psychiatry 41:959–967, 1984

Nemeroff CB, Widerlov E, Bissette G, Walleus H, Karlsson I, Eklund K, Kilts CD, Lossen PT, Yale W: Elevated concentrations of CSF corticotropin-releasing factor-like immunoreactivity in depressed patients. Science 226:1342–1343, 1984

NIH Consensus Development Panel on Depression in Late Life: Diagnosis and treatment of depression in late life. JAMA 268(8):1018–1024, 1992

Pardes H, Kaufmann CA, Pincus HA et al: Genetics and psychiatry: Past discoveries, current dilemmas, and future directions. Am J Psychiatry 146:435–443, 1989

Post RM: The transduction of psychosocial stress into the neurobiology of recurrent affective disorder. Am J Psychiatry 149(8):999–1010, 1992

Post RM, Ballenger JC, Uhde TW, Putman TW, Bunney WE: Kindling and Drug Sensitization: Implications for the Progressive Development of Psychopathology and Treatment with Carbamazepine. In Sadler M (ed): The Psychopharmacology of Anticonvulsants, pp 27–53. Oxford, Oxford University Press, 1981

Post RM, Gerner RH, Carman JS, Gillin JC, Jimerson DC, Goodwin FK, Bunney WE: Effects of a dopamine against piribedil in depressed patients. Arch Gen Psychiatry 35:609–615, 1978

Potter WZ, Rudarfer MV, Goodwin FK: Biological findings in bipolar disorders. Washington, DC, American Psychiatric Association Annual Review, Vol 6, 1987

Preskorn SH, Burke M: Somatic therapy for major depressive disorder: Selection of an antidepressant. J Clin Psychiatry 53(suppl 9):5–18, 1992

Quitkin F, Rifkin A, Klein DF: Monoamine oxidase inihibitors. Arch Gen Psychiatry 36:749–759, 1979

Redmond DE, Katz MM, Mass JW, Swann A, Casper R, David JM: Cerebrospinal fluid amine metabolites. Arch Gen Psychiatry 43:939–947, 1986

Reynolds CF, Kupfer DJ: Sleep research in affective illness: State of the art circa 1987. Sleep 10:199–215, 1987

Rickels K, Schweizer E: Clinical overview of serotonin reuptake inhibitors. J Clin Psychiatry 51(suppl B, 12):9–12, 1990

Risch SC, Cohen PM, Janowsky CS, Kalin NH, Insel TR, Murphy DL: Physostigmine induction of depressive symptomatology in normal volunteer subjects. J Psychiatry Res 4:89–94, 1981

Risch SC, Nemeroff CB. Neurochemical alterations of serotonergic neuronal systems in depression. J Clin Psychiatry 53(suppl 10):3–7, 1992

Robins LN, Regier DA (eds.): Psychiatric Disorders in America: The Epidemiologic Catchment Area Study. New York, The Free Press, 1991

Robinson DS, Nies A, Ravaris CL, Lamborn RR: The monoamine oxidase inhibitor, phenelzine, in the treatment of depressive-anxiety states. Arch Gen Psychiatry 29:407–413, 1973

Roose SP, Dalack GW: Treating the depressed patient with cardiovascular problems. J Clin Psychiatry 53(suppl 9):25–31, 1992

Roy A, Pickar D, Linnoila M, Doran AR, Ninan P, Paul SM: Cerebrospinal fluid monoamine metabolite concentrations in melancholia. Psychiatry Res 15:281–292, 1985

Schatzberg AF: Recent developments in the acute somatic treatment of major depression. J Clin Psychiatry 53(suppl 3):20–25, 1992

Schildkraut JJ: Current Status of the Catecholamine Hypothesis of Affective Disorders. In Lipton MA, DiMascio A, Killiam KF (eds.): Psychopharmacology: A Generation of Progress, pp 1223–1234. New York, Raven Press, 1978

Scully RF, Galdabini JJ, McNely BV: Case records of the Massachusetts General Hospital. N Engl J Med 304:1025–1032, 1981

Sedvall G, Fyro B, Gullberg B, Nyback H, Wiesel FA, Wode-Helgot B: Relationships in healthy volunteers between concentrations of monoamine metabolites in cerebrospinal fluid and family history of psychiatric morbidity. Br J Psychiatry 136:366–374, 1980

Shapira B, Yagmur MJ, Gropp C, Newman M, Lerer B: Effect of clomipramine and lithium on fenfluramine-induced hormone release in major depression. Biol Psychiatry 31:975–983, 1992

Sitaram N, Nurnberger JI, Gershon ES, Gillin JC: Faster cholinergic REM induction in euthymic patients with primary affective illness. Science 208:200–202, 1980

Sitaram N, Nurnberger JI, Gershon ES, Gillin JC: Cholinergic regulation of mood and REM sleep: Potential model and marker of vulnerability to affective disorder. Am J Psychiatry 139:571–576, 1982

Smith SB, Garcia-Sevilla JA, Hollingsworth PJ: Adrenoceptors in rat brain are decreased after long-term trycyclic antidepressant drug treatment. Brain Res 210:413–418, 1981

Stoudemire A: Depression. In Lubin MF, Walker HK, Smith RB (eds) Psychiatric Disorders in the Medical-Surgical Patient, Section IV, 3rd ed. Boston, Butterworths, in press.

Stoudemire GA, Fogel BS Gulley LR, Moran MG: Psychopharmacology in the Medical Patient. In Stoudemire A, Fogel BS (eds): Psychiatric Care of the Medical Patient, pp 155–206. New York, Oxford University Press, 1993.

Sulser F, Vetulani J, Mobley PL: Mode of action of antidepressant drugs. Biochem Pharmacol 27:257–261, 1978

Targum SD: Application of serial neuroendocrine challenge studies in the management of depressive disorders. Biol Psychiatr 18:3–19, 1983

Thase ME: Long-term treatment of recurrent depressive disorders. J Clin Psychiatry 53(suppl 9): 32–44 1992

Theohar C, Fischer-Cornelsson K, Akesson HO, Ansari J, Gerlach G, Ohman R, Ose E, Stegink AJ: Bromocryptine as anti-depressant: Double-blind comparative study with imipramine in psychogenic and endogenous depression. Curr Ther Res 30:830–842, 1981

Van Praag HM, DeHaan S: Central serotonin metabolism and frequency of depression. Psychiatr Res 1:219–224, 1979

Van Scheyen JD, Van Praag HM, Korf J: Controlled study comparing nomifensine and chlomipramine in unipolar depression, using the probeneced technique. Br J Clin Pharmacol 4:1795–1845, 1977

Veith RC, Raskind MA, Caldwell JH: Cardiovascular effects of tricyclic antidepressants in depressed patients with chronic heart disease. N Engl J Med 306:954–959, 1982

Vetulani J, Stawarz RJ, Dingell JV, Sulser F: A possible common mechanism of action of antidepressant treatments: Reduction in the sensitivity of the noradrenergic cycle AMP generating system in the rat limbic forearm. Naunyn-Schmiedeberg's Arch Pharmacol 293:109–114, 1976

Waehrens J, Gerlach J: Bromocryptine and imipramine in endogenous depression: A double-blind controlled trial in outpatients. J Affect Disord 3:193–202, 1981

Weisler RH. A profile of bupropion: A nonserotonergic alternative. J Clin Psychiatry Monograph 9(1):29–35, 1991

Weissman MM, Boyd JH: The Epidemilogy of Affective Disorders. In Post RM, Ballenger JC (eds): Neurobiology of Mood Disorders. Baltimore, Williams & Wilkins, 1984

Weissman MM, Klerman GL: Depression: Current understanding and changing trends. Annu Rev Publ Health 13:319–39, 1992

Williams AW, Ware JE, Donald CA: A model of mental health, life events, and social supports applicable to general populations. J Health Soc Behav 22:324–336, 1981

Willner P: Depression: A Psychobiological Synthesis. New York, A Wiley-Interscience Publication, 1985

Alan Stoudemire (ed). *Clinical Psychiatry for Medical Students*, Second Edition. Copyright © 1994, 1990 by J. B. Lippincott Company.

8 *Anxiety Disorders*

Linda M. Nagy, John H. Krystal, and Dennis S. Charney

The anxiety disorders discussed in this chapter are those included in the *Diagnostic and Statistical Manual of Mental Disorders*, Fourth Edition (DSM-IV): panic disorder and agoraphobia, social phobia, specific phobia, obsessive–compulsive disorder, posttraumatic stress disorder, generalized anxiety disorder, and acute stress disorder (APA 1993, in press [1994]). For each disorder, epidemiologic data, a basic description of the syndrome, similarity to and differences from other psychiatric or nonpsychiatric medical disorders, current models and theories of etiology, and treatment approaches are reviewed. It is crucial that physicians be able to properly recognize anxiety disorders and be aware of their appropriate treatments. These conditions are among the most common in the general population, lead to high utilization of health care services, and, when untreated, produce significant distress and disability.

ADJUSTMENT DISORDER WITH ANXIETY

The general category of *adjustment disorder* has been mentioned in Chapter 7 by Drs. Risby, Risch, and Stoudemire in reference to depressive reactions. In the context of anxiety, an adjustment disorder with anxiety would be defined as a *maladaptive* reaction to an identifiable environmental or psychosocial stress, accompanied predominantly by symptoms of anxiety, that interferes with the patient's functioning. Although the degree of anxiety-related stress can be disabling, the anxiety is expected to remit after the stress remits or an adaptation is made. Patients can also be designated as having "mixed anxiety and depressed mood" if symptoms of anxiety and depression appear enmeshed.

These types of stress-related reactions often bring patients to physicians' offices with a variety of physiological symptoms of their anxiety. Short-term use of low-dose benzodiazepines may be of benefit as long as the patient is helped to identify the stress that may have caused the symptoms and means of managing it more effectively are discussed. If the stress appears to be chronic or unmanageable by the patient, the patient may require further evaluation and possibly some form of psychotherapy. Referral for a thorough psychiatric evaluation should be made well before the long-term use of benzodiazepines becomes the only alternative for managing chronic anxiety.

PANIC DISORDER AND AGORAPHOBIA

Panic disorder is characterized by recurrent discrete attacks of anxiety accompanied by several somatic symptoms, such as palpitations, paresthesias, hyperventilation, diaphoresis, chest pain, dizziness, trembling, and dyspnea. Usually the condition is accompanied by agoraphobia, which consists of excessive fear (and often avoidance) of situations, such as driving, crowded places, stores, or being alone, in which escape or obtaining help would be difficult. Current DSM-IV classifications include "panic disorder without agoraphobia," "panic disorder with agoraphobia," and "agoraphobia without history of panic disorder."

Epidemiology

The Epidemiologic Catchment Area Study (ECA) reports prevalence estimates based on DSM-III diagnoses, which were separated into agoraphobia and panic disorder. Lifetime prevalence rates at the three sites varied between 7.8 and 23.3% for all phobias (including social and simple) and between 1.4 and 1.5% for panic disorder. Six-month prevalence rates were 2.7 to 5.8% for agoraphobia and 0.6 to 1.0% for panic disorder. The lifetime rate for females was 2.4 to 4.3 times greater than that for males for agoraphobia and 1.3 to 3.5 times greater for panic disorder; however, 6-month prevalence rates for panic disorder were either similar between sexes or increased in males (Robins et al, 1984; Myers et al, 1984). It is generally felt that there may be underreporting of these disorders by men either due to reluctance to admit to having these symptoms or through disguise by alcoholism. Alternatively, there may be true higher rates in females because of hormonal, social, or other types of gender-related differences.

Age of onset is typically in the late teens to early thirties and is unusual after the age of 40 years. *The majority (78%) of patients describe the initial panic attack as spontaneous* (occurring without an environmental trigger). In the remainder the first attack is precipitated by confrontation with a phobic stimulus or use of a psychoactive drug. Onset of the disorder often follows within six months of a major stressful life event, such as marital separation, occupational change, or pregnancy (Breier et al, 1986).

These disorders appear to be less prevalent in the elderly. Both six-month and lifetime rates are lower in the over-65 age group, suggesting possible underreporting, decreased survival of those with the disorder, or a cohort effect, such that the frequency of the disorder is increased in the middle-age groups. Rates are generally similar for blacks and whites, and higher for noncollege graduates and unmarried individuals. It is not yet established whether these differences reflect predisposing factors, noncausal associations, or consequences of the disorder. Panic disorder is increased among family members of those with the disorder (see Etiology, below). A history of childhood separation anxiety disorder is reported by 20 to 50% of patients. Preliminary findings of high rates of behavioral inhibition in the offspring of patients with panic disorder are consistent with the hypothesis that the disorder may have developmental antecedents.

Description and Differential Diagnosis

Panic disorder usually begins with a spontaneous panic attack that often leads the individual to seek medical treatment, such as presenting to an emergency room believing that he or she is having a heart attack, stroke, losing his or her mind, or experiencing some other serious medical event (Table 8–1). Some time may pass before subsequent attacks, or the patient may continue to get frequent attacks. Patients may feel constantly fearful and anxious after the first attack, wondering what is wrong and fearing it will happen again. Some patients experience nocturnal attacks that awaken them from sleep. Usually patients gradually become fearful of situations (1) that they associate with the attacks; (2) in which they would be unable to flee if the attack occurred; (3) in which help would not be readily available; or (4) in which they would be embarrassed if others should notice they are experiencing an attack (although attacks are not usually evident to others). Typical agoraphobic situations are

Table 8–1 **Symptoms of a Panic Attack***

A discrete period of intense fear or discomfort, in which at least four of the following symptoms developed abruptly and reached a peak within 10 minutes:
1. palpitations, pounding heart, or accelerated heart rate
2. sweating
3. trembling or shaking
4. sensations of shortness of breath or smothering
5. feeling of choking
6. chest pain or discomfort
7. nausea or abdominal distress
8. feeling dizzy, unsteady, lightheaded, or faint
9. derealization (feelings of unreality) or depersonalization (being detached from oneself)
10. fear of losing control or going crazy
11. fear of dying
12. paresthesias (numbness or tingling sensations)
13. chills or hot flushes

* Adapted from DSM-IV (APA 1993, in press [1994])

listed in Table 8–2. Less frequently, a history of phobia may precede the first panic attack. Before patients are educated about the symptoms of the disorder they believe they are suffering from a serious medical condition. They are often embarrassed about their symptoms and will try to hide them from others, often making excuses not to attend functions or enter phobic situations.

The differential diagnosis of panic disorder and agoraphobia includes anxiety disorders due to general medical conditions; anxiety due to substances such as caffeine, cocaine, or amphetamines; withdrawal from alcohol, sedative-hypnotics and benzodiazepines; as well as other phobic conditions, generalized anxiety disorder, and

Table 8–2 **Features of Agoraphobia***

A. **Panic Disorder with Agoraphobia:** Anxiety about being in places or situations in which escape might be difficult (or embarrassing) or in which help may not be available in the event of having an unexpected or situationally predisposed panic attack.

Agoraphobia Without History of Panic Disorder: The patient has never met criteria for panic disorder and the anxiety may occur in situations in which help may not be available in the event of suddenly developing panic-like symptoms that the individual fears could be incapacitating or extremely embarrassing, for example, fear of going outside because of fear of having a sudden episode of dizziness or a sudden attack of diarrhea. If a general medical condition is present, this fear described in the latter diagnosis, is clearly in excess of that usually associated with the condition.

B. Agoraphobic fears typically involve characteristic clusters of situations that include

TRAVEL:	PROXIMITY OF SAFETY:
Airplane*	May have a safe perimeter**
Car	Far from medical help
Bus	Being home alone or outside the home
Subway	PUBLIC PLACES:
Train	Stores
DRIVING:	Malls
Alone	Restaurants
Highways	Theaters
Bridges	Church/Temple
Tunnels	Crowds
Heavy traffic	OTHER:
Inner lane of highway	Sitting in a meeting
	Waiting in line
	Sitting far from an exit***

   *Fear is of being trapped, not that plane will crash.
  **A specific distance from home; in severe form can become housebound.
 ***Prefer last row, aisle seat in theater, auditorium, or classroom.

C. Agoraphobic situations are avoided (e.g., restricts travel), or else endured with marked distress or with anxiety about having a panic attack (or panic-like symptoms), or require the presence of a companion.

D. The anxiety or phobic avoidance is not better accounted for by another mental disorder, such as Specific Phobia (e.g., avoidance limited to a single situation like elevators), Separation Anxiety Disorder (e.g., avoidance of school), Obsessive–Compulsive Disorder (e.g., fear of contamination), Posttraumatic Stress Disorder (e.g., avoidance of stimuli associated with a traumatic event), or Social Phobia (e.g., avoidance limited to social situations because of fear of embarrassment unrelated to panic attacks).

* Adapted from DSM-IV (APA 1993, in press [1994])

psychosis. Medical illness that may produce symptoms similar to panic attacks must be excluded. Endocrine disturbances, such as pheochromocytoma, thyroid disorder, or hypoglycemia, may produce similar symptoms and can be excluded with appropriate clinical history and laboratory evaluations. When gastrointestinal symptoms of attacks are prominent one may need to exclude the diagnosis of colitis. Symptoms of tachycardia, palpitations, chest pain or pressure, and dyspnea may be confused with cardiac or respiratory conditions. Lightheadedness, faintness, dizziness, derealization, shaking, numbness, and tingling may suggest a neurologic condition. The association between mitral valve prolapse and panic disorder is controversial. The presence of mitral valve prolapse in panic disorder patients does not appear to alter treatment response or course, so the diagnosis of panic disorder should be made independently of mitral valve prolapse.

Panic disorder differs from generalized anxiety disorder in that the panic attacks are distinguished by recurrent discrete, intense episodes of panic symptoms, although in both disorders anticipatory anxiety and generalized feelings of anxiety may be present. Although some of the same situations may be feared, agoraphobia differs from social and simple phobias in that the fear is related to feeling trapped or being unable to escape and that the fears often become generalized. Agoraphobics may additionally have a history of other phobias.

Panic disorder is frequently associated with major depression, other anxiety disorders, and alcohol and substance dependence. In clinical samples as many as two-thirds of panic patients report experiencing a major depressive episode at some time in their lives. Similarly, studies of patients seeking treatment for major depression report high rates of panic in these patients and their relatives. Once symptoms begin, patients often describe becoming demoralized as a result of fear related to the symptoms and imagined causes, and resulting from impairment when their activities are restricted by their agoraphobia. Unlike depressed patients, panic disorder patients usually lack vegetative symptoms and have a normal desire to engage in activities but avoid them because of their phobias.

The disorder may cause personality changes. Patients' premorbid personalities may be highly independent, outgoing, and active, but while symptoms are active they can become very dependent, passive, overly agreeable, with an extreme need to please others, and may resist making appointments or social engagements.

Attempts to self-medicate the intolerable anxiety may increase the risk of alcoholism and substance abuse. Patients may require a drink before entering phobic situations. Approximately 20% of patients report a history of alcohol abuse, but the onset of alcoholism precedes the first attack in almost all patients (Breier et al, 1986). Alcoholism may also alter the course of the disorder. Preliminary data suggest panic disorder precipitated by cocaine use may be less likely to respond well to the usual pharmacologic treatments and may have less association with a family history of panic disorder.

Etiologic/Pathophysiologic Theories

Familial/Genetic Theories

Genetic epidemiologic studies have consistently demonstrated increased rates of panic disorder among first- and second-degree relatives of panic disorder probands.

This observation could result from genetic, nongenetic biological, and/or cultural factors shared by family members. The reported recurrence risk of illness in first-degree relatives of panic disorder probands is 15 to 18% by patient report vs. 0 to 5% in controls, and is 20 to 50% by direct interview of relatives of panic probands vs. 2 to 8% in relatives of controls (Crowe, 1985). Segregation analysis indicates the pattern of familial transmission is consistent with single-locus autosomal dominant transmission with incomplete penetrance, although a multifactorial mode of inheritance (additive effects of more than one gene) or genetic heterogeneity (different gene defects producing similar clinical syndromes) have not been excluded as possibilities (Pauls et al, 1980). Comparison of concordance rates in monozygotic vs. dizygotic twins is used to differentiate between genetic and environmental factors in families, since monozygotic twins share 100% of their genetic material and dizygotic twins on average share half. Torgersen (1983) found concordance for anxiety disorder with panic attacks in 4 of 13 monozygotic and 0 of 16 dizygotic twin pairs. Other preliminary reports suggest identical HLA genotypes in sibling pairs concordant for panic disorder; genetic linkage studies thus far have been negative (Crowe et al, 1990).

Other Biologic Theories

Investigation of biologic systems in panic disorder includes examination of adrenergic, benzodiazepine, serotonergic, and opiate neurotransmitter systems; anxiogenic response to caffeine, lactate, and CO_2; models of locus ceruleus involvement; and brain imaging studies. Yohimbine, an alpha-2 adrenergic receptor antagonist, produces greater increases in anxiety (resembling panic attacks), blood pressure, and plasma levels of the norepinephrine metabolite MHPG in panic disorder patients than in healthy subjects. This responsiveness appears to be specific to panic disorder patients; it is not observed in generalized anxiety disorder, obsessive–compulsive disorder, major depression, or schizophrenia. However, posttraumatic stress disorder patients have similar responses (see below). Panic patients exhibit panic attacks and a blunted heart rate response to isoproterenol, a beta-adrenergic agonist, as well as decreased lymphocyte beta-adrenergic receptors. It is hypothesized that downregulation of beta-adrenergic receptor function is due to chronic or episodically increased presynaptic noradrenergic activity.

The benzodiazepine inverse agonist FG-7142 precipitated severe anxiety states comparable to panic attacks in healthy individuals; this is consistent with animal studies in which beta carboline produces an acute fear state. The benzodiazepine antagonist flumazenil precipitated a modest level of anxiety and panic attacks in some panic disorder patients. Further evidence for benzodiazepine system involvement is the finding of a blunted saccadic eye movement response in panic patients.

Preclinical studies have suggested possible serotonergic involvement in anxiety and in the mechanisms of action of medications used to treat anxiety. However, the prolactin response to the serotonin precursor tryptophan is not altered in panic disorder. The serotonin agonist m-chlorophenylpiperazine (MCPP) may elicit greater anxiety responses in panic disorder patients, but the response is not as pronounced or consistent as that observed with yohimbine or lactate. Fenfluramine (a serotonin release and reuptake blocker) can also produce panic in panic disorder patients.

Neuropeptides are receiving increasing attention. CCK is anxiogenic in healthy controls as well as panic patients. Neuropeptide Y is anxiolytic in animals but has not been studied in panic patients. Interactions between opiate and adrenergic systems were studied using yohimbine and naloxone, an opiate antagonist. The combination produced a synergistic effect of increasing anxiety symptoms and plasma cortisol. This is postulated to occur through opiate-noradrenergic interactions in the locus ceruleus, amygdala, cerebral cortex, or hypothalamus.

Although provocation of panic attacks with sodium lactate is the best-replicated of the provocation procedures in panic, the mechanism by which lactate causes panic attacks is not established. Effects on noradrenergic activity, calcium, and regulation of intracellular pH and ion channels have been explored. Panic patients also demonstrate an increased anxiogenic response to breathing a mixture of air and CO_2 as compared with controls. Effective antianxiety medications appear to block lactate-, yohimbine-, or CO_2-induced attacks.

Caffeine produces significantly greater anxiety symptoms in panic disorder patients than in controls. Therefore, patients are usually advised to eliminate caffeine from their diet. The most likely mechanism of caffeine's anxiogenic effect is antagonism of central adenosine receptors, which have neuromodulatory effects on acetylcholine, norepinephrine, and firing rates of locus ceruleus and other neurons. In animal studies of the locus ceruleus, the major norepinephrine-containing nucleus in the brain, stimulation produces a marked fear and anxiety response and ablation diminishes fear response to threatening stimuli. Additionally, many drugs which increase locus ceruleus firing in animals are anxiogenic in humans, whereas several drugs that decrease locus ceruleus discharge are anxiolytic in humans (Gorman and Liebowitz, 1986).

Unlike major depression, panic disorder patients fail to show nonsuppression of cortisol following dexamethasone and worsen rather than improve with sleep deprivation (reviewed in Roy-Byrne and Cowley, 1988).

Behavioral Theories

Behavioral theories (learning theory) have mainly been applied to the development of agoraphobia. This involves contiguity learning, the paired association of events that have occurred together (e.g., a panic attack and driving over a bridge), together with instrumental learning or operant conditioning, the modification of behavior to avoid future negative events and invite future positive events (e.g., by avoiding bridges, avoid the discomfort of an attack). Stimulus generalization may occur or subsequent attacks may occur in different situations and become associated with those situations (Millon, 1986). Panic disorder has also been viewed as a phobia in which the feared stimuli are internal rather than external. Patients associate somatic sensations with immediate threat and respond with anxiety and fear. After the first panic attack, subsequent attacks begin with unexpected peripheral somatic sensations to which the patient responds with anxiety, resulting in additional somatic symptoms and a spiralling increase in anxiety and symptoms. This theory has led to the application of relaxation, cognitive, and exposure techniques to the treatment of the attacks themselves (Rapee and Barlow, 1988).

Psychoanalytic Theories

Psychoanalytic theory stems from Freud's hypothesis that panic attacks result from incomplete repression of unacceptable impulses. Later he revised this theory to conceptualize anxiety as a signal to the ego that it is in a dangerous situation. The patient then develops neurotic symptoms to reduce the signal anxiety and avoid danger. In any case, unconscious psychological conflict is believed to be the root cause. Freud also felt agoraphobia was due to the recollection of an anxiety attack along with fear of a future attack occurring in a situation in which the patient believed he or she could not escape it. He observed constitutional variability in individuals' capacities to experience anxiety and predicted that the mechanisms of biological predispositions would be better elucidated with advancing knowledge of brain neurochemistry.

Treatment

Pharmacologic Treatment

Imipramine is the most well-established medication for panic, but most tricyclic antidepressants (TCAs) probably have similar efficacy. Monoamine oxidase inhibitors (MAOIs) can be very effective medications for anxiety patients but are not necessarily the drugs of choice, because they necessitate a low-tyramine diet to minimize the risk of hypertensive crisis. Anxiety patients are especially fearful and need extra education and reassurance to take this medication. Preliminary reports suggest various selective serotonin reuptake inhibitors (SSRIs), including fluvoxamine, fluoxetine, clomipramine and citalopram, may also be effective. Despite efficacy in depression, trazodone and buproprion appear to be ineffective in panic disorder.

With all TCAs, MAOIs, and SSRIs, roughly 20% of panic patients will experience a stimulant-like reaction (with jitteriness, insomnia, and possibly increased panic attacks) during initial treatment. We recommend the following: (a) explain to the patient that this may occur, they need not be alarmed, and encourage them to call to discuss problems (rather than abruptly and unnecessarily discontinue treatment); (b) start with the lowest available dose (e.g., 10 mg imipramine, 5 mg fluoxetine); (c) if activation occurs, decrease to the dose that was previously tolerated until symptoms subside, then increase slowly. Some patients will habituate to the activation syndrome but symptoms may reemerge with each dose increment. As in depression, antipanic effects are delayed for 2–6 weeks after reaching a therapeutic dose. Extra reassurance and encouragement are often needed when treating patients with this disorder.

Although alprazolam is the best studied of the benzodiazepines in panic disorder, other benzodiazepines, including lorazepam, clonazepam, and diazepam, are also effective when adequate doses are used. Onset of therapeutic effects is fairly rapid. Some respond to low doses (i.e., 0.25 mg t.i.d. of alprazolam or equivalent) but 3.0 to 6.0 mg/day in divided doses is common. Benzodiazepines are usually used after other treatments have failed for panic because of concerns about difficulty with discontinuation. Benzodiazepines should be avoided in patients with a history of alcohol or substance-abuse problems or personality disorder. Benzodiazepines with an intermediate elimination half-life (see Table 8–11) are sometimes preferred due to the need for less frequent dosing. Very long acting benzodiazepines such as diazepam can lead to problems with dose accumulation, particularly in older or medically compromised patients.

To initiate pharmacologic treatment, begin with a low dose and gradually increase to therapeutic range (see Table 8–3 and Chapters 7 and 18). Reduction of phobic symptoms in particular may require maximal dosages. Once remission is achieved (1–3 months), lower maintenance doses may be adequate (up to 8–12 months) during which time patients should consolidate treatment improvements and return to a normal lifestyle. Discontinuation of medication should be gradual for both pharmacological and psychological reasons. Symptoms may reemerge shortly after benzodiazepine discontinuation and up to 2–3 months after discontinuation of antidepressants. Benzodiazepine withdrawal symptoms can be minimized by tapering slowly (e.g., 0.25–0.5 mg alprazolam every 3 to 7 days) and even more gradually for the last 1.5 mg. Patients need to understand that they may be asked to tolerate mild to moderate symptoms that are not dangerous for 4–10 days and the doctor should be available for guidance and support through this period (Ballenger, 1992). If symptoms persist 3 weeks after a benzodiazepine is discontinued, additional treatment should be considered. (For additional information on long-term treatment, see Nagy, 1989; 1993).

Despite its usefulness in treating generalized anxiety disorder, the nonbenzodiazepine anxiolytic buspirone is probably ineffective in treating panic. Beta-blockers may block symptoms of palpitations or tremor but generally are not as effective against panic attacks as tricyclic antidepressants, MAOIs, or benzodiazepines. Occasionally a combination of a tricyclic antidepressant and benzodiazepine is required. If both medications are initiated together, there is some possibility that the benzodiazepine blocks the therapeutic effect of the tricyclic antidepressant, based on reemergence of symptoms on attempts to withdraw the benzodiazepine (Woods et al, 1992). An alternative explanation is that benzodiazepine discontinuation itself induces symptoms of panic. The combination of pharmacologic treatment with behavioral or supportive psychotherapy is very important, especially when phobias are present. Table 8–3 summarizes pharmacologic approaches for panic disorder/agoraphobia.

Behavioral Treatment

Prolonged exposure in vivo (see behavioral therapies in Chapter 17) appears to be the most effective behavioral treatment for agoraphobia. The usual procedure is to develop a hierarchical list of phobias, gradually enter the least phobic situations repeatedly, then work up the hierarchy to more strongly feared situations. Prolonged (2 hours), in vivo, and frequent (daily) exposure sessions are superior to brief (0.5 hour), imaginal, and spaced (weekly) exposure sessions. Good results can be achieved in groups, individually, or as a self-help or spouse-assisted program. Group therapy may have the additional advantages of being cost effective, providing the patient with coping models, and leading to fewer dropouts. It is not essential to evoke anxiety during exposure. Follow-up studies report enduring effects several years after treatment.

Cognitive therapy appears to reduce irrational beliefs but by itself may not reduce anxiety or avoidance. The focus is to identify distorted patterns of thinking,

Table 8–3 **Pharmacotherapy for Anxiety Disorders**

	ALPRAZOLAM*‡/ BENZODIAZEPINES	BUSPIRONE	IMIPRAMINE‡/TCA	PHENELZINE‡/MAOI	FLUOXETINE/SSRI
Main indications†	PD, GAD, SP	GAD, refractory OCD(?)	PD, PTSD, GAD(?), OCD(?)	PD, PTSD, SP, OCD(?)	OCD, PD(?), SP(?), PTSD(?)
Starting dose	0.25–0.5 mg TID	5 mg TID	10 mg qhs	15 mg q AM	5–20 mg/day
Initial side effects	Sedation, ataxia, memory impairment	Dizziness, nausea, diarrhea, headache, nervousness	Sedation, orthostatic hypotension, dry mouth, anxiety	Orthostatic hypotension, stimulant, tyramine reaction	Gastrointestinal, anorexia, insomnia, anxiety, drowsiness
Onset of effect	Immediate	2–4 wk delay	2–4 wk delay	2–4 wk delay	3–6 wk delay
Common target dose	.25–2.0 mg TID	5–20 mg TID	25–300 mg qhs (or divided dose)	15–30 mg TID	20–80 mg/d
Long-term side effects	Physical dependence	None known at this time	Weight gain	Tyramine reaction	Unknown
Rate of discontinuation	0.25 mg/wk	No need to taper	50 mg/1–2 wk	15–45 mg/wk	No need to taper
Symptoms of abrupt discontinuation	Increased sensitivity to sound/light/touch, autonomic arousal, confusion, seizures	None known at this time	Flulike symptoms, anxiety, nightmares	Hypertension, anxiety, nightmares, autonomic arousal, psychosis	None known at this time

* Benzodiazepine dose equivalents: 1 mg alprazolam = 0.5 mg clonazepam = 2 mg lorazepam = 10 mg diazepam; intermediate-acting benzodiazepines may have advantages. See text regarding discontinuation guidelines.
† PD = panic disorder; SP = social phobia; OCD = obsessive-compulsive disorder; GAD = generalized anxiety disorder; PTSD = posttraumatic stress disorder
‡ Alprazolam, imipramine, phenelzine and fluoxetine are listed as prototypical drugs in their respective classes for purposes of dosage guidelines. Other drugs in the same class may be effective.
(Adapted from Krystal JH, Charney DS: Advances in anxiety therapy. Internal Medicine for the Specialist 9:93–111, 1988)

interrupt the thought with self-instruction to stop, and substitute either distraction or positive thoughts. There is some evidence favoring the combination of relaxation training and biofeedback with cognitive therapy in the treatment of panic attacks. A newer form of cognitive-behavioral therapy—panic control treatment (PCT), which is comprised of breathing retraining, cognitive restructuring, and exposure to somatic cues—can be effective for desensitizing to symptoms of panic attacks in patients with no or mild agoraphobia. A multicenter trial is under way comparing PCT with imipramine and their combination.

Assertiveness training can help with dependency, passivity, and suppressed anger, which commonly result from patients' attempts to deal with panic and phobias. Aggressive individuals can be taught to recognize their aggressive behavior and substitute assertiveness.

Psychoeducation plays a very important role in the management of these patients. Knowing their diagnosis is enormously reassuring to many patients, who tend to believe they have a rare, perhaps life-threatening condition that doctors have failed to recognize. It is important to emphasize that although they feel they will die, faint, lose control, or go crazy during attacks, this will not happen. They also should understand current theories of etiology and that, with treatment, the prognosis for a significant reduction in symptoms and improvement in functioning is very good. Also, *group treatment* is helpful for patients to recognize that others suffer from the same syndrome. These groups can provide very beneficial understanding, support, and encouragement from peers. Many communities have self-help groups for panic/agoraphobic patients.

Combinations of behavior therapies or medication together with behavior therapy are commonly employed. It is important to emphasize alternative treatments to patients expecting to receive only one form of treatment, such as individuals who are "phobic" of medications or patients expecting complete relief from a "magic pill." The possibility of noncompliance with treatment recommendations should be considered in treatment failure.

Psychodynamically oriented psychotherapy may be an important adjunctive treatment for individuals with significant interpersonal difficulties but has no proven specific effect in alleviating panic attacks or agoraphobia.

Role of the Nonpsychiatric Physician in Patient Management

Nonpsychiatric physicians play a crucial role in the initial evaluation and recognition of panic disorder since patients will most frequently present with symptoms of panic attacks in medical settings. Following a negative workup for medical pathology, it is insufficient to attribute the patient's symptoms to "anxiety" or "stress." As stated above, it is very important that patients receive the appropriate diagnosis and treatment.

In ongoing pharmacologic treatment (especially with benzodiazepines), it is important to differentiate the patient's desire to alleviate symptoms with effective medication from the drug-seeking behavior of substance abusers. Once symptoms are relieved, panic patients usually do not request dose increases. On the contrary, they typically fear "addiction" and have the long-term goal of dose reduction or being medication-free. However, due to the chronic nature of the disorder, and because medications provide treatment without necessarily a cure, prolonged pharmacologic treatment or repeated courses of treatment may be necessary.

Indications for Psychiatric Consultation and Referral

In cases that are not straightforward, psychiatric evaluation can aid in establishing the diagnosis, comprehensively assessing co-morbid disorders, and selecting appropriate treatments. When a patient's response to initial treatment is inadequate, psychiatrists experienced in treatment of panic and agoraphobia may facilitate a treatment response with dosage adjustment, management of side effects, addressing resistance to treatment recommendations, and ensuring the adequacy of nonpharmacologic treatments.

CLINICAL PEARLS FOR PANIC DISORDER

- Suspect panic attacks in patients without physical pathology who present with somatic symptoms suggestive of cardiac, endocrine, and neurologic disorders.
- In establishing the diagnosis of panic attacks, ask how quickly the symptoms reach their peak, not how long they last. Ask also if any attacks were unexpected.
- When using antidepressants be sure to warn patients about a possible initial "activation syndrome" and use small doses to begin treatment.
- Benzodiazepines may be required in higher dosages and for longer periods than indicated for other disorders; tricyclics, MAOIs, and SSRIs should be considered first lines of treatment.
- Be alert for coexisting anxiety disorders, major depression, alcoholism, and substance abuse, and address them as indicated.

SOCIAL PHOBIA

Social fears are commonly experienced by healthy individuals, especially in initial public-speaking experiences. For some people, this fear becomes persistent and overwhelming, limiting their social or occupational functioning because of intense anxiety and, often, avoidance. Social phobia is an area of active research; therefore, our knowledge base will be expanding rapidly in the next several years.

Epidemiology

Preliminary estimates of six-month prevalence rates of social phobia ascertained by screening questionnaire in the ECA Study are 1.2 to 2.2% (0.9 to 1.7% in men, 1.5 to 2.6% in women). The distribution is fairly even across the age span although rates may be lower in the over-65 age group. Onset is usually between 15 and

20 years of age, and the course tends to be chronic and unremitting. Complications include interference with work or school, social isolation, and abuse of alcohol or drugs. In inpatient alcoholism treatment programs, 20 to 25% report social phobia beginning before the onset of alcoholism or persisting after 1 year of abstinence. Significant depressive symptoms may also occur in social phobia; in one study, one-third of social phobia patients reported a history of major depression.

Description and Differential Diagnosis

Social phobia is characterized by a persistent and exaggerated fear of humiliation or embarrassment in social situations, leading to high levels of distress and possibly avoidance of those situations (Table 8–4) Patients may become fearful that their anxiety will be evident to others, which may intensify their symptoms or even produce a situational panic attack. The fear may be of speaking, meeting people, eating, or writing in public, and relates to the fear of appearing nervous or foolish, making mistakes, being criticized, or being laughed at. Often physical symptoms of anxiety such as blushing, trembling, sweating, and tachycardia are triggered when the patient feels under evaluation or scrutiny. Subtypes that may predict differential treatment response may be proposed in DSM-IV, such as phobia in which the focus of concern is on *performing* in front of others rather than on social interactions and phobia that is *limited* to one or a few socially interactive situations or is *generalized* to most social situations.

Table 8–4 **Criteria for Social Phobia**

A. A marked and persistent fear of one or more social or performance situations in which the person is exposed to unfamiliar people or to possible scrutiny by others. They fear that they may act in a way that will be humiliating or embarrassing. Examples include being unable to continue talking while speaking in public, choking on food when eating in front of others, being unable to urinate in a public lavatory, hand-trembling when writing in the presence of others, and saying foolish things or not being able to answer questions in social situations.

B. Exposure to the feared social situation almost invariably provokes anxiety, which may take the form of a situationally bound panic attack.

C. The person recognizes that his or her fear is excessive or unreasonable.

D. The feared social or performance situations(s) avoided, or else endured with intense anxiety or distress.

E. The avoidance, anxious anticipation, or distress in the feared social or performance situations interfere significantly with person's normal routine, occupational (academic) functioning, or with social activities or relationships with others, or there is marked distress about having the phobia.

F. The fear or avoidance is not due to a Substance-Induced or Anxiety Disorder Due to a General Medical Condition, and is not better accounted for by Panic Disorder With or Without Agoraphobia, Separation Anxiety Disorder, Body Dysmorphic Disorder, a Pervasive Developmental Disorder, or Schizoid Personality Disorder.

G. If another nonanxiety condition is present (e.g., Stuttering, Parkinson's disease, or Anorexia Nervosa), anxiety about the social impact of the disorder is clearly in excess of that usually associated with the disorder.

Adapted from DSM-IV (APA 1993, in press [1994])

Two case vignettes of social phobia follow:

CASE 1:

A 29-year-old single businessman stated that at age 12 his voice "cracked" during an audition and people laughed at him. A few years later he became very anxious when he had to speak in class. He gradually became very anxious or avoided any situation in which he might be called upon or observed, even to answer a roll call. His avoidance of professional meetings was interfering with his work.

CASE 2:

A 33-year-old single female chemist described how, during the rehearsal dinner for her best friend's wedding, she became very anxious and broke into a cold sweat. She began anticipating that she would perspire excessively when encountering people, which then would occur. She began avoiding any organized social event and was frustrated about this limitation on her life.

Probably the most difficult diagnostic distinctions are between social phobia and normal performance anxiety, or social phobia and panic disorder. Normal fear of public speaking usually diminishes as the individual is speaking or with additional experience, whereas in social phobia the anxiety may worsen or fail to attenuate with rehearsal. Social phobics may experience situational panic attacks resulting from anticipation or exposure to the feared social situation. Some panic disorder/agoraphobia patients avoid social situations due to fear of embarrassment if a panic attack should occur, but usually their initial panic attack is unexpected (occurs in a situation they previously did not fear), and the subsequent development of phobias is generalized beyond social phobia situations. Sometimes social phobia and panic disorder coexist. Social phobia can be differentiated from simple phobias in that the latter do not involve social situations involving scrutiny, humiliation, or embarrassment. In major depression, social avoidance may develop from apathy rather than fear and resolves with remission of the depressive episode. In schizoid personality disorder, social isolation is due to lack of interest rather than fear. In avoidant personality disorder, the avoidance is of personal relationships; however, if the patient develops a marked anxiety about and avoidance of most social situations, the additional diagnosis of social phobia should be given.

Etiology

Familial/Genetic Theories

Animal studies demonstrate heritability of various fear, anxiety, and exploratory, escape, or avoidant behaviors, often mediated by combinations of genes. These are reviewed by Marks (1986) and may be relevant to social phobia and other anxiety disorders. Human studies of general population samples have suggested some genetic heritability for traits such as fear of strangers, shyness, social introversion, and fear of social criticism. Torgersen found greater monozygotic than dizygotic twin concordance for social phobic features such as discomfort when eating with strangers, or when being watched while eating, writing, working, or trembling. The strong heritability of blood-injury phobia has led to the hypothesis that blushing, for example, may be an autonomic response under genetic influence that is tied to social cues and might lead to social phobia. A family history study found familial aggregation of social phobia and a direct-interview family study found that relatives of social phobics without other anxiety disorders had a threefold increased risk for social phobia but not for other anxiety disorders (Fyer et al, 1993). A study of female twins found higher concordance for social phobia among monozygotic as compared with dizygotic twins and support for the role of both genetic and random environmental factors (Kendler et al, 1992).

Other Biological Theories

Symptoms reported by social phobia patients in phobic situations suggest heightened autonomic arousal. When placed in a phobic situation, social phobics experience significant increases in heart rate that are highly correlated with self-perceived physiologic arousal, in contrast to claustrophobics, who experience less heart rate increase and negative correlations between perceived and actual physiologic arousal. In social role-playing situations, the generalized subtype is associated with a moderate, consistent increase in heart rate whereas those with public speaking-type (performance) show an initial marked increase in heart rate that adapts relatively quickly. Stressful public speaking results in two- to threefold increases in plasma epinephrine levels in normal individuals. It is not known whether social phobia patients have greater or more sustained epinephrine increases or are more sensitive. Epinephrine infusions do not appear to cause social anxiety in social phobia patients. Baseline norepinephrine levels may be elevated. Social phobia patients may lack normal habituation to anxiety in social situations, but this has not been studied systematically. The response of social phobia patients to lactate challenge appears to be more similar to normal controls than to panic patients.

Behavioral Theories

It is suggested social phobia may result from a lack of social skills (skills-deficit model), faulty evaluation of one's performance in social situations (cognitive inhibition model), hypersensitivity to criticism or rejection, or early unpleasant social or performance experiences (conditioned-anxiety model). These models have led to application of various behavioral techniques to the treatment of social phobia (see below).

Psychoanalytic Theories

Psychoanalytic theories do not differentiate between phobias, and so would explain social phobias in a manner similar to agoraphobia (see above). A number of traits have been observed in social phobia, such as rigid concepts of appropriate social behavior, an unrealistic tendency to experience others as critical or disapproving, increased awareness and fear of scrutiny by others, exaggerated awareness and tendency to overreact to minimal somatic symptoms, but the relevance of these traits to social phobia and whether they cause or result from the disorder have not been studied. As adults, social phobia patients retrospectively rate their parents as less caring, more rejecting, and overprotective as compared with healthy adults' perceptions of their parents; however, the accuracy of retrospective reporting and the specificity of this finding in social phobia are not established.

Treatment

Pharmacologic Treatment

Most pharmacologic studies have been performed on mixed phobic groups or have examined social anxiety in nonpatient (subclinical analogue) populations. Studies specific to social phobic patients are now beginning to be published. In one study of social phobia, the monamine oxidase inhibitor phenelzine (45–90 mg/day) was superior to both the beta blocker atenolol (50–100 mg/day) and placebo; however, atenolol may have specific efficacy for discrete performance anxiety (Liebowitz et al, 1992). Another trial suggested that phenelzine with exposure instructions may have a higher rate of full responders and greater maintenance of treatment 2 months after treatment discontinuation as compared with alprazolam or cognitive-behavioral therapy. However, all three treatment conditions demonstrated significant improvement (Gelernter et al, 1991). Treatment response is typically assessed after 8 weeks. Several studies of performance anxiety in nonclinical populations support the use of beta-blockers to reduce subjective anxiety, physical symptoms, and observed anxiety during performance. In most trials, single doses of the beta blockers propranolol 40 mg, oxyprenolol 40 mg, alprenolol 50 to 100 mg, or pindolol 5 mg were administered prior to the performance situation; one study used a maintenance dose of oxprenolol 40 mg b.i.d. (reviewed in Liebowitz et al, 1985).

Tricyclic antidepressants have not received much study in social phobia. A few studies report efficacy of clomipramine in mixed phobic samples. Comparison trials of MAOIs and tricyclic antidepressants in depressed outpatients suggest MAOIs may be more effective in reducing social anxiety.

Two case studies suggest possible efficacy of fluoxetine; most had generalized subtypes but those with the performance type also responded. Thus far, we are not aware of any published trials of the non-benzodiazepine anxiolytic buspirone for social phobia.

Behavioral Treatment

Recent behavioral literature (Heimberg and Barlow, 1991) supports certain combinations of behavioral techniques and matching treatment to patient characteristics. The combination of exposure and cognitive-restructuring techniques are superior to either treatment alone, and patients are more likely to continue to improve after treatment. It is recommended that these treatments be integrated. Some authors have discussed why exposure therapy may be harder to implement in social phobia (as compared with other phobias) due to the nature of the phobic situations. Anxiety

Management Training (relaxation + distraction + rational self-talk) also may augment exposure therapy.

One study showed that "behavioral reactors" (poor social behavior but little increase in heart rate) improved most with social skills training; they also responded to group exposure therapy. "Physiologic reactors" (no social skill deficit, but increased heart rate on exposure to phobia) improved most with applied relaxation. The comparative efficacy of behavioral or pharmacologic treatments with their combination has not been studied.

Psychodynamic Treatments

Psychodynamic treatments or other psychotherapies may be useful in social phobia but systematic studies have not been conducted.

Patient Management and Indications for Psychiatric Consultation and Referral

Consultation with a psychiatrist may help in establishing the diagnosis, especially when features of other psychiatric disorders may be present. After identification of the disorder, a trial of beta-blockers for performance subtype, or an MAOI for other social phobias may be considered. Behavioral treatments may be used alone, but are probably enhanced when used concurrently with medication.

CLINICAL PEARLS FOR SOCIAL PHOBIA

- Social phobia is differentiated from normal social or performance anxiety by the degree of distress resulting from the fear or by the presence of social or occupational impairment. Anxiety often increases rather than attenuates in the phobic situation.
- As currently defined, social phobia patients have never experienced a spontaneous panic attack; situational panic attacks are confined to the social phobic situations.
- Consider phenelzine (MAOIs) first-line treatment for social phobia; beta-blockers may help limited performance anxiety; initial reports suggest benzodiazepines or SSRI's may have some benefit as well.
- Behavioral treatment with a combination of exposure and cognitive-restructuring techniques is effective and likely to result in continued improvement. Patients with poor social behavior may respond best to social skills training or group exposure therapy, whereas those with increased heart rate on exposure to their phobia respond to applied relaxation.

SPECIFIC PHOBIA

The DSM-III name for this disorder, "simple phobia," has been changed to "specific phobia" in DSM-IV, and differentiation from other anxiety disorders is emphasized in that the anxiety or avoidance in this phobic disorder is not better accounted for by obsessive–compulsive disorder, posttraumatic stress disorder, panic disorder with agoraphobia, agoraphobia without history of panic disorder, or social phobia. Subtypes of "natural environment" (animals, insects, storms, water), "blood/injection/injury," "situational" (heights, elevators, planes), or "other" may be proposed.

Epidemiology

Six-month prevalence rates of specific phobia reported in the ECA Study are between 4.5 and 11.8%; rates are higher for females than for males. The onset of animal phobia is usually in childhood. Blood-injury phobia usually begins in adolescence or early adulthood and may be associated with vasovagal fainting on exposure to the phobic stimulus. Age of onset may be more variable for other specific phobias. Many childhood-onset phobias may remit spontaneously. Impairment depends on the extent to which the phobic object or situation is routinely encountered in the individual's life. Specific phobias may coexist with social phobia and panic disorder, but are believed to be unrelated.

Table 8–5 **Features of Specific Phobia**

A. Marked and persistent fear that is excessive or unreasonable, and is cued by the presence or anticipation of a specific object or situation (e.g., flying, heights, water, animals, receiving an injection, seeing blood).

B. Exposure to the phobic stimulus almost invariably provokes an immediate anxiety response, which may take the form of a situationally bound or predisposed panic attack.

C. The person recognizes that the fear they are experiencing is excessive or unreasonable.

D. The phobic situation(s) is avoided, or else endured with intense anxiety or distress.

E. The avoidance, anxious anticipation, or distress in the feared situation interferes significantly with the person's normal routine, occupational (academic) functioning, or with social activities or relationships with others. The person experiences marked distress about having the phobia.

F. The anxiety, panic attacks, or phobic avoidance associated with the specific object or situation is not better accounted for by another mental disorder, such as Obsessive–Compulsive Disorder (e.g., fear of contamination), Posttraumatic Stress Disorder (e.g., avoidance of stimuli associated with a traumatic event), Separation Anxiety Disorder (e.g., avoidance of school), Social Phobia (e.g., avoidance of social situations because of fear of embarrassment), Panic Disorder with Agoraphobia, or Agoraphobia Without History of Panic Disorder.

Adapted from DSM-IV (APA 1993, in press [1994])

Description and Differential Diagnosis

Specific phobia is usually a circumscribed fear of a focal object or situation (Table 8–5). As with the other phobias, the fear is excessive and unrealistic, exposure to the phobic stimulus produces an anxiety response, expectation of exposure may produce anticipatory anxiety, and the object or situation is either avoided or endured with considerable discomfort. However, unlike social phobia, the fear does not involve scrutiny or embarrassment and, unlike agoraphobia, the fear is not of being trapped or of having a panic attack. The nature of the fear is specific to the phobia, such as a fear of falling or loss of visual support in height phobia, or fear of crashing in a flying phobia. Isolated fears are common in the general population; a diagnosis of simple phobia is reserved for situations in which the phobia results in marked distress or some degree of impairment in activities or relationships.

Etiology

A family study of specific (simple) phobia demonstrated a high degree of familial transmission of specific phobia, but not of subclinical fears, and supports separation from other anxiety disorders, including other phobic disorders (Fyer et al, 1990). A study of female twins found higher monozygotic than dizygotic concordance for animal phobia (Kendler et al, 1992). Blood-injury phobia has a strong family history; 68% of probands have relatives with blood phobia. Concordance rates are higher in monozygotic than dizygotic twins. When blood-injury phobics are exposed to their phobic stimuli they exhibit a biphasic cardiovascular response with initial tachycardia followed by extreme bradycardia, which can produce syncope. It is presumed that this autonomic response is genetically determined and present at an early age (Marks, 1988).

In behavior theory, the classic case study of "Little Albert" illustrates how operant learning may produce specific phobia. A 2-year-old boy experienced a loud noise while playing with a white rat and became fearful of rats and objects resembling rats. In this example, the loud noise is the unconditioned stimulus, the fear reaction to the noise is the unconditioned response. The white rat, the conditioned stimulus, is paired with the loud noise and elicits a similar fear response, the conditioned response.

Freud's psychoanalytic theory of phobias is portrayed in the classic analytic study of "Little Hans," a 5-year-old boy who developed a fear of horses. Freud hypothesized that the phobia was a symptom of an unresolved unconscious Oedipal conflict in which the boy had sexual longings for his mother but felt guilt and feared retribution from his father in the form of castration. The libidinal impulse was repressed into the unconscious and the threat of danger displaced onto the horse, an avoidable object. However, the love for and desire to marry one's opposite-sexed parent is also believed to be a normal developmental stage and it is not clear why this dynamic might result in phobic symptoms in some individuals and not others.

Treatment

The standard treatment for specific phobias is exposure, to achieve habituation to or extinction of the fear response. The types of phobias in which efficacy is documented include height, darkness, animals, blood-injury, and claustrophobia. Cognitive therapy has been attempted but does not appear to add any benefit. There is some evidence supporting the use of applied relaxation techniques in patients with strong physiological reactions. When exposure to the phobic stimulus is infrequent, predictable, and difficult to practice repeatedly, such as in flying phobia, benzodiazepines on a "prn" basis may be considered. Self-medication with alcohol is common.

OBSESSIVE–COMPULSIVE DISORDER

Obsessions are recurrent distressing thoughts, ideas, or impulses experienced as unwanted and senseless but irresistible. Compulsions are repetitive, purposeful, intentional behaviors, usually performed in response to an obsession, which are recognized as unrealistic or unreasonable, but again irresistible. What was considered a rare disorder with poor response to treatment has recently received more attention. Advances in treatment and exploration of the underlying etiology and pathophysiology have increased the importance of recognizing obsessive–compulsive disorder. Public awareness and decreased stigma have been fostered by the media (television talk shows, radio and newspaper features), and advocacy for obsessive–compulsive disorder sufferers is accomplished through organizations such as the OCD Foundation and the National Alliance for the Mentally Ill.

Epidemiology

Obsessive–compulsive disorder was previously thought to be a rare disorder affecting only 0.05% of the population. However, with increased awareness and detection, recent estimates of population rates have been higher. The ECA Study found lifetime population prevalence rates of 2 to 3% and six-month prevalence rates of 1.3 to 2.0% (Robins et al, 1984; Myers et al, 1984). Although there were problems with the accuracy of ECA diagnosis, 1% prevalence rates have been confirmed in other surveys. The risk in females may be increased as much as twofold over males, but some samples have reported higher rates in males. Rates of obsessive–compulsive traits and disorder are increased in family members of patients (see Etiology, below). Age of onset is usually in adolescence or early adulthood (70% between ten to 23 years old). Several years may pass between onset and when a patient first seeks treatment. Obsessive traits are commonly present before onset of the disorder. Most patients are unable to identify an environmental trigger as a precipitant to onset of the disorder, but once the disorder is established, many individuals experience an increase in symptoms with stressful life events.

The majority of obsessive–compulsive disorder patients report depressive symptoms after experiencing impairment from obsessive–compulsive disorder symptoms (Rasmussen and Tsuang, 1986). Obsessive–compulsive disorder can also co-exist with panic disorder in up to 15 to 20% of patients (Breier et al, 1986). Other co-occurring disorders include other anxiety disorders, eating disorders, Gilles de la Tourette's syndrome, and schizophrenia. Separation anxiety disorder in childhood is also occasionally reported by obsessive–compulsive disorder patients (see Chapter 16).

Description and Differential Diagnosis

Obsessive–compulsive disorder is defined as the presence of obsessions or compulsions that produce discomfort or impairment (Table 8–6). Obsessions are thoughts, impulses, or images that are recurrent, persistent, intrusive, and recognized as senseless (at least initially). Compulsions are behaviors (rituals) that are repetitive, purposeful, and intentional; are in response to an obsession; are performed in a stereotyped fashion or according to certain rules to prevent discomfort or a dreaded event; and are initially recognized as excessive or unreasonable. Obsessions and compulsions are not in themselves pleasurable, and patients usually attempt to ignore, suppress, or neutralize obsessions. In clinical samples both obsessions and compul-

---

Table 8–6 **Symptoms of Obsessive–Compulsive Disorder**

A. Either obsessions or compulsions:
   Obsessions (1), (2), (3), and (4):
   1. Recurrent and persistent, thoughts, impulses, or images that are experienced, at sometime during the disturbance, as intrusive and inappropriate, and cause anxiety or distress: e.g., a parent's having repeated impulses to kill a loved child, a religious person's having recurrent blasphemous thoughts
   2. The thoughts, impulses, or images are not simply excessive worries about real life problems.
   3. The person attempts to ignore or suppress such thoughts or impulses or to neutralize them with some other thought or action
   4. The person recognizes that the obsessions are the product of their own mind (not imposed from without as in thought insertion)
   Compulsions (1), (2), and (3):
   1. Repetitive behaviors or mental acts that the person feels driven to perform in response to an obsession, or according to rigid rules.
   2. The behavior or mental act is aimed at preventing or reducing distress or preventing some dreaded event or situation; however, these behaviors or mental acts are either not connected in a realistic way with what they are designed to neutralize or prevent, or are clearly excessive
   3. The person recognizes that his or her behavior is excessive or unreasonable (this may not be true for young children; it may no longer be true for people whose obsessions have evolved into overvalued ideas)
B. At some time during the course of the disorder, the person has recognized that the obsessions and compulsions are excessive and unreasonable (may not apply to children).
C. The obsessions or compulsions cause marked distress, are time consuming (take more than an hour a day), or significantly interfere with the person's normal routine, occupational functioning, or usual social activities or relationships with others.
D. If another Axis I disorder is present, the content of the obsessions or compulsions is not restricted to it: e.g., the ideas, thoughts, impulses, or images are not about food in the presence of an Eating Disorder, about drugs in the presence of a Psychoactive Substance Use Disorder, or guilty thoughts in the presence of a Major Depression.
E. Not due to a substance-induced or an anxiety disorder due to a general medical condition.

Adapted from DSM-IV (APA 1993, in press [1994])

sions are almost always present and multiple obsessions and/or compulsions are common. Changes in DSM-IV more clearly delineate obsessive–compulsive disorder from other disorders and may include subtypes based on level of insight (e.g., with insight, overvalued ideas, or delusions) and on the predominance of obsessions, compulsions, or their combination.

Patients are often reluctant to spontaneously divulge their symptoms, so these must be inquired about directly. Reasons for the patient's difficulty in discussing symptoms include embarrassment over content that is perceived as socially unacceptable, recognition of the strangeness of the thoughts and behaviors, fear of being viewed as "crazy," and content that is disturbing to the patient. In addition, long-standing symptoms may be incorporated into the patient's lifestyle and no longer be recognized as abnormal. One study found that unrecognized obsessive–compulsive disorder was common among patients presenting to a dermatology clinic with dermatitis because they did not divulge their obsessive–compulsive symptoms.

Obsessive thoughts may take the form of images of a child being killed, counting rituals, or mental list-making that can occupy hours or entire days, or repeated thoughts of having sex with a dead person, which the patient finds disgusting and distressing yet is unable to dismiss. Compulsive cleaners may spend hours meticulously dusting, vacuuming, and so on. Compulsive hoarders are unable to discard useless objects, resulting in a home cluttered with mail, bags of used containers, dustballs, and so on. Some patients need to repeat tasks over and over to "get it right" or repeatedly rearrange objects so that they assume an exact pattern. Fear of contamination can result in avoidance of any contact with dirt or of any object that could possibly have come in contact with the feared contaminant or was sold in the same store as the contaminant. While driving, the thought that they hit someone may come to mind, followed by the need to repeatedly return to a location to check, despite the virtual certainty that no accident occurred. One individual feared losing his daughter and repeatedly checked billboards and envelopes for her presence, knowing that this was absurd yet being unable to pass a billboard or discard an envelope without repeated checking. Common obsessions and compulsions are listed in Table 8–7.

Symptoms may result in lateness due to time spent repeating rituals or in chapped and thickened skin from repeated washing. In one extreme case, a woman

Table 8–7 **Common Obsessions and Compulsions**

Obsessions	**Compulsions**
Contamination/illness	Checking
Violent images	Cleaning/washing
Fear of harming others/self	Counting
Perverse/forbidden sexual thoughts, images, or impulses	Hoarding/collecting
	Ordering/arranging
Symmetry/exactness	Repeating
Somatic	
Religious	

had a compulsion to lie down in the street in a north-south and then an east-west direction. She was unable to get up in time to avoid oncoming traffic and lost both legs.

The disorder may cause isolation and dependence on others; patients may make demands on family and treaters to decontaminate objects, check for them, and so on. Suicide risk must be considered since death may be perceived as the only escape from chronic symptoms.

In clinical samples, symptoms are present continuously from the time of onset until the patient seeks treatment. Occasionally, there is a chronic deterioration in which the obsessions and compulsions become more pronounced and more difficult to resist; they may consume all of the individual's time so that he or she is unable to function outside of performing rituals. An episodic course of illness is uncommon (2%) in clinical samples but may be more frequent in individuals who do not seek treatment (or go undiagnosed).

The differential diagnosis of obsessive–compulsive disorder may include schizophrenia, major depression, phobias, Tourette's syndrome, amphetamine intoxication, obsessive–compulsive personality, and normal thoughts and behavior. In obsessive–compulsive disorder, behavior can be bizarre and can have an impact on social and occupational functioning similar to schizophrenia. However, the behaviors are limited to the execution of compulsive rituals. When reality testing is lost, the loss is limited to convictions regarding obsessive ideas and does not extend to other areas of thinking. Occasionally, the depressive ruminations seen in major depressive episodes may be mistaken for obsessions, but the brooding has a clear depressive or guilty quality and resolves with recovery from the episode. Avoidance of contaminants or other objects and situations may resemble the avoidance seen in phobic disorders, but the fear is not of being trapped as in agoraphobia, or social embarrassment as in social phobia, but is directly related to the obsessional thought. It is distinguished from generalized anxiety disorder in that these patients worry excessively about realistic concerns, as opposed to the senseless and ego-dystonic nature of obsessions. The repetitive, irresistible movement or utterances of Tourette's syndrome may be difficult to differentiate from obsessive–compulsive disorder, and the disorders may coexist. The repetitive, stereotyped behavior seen in amphetamine (or cocaine) intoxication usually is mechanical, without the intellectual quality and intention of obsessive–compulsive disorder.

Obsessive–compulsive personality (see Chapter 6), although similar in name, consists of ego-syntonic attitudes and behaviors that are not resisted or experienced as intrusive. Other repetitive behaviors, such as gambling, addiction, sexual behavior, and eating, are to some degree inherently pleasurable, resisted only due to deleterious consequences, and lack the senseless, unrealistic nature of obsessive–compulsive disorder symptoms. Normal checking or meticulousness is not intrusive, senseless, distressing, difficult to resist, or time consuming to the extent of interference with usual activities.

Etiology and Pathophysiology

Familial and Genetic Theories

Reports of the prevalence rates of obsessive–compulsive disorder in first-degree relatives of obsessive–compulsive disorder probands range from 0 to 37%; of obsessive–compulsive personality, from 3 to 33%; of mood disorder, from 3 to 11%; and of any psychiatric disorder, from 9 to 73% (for review, see Marks, 1986; Insel, 1985). Although these rates of obsessive–compulsive illness in family members of obsessive–compulsive disorder probands are clearly elevated, interpretation of these findings would be strengthened by comparison to rates of obsessive–compulsive disorder in relatives of nonobsessive–compulsive disorder probands using the same methodology, since estimates of population prevalence vary widely. Concordance rates summarized across three twin studies are 75% for monozygotic and 32% for dizygotic twin pairs. Only the two studies reporting obsessional features in co-twins of obsessive–compulsive disorder probands showed any concordance. The hypothesis that milder obsessional tendencies may be inherited is supported by the high proportion of the variance (45%) for obsessive traits and symptoms that is hereditary in normal twin pairs, as measured by the Leyton Obsessional Inventory. In probands with Tourette's syndrome (with or without obsessive–compulsive disorder), rates of both disorders are increased in biologic relatives, suggesting that in these families, obsessive–compulsive disorder and Tourette's may be alternative phenotypic expressions of the same underlying genetic defect (a highly penetrant, sex-influenced, autosomal dominant trait).

Psychoanalytic Theories

Psychoanalytic theories of obsessive–compulsive disorder attribute symptoms to a disturbance in the anal-sadistic phase of development. A conflict (such as the oedipal-genital impulse) may lead to regression to use of earlier defenses, including isolation, undoing, displacement, and reaction formation, resulting in ambivalence and magical thinking.

Cognitive Theories

Obsessive–compulsive disorder patients appear to have a defect in their cognitive information-processing mechanism, with frequent mismatch between beliefs and sensory data (e.g., a patient may continue rinsing his hands because he feels the soap is not washed off or restack dishes because they do not appear to be straight).

Behavioral Theories

Psychiatrists working from a behavioral perspective have suggested a two-stage classical instrumental conditioning model of obsessive–compulsive disorder. Obsessions are thought to result from pairing mental stimuli with anxiety-provoking thoughts. Compulsions are neutral behaviors that have been associated with anxiety reduction and thereby reinforced. Avoidance of anxiogenic stimuli may also be reinforced, as in phobic disorders.

Neurobiological Theories

The predominant neurobiological hypothesis of the etiology of obsessive–compulsive disorder involves dysfunction of brain serotonin neuronal systems. These systems have been the subject of much investigation in obsessive–compulsive disorder since the potent serotonin (5-HT) reuptake blocker clomipramine was found to have therapeutic efficacy. Clomipramine was found to have greater efficacy than other antidepressants having less serotonergic selectivity or potency, and its efficacy correlated with levels of the serotonergically selective compound clomipramine rather than with desmethylclomipramine, the noradrenergically active metabolite. In one study, higher baseline CSF 5-HIAA (5-hydroxyindoleacetic acid, a serotonin metabolite) and platelet 5-HT concentrations and greater drug-induced decreases of these measures correlated with treatment response. Other treatments with serotonergic effects (L-tryptophan, lithium augmentation of tricyclic antidepressants, fluoxetine, sertraline, and fluvoxamine) have also been used to decrease obsessive–compulsive symptoms. Whole-blood 5-HT levels were decreased in obsessive–compulsive disorder patients in one study, whereas the opposite finding was reported in patients with a family history of obsessive–compulsive disorder in another study. Studies of peripheral 5-HT receptors have produced conflicting findings. Initial reports of elevated CSF 5-HIAA have not been confirmed thus far in a large replication study. The identification of several different 5-HT receptor subtypes has highlighted the need for greater sophistication in pharmacologic studies. Obsessive–compulsive disorder patients may have a blunted neuroendocrine response and behavioral hypersensitivity to 5-HT agonists but results are inconsistent. The absence of robust or consistent findings despite the number of studies of the 5-HT system have led investigators to question if changes seen in 5-HT function are compensatory rather than primary abnormalities in obsessive–compulsive disorder (Barr et al, 1992). The role of serotonin function in habituation has been explored in animal studies. Experimentally induced lesions of 5-HT systems in rats exacerbated amphetamine-induced preservative behavior, which may be analogous to compulsions.

Neurobiologic systems believed to be involved in other anxiety disorders have been examined in obsessive–compulsive disorder. Yohimbine, an alpha-2 antagonist, produced no consistent change in MHPG, cortisol, or behavior. Caffeine and lactate did not produce anxiogenic responses such as those in panic disorder. It has been suggested that the opiate system may mediate "drive reward reduction," and it has been further hypothesized that a deficit in an opiate-mediated capacity to register reward may be manifested as a cognitive deficit in reaching certainty in obsessive–compulsion patients with ruminative doubt and compulsive checking behavior. To test this hypothesis, an opiate antagonist was administered and found to exacerbate obsessions in one study but produced no consistent behavioral change in another.

Possible involvement of dopamine and serotonin systems is implied by PET-scan findings of increased metabolic activity in the heads of the caudate nuclei and orbital gyri. It has been hypothesized that in obsessive–compulsive disorder, functional activity in the cortex and orbital gyrus has increased beyond the caudate's ability to maintain integrative function. After successful treatment, the increase in caudate activity relative to the structures with which it interacts may represent a reestablishment of the caudate nucleus' integrative capacity (Baxter et al, 1987). Further questions of dopaminergic involvement are raised by the observation of obsessions and compulsions in postencephalitic parkinsonism. The role of dopamine dysfunction in the pathogenesis of obsessive–compulsive disorder deserves further study.

Treatment

Psychodynamic Treatment

If psychotherapy is undertaken, caution may be advisable as a searching, interpretive, in-depth approach may exacerbate introspective obsessional thinking. There are individual anecdotal reports of successful analytic treatment (Shear and Frosch, 1986).

Behavioral Treatment

A variety of behavioral techniques have been applied to obsessive–compulsive disorder and are often beneficial; however, absence of compulsions, severe symptoms, significant depression, use of CNS-depressing drugs, and poor motivation can limit the effectiveness of behavior therapy. The specific elements responsible for treatment efficacy that have been identified are prolonged exposure to ritual-eliciting stimuli together with prevention of the compulsive response. Flooding is less well tolerated and no more effective than gradual exposure. Therapist modeling and self-instructional training do not seem to enhance treatment. Home-based treatment administered by the patient, alone or with the assistance of a partner, may improve maintenance of therapeutic gains. Prolonged rather than short exposure sessions and attention focusing instead of distraction improve outcome. Behavior therapy may be enhanced by pharmacologic treatment and assertiveness training. Obsessions appear less responsive to behavioral treatment, but prolonged exposure to obsessive material in imagination may have some benefit.

Most improvement occurs in the first month of treatment but improvement may continue with additional treatment up to 6 months. Treatment gains have been maintained at 2- to 6-year follow-up. Earlier age of onset is associated with better long-term outcome; higher initial anxiety and depression are associated with poorer short-term but similar long-term outcome (for review, see Emmelkamp, 1986).

Pharmacologic Treatment

Clomipramine (CMI) was the first medication discovered to have an effect on obsessive–compulsive disorder symptoms and is the best studied. It is believed that clomipramine's serotonergic effects are responsible for somewhat specific treatment for obsessive–compulsive disorder symptoms, since it has greater efficacy than antidepressants with less potent serotonergic activity. Other selective serotonin reuptake inhibitors (SSRIs) also reduce obsessive–compulsive disorder symptoms. These include fluvoxamine, a selective and potent serotonin reuptake inhibitor, and preliminary studies support the use of fluoxetine and sertraline. If one SSRI is unsuccessful at maximal dose after 12 weeks, another SSRI should be tried.

Pharmacologic treatment response in obsessive–compulsive disorder differs from major depression in having later onset of therapeutic effect (3 to 4 weeks), lower response rate (40–60%), more gradual improvement, and significant reduction of symptoms and disability usually without complete remission. Return of symptoms is common when effective medication is decreased or discontinued. Higher doses of SSRIs than typically used to treat depression may be required but lower maintenance doses are often adequate.

MAO inhibitors may be especially helpful in obsessive–compulsive disorder patients with a history of panic attacks. Lithium augmentation of antidepressant treatment has been used as a result of evidence that lithium increases presynaptic serotonin release onto postsynaptic serotonin receptors that were sensitized by prior treatment with antidepressant medications. Reports indicate lithium added to CMI, trazodone, or fluvoxamine and probably fluoxetine may further reduce obsessions and compulsions. Fenfluramine added to an SSRI may also be helpful. Buspirone, despite efficacy in generalized anxiety and partial serotonin agonist properties, fails to decrease obsessive–compulsive disorder symptoms, but has been used to augment SSRIs in treatment refractory patients. Benzodiazepines may reduce anxiety associated with obsessive–compulsive symptoms but do not appear to alleviate the central symptoms of the disorder.

Current evidence does not support the use of neuroleptics alone in obsessive–compulsive disorder. Preliminary reports suggest that addition of a neuroleptic (e.g., pimozide) to an antidepressant drug may have benefit when schizotypal features, delusions, or tics are present.

Psychosurgical Treatment

In severe, debilitating cases that have failed all attempts at more conservative treatment, psychosurgical techniques such as cingulotomy, subcaudate tractotomy, stereotactic limbic leukotomy, or anterior capsulotomy can be beneficial. The effectiveness of these procedures is believed to be the disruption of efferent pathways from frontal cortex to basal ganglia. In general, electroconvulsive therapy (ECT) is not effective in obsessive–compulsive disorder but symptom response is reported in individual cases (for review see Goodman et al, 1992).

Role of the Nonpsychiatric Physician in Patient Management

Initial treatment of obsessive–compulsive disorder is usually best accomplished by psychiatrists who have familiarity and experience in treating this disorder. Supportive or behavioral psychotherapies are usually necessary in addition to pharmacotherapy. Once satisfactory treatment has been initiated, ongoing pharmacologic treatment can at times be managed by a nonpsychiatric physician.

Indications for Psychiatric Consultation and Referral

Consultation with a psychiatrist can assist in establishing the diagnosis of obsessive–compulsive disorder and forming an appropriate treatment plan. In individuals with severe persistent symptoms who are unable to tolerate the distress resulting from their illness, or when concurrent depression is present, assessment of suicide potential and indications for hospitalization may require evaluation by a psychiatrist. Any patient requesting psychosurgery should have careful psychiatric evaluation to determine if less-invasive treatment options have been exhausted. Obsessive–compulsive disorder patients may also benefit from involvement in support groups; the Obsessive–Compulsive Disorder Foundation (P.O. Box 9573, New Haven, CT 06535) is a useful resource formed by obsessive–compulsive disorder sufferers in 1987.

CLINICAL PEARLS FOR OBSESSIVE–COMPULSIVE DISORDER

- Recognition of obsessive–compulsive disorder can be difficult; if the specific obsessions or compulsions the patient experiences are not directly inquired about, the diagnosis can be missed. Therefore, when you suspect obsessive–compulsive disorder, question the individual about each of the common obsessions or compulsions.
- The course of the illness is usually chronic and exacerbated by stressful life events, and treatment response is often gradual and incomplete.
- The combination of pharmacotherapy and behavioral therapy is considered optimal treatment for obsessive–compulsive disorder. Serotonin reuptake inhibitors are specifically effective for this disorder, whereas most other agents are ineffective. Behavioral therapy consisting of exposure to ritual-eliciting stimuli and prevention of the compulsive response is beneficial in most cases.
- Depression, panic attacks, schizotypal features, delusions, and Tourette's syndrome may coexist with obsessive–compulsive disorder symptoms.

POSTTRAUMATIC STRESS DISORDER

Posttraumatic stress disorder (PTSD) can be an immediate or delayed response to a catastrophic life event. This disorder has become the focus of intensive research, which will lead to a rapid growth of information. One difficulty in establishing PTSD has been the frequent complication of compensation and legal issues. Therefore, although this disorder clearly occurs in the absence of secondary gain, research in populations where these issues are not present will help to exclude a potential source of inaccuracy or bias (Table 8–8).

Epidemiology

Posttraumatic stress disorder was not recognized as an independent diagnosis until the publication of DSM-III in 1980, although descriptions of the syndrome date at least to the Crimean and American Civil Wars. In a remarkable epidemiologic survey, the National Vietnam Veterans Readjustment Study (NVVRS; Kulka et al, 1990) examined PTSD in Vietnam theater and era veterans and matched civilian controls. The lifetime rate of PTSD in male theater veterans was 31%, and 15% had current PTSD. Rates in females were 26.9% and 8.5%, respectively. There was a direct relationship between level of combat and risk for PTSD, even when premilitary factors were taken into account; Hispanic race also increased risk. Future analyses will evaluate pre-trauma and post-trauma risk factors and aspects of the trauma. Rates of most other psychiatric disorders were elevated among those with PTSD. An epidem-

Table 8–8 **Criteria for Posttraumatic Stress Disorder**

A. The person has experienced or witnessed an event that involves death, threat to life, or serious injury to himself or others that was experienced with intense fear, helplessness or horror.
B. The traumatic event is persistently reexperienced in at least one of the following ways:
    1. Recurrent and intrusive distressing recollections of the event (in young children, repetitive play in which themes or aspects of the trauma are expressed)
    2. Recurrent distressing dreams of the event
    3. Sudden acting or feeling as if the traumatic event were recurring (includes a sense of reliving the experience, illusions, hallucinations, and dissociative [flashback] episodes, even those that occur upon awakening or when intoxicated)
    4. Intense psychological distress at exposure to events that symbolize or resemble an aspect of the traumatic event, including anniversaries of the trauma
    5. Physiologic reactivity upon exposure to internal or external cues that symbolize or resemble an aspect of the traumatic event (e.g., a woman who was raped in an elevator breaks out in a sweat when entering any elevator)
C. Persistent avoidance of stimuli associated with the trauma or numbing of general responsiveness (not present before the trauma), as indicated by at least three of the following:
    1. Efforts to avoid thoughts or feelings associated with the trauma
    2. Efforts to avoid activities, situations, or people that arouse recollections of the trauma
    3. Inability to recall an important aspect of the trauma (psychogenic amnesia)
    4. Markedly diminished interest in significant activities (in young children, loss of recently acquired development skills such as toilet training or language skills)
    5. Feeling of detachment or estrangement from others
    6. Restricted range of affect: e.g., unable to have loving feelings
    7. Sense of a foreshortened future: e.g., does not expect to have a career, marriage, or children, or a long life
D. Persistent symptoms of increased arousal (not present before the trauma), as indicated by at least two of the following:
    1. Difficulty falling or staying asleep
    2. Irritability or outbursts of anger
    3. Difficulty concentrating
    4. Hypervigilance
    5. Exaggerated startle response
E. Duration of the disturbance (symptoms in *B, C,* and *D*) of at least 1 month.
F. The disturbance causes marked distress or significant impairment in social or occupational functioning.

Specify delayed onset if the onset of symptoms was at least 6 months after the trauma.

Adapted from DSM-IV (APA 1993, in press [1994])

iologic survey of adult women (Kilpatrick, 1985) revealed alarmingly high rates of traumatic events, particularly being the victim of a crime; lifetime and current prevalence estimates of PTSD were 13 and 3%, respectively. Victims of sexual assault were at especially high risk for subsequent mental health problems and suicide. One site of the ECA Study estimated a population prevalence of 1 to 2%, which may be an underestimate. A survey of 20- to 30-year-olds in a large HMO (Breslau et al, 1991) found that 39.1% had been exposed to a traumatic event and the lifetime rate of PTSD in those exposed was 23.6% (i.e., lifetime population prevalence 9.2%). Risk factors for exposure to traumatic events included family history of any psychiatric disorder, history of conduct disorder symptoms, male sex, extroversion, and neuroticism. Risk factors for PTSD following exposure to trauma included separation from parents during childhood, family history of anxiety, preexisting anxiety or depression, family history of antisocial behavior, female sex, and neuroticism.

A latent period of months or years may intervene between the trauma and the onset of symptoms, or an exacerbation or relapse can occur after a period of remission. The disorder can occur in childhood. Individuals with posttraumatic stress disorder may be at increased risk for impulsive behavior or suicide.

Description and Differential Diagnosis

The mental status examination should routinely include questions about exposure to trauma or abuse. Examples of traumatic events are listed in Table 8–9. The symptoms are clustered into three categories: reexperiencing the trauma, psychic numbing or avoidance of stimuli associated with the trauma, and increased arousal (see Table 8–8). Reexperiencing phenomena include intrusive memories, flashbacks, nightmares, and psychological or physiological distress in response to trauma reminders. Intrusive memories are spontaneous, unwanted, distressing recollections of the traumatic event. Repeated nightmares contain themes of the trauma or a highly accurate and detailed re-creation of the actual event(s). Flashbacks are dissociative states in which components of the event are relived, and the person feels as if he or she is experiencing the event for a few seconds to as long as days. Reactivity to trauma-related stimuli can involve intense emotional distress or physical symptoms similar to those of a panic attack when exposed to sights, sounds, smells, or events that were present during the traumatic event. Avoidance may include thoughts, feelings, situations, or activities that are reminders of the trauma. Numbing may occur through amnesia, emotional detachment, restricted affect, or loss of interest in activities. Increased arousal may include insomnia, irritability, hypervigilance, increased startle response, or impaired concentration. This disorder can have pervasive effects on an individual's interpersonal behavior and all spheres of her or his life. Since events of this magnitude would be markedly distressing to anyone and are commonly followed by transient PTSD symptoms, distinguishing between a normal reaction and clinically relevant symptoms can be difficult. The level of distress, impairment, and duration of

Table 8–9 **Typical Traumatic Events in PTSD**

Combat or other war experiences
Serious accidents (e.g., crash, fire, explosion, etc.)
Natural disaster (e.g., tornado, hurricane, flood, earthquake, etc.)
Physical assault (e.g., rape, physical or sexual abuse, mugging, torture)
Other serious danger of death or severe injury to oneself
Witnessing the mutilation, serious injury, or violent death of another person
Receiving news of above in someone close to you

(Adapted from National Vietnam Veteran Readjustment Study interview, traumatic events booklet.)

the symptoms are key. Recent research suggests that a three-month duration may be a threshold between "acute" and "chronic" PTSD. However, a one-month duration is the threshold for diagnostic criteria at the time of this writing.

In adjustment disorder, the stressor is usually less severe, and the characteristic symptoms of posttraumatic stress disorder, such as reexperiencing and avoiding, are not present. Avoidance of trauma-associated stimuli may resemble a phobia; however, in posttraumatic stress disorder the avoidance is limited to reminders of the trauma. The physiological response to events symbolizing the trauma may resemble panic attacks but in pure posttraumatic stress disorder no spontaneous attacks occur, nor do attacks occur apart from trauma-related stimuli. Many of the symptoms of post-traumatic stress disorder resemble those of major depression. If a full depressive syndrome also exists both diagnoses should be made; the same is true of coexisting anxiety disorders. The amnesia and impaired concentration may resemble a neuro-logic disorder; if the trauma involved head injury, brain impairment should be consid-ered. Reexperiencing phenomena, such as flashbacks, can be mistaken for psychosis. Very commonly, patients are referred for medication to help with sleep. It is important to inquire about nightmares and other trauma-related symptoms in order to recognize the underlying disorder and not mistake it for other causes of insomnia (see Treat-ment, below).

Etiology

Posttraumatic stress disorder is unique among psychiatric disorders in that a specific triggering event can be identified for the psychological, behavioral, and physiologic symptoms that comprise this syndrome. Early psychodynamic theories focused on the function of traumatic experiences in reactivating latent conflicts originating in infancy. Subsequent theories suggest that PTSD is related to a failure to integrate the trauma with one's self-concept, world image, and meaning of life. A conflict between internal and external information is expressed through defenses, such as intrusion and avoidance symptoms.

Psychobiological Theories

A series of psychophysiologic studies of PTSD have found heightened autonomic or sympathetic nervous system (NS) arousal in response to trauma reminders. Other studies have focused on dysregulation of sympathetic NS activity, including elevated urine NE excretion and decreased alpha-2 adrenergic receptor density. The alpha-2 antagonist, yohimbine, produced panic attacks and flashbacks in patients with combat PTSD, as well as heightened biochemical and cardiovascular responses, which could not be accounted for by co-morbid panic disorder. Involvement of opiate systems is supported by finding that naloxone reverses the stress-induced analgesia from watch-ing combat films in combat PTSD patients. Abnormalities of the hypothalamic-pituitary-adrenal axis have been investigated, suggesting that central inhibition of CRF and ACTH may be increased in PTSD, consistent with HPA adaptation to chronic stress in preclinical studies. Based on preclinical studies, it is hypothesized that processes involving the locus ceruleus, amygdala, hypothalamus, hippocampus, and prefrontal cortex are involved in the pathophysiology of PTSD (Charney et al, 1993).

Preliminary evidence from family and twin studies suggest genetic and familial factors may play a role in vulnerability to PTSD, which is consistent with preclinical data on genetic vulnerability to stress responses. A possible relationship with other anxiety disorders is being explored.

Behavioral Models

Two-factor learning theory has been applied to PTSD. Classical (aversive) conditioning, in which previously neutral stimuli are paired with reaction to the trauma, and higher order conditioning (additional stimuli become associated and produce anxiety) leads to instrumental learning, whereby behaviors are acquired to avoid anxiety from the conditioned stimuli. A number of factors may interfere with extinction occurring naturally (Keane et al, 1985; Charney et al, 1993).

Treatment

Initiating assessment and treatment quickly after a trauma is hoped to prevent many of the complications and disability associated with prolonged PTSD. As with other anxiety disorders, treatment for posttraumatic stress disorder often is best accomplished with a combination of pharmacologic and nonpharmacologic therapies. It has been proposed that pharmacologic treatment may be required to control the physiological symptoms so that the patient will be able to tolerate working through highly emotional material in psychotherapy. Treatment of PTSD is often complicated by co-morbid disorders. If alcohol or substance abuse is present, these problems should be the initial focus of treatment. Treatment should focus on PTSD even if a coexisting depression is present, because the course, biology, and treatment response are unlike that of classic major depression.

There are still very few controlled medication trials in PTSD. In a double-blind placebo-controlled trial of phenelzine and imipramine (Frank et al, 1988), both agents significantly reduced intrusion (reexperiencing) symptoms but did not affect avoidance items; there was some suggestion of greater efficacy for phenelzine. Usual dose ranges were 60 to 75 mg/day for phenelzine and 200 to 300 mg/day for imipramine. Other controlled trials of TCAs include amitriptyline and desipramine. It appears 8 weeks of treatment is needed to evaluate efficacy. Alprazolam was no more effective than the placebo in a controlled trial. This lack of efficacy, together with a high rate of alcohol- and substance-abuse problems in PTSD, make benzodiazepines a poor choice. Open trials and case reports suggest efficacy for a variety of other medications, but controlled trials are needed to confirm these results. Recent reports suggest some efficacy for all three symptom clusters with fluoxetine (Nagy et al, 1993). Clonidine 0.2 to 0.4 mg/day and propranolol 120 to 180 mg/day relieved startle, explosiveness, nightmares, and intrusive reexperiencing in some patients. Lithium decreased autonomic arousal, reexperiencing of symptoms, and ethanol use in 64% of patients; carbamazepine appeared to have similar effects.

Buspirone may be helpful in some patients, but additional studies are needed. When poor impulse control or psychotic features are prominent, neuroleptics may be considered, but due to the risk of tardive dyskinesia, their use should be limited to specific indications and the lowest dose and shortest duration necessary.

Controlled studies of behavioral therapies, including systematic desensitization and flooding, produce a decrease in reexperiencing and hyperarousal, but not avoidant/numbing symptoms. A controlled trial of cognitive therapy found that stress inoculation training (relaxation, thought stopping, breathing control, communications skills, cognitive restructuring) reduced PTSD symptoms early in treatment; long-term results were best when combined with prolonged exposure. This is consistent with efficacy of cognitive processing therapy, which combines education, exposure, and cognitive therapy. Anecdotally, after successful cognitive-behavioral treatment, a subsequent relapse due to a new trigger of traumatic memories can respond to another course of cognitive-behavioral therapy.

One controlled study compared psychodynamic therapy, hypnotherapy, and systematic desensitization to waiting list controls. Hypnotherapy was similar to desensitization, with more improvement in reexperiencing symptoms and less improvement in avoidance, whereas psychodynamic therapy had a greater effect on avoidance than reexperiencing (reviewed in Solomon et al, 1992).

Acute Stress Disorder

A new disorder, acute stress disorder, was proposed for DSM-IV and will likely be added to our diagnostic nomenclature. Recent surveys of victims of disasters (such as a fire, an earthquake, or witnessing an execution) have identified symptoms in the immediate aftermath of a trauma that are predictive of subsequent problems with PTSD symptoms (Cardena and Spiegel, 1993; Spiegel et al, in press). These acute symptoms are highly correlated with the severity of trauma exposure. Other than being a precursor for PTSD, little is known about this disorder. In particular, optimal treatment strategies have not been studied since data are primarily from anonymous surveys rather than clinical samples. The identification of this disorder is hoped to facilitate early detection and treatment and reduce long-term complications.

As for PTSD, the A criterion specifies that the individual has been exposed to a traumatic event (see Table 8–8, Item A). In addition, this syndrome is characterized by several numbing or dissociative symptoms, such as numbing of emotional responsiveness or detachment, decreased awareness of one's surroundings (e.g., "in a daze"), derealization, psychogenic amnesia, and depersonalization. One or more reexperiencing symptoms (see Table 8–8, Item B) or distress when exposed to reminders of the event is typical, as well as avoidance of stimuli that provoke memories of the trauma. Other symptoms of hyperarousal (see Table 8–8, Item D) or restlessness may also occur. The diagnosis of acute stress disorder is made when the level of distress is clinically significant, when there is impairment in functioning, or when the individual fails to pursue a necessary task, such as obtaining medical, legal, or social assistance. The duration of acute stress disorder is from 2 days to 4 weeks; if symptoms persist beyond 4 weeks after the trauma, consider the diagnosis of PTSD.

GENERALIZED ANXIETY DISORDER

Generalized anxiety disorder (GAD) is characterized by excessive and uncontrollable worry about multiple life circumstances accompanied by symptoms of muscle tension, restlessness, fatigue, concentration problems, difficulty falling or staying asleep, and irritability. The anxiety is unrelated to panic attacks, phobic stimuli, obsessions, having an illness, or traumatic events (in PTSD). The validity of GAD as a diagnosis distinct from other anxiety disorders or depression, or whether a homogeneous category, is still being examined.

Epidemiology

An epidemiologic study in New Haven, Connecticut, estimated a 2.5% one-month prevalence rate for GAD using research diagnostic criteria. Of the patients with GAD, 80% had at least one other anxiety disorder in their lifetime, and 7% had major depression. In this study GAD was slightly more common in young to middle-aged females, nonwhites, those not currently married, and those of lower socioeconomic status. Rates for GAD were not reported in the ECA Study. Age at onset is variable but is usually in the 20s to the 30s. GAD may begin as childhood overanxious disorder. In clinical samples the prevalence in males and females appears to be equal and the course tends to be chronic (Merikangas and Weissman, 1986).

Description and Differential Diagnosis

The most common diagnostic error made by beginning students is to misdiagnose GAD when another anxiety disorder is present, which leads to inappropriate and ineffective treatment decisions. The *symptom* of anxiety is prominent in a number of conditions, including depressive, psychotic, substance use, and somatoform disorders as well as some medical conditions (particularly those associated with dyspnea) and medication side effects (e.g., sympathomimetic), so careful questioning is necessary to differentiate between the multiple causes of anxiety.

GAD is characterized by chronic excessive anxiety about life circumstances accompanied by symptoms of motor tension, autonomic hyperactivity, vigilance, and scanning (Table 8–10). The individual often "awakens with" apprehension and unrealistic concern about future misfortune. One patient described experiencing the anxiety of a final exam with every task he was assigned at work. The current diagnostic criteria require 6-month duration of symptoms to differentiate the disorder from more transient forms of anxiety, such as adjustment disorder with anxious mood. GAD is no longer a residual diagnosis covering a heterogeneous group of anxiety conditions that do not fit other diagnoses. Recently an attempt has been made to refine the definition of this syndrome and evaluate if and how it is distinct from other diagnoses.

The DSM-IV criteria emphasize that the worry is out of proportion to the likelihood or impact of the feared events, is pervasive (focused on many life circumstances), is difficult to control, is not related to hypochondriacal concerns or part of PTSD, and that anxiety secondary to substance-induced or medical etiologies will be excluded. Tension or nervousness may be manifested by three of the following: restlessness, easily fatigued, feeling keyed up or on edge, difficulty concentrating/mind going blank, and irritability. In addition, significant functional impairment or marked distress is required for the diagnosis.

Generalized persistent anxiety may develop between attacks in panic disorder. GAD symptoms are often present in episodes of depression. In patients with somatiza-

Table 8–10 **Major Features of Generalized Anxiety Disorder***

A. Excessive anxiety or worry (apprehensive expectation) about several life events or activities: e.g., worry about possible misfortune to one's child (who is in no danger) or worry about finances (for no good reason), for a period of 6 months or longer, during which the person has been bothered more days than not by these concerns. In children and adolescents, this may take the form of anxiety and worry about academic, athletic, and social performance.
B. The person finds it difficult to control the worry.
C. At least 3 of the following 6 symptoms are often present when anxious:
   1. muscle tension
   2. restlessness or feeling keyed up or on edge
   3. easy fatigability
   4. difficulty concentrating or "mind going blank" because of anxiety
   5. trouble falling or staying asleep
   6. irritability
D. If another Axis I disorder is present, the focus of the anxiety and worry in *A* is unrelated to it: e.g., the anxiety or worry is not about having a panic attack in the presence of panic disorder; being embarrassed in public in the presence of social phobia; being contaminated in the presence of obsessive–compulsive disorder; gaining weight in the presence of anorexia nervosa; having an illness (as in hypochondriasis or somatization disorder), and is not part of post-traumatic stress disorder.
E. The anxiety, worry, or physical symptoms significantly interfere with the person's normal routine or usual activities, or cause marked distress
F. Not due to a substance-induced or anxiety disorder due to a general medical condition and does not occur only during a mood disorder, psychotic disorder, or pervasive developmental disorder.

* Adapted from DSM-IV (APA 1993, in press [1994])

tion disorder, the focus of worry is about health concerns and physical symptoms rather than apprehensive worry about life circumstances. As with panic disorder, medical conditions that may produce anxiety symptoms, such as hyperthyroidism or caffeinism, must be excluded. If an anxiety disorder is present that does not fit the criteria of any of the anxiety disorders, somatization, psychoactive substance related, or medical conditions, then the diagnosis of anxiety disorder, not otherwise specified, may be considered. However, careful assessment will usually lead to a more specific diagnosis. If in doubt, obtain consultation from an anxiety disorders specialist.

Etiology

Torgersen's twin study found no evidence for genetic transmission of GAD. Diagnostic heterogeneity of GAD is suggested by the high frequency of nonanxiety psychiatric disorders in co-twins. However, a family study of GAD probands reports an increased rate of GAD but not other anxiety disorders in first-degree relatives, suggesting some degree of familial transmission and separation of GAD from panic disorder and agoraphobia (Noyes et al, 1987).

Psychodynamic theories are based on "neuroses," which do not directly correspond to current diagnostic classification. As stated above, unconscious conflict is felt to be the underlying cause of anxiety, which as a symptom is a "signal" to the ego of the danger of expressing unacceptable impulses.

Behavioral theories consider anxiety, like panic disorder, a conditioned response to a stimulus that the individual has come to associate with danger. However, in GAD it is difficult to identify specific anxiogenic stimuli. There is some suggestion that the onset of GAD may be related to the cumulative effects of several stressful life events.

Biological theories relating to GAD stem from preclinical animal models, basic and clinical pharmacologic studies, and pharmacologic properties of effective anxiolytic treatments in humans. Since GAD is a heterogeneous disorder, it is likely that dysfunction of many brain neurochemical systems can account for the observed symptoms. There is preclinical and clinical evidence suggesting that neuronal systems involving noradrenergic, serotonergic, dopaminergic, corticotropin releasing factor, and endogenous benzodiazepine ligands may be involved. There is particular interest in the endogenous benzodiazepine system because of the marked efficacy of benzodiazepine drugs in this disorder. An endogenous anxiogenic substance with strong affinity for benzodiazepine receptors in animal and human brain (DBI—diazepam binding inhibitor) has been identified (Ferrero et al, 1986). Acute anxiety and genetically determined anxiety appear to be associated with changes in benzodiazepine receptor density. Betacarbolines, which are benzodiazepine inverse agonists, produce an acute anxiety state in animals and humans. Studies of benzodiazepine function in GAD patients are needed. The efficacy in GAD of buspirone, a $5\text{-}HT_{1A}$ agonist that reduces serotonin function, has led to interest in the role of serotonergic systems. Studies of serotonergic function using tryptophan and MCPP are being conducted. The available data suggest that noradrenergic function in GAD patients may be normal.

Treatment

Psychotherapy may be indicated for cases of GAD in which the clinician feels unresolved unconscious conflict causes or perpetuates a patient's chronic anxiety (see Chapter 17).

Preliminary studies of behavioral treatment of GAD suggest positive results with live presentation of progressive muscle relaxation to community volunteers and anxiety management (application of relaxation in response to physiologic cues of tension) in anxious outpatients. Biofeedback does not appear to have a specific value. Cognitive therapy combined with systematic desensitization in imagination or relaxation improves GAD symptoms, but cognitive therapy alone is not effective. A treatment combination of biofeedback, relaxation, and cognitive therapy resulted in improvement in subjective and physiologic measures of anxiety, but it is not known which element(s) of treatment are necessary.

The most commonly used pharmacologic agents for GAD are benzodiazepines such as diazepam, alprazolam, lorazepam, and clonazepam (Table 8–11). Advantages include rapid onset of efficacy and long-term safety. Disadvantages include memory impairment, sedation, difficulty with discontinuation dependence and abuse potential. Antidepressant medications were believed to be ineffective in treating GAD, but some studies suggest imipramine may be of some benefit.

Table 8–11 **Commonly Used Benzodiazepines**

TYPE	PRIMARY ROUTE OF BIOTRANSFORMATION	ELIMINATION HALF-LIFE (HOURS)
Diazepam (Valium)	oxidation	36–200
Flurazepam (Dalmane)	oxidation	50–120
Halazepam (Praxipam)	oxidation	36–200
Chlordiazepoxide (Librium)	oxidation	30–90
Alprazolam (Xanax)	oxidation	12–15
Triazolam (Halcion)	oxidation	3–5
Clorazepate (Tranxene)	oxidation	36–200
Prazepam (Centrax, Vestran)	oxidation	36–200
Midazolam (Versed)*	oxidation	2–4
Lorazepam (Ativan)	conjugation	10–20
Temazepam (Restoril)	conjugation	8–12
Oxazepam (Serax)	conjugation	8–12
Clonazepam (Klonopin)	nitroreduction	30–60

* IM or IV route only
(Reprinted with permission from Stoudemire A, Fogel BS, Gulley LR, Moran MG: Psychopharmacology in the medical patient. In Stoudemire A, Fogel BS (eds): Psychiatric Care of the Medical Patient, p 188. New York, Oxford University Press, 1993)

Buspirone, a nonbenzodiazepine anxiolytic, may become the treatment of choice for GAD. The mechanism of action is not established, but pharmacologic activity includes decrease in serotonin and increase in dopamine and norepinephrine cell firing. In contrast to benzodiazepines, therapeutic effects are delayed from 1 to 4 weeks. Side effects are usually mild and transient but may include dizziness, nausea, diarrhea, headache, or nervousness. Buspirone does not produce drowsiness or impair driving skill, and thus far appears to lack abuse potential or withdrawal symptoms with abrupt discontinuation (Sussman, 1987). The drug is not sedating. Consider buspirone as the first-line treatment in patients with an alcohol- or drug-abuse history. It is important to note that buspirone does not block alcohol or benzodiazepine withdrawal symptoms, so in patients exposed to these agents withdrawal symptoms should not be confused with lack of efficacy of anxiolytic therapy. Other serotonergic agents and mixed agonist-antagonist benzodiazepines are being studied.

As with the other anxiety disorders, optimal treatment may involve a combination of psychotherapy, behavioral therapy, and/or pharmacotherapy. Comparative trials are needed to establish the relative efficacies of these treatment modalities or their combination.

Role of the Physician in Patient Management and Indications for Psychiatric Consultation and Referral

The initial step in evaluating an anxious patient is to exclude medical conditions that produce anxiety syndromes. If another anxiety disorder (such as panic attacks or phobias) or another Axis I disorder (such as major depression or psychosis) is present, more specific treatments are usually indicated for these disorders. When GAD is the sole diagnosis or a residual condition, the treatments outlined above may be implemented. Psychiatric consultation can assist in excluding other diagnoses and choosing the optimal treatment.

CLINICAL PEARLS FOR GENERALIZED ANXIETY DISORDER

- Exclude medical conditions that cause anxiety.
- Exclude other psychiatric disorders, particularly other anxiety disorders.
- Inquire about use of ethanol or other substances, *especially* caffeine. If a history of substance abuse exists, avoid use of benzodiazepines.
- Consider buspirone, antidepressant medications, or benzodiazepines (at lowest effective dose and shortest duration necessary).
- Consider psychotherapy or behavioral therapy, alone or with medication.

ANXIETY DISORDERS DUE TO GENERAL MEDICAL CONDITIONS AND SUBSTANCE-INDUCED ANXIETY DISORDERS

Anxiety caused by general medical disorders (hyperthyroidism) and substances (such as caffeine) are frequently overlooked. A high index of suspicion, a rigorous history in regards to the use of medications and drugs, as well as a good physical evaluation will usually reveal the most common causes of anxiety syndromes caused by medical conditions and substances. Chapter 20 by Dr. Levenson discusses in more detail general medical conditions that cause psychiatric symptoms including anxiety.

ANNOTATED BIBLIOGRAPHY

Barr L, Goodman W, Price L, McDougle C, Charney D: The serotonin hypothesis of obsessive–compulsive disorder: Implications of pharmacologic challenge studies. J Clin Psychiatry 1992 54:(Suppl 4) 17–28.

> Excellent scholarly discussion of our current understanding of the neuropharmacology of OCD.

Emmelkamp PMG: Behavior therapy with adults. In Garfield SL, Bergin AE (eds): Handbook of Psychotherapy and Behavior Change, 3rd ed. New York, John Wiley & Sons, 1986.

> Provides a critical review of behavioral and cognitive treatment studies in each of the anxiety disorders with the exception of posttraumatic stress disorder. Information is well documented and conclusions clearly stated.

Goodman WK, McDougle J, Price LH: Pharmacotherapy of obsessive–compulsive disorder. J Clin Psychiatry 1992;54[4, suppl]:29–37.

An excellent review of pharmacologic treatment issues and practical treatment suggestions in OCD.

Krystal JH, Goodwin WK, Woods SW, Charney DS: Anxiety Disorders. In Lazare A (ed): Outpatient Psychiatry, Diagnosis, and Treatment, 2nd ed., pp 416–454. Baltimore, Williams & Wilkins, 1989.

> A comprehensive overview of anxiety disorders containing both practical and theoretical information. Integration of the various etiologic constructs is emphasized in understanding the development of these disorders.

Liebowitz MR, Gorman JM, Fyer AS, Klein DF: Social phobia: Review of a neglected anxiety disorder. Arch Gen Psychiatr 42:729–736, 1985.

> A very helpful summary of social phobia discussing diagnostic validity, epidemiology, pathophysiology, and etiology, and summarizing methods and findings of early treatment studies of social phobia and performance anxiety.

Marks IM: Genetics of fear and anxiety disorders. Br J Psychiatr 149:406–418, 1986.

> Reviews animal and human genetic studies of fear and anxiety and summarizes earlier family and twin studies of panic disorder, phobic disorders and obsessive–compulsive disorder.

Nemiah JC: Foundations of Psychopathology. New York, Oxford University Press, 1961

> Chapters 7, 8, and 9 discuss anxiety as a symptom and anxiety syndromes from a psychoanalytic perspective.

Rickels K, Schweizer E: The clinical course and long-term management of generalized anxiety disorder. J Clin Psychopharm 10[3 Suppl]:101–110, 1990.

> An excellent overview of studies of GAD and possibly related anxiety conditions by two of the foremost authors in this area.

Roy-Byrne PP, Cowley DS: Panic disorder: Biological aspects. Psychiatr Ann 18:457–463, 1988

> A concise, comprehensive, and clearly written review of biological studies in panic disorder.

Solomon SD, Gerrity DT, Muff AM: Efficacy of treatments for posttraumatic stress disorder: An empirical review. JAMA 268:633–638, 1992.

> An excellent and concise review of PTSD treatment studies and their rationale.

REFERENCES

American Psychiatric Association: DSM-IV Draft Criteria 3/1/93. Washington DC, American Psychiatric Association, 1993

American Psychiatric Association: Diagnostic and Statistical Manual of Mental Disorders, 4th Ed., Revised. Washington, DC, American Psychiatric Association, in press [1994]

Ballenger JC: Medication discontinuation in panic disorder. J Clin Psychiatry 53 (suppl 3):31, 1992

Barr L, Goodman W, Price L, McDougle C, Charney D: The serotonin hypothesis of obsessive compulsuive disorder: Implications of pharmacologic challenge studies. J Clin Psychiatry 1992 54:(Suppl 4) 17–28

Baxter LR, Phelps ME, Mazziotta JC et al: Local glucose metabolic rates in obsessive–compulsive disorder. Arch Gen Psychiatry 44:211–218, 1987

Breier A, Charney DS, Heninger GR: Agoraphobia with panic attacks: Development, diagnostic stability, and course of illness. Arch Gen Psychiatry 43:1029–1036, 1986

Breslau N, Davis GC, Andreshi P, Peterson E: Traumatic Events and Posttraumatic Stress Disorder in an Urban Population of Young Adults. Arch Gen Psychiatry 48:216–222, 1991

Britton KT: The neurobiology of anxiety. In Cavenar JO (ed): Psychiatry, vol 3. Philadelphia, JB Lippincott, 1986

Cardena E, Spiegel D: Dissociative reactions to the San Francisco Bay area earthquake of 1989. Am J Psychiatry 150:474–478, 1993

Charney DS, Deutch AY, Krystal JH, Southwick SM, Davis M: Psychobiologic mechanisms of posttraumatic stress disorder. Arch Gen Psychiatry 50:294–305, 1993

Crowe RR: The genetics of panic disorder and agoraphobia. Psychiatric Developments 2:171–186, 1985

Crowe RR: Panic disorder: Genetic considerations. J Psychiat Res 24 (suppl 2):129–134, 1990

Emmelkamp PMG: Behavior therapy with adults. In Garfield SL, Bergin AE (eds): Handbook of Psychotherapy and Behavior Change, 3rd ed. New York, John Wiley & Sons, 1986

Ferrero P, Costa E, Conti-Tronconti B, Guidotti A: A diazepam binding inhibitor (DBI)-like neuropeptide is detected in human brain. Brain Res 399:136–142, 1986

Frank JB, Kosten TR, Giller EJ et al: A randomized clinical trial of phenelzine and imipramine for post-traumatic stress disorder. Am J Psychiatry 145:1289–1291, 1988

Fyer AJ, Klein DF: Agoraphobia, social phobia, and simple phobia. In Cavenar JO (ed): Psychiatry, vol 1. Philadelphia, JB Lippincott, 1986

Fyer AJ, Mannuzza S, Chapman TF, Liebowitz MR, Klein DF: A direct interview family study of social phobia. Arch Gen Psychiatry 50:286–293, 1993

Fyer AJ, Mannuzza S, Gallops MS, Martin LY, Aaronson C, Gorman JM, Liebowitz MR, Klein DF: Familial transmission of simple phobias and fears: A preliminary report. Arch Gen Psychiatry 47:252–256, 1990

Gelernter CS, Uhde TW, Cimbolic P, Arnkoff DB, Vittone BJ, Tancer ME, Bartko JJ: Cognitive-behavioral and pharmacological treatments of social phobia: A controlled study. Arch Gen Psychiatry 48:938–945, 1991

Gorman JM, Liebowitz MR: Panic and anxiety disorders. In Cavenar JO (ed): Psychiatry, vol 1. Philadelphia, JB Lippincott, 1986

Heimberg RG, Barlow DH: New developments in cognitive-behavioral therapy for social phobia. J Clin Psychiatry 52:(suppl 11):21–30, 1991

Insel TR: Obsessive–compulsive disorder. Psychiatr Clin North Am 8:105–117, 1985

Keane TM, Fairbank JA, Caddell JM, Zimering RT, Bender ME: A behavioral approach to assessing and treating posttraumatic stress disorder in Vietnam veterans. In Figley CR (ed): Trauma and its Wake. New York, Brunner/Mazel, 1985

Kendler KS, Neale MC, Kessler RC, Heath AC, Eaves LJ: The genetic epidemiology of phobias in women. Arch Gen Psychiatry 49:273–281, 1992

Kilpatrick DG, Best CL. Veronen LJ, Amick AE, Villeponteaux LA, Ruff GA: Mental health correlates of criminal victimization: A random community survey. J Consult Clin Psychology 53:866–873, 1985

Krystal JH, Charney DS: Advances in anxiety therapy. Internal Medicine for the Specialist 9:93–111, 1988

Krystal JH, Goodman WK, Woods SW et al: Anxiety disorders. In Lazare A (ed): Outpatient Psychiatry, Diagnosis and Treatment, 2nd ed. Baltimore, Williams & Wilkins, 1989

Kulka RA, Schlenger WE, Fairbank JA, Hough RL, Jordan BK, Marmar CR, Weiss DS: Trauma and the Vietnam War Generation. New York, Brunner/Mazel, 1990

Liebowitz MR, Gorman JM, Fyer AJ, Klein DF: Social phobia: Review of a neglected anxiety disorder. Arch Gen Psychiatry 42:729–736, 1985

Liebowitz MR, Schneier F, Campeas R, Hollander E, Hatterer J, Fyer A, Gorman J, Papp L, Davies S, Gully R, Klein D: Phenelzine vs atenolol in social phobia: A placebo-controlled comparison. Arch Gen Psychiatry 49:290–300, 1992

Marks IM: Genetics of fear and anxiety disorders. Br J Psychiatry 149:406–418, 1986

Marks I: Blood-injury phobia: A review. Am J Psychiatry 145:1207–1213, 1988

Merikangas KM, Weissman MM: Epidemiology of anxiety disorders in adulthood. In Cavenar JO (ed): Psychiatry, vol 3. Philadelphia, JB Lippincott, 1986

Millon T: Social learning models. In Cavenar JO (ed): Psychiatry, vol 1. Philadelphia, JB Lippincott, 1986

Myers JK, Weissman MM, Tischler GL et al: Six-month prevalence of psychiatric disorders in three communities: 1980 to 1982. Arch Gen Psychiatry 41:959–967, 1984

Nagy LM, Krystal JH, Woods SW, Charney DS: Clinical and medication outcome after short-term alprazolam and behavioral group treatment in panic disorder: 2.5-year naturalistic follow-up study. Arch Gen Psychiatry 46:993–999, 1989

Nagy LM, Krystal JH, Charney DS, Merikangas KR, Woods SW: Long-term outcome of panic disorder after short-term imipramine and behavioral group treatment: 2.9-year naturalistic follow-up study. J Clin Psychopharm 13:16–24, 1993

Nagy LM, Morgan CA, Southwick SM, Charney DS: Open prospective trial of fluoxetine for posttraumatic stress disorder. J Clin Psychopharm, 13:107–113, 1993

Noyes R, Clarkson C. Crowe RR et al: A family study of generalized anxiety disorder. Am J Psychiatr 144:1019–1024, 1987

Pauls DL, Bucher KD, Crowe RR et al: A genetic study of panic disorder pedigrees. Am J Hum Genet 32:639–644, 1980

Rapee RM, Barlow DH: Panic disorder: cognitive-behavioral treatment. Psychiatr Ann 18:473–477, 1988

Rasmussen SA, Tsuang MT: Clinical characteristics and family history in DSM-III obsessive-compulsive disorder. Am J Psychiatry 143:317–322, 1986

Robins LN, Helzer JE, Weissman MM et al: Lifetime prevalence of specific psychiatric disorders in three sites. Arch Gen Psychiatry 41:949–958, 1984

Roy-Bryne PP, Cowley DS: Panic disorder: Biological aspects. Psychiatr Ann 18:457–463, 1988

Shear KM, Frosch WA: Obsessive–compulsive disorder. In Cavenar JO (ed): Psychiatry, vol 1. Philadelphia, JB Lippincott, 1986

Solomon SD, Gerrity DT, Muff AM: Efficacy of treatments for posttraumatic stress disorder: An empirical review. JAMA 268:633–638, 1992

Spiegel D, Koopman C, Cardena E, Classen C: Diagnosis of brief reactive dissociative disorder, in press

Sussman N: Treatment of anxiety with buspirone. Psychiatr Ann 17:114–120, 1987

Torgersen S: Genetic factors in anxiety disorders. Arch Gen Psychiatry 40:1085–1089, 1983

Van der Kolk BA (ed): Psychological Trauma. Washington DC, American Psychiatric Press, 1987

Woods SW, Nagy LM, Koleszar AS, Krystal JH, Heninger GR, Charney DS: Controlled trial of alprazolam supplementation during imipramine treatment of panic disorder. J Clin Psychopharm 12:32–38, 1992

Alan Stoudemire (ed). *Clinical Psychiatry for Medical Students,* Second Edition. Copyright © 1994, 1990 by J. B. Lippincott Company.

9 Somatoform Disorders, Factitious Disorders, and Malingering

David G. Folks, Charles V. Ford, and Carl A. Houck

Somatoform disorders, factitious disorders, and malingering represent various degrees of illness behavior characterized by the process of somatization. These distinct diagnostic categories are often conceptualized as a continuum of abnormal illness behavior. Particular attention is given to the question of whether symptoms are consciously or unconsciously produced. This chapter will cover many of the current concepts of the epidemiology, diagnosis, etiology, and clinical management of each diagnostic group. The management of chronic pain is not thoroughly covered in this chapter, which rather addresses aspects of pain relevant to somatization; the reader is referred to Chapter 23 by Dr. Goldberg for more extensive coverage of pain management.

THE PROCESS OF SOMATIZATION

Somatization is a process by which an individual consciously or unconsciously uses the body or bodily symptoms for psychological purposes or personal gain. The observed prevalence of abnormal illness behavior characterized by somatization varies according to the clinical setting and the medical specialty, with reported figures ranging between 5 and 40% of patient visits (Ford, 1983). Somatization is more prevalent among clinical populations presenting to primary care clinicians. Somatizing disorders undoubtedly result in increased use of medical services and significantly affect the cost of medical care. Conservative estimates indicate that at least 10% of all medical services are provided for patients who have no evidence of physical disease;

these figures do not include services provided for patients with identified psychiatric syndromes (Smith et al, 1986).

Somatization is facilitated in cultures that accept physical disease as an excuse for disability but reject psychological symptoms as acceptable for entry into the "sick role." Similarly, governmental agencies, insurance companies, and other third-party payers may allow financial restitution for medical expenses, or approve disability payments for physical disease, but deny benefits for disturbances that are psychiatric. Thus, many somatizing individuals receive secondary gain for illness behavior. Ford (1986) has elucidated other specific motivations for somatization as follows: (1) the manipulation of interpersonal relationships; (2) the privileges of the sick role, including sanctioned dependency; (3) financial gain; (4) communication of ideas or feelings that are somehow blocked from verbal expression; and (5) the influence of intrapsychic defense mechanisms.

Perhaps the major conscious or unconscious motivation for somatization is the achievement of the *sick role*. The sick role, first examined by Parsons (1951), enables release from the normal and usual obligations of society while absolving the affected person from blame for the condition. When considering etiologic factors relevant to the process of somatization, one must also appreciate the distinction between the concepts of illness and disease (Eisenberg, 1977). *Disease* is defined as objectively measurable anatomic deformations and pathophysiologic states presumably caused by such varied factors as degenerative processes, trauma, toxins, and infectious agents. *Illness* refers to those experiences associated with disease that ultimately impact on an individual's state of being and social functioning. Therefore, illness takes into account the personal nature of suffering, alienation from one's usual gratifying activities, and a decreased capacity to participate in society, all of which significantly affect life quality itself.

Irrespective of the underlying motivation(s), all of the possible explanations for somatization encourage a thorough diagnostic investigation and therapeutic approach that focuses on the psychosocial history while formulating the extent of the patient's disease, the magnitude of the illness, and the degree to which the patient is suffering and unable to engage in his or her usual activities. Also worthy of consideration is the appropriateness of an individual's illness behavior in the context of existing disease and the extent to which a patient's symptoms could serve to resolve life problems or represent psychological conflicts. In this regard, Brodsky (1984) has identified family factors that predispose to somatization as follows: (1) growing up in a family of somatizers; (2) being raised by parents who were demanding and unrewarding when the child was well, but caring and loving when the child was ill; (3) experiencing an environment in which one or both parents suffered illness; (4) living in an environment in which other coping mechanisms for dealing with a psychosocial crisis are unavailable; (5) developing a repertoire of reactions used to withdraw from usual life activities or to engage or punish others; and (6) consciously feigning illness to obtain something or to avoid punishment, responsibility, or required duties. *One must also consider the possibility that somatization is primarily or secondarily associated with an underlying psychiatric syndrome, a coexisting personality disorder, or a psychosocial stressor that has diagnostic significance with respect to the interpersonal or intrapsychic features of the case* (Miranda et al, 1991). For example, psychiatric disorders and medical symptoms are common in women with histories of severe childhood sexual abuse (Walker et al, 1992). Another study suggested that among individuals with or without diagnosed psychiatric disorder in the community, those with panic anxiety were among the highest utilizers of ambulatory services for unexplained medical symptoms (Katon et al, 1992).

Psychiatric referral is infrequent with somatization, probably because cases are not recognized as such or these patients lack the psychological capacity and motivation to cooperate with a psychiatric consultant. Fortunately several very helpful recommendations have evolved regarding the general therapeutic approach outlined in Table 9–1.

Somatothymia

Some individuals have a limited capacity to articulate their feelings and intrapsychic conflicts in psychologically based verbal language. Research has shown that the capability to use abstract psychological terms varies among cultures and individuals within a given culture. The ability to use psychological language (as defined by Western standards) may be determined by a variety of developmental, familial, educational, and linguistic factors. In many non-Western cultures somatically or physically based terms still are the predominant mode of communicating emotional distress.

When examining the development of affective language in children, it may be observed that children first appear to experience affective states such as anxiety and fear physically long before they have verbal language either to conceptualize or label these feelings and communicate them to others. It is only later in development that

Table 9–1 **Somatization: Principles of Clinical Management**

1. The presentation is considered in the context of psychosocial factors, both current and past.
2. The diagnostic procedures and therapeutic interventions are based on objective findings.
3. A therapeutic alliance is fostered and maintained involving the primary care and/or psychiatric physician.
4. The social support system and relevant life quality domains* are carefully reviewed during each patient contact.
5. A regular appointment schedule is maintained for outpatients, irrespective of clinical course.
6. The patient dialogue and examination and the assessment of new symptoms or signs are engaged judiciously, and usually primarily address somatic rather than psychologic concerns.
7. The need for psychiatric referral is recognized early, especially for cases involving chronic symptoms, severe psychosocial consequences, or morbid types of illness behavior.
8. Any associated, coexisting, or underlying psychiatric disturbance is assiduously evaluated and steadfastly treated.
9. The significance of personality features, addictive potential, and self-destructive risk is determined and addressed.
10. The patient's case is redefined in such a way that management rather than cure is the goal of treatment.

* Quality of life is an elusive concept but includes the psychosocial domains of occupation; leisure; family, marital, and health; and sexual and psychological functioning.

children "learn" to label their feelings and to communicate them to others in verbal terms. Even in our own culture, many individuals as adults may be observed to have a limited capacity to communicate their inner experience and feelings using abstract psychological language.

It is often the task of the astute physician to interpret physical symptoms (or psychosomatic illness) as the patient's characteristic means of expressing and communicating the presence of internal emotional distress. Some individuals may be able to recognize their physical distress as related to or as a manifestation of emotional distress yet others may have limited insight to make such connections.

The phenomenon of communicating emotional distress in physical language has been termed "somatothymia" or "somatothymic language." Some patients with somatoform disorders may be understood as using a somatic or somatothymic language in which their physical symptoms are a manifestation of emotional distress and intrapsychic conflict. Somatothymic language is the earliest form of affective communication in the developing human and in many cultures and, in some patients with somatoform disorders, remains the predominant mode of "psychological communication." The somatoform disorders may be, at least in part, understood as *clusters of behavior* in which the predominant language used by the patient is somatothymic (Stoudemire, 1991a, 1991b). The concept of somatothymia is also discussed in Chapters 1 (by Drs. Yates, Kathol, and Carter) and 7 (by Drs. Risby, Risch, and Stoudemire).

SOMATOFORM DISORDERS

Somatoform disorders are characterized by physical complaints lacking known medical basis or demonstrable physical findings in the presence of psychological factors judged to be etiologic or important in the initiation, exacerbation, or maintenance of the disturbance. A comparison of the individual subtypes of somatoform disorder is presented in Table 9–2. These clinical features are fundamentally important and serve to facilitate the discussion that follows.

Somatization Disorder

Formerly "hysteria" or Briquet's syndrome, somatization disorder represents a polysymptomatic disorder beginning in early life, affecting mostly women, and characterized by recurrent, multiple somatic complaints reflected in a diffusely positive review of systems. Cases date back more than 3,000 years, with the first systematic evaluation being reported by Briquet, for whom the condition was originally named (Guze, 1975). Certain diagnostic aspects of the syndrome have been refined, resulting in the more reliable diagnostic criteria ultimately included in the DSM-IV nomenclature.

Epidemiology

Estimates from the Epidemiologic Catchment Area Study (ECA) show an estimated lifetime prevalence of approximately 0.4% for somatization disorder (Swartz et al, 1986). Although accurate point prevalence figures are not readily available, 1 to 2%

Table 9–2 Somatoform, Factitious or Malingering: A Comparison of Clinical Features

Somatoform Disorders

DIAGNOSTIC SUBTYPE	CLINICAL PRESENTATION	DEMOGRAPHIC/ EPIDEMIOLOGIC FEATURES	DIAGNOSTIC FEATURES	MANAGEMENT STRATEGY	PROGNOSTIC OUTLOOK	ASSOCIATED DISTURBANCES	PRIMARY DIFFERENTIAL PRESENTATION	PSYCHOLOGIC PROCESSES CONTRIBUTING TO SYMPTOMS	MOTIVATION FOR SYMPTOM PRODUCTION
Somatization disorder	Polysymptomatic Recurrent/ chronic "Sickly" by history	Younger age Female predominance 20 to 1 Familial pattern 5–10% incidence in primary care populations	ROS profusely positive Multiple clinical contacts Polysurgical	• Therapeutic alliance • Regular appointments • Crisis intervention	Poor to fair	Personality disorder Sociopathy Substance/ alcohol use Many life problems Conversion	Physical disease Depression	Unconscious Cultural/ developmental	Unconscious psychologic factors
Conversion disorder	Mono-symptomatic Mostly acute Simulates disease	Highly prevalent Female predominance younger age Rural/lower social class Less educated/ psychologically unsophisticated	Simulation incompatible with known physiologic mechanisms or anatomy	• Suggestion and persuasion • Multiple techniques	Excellent except chronic conversion	Drug/alcohol dependence Sociopathy Somatization disorder Histrionic personality	Depression Schizophrenia Neurologic disease	Unconscious Psychologic stress or conflict may be present	Unconscious psychologic factors
Pain Disorder	Pain syndrome simulated or magnified by psychological factors	Female predominance 2 to 1 Older: 4th or 5th decade Familial pattern Up to 40% of pain populations	Simulation or intensity incompatible with known physiologic mechanisms or anatomy	• Therapeutic alliance • Redefine goals of treatment • Antidepressant medications	Guarded, variable	Depression Panic disorder Substance/ alcohol use Dependent/ histrionic personality	Depression Psycho-physiologic Physical disease Malingering/ disability syndrome	Unconscious Acute stressor/ developmental Physical trauma may predispose	Unconscious psychologic factors
Hypochondriasis	Disease concern or preoccupation	Previous physical disease Middle or older age Male/female ratio equal	Disease conviction amplifies symptoms Obsessional	• Document symptoms • Psychosocial review • Psychotherapeutic	Fair to good Waxes and wanes	Depression Panic disorder Obsessive-compulsive disorder	Depression Physical disease Personality disorder Delusional disorder	Unconscious Stress— bereavement Developmental factors	Unconscious psychologic factors
Body dysmorphic disorder	Subjective feelings of ugliness or concern with body defect	Adolescence or young adult ? Female predominance Largely unknown	Pervasive bodily concerns	• Therapeutic alliance • Stress management • Psychotherapies • Antidepressant medications	Fair to good	Obsessive-compulsive disorder Anorexia nervosa Psychosocial distress Avoidant/ compulsive personality disorder	Delusional psychosis Depression Somatization disorder	Unconscious Self-esteem factors	Unconscious psychologic factors

Factitious Disorders

Disorder	Definition	Clinical Features	Management	Prognosis	Associated Disorders	Differential Diagnosis	Psychodynamics	Motivation
Factitious with predominantly physical symptoms	Feigned or simulated physical symptoms or signs or disease	Feigned illness No external goal of simulation is obvious Organ mode of presentation varies but is physical	Female, younger, socially conforming Employed in medical field Social supports often available	• Confront as appropriate • Redefine illness as psychiatric • Psychiatric referral	Fair to good except Munchausen's subtype	Depression Borderline or other personality disorder	Malingering Conversion disorder Hypochondriasis Depression Schizophrenia	Unconscious Developmental/family factors Masochism, dependency, and mastery are utilized	Conscious effort to assume patient status
Factitious with predominantly psychological symptoms	Multiple hospitalizations	Feigned illness No external goal of simulation is obvious Mode of presentation varies but is psychiatric	Female, younger, socially conforming Employed in medical field Social supports often available	• Confront as appropriate • Redefine illness as psychiatric • Psychiatric referral	Fair to good except Munchausen's subtype	Schizophrenia Borderline or other personality disorder	Malingering Conversion disorder Hypochondriasis Depression Schizophrenia	Unconscious Developmental/family factors Masochism, dependency, and mastery are utilized	Conscious effort to assume patient status
Munchausen's syndrome	Multiple hospitalizations	Feigned illness Pathologic liar Geographic wandering Antisocial features Frequently leaves against medical advice	Male, younger, socially nonconforming Social supports often unavailable	• Recognize • Confront • Avoid invasive or iatrogenic procedures or treatments • Social work referral	Poor	Antisocial, histrionic, or borderline personality	Malingering Conversion disorder Hypochondriasis Depression Schizophrenia	Unconscious Developmental/family factors Masochism, dependency, and mastery are utilized	Conscious effort to assume patient status

Malingering

Disorder	Definition	Clinical Features	Management	Prognosis	Associated Disorders	Differential Diagnosis	Psychodynamics	Motivation
Malingering	Feigned or simulated with physical or psychological symptoms	Feigned illness External incentives for disease present	? Male predominance Psychosocial stress or failure present	• Confront • Consider psychiatric or psychosocial problems	N/A	Antisocial personality Substance abuse/dependence	Factitious disorder Personality disorder Ganser syndrome Münchausen syndrome Major psychosis Disability syndrome	Conscious but may display other psychopathology	Conscious response to external incentives

prevalence is suggested for women with a female-to-male predominance of approximately 20 to 1. Somatization disorder is more commonly observed in lower socioeconomic groups. Between 5 and 10% of a primary care ambulatory population will meet diagnostic criteria for somatization disorder, suggesting that somatization is the fourth most common diagnostic group seen in an ambulatory medical setting. A relationship between somatization disorder and polysurgery is also well documented. A familial pattern is observed affecting 10 to 20% of female first-degree biologic relatives of females with somatization disorder; male relatives of females with this disorder show an increased risk of antisocial personality disorder and/or substance-use disorder (Bohman et al, 1984). Adoption studies have indicated that both genetic and environmental factors contribute to the risk for the disorder. Several investigators have reported the tendency for somatization disorder to be associated with sociopathy, alcoholism, and drug addiction. Although no specific data exist to establish the economic impact of somatization, the prevalence and tendency to use surgery and advanced technology in diagnosis or treatment undoubtedly represents a significant cost.

Diagnosis and Differential Diagnosis

The most important diagnostic feature of somatization disorder is recurrent, multiple somatic complaints of several years duration for which medical attention has been sought. The diagnostic criteria are summarized in Table 9–3. A specific pattern of complaints not fully explained by a known medical condition may include (1) at least four pain symptoms involving multiple sites or functions, (2) gastrointestinal symptoms (at least one), (3) sexual or reproductive symptoms other than pain (at least one), or (4) pseudoneurologic symptoms or deficits (APA, 1991). The diagnosis has been shown to possess criterion stability, with a high degree of reliability and validity. Liskow observed that the disorder is quite heterogeneous and that other psychiatric illness is likely to coexist (Liskow et al, 1986). Personality disorders are more frequently associated and may appear in conjunction with anxiety or depressed mood, as well as substance abuse. Interestingly, recent reports suggest that avoidant, paranoid, self-defeating, and compulsive personality disorder occur with greater frequency than do histrionic and antisocial disorders (Rost et al, 1992; Smith et al, 1991). Conversion symptoms may also be a prominent clinical feature with somatization disorder. Antisocial behavior and occupational, interpersonal, or marital difficulties are also frequently observed.

The differential diagnosis includes schizophrenia, panic disorder, conversion disorder, factitious disorder, and psychological factors affecting physical illness in addition to medical disorders that presents with confusing, vague, and somatic symptoms. Patients with somatization disorder may present in the context of acute illness, psychophysiologic symptoms, or other chronic medical conditions. A history of depression, panic, suicide attempt, and divorce is also common (Tomasson et al, 1991). Thus, a mix of primarily psychogenic and physical symptoms is the rule rather than the exception, making these cases extraordinarily challenging diagnostically.

Etiology and Pathogenesis

The etiologic foundations of somatization disorder are not readily discernible, although familial incidences and association with antisocial and histrionic personality

Table 9–3 **Summary of Diagnostic Criteria for Somatization Disorder***

- Multiple physical complaints with onset prior to age 30, and long-standing occurrence for several years. Results in medical intervention and significant impairment in social or occupational functioning.
- Symptoms have occurred within each of the following categories that are not fully due to a known medical condition or are not fully explained by clinical findings:
  —Pain symptoms in four different sites, e.g., head, abdomen, back, joints, extremities, chest, rectum, or pelvis (with intercourse, menstruation, or elimination).
  —Gastrointestinal symptoms (two or more), e.g., nausea, diarrhea, bloating, vomiting, or food intolerance.
  —Sexual symptom(s), e.g., indifference, erectile or ejaculatory dysfunction, irregular menses or excessive bleeding, or vomiting throughout pregnancy.
  —Pseudoneurologic symptoms, i.e., conversion symptom or dissociative symptom.

Adapted from DSM-IV (APA 1993, in press [1994])

disorder, as well as substance- and alcohol-abuse disorders, suggest a biologic predisposition. Undoubtedly, a learning model or behavioral theory is applicable, because the general use of somatizing behavior in the family of origin or culture may predispose to the syndrome (Brodsky, 1984). Furthermore, the disorder begins early in life (before age 30).

Clinical Management

The first step in the management of somatization disorder is simply to recognize the syndrome and initiate a therapeutic strategy in keeping with the principles outlined in Table 9–1. These patients see themselves as functionally disabled and readily use medical services despite the fact that no objective measures support that they are physically sick. The following case is illustrative:

A CASE STUDY

A 40-year-old woman presented to the emergency room with a complaint of chest pain. A preliminary evaluation revealed no obvious cause, but because she reported numerous symptoms in her systems review, she was admitted for a more complete evaluation. Her diagnostic workup ultimately included cardiac catheterization, which yielded totally normal results. The medical student involved in her case learned that her twin children who had "always helped" her in illness, had recently left to attend college. Furthermore, a review of her complaints in view of the negative findings seemed to indicate that the patient was "psychosomatic." At this point a psychiatric consultant was asked to see the patient and obtained a thorough psychosocial history revealing that the patient had been sickly since about age 15, with numerous chronic symptoms aris-

ing in different organ systems: nausea, bloating, back pain, dysuria, pain in her knees, palpitations, dizziness, dyspnea, double vision, gait unsteadiness, weakness of her arms, trouble swallowing, dyspareunia, and dysmenorrhea were all related at various times throughout the interview. She dramatically related that she was "tired of suffering" and was "frustrated" with her doctors, who had been unable to diagnose her case or satisfactorily explain the disabling symptoms. The psychiatrist, who recognized her problem as somatization disorder, suggested psychotherapy as a means to help her cope with the rather obvious family stresses that had precipitated her pain, but she declined, saying that she preferred to see "a real doctor who can understand me better."

As represented in the case above, many patients are highly resistant to psychiatric referral, thus the recommendations for treatment must first consider the general principles outlined in Table 9–1. A cure is seldom achieved, but recurrent debilitating symptoms can be relinquished and perhaps exchanged for controlled dependence on a clinic or physician. Again, the psychiatric consultant's role usually involves crisis intervention or attention to associated disturbances, with the key therapeutic interventions resulting from a developing therapeutic relationship with the primary clinician.

Conversion Disorder

Conversion symptoms have been described since antiquity and represent a type of somatoform disorder in which there is a loss or alteration in physical functioning suggesting a physical disorder but which cannot be explained on the basis of known physiologic mechanisms (Table 9–4). Conversion disorder is usually seen in ambulatory settings or emergency departments, and frequently runs a rather short-lived course, responding to nearly any therapeutic modality that offers a suggestion of cure.

Table 9–4 **Summary of Diagnostic Criteria for Conversion Disorder*†**

- Symptom(s) or deficit(s) under voluntary control affecting motor or sensory function, which suggests a medical condition.
- The initiation or exacerbation of the symptom(s) or deficit(s) is preceded by conflicts or stressors, i.e., psychologic factors are prominent.
- Symptom(s) or deficit(s) is not consciously or intentionally produced.
- Symptom(s) or deficit(s) is not fully explained, after clinical assessment, as a medical condition or culturally sanctioned phenomenon.
- Symptom(s) or deficit(s) impairs social or occupational function, creates significant distress, or requires medical intervention.
- Symptom(s) or deficit(s) is not limited to pain or sexual dysfunction or is not a component of somatization disorder or other psychiatric syndrome.

* The symptom(s)/deficit(s) may be designated as motor, convulsive, sensory, or mixed.

† Adapted from DSM-IV (APA 1993, in press [1994])

Epidemiology

Conversion symptoms are exceedingly common in medical practice; estimates of 20 to 25% prevalence are given for patients admitted to a general medical setting (Ford, 1983). General hospital patients have consistently shown conversion symptoms in between 5 and 14% of all psychiatric consultations (Folks et al, 1984). Conversion symptoms are also ubiquitous among randomly selected psychiatric clinic patients, and particularly prevalent among patients with drug addiction, sociopathy, alcoholism, and somatization disorder or "hysteria." The disorder more typically occurs in women. In men the disorder tends to be associated with a history of industrial accidents or, more typically, military duty. Conversion disorder reportedly encompasses ages ranging from early childhood into the ninth decade. The disorder appears more frequently in lower socioeconomic groups and in rural or less psychologically sophisticated populations. The more primitive and grossly nonphysiologic conversion symptoms are observed in patients of rural background; by contrast, conversion symptoms observed in better-educated populations will more closely simulate known disease.

Diagnosis and Differential Diagnosis

Diagnostic descriptions and terminology relating to conversion phenomena have changed markedly over the past 30 years. Diagnostic criteria are depicted in Table 9–4. The diagnosis is unique, implying that specific psychodynamic mechanisms account for the disturbance. In contrast with somatization disorder, which is chronic and polysymptomatic, involving many organ systems, conversion disorder is generally sporadic and monosymptomatic with a symbolic relationship between the underlying psychological conflict and the disturbance in physical functioning. *A number of traditional clinical features previously associated with conversion— for example, secondary gain, histrionic personality, and* la belle *indifference— appear to have no diagnostic significance; these are regarded as "soft signs," supportive of the diagnosis and having no firm diagnostic validity.* The diagnosis of conversion must ultimately rest upon positive clinical findings clearly indicating that the symptom does not derive from physical disease, such as demonstration of normal motor function in patients with "paralysis." Common examples of conversion symptoms include paralysis, abnormal movements, aphonia, blindness, deafness, or pseudoseizures, the last of which is illustrated by a case vignette:

A CASE STUDY

A 42-year-old woman was admitted to the neurology service for evaluation of seizures beginning 1 month earlier. The seizures consisted of abrupt onset of tonic-clonic movements, lasting about 10 minutes, resolving equally abruptly, with no postictal confusion or diminished consciousness. An intensive neurological evaluation revealed no abnormal physical findings: neurological exam, routine physical exam, routine laboratory exam, head CT scan, magnetic resonance imaging of the brain, lumbar puncture, and routine electroencephalogram were all normal. The patient's brain electrophysiologic activity was then monitored continuously and showed no abnormal EEG patterns despite the occurrence of several "seizure" episodes. A psychiatric consultant was called

*who learned that the seizure activity—now thought to represent a con-
version disorder—began within a week of learning that her husband
had been unfaithful. An amobarbital interview revealed that the patient
had been considering a divorce although such an alternative was unacceptable to her or her family of origin's value system.*

As suggested by the case, conversion symptoms will usually conform to the
patient's concept of disease rather than to typical pathophysiologic mechanisms or
anatomical patterns. When the symptom occurs in isolation, it is appropriate to assign
a diagnosis of conversion disorder; however, conversion symptoms may also occur as a
part of other major syndromes, such as somatization disorder, schizophrenia, depression, and even medical or neurological disease.

Etiology and Pathogenesis

Clinical descriptions of conversion phenomena date back to at least 1900 BC, at
which time the Egyptian papyri attributed symptoms to "wandering of the uterus."
Conversion symptoms result from stressful environmental events acting on the *affective* part of the brain in predisposed individuals. Some patients' symptoms conform to
Freud's concept of "conversion" in reference to the concept that conversion results
from the substitution of a somatic symptom for a repressed idea or psychological
conflict. Conversion may also be a means of express forbidden feelings or ideas, as a
kind of communication via pantomime or mimicry when direct verbal communication
is blocked, or may simply serve as an acceptable means of enacting the sick role or as
an acute entry into illness behavior. The individual with conversion avoids certain
responsibilities or noxious situations and is frequently able to control or manipulate
the behavior of others. Classical conditioning paradigms have provided other possible
explanations for conversion phenomena. Learned symptoms of illness are then later
used as a means of coping with particularly stressful situations. More recent theories
have proposed social, communication, and sophisticated neurophysiologic mechanisms (Folks et al, 1984).

Clinical Management

A wide variety of treatment techniques have been successfully used for conversion disorder. Brief psychotherapy focusing on stress and coping, and suggestive
therapy—sometimes using hypnosis or amobarbital interviews that focus on symptom removal—are commonly employed with amazing efficacy. A short hospital admission also may be helpful, particularly when symptoms are disabling or alarming.
Hospitalization may serve to remove the patient from the stressful situation, demonstrate to the family that the matter is important, or facilitate resolution of the
psychological trauma. Many patients experience spontaneous remission of symptoms
or demonstrate marked or complete recovery after a brief therapeutic intervention. In
fact, prompt recovery is the rule, and few patients will need long-term management.
For example, a case seen in our facility involved a healthy 29-year-old farmer who
experienced acute blindness when confronted with a mortgage foreclosure notice and

was ultimately "cured" with saline drops. The psychiatric consultant merely told the patient that the "special" eye drops had "cured several others in a matter of days."

Unfortunately, chronic conversion disorder carries a poorer prognosis and is notoriously difficult to treat, resembling somatization disorder. Behavior modification can be used in the approach to recalcitrant conversion symptoms maintained by secondary gain. The therapeutic principles outlined in Table 9–1 are particularly relevant to these chronic cases, and psychiatric consultants are often required.

Pain Disorders Associated with Psychological Factors

The general category of "pain disorder" in DSM-IV has the four following major criteria: (a) the pain should be present in one or more anatomical sites and of sufficient importance to warrant clinical attention; (b) the pain causes significant distress or impairment in the patient's social or occupational functioning; (c) psychological factors appear to be operative in the onset, severity, exacerbation or maintenance of the pain; and (d) the patient's pain is not primarily due to a mood, anxiety, or psychotic disorder (see Table 9–5).

The DSM-III-R term "somatoform pain disorder" has been eliminated in DSM-IV. Pain syndromes in which psychological factors are believed to have a primary role in the onset, severity, exacerbation, or maintenance of a patient's pain complaints are now classified under the subcategory "pain disorder associated with psychological factors." If the patient has a medical condition, the medical condition should not have a major role in the manifestation of pain for this subcategory to be assigned.

In many situations, however, the patient may have a bona fide physical illness (such as lumbar disk disease) but psychological factors appear to magnify their clinical pain symptoms. If the medical disorder appears to be present and making a significant role in the patient's pain complaints, and these complaints are magnified in severity by psychological factors, then the patient may be diagnosed with "pain disorder associated with *both* psychological factors *and* a general medical condition." This section will primarily focus on pain syndromes in which psychological factors appear to predominate and there are minimal contributions from bona fide medical

---

Table 9–5 **Summary of Diagnostic Criteria for Pain Disorder*†**

- Pain as the prominent clinical presentation of sufficient severity to require assessment.
- Pain resulting in social, occupational or functional impairment or clinically significant distress.
- Psychologic factors precipitate, exacerbate, maintain the pain, or contribute to the severity of the pain.
- Pain is not a component of somatization disorder or other psychiatric disorder including sexual dysfunction.

* Pain per se may be associated with psychologic factors and/or a general medical condition; it may be acute with a duration of less than six months or chronic. The anatomical site(s) is coded on Axis III of DSM-IV.
† Adapted from DSM-IV (APA 1993, in press [1994])

and neurological factors. (The treatment of more routine pain syndromes not complicated by major psychological factors is discussed by Dr. Goldberg in Chapter 23.) As
noted above, this discussion is primarily in reference to "pain disorders associated
with psychological factors." As many as 75 million Americans are afflicted with chronic
pain, at a cost of some $40 billion per annum (Bonica, 1976). Multidisciplinary pain
clinics have developed in which patients can be effectively evaluated and treated by
consultants from a variety of disciplines—anesthesia, neurology, neurosurgery, ortho-
pedics, psychiatry, psychology, and social work. Various diagnostic categories of pain
are encountered. This chapter is confined to the diagnosis and clinical management of
certain aspects of pain associated with psychological factors.

Epidemiology

As much as 40% of pain patients exhibit pain that is psychogenic in origin
(Stoudemire, Sandhu, 1987). Pain typically presents in the fourth or fifth decade,
usually as acute pain increasing in severity over time. Pain that is associated with
prominent psychological features is diagnosed in women twice as frequently as in
men. Evidence exists to suggest a familial pattern, with first-degree biologic relatives
being at higher risk for developing the disorder. A known familial pattern that includes
a history of anxiety, depression, or alcohol dependence occurs at a greater frequency
than might be expected within the general population.

Diagnosis and Differential Diagnosis

Pain may involve one or more clinical sites and cause significant problems with
social, occupational or relationship functioning. Psychological factors are judged to
have a significant role in accounting for the pain (APA, 1991).

A CASE STUDY

*A 29-year-old radiologist complained to his family physician of constant
abdominal pain so severe that he had used up all of his sick leave and
was now strongly having to consider quitting his prestigious new position. An admission to the hospital led to a comprehensive but fruitless
evaluation of the pain, culminating in an unremarkable exploratory
laparotomy. On learning that the surgery was unrevealing, the patient
appeared surprised, frustrated, and distraught, proclaiming that he was
"afraid" that he would be unable to return to work with his boss, his
father, the division chief.*

The differential diagnosis of pain must take into consideration other psychiatric
syndromes, such as somatization disorder, depressive disorder, or schizophrenia, in
which complaints of pain are common. Of course, a significant minority of these
patients are ultimately found to be malingering (as is discussed below), and the
symptoms are manifested for the sole purpose of obtaining an obviously explainable or
recognizable goal, or in an attempt to secure narcotic analgesics or other addictive
substances. Another important differential diagnosis is psychophysiologic disorders,
such as muscle contraction headache, muscular spasm back pain, proctalgia fugax

affecting the musculature of the anus, or other syndromes that may involve a clear pathophysiologic mechanism that reasonably accounts for the pain syndrome.

Anxiety, especially panic, or depressive symptoms are often present as an underlying or coexisting disorder (Kuch et al, 1991; Smith, 1992). The changes in mood and in personality that accompany chronic pain are also frequently seen in depression (Reuler et al, 1980). Indeed, all pain patients seem to report symptoms or changes in their physiologic response, with the emergence of vegetative symptoms similar or identical to those that accompany anxiety or depression. The observed personality disorders that most frequently accompany somatoform pain are histrionic and dependent (Reich et al, 1983). For a discussion of more specific pain syndromes, the reader is referred to Ford (1983), where the clinical features of psychogenic aspects of pelvic pain, phantom pain, low back pain, and atypical facial pain are discussed.

Etiology and Pathogenesis

Pain disorders are sometimes diagnosed only on the basis of psychosocial features identified by history; evidence of past somatization, the presence of a symptom model, prominent guilt, or a history of physical or psychogenic abuse by either a parent or a spouse. However, these "soft" findings together with negative physical or laboratory or radiographic findings do not necessarily imply that pain is attributable to psychosocial forces. Moreover, as with all forms of somatization, a complete separation of etiology into physical or psychogenic may be difficult and in some ways unnecessary.

Full appreciation of the etiologic factors involved in any form of pain that appears to be exacerbated by psychological factors is complicated, since the clinician must account for the economy of secondary gain or reinforcement, understand abnormal illness behavior, and evaluate the role of unconscious motivations and primary gain. Those individuals receiving compensation are prone to confound their management; compensation neurosis or disability syndromes (not covered in this chapter) are perhaps the best studied etiologic and consequential factors resulting in patients with pain syndromes.

Psychological tests, most popularly the Minnesota Multiphasic Personality Inventory (MMPI), are used routinely in pain clinics to identify psychological factors. An elevation of scores on the three scales labeled hypochondriasis (Hs), depression (D), and hysteria (Hy), referred to as the "conversion V profile," purportedly provides evidence that the patients are "neurotic," representing themselves as physically ill and obtaining appreciable secondary gain from their symptoms. These psychological tests should not be carried out or interpreted in a vacuum and are unlikely to be useful diagnostically without other means of supporting data. In short, correlations do *not* distinguish organic from nonorganic patients for whom "conversion" or psychogenic forces are assumed to account for the pain.

Clinical Management

A multiplicity of treatments for pain syndromes influenced or magnified by psychologic factors have been suggested in the literature (Stoudemire and Sandhu, 1987; Reich et al, 1983). Generally, a systems approach and a variety of therapeutic techniques are necessary. The therapeutic strategy is to initially minimize the doctor-shopping and other interpersonal "games" while establishing a strong therapeutic alliance assuring the patient that complete relief is unlikely. The therapeutic principles outlined in Table 9–1 are effective. A major task is to convince patients that they must work to modify their therapeutic expectations and attempt to manage or live with their pain. A therapeutic contract can usually be initiated and the clinician quickly discerns whether the patient is really motivated to get "better." Because stress and psychological problems are always a component of pain cases, the psychiatric consultant is an invaluable participant in the psychological treatment and should be involved early. Moreover, the possible role of psychosocial or psychological factors and the impact of stress are better considered during the initial evaluation process. Specifically, many experienced clinicians recommend involving the psychiatric consultant at the outset of the diagnostic evaluation to minimize any feelings of rejection or abandonment that may otherwise emerge when psychiatric consultation is deemed necessary.

A number of nonpharmacologic treatments are useful in pain patients: transcutaneous nerve stimulation, nerve blocks, biofeedback, and other forms of behavioral or psychotherapy. Irrespective of the selected intervention, attention must be given to the patient's psychosocial, marital, and family situation, and to the meaning and significance of the pain itself. Regarding pharmacologic modalities, narcotics or other addicting substances are rarely indicated, but the psychotropics may serve as adjuvants. The cyclic antidepressants often afford pain relief (i.e., 50 to 75 mg daily of nortriptyline). MAO inhibitors have also been suggested as reasonable when combined with some of the aforementioned nonpharmacologic therapies.

Hypochondriasis

Epidemiology

The actual prevalence of hypochondriasis as a disorder distinct from other somatoform disorders is unknown, with estimates varying with culture and diagnostic criteria. Only a few twin studies have been reported, and inadequate evidence exists for conclusions about the importance of genetic factors. Developmental or other predisposing factors include parental attitudes toward disease, previous physical disease, lower social class, and culturally acquired attitudes relevant to the epidemiology and etiology of the disorder. Hypochondriasis typically begins in middle or older age and is equally common in men and women—features that serve to distinguish it from somatization and conversion disorder.

Diagnosis and Differential Diagnosis

Pilowsky (1970) defines hypochondriasis as "a concern with health or disease in one's self which is present for the major part of the time." The preoccupation must be unjustified by the amount of physical pathology and must not respond more than temporarily to clear reassurance given after a thorough examination. The core features of hypochondriasis appear to consist of a complex of attitudes: disease fear, disease conviction, and bodily preoccupation associated with multiple somatic complaints. These diagnostic features are reflected in Table 9–6. On presentation, the

Table 9–6 **Summary of Diagnostic Criteria for Hypochondriasis*†**

- Preoccupation or fear of serious disease with misinterpretation of bodily symptoms for six months or more.
- Medical evaluation and reassurance are ultimately not therapeutic.
- The preoccupation is not delusional or is not consistent with body dysmorphic disorder or is not a component of another psychiatric disorder.
- Significant social, occupational, or functional impairment occurs together with clinically significant distress.

* The patient's level of insight is of prognostic significance and may be specified.
† Adapted from DSM-IV (APA 1993, in press [1994])

medical history is often related in great detail in the context of doctor-shopping, deteriorating doctor–patient relationships, and associated feelings of frustration and anger. Anxiety, depression, and obsessive personality features are frequently encountered (Holmlund, 1992). The clinical course is chronic with waxing and waning of symptoms. Complications may arise secondary to numerous exposures to medical care and the dangers of repeated diagnostic procedures. The possible evolution of this pattern is illustrated by the following case:

A CASE STUDY

A 35-year-old accountant presented to a gastroenterologist with a request to be "checked for colon cancer." The patient stated that, in contrast to his usual pattern of daily bowel movements, he had been constipated for the past 3 weeks. He also stated that 6 months previously, he had been constipated and an evaluation had revealed nothing wrong. However, a family history of colon cancer and fears relating to his dietary habits were elaborated. The current episode was not associated with rectal bleeding, abdominal pain, or other symptoms. Subsequently, a thorough outpatient evaluation, including digital rectal exam, flexible sigmoidoscopy, and barium enema revealed no significant abnormalities. While exploring psychological possibilities, a personal history revealed some occupational distress related to his not yet becoming a full partner in the accounting firm, which in the same breath was compared to the rather glowing career observed in his brother, recently promoted to vice president at the local bank. The patient seemed quite irritated by the questions pertaining to his personal life and emotional well-being. Reluctantly he stated that he would "just have to accept the fact that everything's okay" but proceeded to question the doctor's credentials and the diagnostic validity of the completed procedures. Within 2 weeks, a letter from a gastroenterology colleague across town requested the patient's records, implying that the same complaints had been offered with a request for a "more thorough evaluation."

The most important step in the differential diagnosis of hypochondriasis is the exclusion of physical disease. A number of medical disorders can be difficult to identify in their early course, including myasthenia gravis, multiple sclerosis, slowly deteriorating degenerative diseases of the neurologic system, endocrinopathies, or systemic diseases such as systemic lupus erythematosus or occult neoplastic disorders. However, the diagnosis should not be one of exclusion; a positive diagnosis can be made by careful history in the absence of objective physical findings and on recognition that an emotional component contributes to the symptoms.

Among psychiatric diagnoses, the most important are anxiety disorders or major depression; the entity of "secondary hypochondriasis" is repeatedly cited in the literature (Pilowsky, 1970; Barsky et al, 1992; Kellner et al, 1992). One must also carefully consider the existence of other somatoform disorders, factitious disorders, or malingering, and of psychotic disorders for cases manifesting hypochondriacal delusions. Investigators have consistently reported syndromes of hypochondriasis that qualify as a delusional state.

Patients with hypochondriasis seem to perceive their bodily functions more acutely than others. Barsky's suggested term "amplifying somatic style" emphasizes that these individuals selectively perceive bodily functions and attribute their symptoms to physical disease (Barsky, 1979); *why* patients develop this type of behavior is unknown. Worry about disease and absorption in their health can be a powerful motive for attending selectively to a bodily sensation. Anxiety escalates and further serves as a motive for selective perception. Depression or dysphoria exists since the patient suffers and feels helpless or hopeless as the illness evolves. Anger may also arise as a result of unmitigated distress, conflicting diagnoses, ineffective treatments, and experiences of encountering impatient, rejecting, or hostile physicians. These emotions are compounded by doctor-shopping, medication problems, conflicting opinions from physicians, and iatrogenic phenomena, as well as the specific personality features in any individual case (Kellner, 1987).

Clinical Management

The most crucial management technique in caring for the hypochondriacal patient is the inclusion of a legible psychosocial history in a prominent place in the patient's record (Brown and Vaillant, 1981). The general therapeutic principles described in Table 9–1 are applicable to the vast majority of cases. Moreover, the effective strategy for the treating physician is to appreciate the obsessional features with respect to bodily complaints and to intellectually understand the fascinating displacement of psychodynamics involved in the symptom formation while appreciating the psychosocial history.

Generally, effective treatment takes place in the context of collaboration by a consulting psychiatrist and the primary physician, who continues to offer regular appointments to the patient. The possibility of concurrent medical disease or intercurrent illness exists—indeed, these will eventually occur as life progresses. Adequate physical examination on a regular and reasonable basis is helpful, and the judicious and coordinated use of other medical consultants is also appropriate in order to evaluate new or justifiable physical complaints. Hypochondriacal patients are best managed in a primary care or medical setting, but psychiatric consultation should be considered when the patient requests adjunctive psychiatric treatment—usually for anxiety, depression, or psychosocial distress—or when the primary physician becomes concerned about suicide or overt symptoms of depression or is unable to manage his or her own emotional response to the hypochondriacal patient. Surprisingly, the prognosis for hypochondriasis is good in a substantial portion of patients.

Body Dysmorphic Disorder

Body dysmorphic disorder, or dysmorphophobia, has been included as a separate disorder in the nomenclature. This syndrome had been regarded as a hypochondriacal subtype or unspecified somatoform syndrome in past literature.

Epidemiology

Because the vast majority of references involve case reports, descriptive accounts of body dysmorphic disorder offer little substantial information regarding epidemiologic or etiologic factors. Onset typically occurs in adolescence, but the initial presentation can be as late as the third decade. The condition can persist for years and significantly affect social or occupational functioning. Polysurgery or unnecessary surgical procedures complicate the cases, but currently no information is available on the predisposing factors, sex ratio, or familial pattern.

Diagnosis and Differential Diagnosis

The fundamental diagnostic feature is primarily a pervasive subjective feeling of ugliness or physical defect; the patient genuinely feels that changes are readily apparent to others (Munro and Stewart, 1991; Thomas, 1984). The diagnostic criteria for body dysmorphic disorder are outlined in Table 9–7. Commonly, the symptoms of body dysmorphic disorder involve facial flaws such as wrinkles; spots on the skin; excessive facial hair; the shape of the nose, mouth, jaw, or eyebrows; and swelling of the face. Rarely, they may include complaints involving the feet, hands, breast, back, or some other body part. A slight physical defect may actually be present, but the concern expressed is grossly in excess of what might be considered appropriate. This disorder is also characterized by much distress but is not to be confused with those transient feelings commonly experienced by adolescents. A case illustration can better distinguish the pathologic state:

Table 9–7 **Summary of Diagnostic Criteria for Body Dysmorphic Disorder***

- Preoccupation with an imagined or grossly exaggerated bodily defect.
- Clinically significant distress together with social, occupational, or functional impairment.
- Anorexia nervosa, psychotic, or other disorder cannot account for the preoccupation and impairment.

* Adapted from DSM-IV (APA 1993, in press [1994])

A CASE STUDY

A 19-year-old college student approached her campus physician with a request for him to "remove some of the bone" from her nose. She described the end of her nose as "too large," and believed that she could not attract a date because her nose was "repugnant." She conceded that perhaps her nose was really not too excessively large, but continued to worry about its impact on her social life and presented again and again wanting it "fixed." She was reluctantly referred to a plastic surgeon, who concurred that indeed no appreciable defect existed and that a surgical procedure was not justifiable. However, the surgeon was familiar with such presentations and suggested that a psychiatric colleague could "help her cope with her distress." The patient, who was somewhat compulsive, felt obliged to accept psychiatric referral. She was evaluated and ultimately became involved in group psychotherapy, which was therapeutic in helping her correct her distorted self-perceptions.

The differential diagnoses entertained with hypochondriasis are equally applicable to body dysmorphic disorder. However, the differential diagnosis must also consider phobias; personality disorders, especially avoidant and compulsive types; major depression; delusional disorder (somatic subtype); and the other somatoform disorders. Body dysmorphic disorder may also accompany anorexia nervosa and transsexualism, in which the patient displays unfounded beliefs about body weight and/or gender-related physical characteristics.

Etiology and Pathogenesis

Individuals with body dysmorphic disorder who indeed appear normal develop a low sense of aesthetic perception, whereas those who are somewhat abnormal regard their appearance in the context of a high sense of aesthetic perception. Avoidance of social or occupational situations due to anxiety or apprehension about the defect is the rule. Thus, a "neurotic" syndrome is operating with secondary features of anxiety and depression. Some authors have regarded this syndrome as rather ominous, a prodrome of schizophrenia. Furthermore, the belief in the physical defect of appearance can sometimes be delusional in its intensity. In some cases, it is unclear whether two different disorders can be clearly distinguished on the basis of whether the belief is quasidelusional or a clear delusion. Symptoms bordering on psychosis are presumed to develop more often in individuals with schizoid, narcissistic, or obsessional personality traits.

Clinical Management

Persons with body dysmorphic disorder frequently visit primary care physicians, dermatologists, or plastic surgeons repeatedly in an effort to correct the defect; depressive and obsessive personality traits and psychosocial distress frequently coexist with the disorder and require treatment. Psychiatric consultation may be useful in identifying and treating depression, anxiety, and other disturbances that require pharmacologic or psychotherapeutic intervention. Brotman and Jenike (1984) have suggested that patients with persistent anxiety or depressive symptoms be started on a trial of antidepressant therapy, either a cyclic antidepressant with serotonin-active properties or an MAO inhibitor. Similarly, a recent report suggests the responsiveness to the selective serotonin reuptake inhibitors (such as fluoxetine), especially with underlying anxiety, e.g., obsessive–compulsive disorder (Filteau et al, 1992). The antipsychotic drug pimozide has also produced startling and sustained improvement, particularly in patients whose neurotic preoccupation has become quasidelusional. However, no other antipsychotic or other pharmacologic agents have proven as effective in the treatment of this disorder. As illustrated in the above case, psychiatric intervention with individual or group therapy may be useful, again focusing on psychosocial functions and body image complaints while supporting the patient's efforts to understand their "use" of the defect to cope and receive secondary gain. Family conferences or therapy are also required in cases where the individual is not yet emancipated from the family of origin, particularly if an eating disorder, personality disorder, or other coexisting disturbance is identified.

Undifferentiated Somatization Disorder (Somatoform Disorders Not Otherwise Specified)

DSM-IV includes an undifferentiated somatoform disorder category for clinical presentations that do not meet the full symptom picture of somatization disorder or one of the other somatizing syndromes. Autonomic arousal disorders or psycho-physiologic disturbances involving cardiorespiratory systems, gastrointestinal systems, the urogenital system, or the skin are being considered as specific types or subtypes. In these cases, psychological factors contribute to symptomatology and/or the disturbance cannot be explained by a known nonpsychiatric medical condition or known pathophysiologic mechanism, e.g., effects of medication, substances of abuse, or injury (APA, 1991). Also, neurasthenia has traditionally been considered as a distinct diagnostic entity. This disturbance is characterized by persistent complaints of mental fatigue, physical fatigue, or body weakness or exhaustion after performing daily activities. The individual does not recover with rest or leisure. Symptoms include dizziness, muscular aches, headache, irritability, sleep disturbance, and gastrointestinal complaints (Katon et al, 1991; APA, 1991). The diagnostic criteria for undifferentiated somatization disorder are illustrated in Table 9–8. This newly added diagnosis was recently assigned in the following case:

A CASE STUDY

A 68-year-old woman presented to her family physician for an evaluation of dysuria and fatigue. She had experienced the symptoms for many years. Complete evaluation produced no evidence of a physical disease to account for her symptoms. Further questioning revealed no other physical symptoms and she did not display a depressive or associated psychiatric disorder. A consulting psychiatrist subsequently learned that the patient lost her parents, both at 65 years of age, due to cancer— leukemia in her father and renal cell carcinoma in her mother.

Table 9–8 **Summary of the Diagnostic Criteria for Undifferentiated Somatoform Disorder***

- Physical complaint not explained by medical/physiologic condition or physical complaint in association with medical/physiologic disturbance in excess of that expected from clinical findings.
- Social, occupational, or functional impairment together with clinically significant distress for at least six months.
- Physical complaint(s) is not a component of another somatoform or psychiatric disorder.

* Adapted from DSM-IV (APA 1993, in press [1994])

As illustrated, these disorders involve a single, circumscribed condition that is not explainable on the basis of demonstrable physical findings or known pathophysiologic mechanisms. In keeping with somatoform disorders, the presentation is apparently linked with psychological factors. The circumscribed symptoms are of 6 months duration or longer and, of course, not a part of another type of somatoform disorder, sexual dysfunction disorder, mood disorder, anxiety disorder, sleep disorder, or one of the other major psychotic syndromes important in differential diagnosis. A diagnosis of somatoform disorder that cannot be otherwise specified is assigned for somatoform symptoms that are of less than 6 months duration, hypochondriacal in nature, nonpsychotic, or presenting with nonstress-related physical complaints.

FACTITIOUS DISORDER

Most clinicians will at some point in their career encounter a case of factitious disorder. These somatizing states are essentially characterized by the voluntary production of signs, symptoms, or disease for no apparent goal other than to achieve the role of being a patient. By contrast, the somatoform disorders are collectively viewed as having symptoms that are manifested unconsciously. Munchausen's syndrome, the most extreme type of factitious disorder, is characterized by a triad of features involving simulation of disease, pathological lying, and wandering. These cases frequently involve men of lower socioeconomic class who have had a lifelong pattern of social maladjustment. Several other clinical features of the Munchausen type are depicted in Table 9–9. However, most authorities concur that the vast majority of factitious disorders involve socially conforming young women of a higher socioeconomic class who are intelligent, educated, and frequently employed in a medically related field. Thus, one will rarely encounter the socially nonconforming "wanderers" who satisfy the Munchausen's syndrome criteria listed in Table 9–9.

Epidemiology

The available literature provides only a few indications of the incidence of factitious illness. These disorders appear to be far more common than was once generally believed, perhaps because of the progress in medical technology and the

Table 9–9 **Munchausen's Syndrome: Diagnostic Features***

Essential Features
Pathologic lying (Pseudologia fantastica)
Peregrination (traveling or wandering)
Recurrent, feigned, or simulated illness

Supporting Features†
Borderline and/or antisocial personality traits
Deprived in childhood
Equanimity for diagnostic procedures
Equanimity for treatments or operations
Evidence of self-induced physical signs
Knowledge of or experience in a medical field
Most likely to be male
Multiple hospitalizations
Multiple scars (usually abdominal)
Police record
Unusual or dramatic presentation

---

* Patients will meet criteria for a chronic factitious disorder or an atypical factitious disorder.
† May also support the diagnosis of other factitious disorders.
(Reprinted with permission from Folks DG, Freeman AM: Munchausen's syndrome and other factitious illness. Psychiatr Clin North Am 8:263–278, 1985)

---

popular medical journalism that is readily available to the lay public. The paucity of systematic studies and disproportionate number of case reports on the Munchausen syndrome have resulted in contradictory data on the age and sex ratio. Patient age averages approximately 30 years and ranges from adolescence to old age. The available epidemiographic data on factitious disorders are inadequate, but again strongly suggest a preponderance of young adults, the majority of whom are female and likely to be employed in the health professions.

Differential Diagnosis

Factitious illness is not real, genuine, or natural. Thus, physical or psychological symptoms are under voluntary control and are simulated to deceive the physician, although the manifestation of symptoms possesses a rather compulsive quality. The characteristic presenting modes and organ system subtypes of factitious disorder are listed in Table 9–10. Factitious disorder with predominantly physical symptoms is the most common subtype (Table 9–11). A dramatic presentation with a history of multiple hospitalizations and, of course, the primary goal of assuming the patient role are the pertinent diagnostic features. Eisendrath (1984) suggests that factitious presentation may be manifested at one of three levels of enactment: (1) a fictitious history, (2) a simulated disease, or (3) the presence of verifiable pathophysiology. The last is illustrated by the following case vignette:

A CASE STUDY

A 32-year-old psychiatric nurse was hospitalized for uncontrolled diabetes mellitus. During her hospitalization, her serum glucose levels fluc-

Table 9–10 **Commonly Presenting Features of Chronic Factitious Illnesses**

ORGAN SYSTEM SUBTYPES	DEMEANOR OR BEHAVIOR
Abdominal*	Bizarre
Cardiac	Demanding
Dermatologic†	Dramatic
Genitourinary	Evasive
Hematologic*†	Medically sophisticated
Infectious	Self-mutilating
Neurologic*	Unruly
Psychiatric	
Self-medication*‡	

* Original subtypes identified
† Recently reported to be more common
‡ Especially insulin, thyroid, vitamins, diuretics, and laxatives
(Reprinted with permission from Folks DG, Freeman AM: Munchausen's syndrome and other factitious illness. Psychiatr Clin North Am 8:263–278, 1985)

tuated markedly despite diligent efforts to regulate her insulin dosage requirements. On the fourth hospital day, the patient suggested that perhaps she needed further diagnostic testing to determine whether any other unrecognized problems might be present. Her physician discouraged further testing. The next morning the ward nurse found the patient lying comatose in her bed. A stat blood sugar showed severe hypoglycemia. During the emergency evaluation, a medical student found a used syringe and a bottle of regular insulin lying behind the patient's nightstand. When the patient recovered and was confronted with the discovery of the covert insulin, she became highly indignant and left the hospital against medical advice.

A diagnosis of inclusion, not exclusion, factitious disorder with either predominantly physical or psychologic symptoms or both requires a high index of suspicion and clinical perseverance once the diagnosis is established. In addition to the possi-

Table 9–11 **Diagnostic Criteria for Factitious Disorder*†**

- Conscious production of clinical signs or symptoms.
- Primary intent is to assume the sick role.
- The patient does not benefit from or have external incentives for the production of signs or symptoms.

* Factitious disorder may occur predominantly with psychologic and/or physical signs and symptoms.
† Adapted from DSM-IV (APA 1993, in press [1994])

bility that a true disease exists and accounts for the presentation, malingering, pseudomalingering, conversion disorder, and hypochondriasis are the leading differential diagnoses. Diagnostic criteria for factitious disorder are depicted in Table 9–11. Cases involving psychological presentations of factitious illness include factitious mourning or grief, or feigned psychosis or posttraumatic stress disorder.

Factitious disorder by proxy may also be encountered; in these cases a parent or caregiver presents with a factitial illness induced within a child or another person who is under their care. Similar to factitious disorder, the motivation for the perpetrator's behavior is a psychologic need to assume the sick role indirectly; the presentation is in the absence of external incentives for the behavior, e.g., economic gain (APA, 1991; Folks and Freeman, 1985). Factitial cases seen in psychiatric consultation may have already been misdiagnosed as a range of psychiatric disorders, including conversion disorder, somatization disorder, malingering, schizophrenia, or other major psychoses. Histrionic, schizotypal, borderline, antisocial, and masochistic personality disorders often, if not always, are concurrently diagnosed on Axis II; borderline personality disorder is the most common type of personality disorder observed (Folks and Freeman, 1985). Poorly defined distinctions between factitious disorder, somatization disorder, and malingering have likely contributed to the diversity of diagnoses included in the differential diagnosis of factitious disorder. Atypical factitious illness not otherwise specified is also an appropriate diagnosis for patients who do not seek hospital admission and for other atypical cases involving simulated illness, such as dermatitis artifacta.

Etiology and Pathogenesis

Any attempt to understand the etiology of factitious disorder requires careful consideration of any developmental disturbance, personal history, and current life stressors and an appreciation of primary psychodynamic mechanisms—masochism, dependency, and mastery. The desire to be the center of interest and attention; a grudge against physicians and hospitals that is somehow satisfied by frustrating and deceiving the staff; a desire for drugs; a desire to escape the police; and a desire to obtain free room and board while tolerating the consequences of various therapeutic investigations and treatment are some of the more frequently listed reasons that might possibly motivate the self-destructive behaviors of patients with a factitious disorder.

Although patients often possess borderline personality traits, one can often obtain a history of childhood emotional insecurity; excluding or rejecting parents; and broken homes leading to foster home placement or adoption and subsequent delinquency, antisocial behavior, or failure in psychosexual development. The possible enactment of past or present developmental disturbances within the medical setting should also be considered. In essence it seems that these patients, through their illness, also may primarily seek to compensate for developmental traumas and secondarily escape from and make up for stressful life situations. Psychodynamic explanations suggest that the factitiously disordered patients experiences satisfaction from manipulating as many aspects of their own medical and surgical care as possible (mastery), receive strong sexual gratification from diagnostic and therapeutic procedures (masochism), and enjoy the warm and personal but ambivalent care inherent in the doctor–patient relationship (dependency), culminating in the excitement of the hospital experience.

Clinical Management

The general therapeutic approach outlined in Table 9–1 is applicable to cases of factitious disorder, and a comparison with the somatoform disorders is presented in Table 9–2. The initial clinical approach also requires a clear recognition of the syndrome or a high index of suspicion that a factitious disorder is indeed present. Psychiatric consultation should be requested for all cases, and if confrontation is advisable, the primary physician (as opposed to the consultant) should confront the patient in a nonpunitive manner (Hollender and Hersh, 1970). Patients are usually less difficult to confront than might be expected and do not show the intense anger, impulsivity, or instability of interpersonal relationships that is commonly reported with the more extreme cases representing Munchausen's syndrome (Reich and Gottfried, 1983). If confronted with the factitious nature of the illness, the patient may deny it, refuse psychiatric intervention, and resume the same behavior; may admit that the factitious illness is present but refuse psychiatric intervention; or may acknowledge the factitial nature of the illness and cooperate with psychiatric intervention (Ford, 1983; Hollender and Hersh, 1970). Confrontation is not necessarily appropriate for all cases; the psychiatrist may simply attempt to build rapport with the patient while the primary physician continues any necessary noninvasive medical treatment. Confrontation is more often favored in the hospitalized patient who has the intelligence, psychosocial supports, and personal attributes necessary for a more mature adaptation. The psychiatric consultant also serves to assist the medical staff with its negative reactions to the factitiously disordered patient. In turn, the medical staff team can protect the patient from himself or herself by avoiding potentially dangerous diagnostic or operative procedures. Family members can be especially therapeutic in providing pertinent history or assisting the medical staff in maintaining acceptable limits on the illness behavior. Treatable psychopathology such as anxiety disorders, depressive syndromes, conversion symptoms, and major psychoses should be assiduously evaluated and steadfastly treated whenever possible (Folks and Freeman, 1985).

The prognosis for factitious illness has generally been considered poor. However, careful exclusion of malingerers, severe borderline personalities, wandering patients with Munchausen's syndrome, and the chronic medically ill can result in a subgroup of potentially treatable patients (Folks and Freeman, 1985; Table 9–12). The prognosis is better for patients with an underlying depression than for those merely possessing a personality disorder. Reich and associates observed that once the diagnosis was established, even some of the more severe and chronic cases responded quite well to a combined medical and psychiatric approach (Reich and Gottfried, 1983). Finally, as noted with other forms of somatization, the possibility of coexisting physical disease or intercurrent illness should be appreciated in all diagnostic and therapeutic endeavors.

Table 9–12 **Aspects of Factitious Illness**
Potentially Amenable to Treatment

1. Presence of treatable psychiatric syndromes, including:
   Mood disorders
   Anxiety disorders
   Psychotic disorders
   Conversion disorders
   Substance abuse disorders
   Neuropsychiatric disorders
2. Personality organization closer to compulsive, depressive, or histrionic rather than borderline, narcissistic, or antisocial.
3. Stability in psychosocial support system as manifested by marriage, stable occupation, and family ties, as opposed to the single, unemployed wanderer.
4. Ability to cope with confrontation or some redefinition of the illness behavior.
5. Capability of establishing and maintaining rapport with the treating clinicians.

(Reprinted with permission from Folks DG, Freeman AM: Munchausen's syndrome and other factitious illness. Psychiatr Clin North Am 8:263–278, 1985)

MALINGERING

The essential clinical feature of malingering is the intentional production of illness or grossly exaggerated physical or psychological symptoms that is motivated by external incentives such as avoiding military duty, obtaining financial compensation through litigation or disability, evading criminal prosecution, obtaining drugs, or simply securing better living conditions (Gorman, 1982). Clinical reports suggest that malingering should be strongly suspected in the following circumstances: (1) a medical/legal context overshadows the presentation, (2) a marked discrepancy exists between the clinical presentation and the objective findings, (3) a lack of cooperation is experienced with diagnostic efforts or in compliance with medical regimen, and/or (4) the psychosocial history suggests the presence of an antisocial personality disorder. No specific patterns or indices reliably identify malingering with regard to psychological testing (Folks and Houck, 1993; Perry and Kinder, 1990). Malingering can be fundamentally viewed as a feigning of illness: the fraudulent simulation or exaggeration of physical or mental disease or defect consciously produced to achieve a specific goal. The reasons for the illness behavior in the individual circumstances can be readily understood by an objective observer. Unlike the patient with factitious disorder, who merely wishes to assume the patient role, a malingering individual has a more clearly external motivation, and the illness behavior is intentional and consciously produced to achieve a consciously desired goal. This distinction is represented in Table 9–2 and illustrated by the following case:

A CASE STUDY

A 57-year-old man appearing thin and disheveled presented to the emergency room one cold wintry night at 2:00 a.m. complaining of chest pain. He stated that he had a history of angina; he stated that only in-travenous morphine could alleviate his pain. The emergency physician, in obtaining a history of the pain, noted that it did not seem to fit the pattern of any of the common causes of chest pain; routine physical exam, laboratory screen, arterial blood gases, and electrocardiogram were surprisingly normal. However, as a precaution, the patient was ad-mitted for further observation and evaluation. The next day, the chest pain persisted and the patient still requested narcotics. A medical stu-dent ascertained that no relatives were available, and that the patient had no reasonable plan for how he might manage following hospital dis-charge. On afternoon rounds, the patient, after being informed that he would be given no narcotics, reported that his pain had disappeared, and despite the physician's willingness to search further for the cause, he insisted on leaving the hospital.

Malingering may be sometimes adaptive (arguable in the case just presented) and is, to a lesser degree, observed in apparently normal children, students, test subjects, and employees; thus malingering behavior does not always represent a maladaptive or malignant form. A few clinicians have promulgated the theory that pure malingering is a mental disease worthy of a therapeutic response. Malingering has also been conceptualized as occurring on a continuum with conversion disorder (Ford, 1986). Briefly, the conscious effort to falsify symptoms may in some cases include rather complex motivations, originating in part from the unconscious. Malin-gering is also likely to arise in individuals with antisocial personality disorder or other various forms of feigned illness, such as Ganser syndrome, or as a component of a neurotic state. These coexisting psychiatric disturbances should be the focus of evaluation and treatment for these "mentally ill" malingerers.

Irrespective of one's views on malingering, some basic legal principles should be considered in examining for the presence or absence of malingering. In particular, before reporting malingering one should steadfastly follow the basic rules of confiden-tiality and privilege. Another important aspect of malingering concerns the way in which physicians perceive such behavior and their moral judgment of it. As a case in point, situations certainly exist in which this extreme form of somatization is regarded as acceptable, constructive, or even praiseworthy, as in the case of the prisoner of war who malingers to protect his country's interests. Therefore, a professional and thera-peutic posture in approaching the malingering patient must initially include an examination of one's own feelings of anger, disgust, or humiliation, recognizing that the malingering behavior often threatens the very foundations of the doctor–patient relationship. Frank, nonjudgmental communication between the physician and the malingerer, and awareness that the behavior may be an ongoing reaction to stress or due to a psychiatric disorder may lead to an open discussion of the patient's needs—which may, in turn, provide a basis for an adequate therapeutic alliance or a solution to the problem (Lande, 1989; Mark et al, 1987).

Finally, a number of authors have described simulation among persons seeking compensation for work-related injuries or disease (Weighill, 1983). However, the psychological difficulties in these cases vary greatly, and the physician must be able to appreciate and assess a number of background factors, such as severity of injury, preexisting personality traits, developmental characteristics, social class, attitudinal response, and the pertinent family, social, and employment factors, as well as the actual progress of the physical condition or legal process of settlement. Unfortunately, these disability syndromes are beyond the scope of this chapter.

As a final note, a number of clinical pearls and suggested readings will serve to expand upon the material presented in this chapter. A thorough review of Tables 9–1 and 9–2 in conjunction with the Clinical Pearls section will aid in the diagnostic and therapeutic approach to each diagnostic type.

CLINICAL PEARLS

General Points

Somatoform disorders, factitious disorders, and malingering represent illness behavior; whether symptoms are consciously or unconsciously produced and whether the motivations for the production of symptoms are conscious or unconscious will determine what particular diagnostic category is assigned.

- Somatization is a process by which an individual consciously or unconsciously uses the body or bodily symptoms for psychological purposes or personal gain.
- Somatizing individuals are primarily motivated and secondarily receive gain for illness behavior, including the privileges of the sick role and sanctioned dependency.
- The presence of somatization encourages a thorough diagnostic investigation and therapeutic approach that focuses on psychosocial history and illness behavior in the context of existing disease, life problems, and psychological conflicts.
- Somatization may be primarily or secondarily associated with an underlying psychiatric syndrome, coexisting personality disorder, or psychosocial stressor of diagnostic significance.
- Some individuals may lack the ability to verbalize their feelings and intrapsychic conflicts in psychological terms. Somatothymia, or somatothymic language, describes the use of physically based language terms to communicate emotional distress.

Somatization Disorder

Somatization disorder is a polysymptomatic disorder that begins in early life, affects mostly women, and is characterized by recurrent multiple somatic complaints and a profusely positive review of systems.

- The disorder is commonly associated with sociopathy, alcoholism, and drug addiction.
- The disorder is heterogeneous and likely to coexist with a psychiatric disturbance or personality disorder.
- Management includes a therapeutic alliance with an empathic primary care physician, regularly scheduled patient visits, appreciation of the psychological significance of symptoms, use of diagnostic or therapeutic procedures or medications based on objective findings, and use of psychiatric consultation for complications, coexisting disturbances, or crisis intervention.

Conversion Disorder

Conversion symptoms are ubiquitous among psychiatric patients with schizophrenia, somatization disorder, alcoholism, sociopathy, and drug addiction.

- Conversion disorder typically occurs in women who are of lower socioeconomic class, psychologically unsophisticated, or of rural background.

- The diagnosis of conversion disorder must ultimately rest on positive clinical findings clearly indicating that the symptom does not derive from physical disease or as a part of another psychiatric disorder.
- Conversion symptoms often accompany degenerative neurological syndromes such as multiple sclerosis, amyotrophic lateral sclerosis, and so on. These and other disorders need to be carefully considered and ruled out before making the diagnosis.
- Acute conversion disorder can usually be etiologically related to psychological conflict and allows an individual to avoid certain responsibilities or noxious situations and secondarily enables control or manipulation of the behavior of others (i.e., secondary gain).
- Treatment usually includes supportive and suppressive approaches that include some element of suggestion or persuasion using the therapeutic principles outlined in Table 9–1; a multitude of treatments have proved successful.

Pain Disorder Associated with Psychological Factors
In as many as 40% of patients presenting with pain, the pain will be assigned as psychogenic or idiopathic.
- Pain disorder with psychological factors is diagnosed when psychological factors are believed by the clinician to have a significant role in the outset, severity, exacerbation, or perpetuation of pain syndromes.
- Psychological factors must be appreciated and may include any of the following:
  - identified precipitants by history
  - avoidance of an activity or responsibility that is unacceptable or noxious
  - acquisition of significant psychosocial support that would not otherwise be forthcoming
- Major depression or anxiety are often present and may be a component of the pain syndrome or represent a coexisting disorder.
- The best therapeutic strategy is to limit doctor-shopping and modify the patient's therapeutic expectations from "cure" to "management" of the pain, while attempting to appreciate the role of psychosocial or psychological factors and the impact of stress on the case, using psychiatric consultation as appropriate.

Hypochondriasis
Hypochondriasis is characterized by a concern or preoccupation with health or disease in oneself that is present most of the time and is not justified by the physical pathology.
- The core features include disease fear, disease conviction, and bodily preoccupation associated with multiple amplified somatic complaints.
- As with pain, the possibility of an underlying or secondary anxiety or depression should be strongly considered, and physical disease should be excluded.
- Treatment is most effective when there is collaboration between a primary physician who continues regular appointments and a consulting psychiatrist who focuses on coping with the pain syndrome and treats symptoms of anxiety, depression, or psychosocial distress.

Body Dysmorphic Disorder
Body dysmorphic disorder typically occurs in adolescence or young adulthood, persists for years, and significantly affects social and occupational functioning.
- The fundamental diagnostic feature is a pervasive feeling of ugliness or physical defect that the patient feels is readily apparent to others.
- Patients frequently consult primary care physicians, dermatologists, and plastic surgeons in an effort to correct the defect.
- Depressive and anxious symptoms, obsessive personality traits and psychosocial distress frequently coexist with the disorder and provide a basis and rationale for psychiatric consultation.
- Individual therapy that focuses on psychosocial distress and group or family therapy as appropriate are the primary interventions, in keeping with the principles outlined in Table 9–1.

Factitious Disorders

Factitious disorders usually involve socially conforming young women of a higher socioeconomic class who are intelligent, educated, and frequently employed in a medically related field.

- A distinction can be drawn between "wanderers," who frequently satisfy the Munchausen's syndrome criteria, and "nonwanderers," who do not. The latter (the majority) are amenable to treatment.
- As opposed to somatoform disorders, factitious disorders are characterized by psychological and/or physical symptoms that are *consciously* produced (or induced by proxy) with the goal of assuming the patient role; thus a patient (or caregiver) may be confronted about the illness behavior. However, unconscious motivations are responsible for the clinical presentation and must be addressed as such (see below).
- The primary therapeutic approach involves an attempt to understand the etiology, including consideration of developmental disturbances, personal history, and current life stressors; appreciation of primary psychodynamic mechanisms (masochism, dependency, and mastery); and an appreciation of any personality disorders that might complicate treatment planning. Usually a borderline personality disorder is involved.
- Clinical management includes confrontation by the primary physician and/or referral to a psychiatric consultant who redefines the illness as primarily psychiatric and offers a psychotherapeutic approach to those patients who do not represent the Munchausen's syndrome.
- The possibility of intercurrent illness or coexisting physical disease should be appreciated in all diagnostic and therapeutic endeavors. Careful follow-up by the primary physician is essential.

Malingering

The essential feature of malingering is the intentional production of illness consciously motivated by external incentives such as avoiding military duty, obtaining financial compensation through litigation or disability, evading criminal prosecution, obtaining drugs, or securing better living conditions.

- Malingering should be suspected in cases where a medical/legal context overshadows the presentation, a marked discrepancy exists between clinical presentation and objective findings, a lack of cooperation is experienced with diagnostic efforts or in compliance with medical regimen, and possibly when the psychosocial history suggests the presence of an antisocial personality disorder.
- The malingering should be confronted in a confidential and empathic but firm manner that leaves an opportunity for constructive dialogue and appreciation of any psychological or psychosocial problems.

ANNOTATED BIBLIOGRAPHY

Folks DG, Freeman AM: Munchausen syndrome and other factitious illness. Psychiatr Clin North Am 8:263–278, 1985

> A thorough review of the factitious disorders distinguishing those that are potentially treatable from Munchausen syndrome and other more refractory factitial syndromes. Includes a section covering Munchausen by proxy encountered in practice.

Ford CV: The somatizing disorders. Psychosomatics 27:327–337, 1986

> Includes an excellent overview of the process of somatization illustrating somatizing behaviors, sociocultural and interactional influences on somatization, and the specific diagnostic categories relevant to the process of somatization.

Ford CV, Folks DG: Conversion disorders: An overview. Psychosomatics 26:371–383, 1985

> An excellent overview of conversion disorder that includes a detailed discussion of its etiology and pathogenesis as well as a review of the diagnostic and treatment approaches.

Gorman WF: Defining malingering. J Forensic Sci 27:401–407, 1982

> An excellent overview that conceptualizes malingering on a continuum from normal to the abnormal to the pathologic forms. Provides the reader with a pragmatic conceptualization for approaching malingers therapeutically.

Kellner R: Hypochondriasis and somatization. JAMA 258:2718–2722, 1987

> A superb discussion of hypochondriasis and of how those affected use somatization in their clinical presentation. An excellent review follows outlining caveats in the management of hypochondriasis.

Quill TE: Somatization disorder: One of medicine's blind spots. JAMA 254:3075, 1985

> An overview of somatization disorder and management strategy in terms of the specific problems encountered in the doctor–patient relationship and in developing a therapeutic alliance.

Stoudemire A, Sandhu J: Psychogenic/idiopathic pain syndromes. Gen Hosp Psychiatr 9:79–86, 1987

> A comprehensive article that reviews the various pain syndromes encountered in clinical practice with special attention to psychogenic or somatoform pain and its evaluation and treatment.

REFERENCES

American Psychiatric Association: DSM-IV Options Book: Work in Progress. Washington, DC, American Psychiatric Association, 1991

American Psychiatric Association: DSM-IV Draft Criteria 3/1/93. Washington, DC, American Psychiatric Association, 1993

American Psychiatric Association: Diagnostic and Statistical Manual of Mental Disorders, 4th ed. Washington, DC, American Psychiatric Association, in press [1994]

Barsky AJ: Patients who amplify bodily sensations. Ann Intern Med 91:63–70, 1979

Barsky AJ, Wyshak G, Klerman GL: Psychiatric comorbidity in DSM-III-R hypochondriasis. Arch Gen Psychiatry 49(2):101–108, 1992

Bohman M, Cloninger R, Von Knorring A-L et al: An adoption study of somatoform disorders: III. Cross-fostering analysis and genetic relationship to alcoholism and criminality. Arch Gen Psychiatry 41:872–878, 1984

Bonica JJ: Organization and Structure of a Multidisciplinary Pain Clinic. In Weisenberg M, Tursky B (eds): Pain: New Perspectives in Therapy and Research. New York, Plenum Press, 1976

Brodsky CM: Sociocultural and interactional influences on somatization. Psychosomatics 25:673–680, 1984

Brotman AW, Jenike MA: Monosymptomatic hypochondriasis treated with tricyclic antidepressants. Am J Psychiatry 141:1608–1609, 1984

Brown HN, Vaillant GE: Hypochondriasis. Arch Intern Med 141:723–736, 1981

Eisenberg L: Disease and illness: Distinctions between professional and popular ideas of sickness. Cult Med Psychiatr 1:9–23, 1977

Eisendrath SJ: Factitious illness: A clarification. Psychosomatics 25:110–116, 1984

Filteau MJ, Pourcher E, Baruch P et al: Can J Psychiatry 37(7):503–509, 1992

Folks DG, Ford CV, Regan WM: Conversion symptoms in a general hospital. Psychosomatics 25:285–295, 1984

Folks DG, Freeman AM: Munchausen syndrome and other factitious illness. Psychiatr Clin North Am 8:263–278, 1985

Folks DG, Houck CA: Somatoform Disorders, Factitious Disorders and Malingering. In Stoudemire A, Fogel B.S. (eds): Psychiatric Care of the Medical Patient, pp. 267–287. New York, Oxford University Press, 1993

Ford CV: The Somatizing Disorders: Illness as a Way of Life. New York, Elsevier, 1983

Ford CV: The somatizing disorders. Psychosomatics 27:327–337, 1986

Gorman WF: Defining malingering. J Forensic Sci 27:401–407, 1982

Guze SB: The validity and significance of the clinical diagnosis of hysteria (Briquet's syndrome). Am J Psychiatry 132:138–141, 1975

Hollender MH, Hersh SP: Impossible consultation made possible. Arch Gen Psychiatr 23:343–345, 1970

Holmlund U: Psychogenic needs and psychiatric symptoms in young Swedish women. Br J Med Psychol 65:27–38, 1992

Katon WJ, Buchwald DS, Simon GE et al: Psychiatric illness in patients with chronic fatigue and those with rheumatoid arthritis (comments). J Gen Intern Med 6(4):378–379, 1991

Katon WJ, Von-Korff M, Lin E: Panic disorder: Relationship to high medical utilization. Am J Med 92(1A):7S–11S, 1992

Kellner R: Hypochondriasis and somatization. JAMA 258:2718–2722, 1987

Kellner R, Hernandez J, Pathak D: Hypochondriacal fears and beliefs, anxiety, and somatization. Br J Psychiatry 160:525–532, 1992

Kuch K, Cox BJ, Woszczyna CB et al: Chronic pain in panic disorder. J Behav Ther Exp Psychiatry 22(4):255–259, 1991

Lande RG: Malingering. J Am Osteopath Assoc 89(4):483–488, 1989

Liskow B, Othmer E, Penick EC et al: Is Briquet's syndrome a heterogeneous disorder? Am J Psychiatry 143:626–629, 1986

Mark M, Rabinowitz S, Zimran A et al: Malingering in the military: Understanding and treatment of the behavior. Military Med 152:260–262, 1987

Miranda J, Perez-Stable EJ, Munoz RF et al: Somatization, psychiatric disorder, and stress in utilization of ambulatory medical services. Health Psychol 10(1):46–51, 1991

Munro A, Stewart M: Body dysmorphic disorder and the DSM-IV: The demise of dysmorphophobia (comments). Can J Psychiatry 36(8):620, 1991

Parsons T: Social structure and dynamic process: The case of modern medical practice. In Parsons T: The Social System, pp 428–479. New York, Free Press, 1951

Perry GG, Kinder BN: The susceptibility of the Rorschach to malingering: A critical review. J Pers Assess 54:47–57, 1990

Pilowsky I: Primary and secondary hypochondriasis. Acta Psychiatr Scand 46:273–285, 1970

Reich P, Gottfried LA: Factitious disorders in a training hospital. Ann Intern Med 99:240–247, 1983

Reich J, Tupin JP, Abramowitz SI: Psychiatric diagnosis of chronic pain patients. Am J Psychiatry 140:1495–1498, 1983

Reuler JB, Girard DE, Nardone DA: The chronic pain syndrome: Misconceptions and management. Ann Intern Med 93:588–596, 1980

Rost KM, Akins RN, Brown FW, Smith GR: The comorbidity of DSM-III-R personality disorders in somatization disorder. Gen Hosp Psychiatry 14(5):322–326, 1992

Smith GR Jr, Monson RA, Ray DC: Psychiatric consultation in somatization disorder: A randomized controlled study. N Engl J Med 314(22):1407–1413, 1986

Smith GR: The epidemiology and treatment of depression when it coexists with somatoform disorders, somatization, or pain. Gen Hosp Psychiatry 14(4):265–272, 1992

Smith GR, Golding JM, Kashner TM, Rost K: Antisocial personality disorder in primary care patients with somatization disorder. Compr Psychiatry 32(4):367–372, 1991

Stoudemire A: Somatothymia: Part I. Psychosomatics 32:365–370, 1991a

Stoudemire A: Somatothymia: Part II. Psychosomatics 32:371–381, 1991b

Stoudemire A, Sandhu J: Psychogenic/idiopathic pain syndromes. Gen Hosp Psychiatry 9:79–86, 1987

Swartz M, Hughes D, George L et al: Developing a screening index for community studies of somatization disorder. J Psychiatr Res 20:335–343, 1986

Thomas CS: Dysmorphophobia: A question of definition. Br J Psychiatry 144:513–516, 1984

Tomasson K, Kent D, Coryell W: Somatization and conversion disorders; Comorbidity and demographics at presentation. Acta Psychiatr Scand 84(3):288–293, 1991

Walker EA, Katon WJ, Hansom J et al; Medical and psychiatric symptoms in women with childhood sexual abuse. Psychosom Med 54(6):658–654, 1992

Weighill VE: "Compensation neurosis": A review of the literature. J Psychosom Res 27:97–104, 1983

Alan Stoudemire (ed). *Clinical Psychiatry for Medical Students*, Second Edition. Copyright © 1994, 1990 by J. B. Lippincott Company.

10 Alcoholism and Substance Abuse

Robert M. Swift

Throughout history, humans have used psychoactive substances for medicinal, social, recreational, and religious purposes. Today, a variety of psychoactive substances continue to be widely used for similar, socially sanctioned purposes. Population surveys suggest that approximately 90% of the American population uses at least some alcohol, 80% use caffeine-containing beverages or medications, and 25% use tobacco products. The 1988 National Household Survey of Drug Abuse estimated that 72.4 million Americans age 12 or older (37% of the population) have used an illicit psychoactive drug at least once in their lifetime. Although the use of illicit drugs appears to have declined over the previous decade, one study estimated that 14.5 million Americans (7% of the population) used at least one illicit psychoactive substance over the month prior to the survey.

The impact of substance-use disorders on society is considerable. A study by D.P. Rice estimated that in 1988, total economic losses to the United States were $85.8 billion from alcohol abuse and $58.3 billion from drug abuse (Rice et al, 1991). Substance-use disorders are a major contributing factor to injuries and medical and psychiatric illnesses. For example, alcohol use is believed to be involved in 20 to 50% of all hospital admissions, but alcohol-use disorders are formally diagnosed less than 5% of the time (Lewis and Gordon, 1983; Holden, 1985). Many people use psychoactive substances to excess, in an uncontrolled fashion, in situations that are not socially approved, or in circumstances that have deleterious effects on health or behavior. Such individuals are considered to have a substance-use disorder. The causes of substance-use problems are complex and involve social, psychological, genetic, and pharmacologic factors.

SPECTRUM OF THE ALCOHOL-RELATED DISORDERS

An estimated 5 to 7% of Americans have alcoholism in a given year; 13% will have it sometime during their life. Simply defined, alcoholism is a "repetitive, but inconsistent and sometimes unpredictable loss of control of drinking which produces symptoms of serious dysfunction or disability" (Clark, 1981). There are marked sex differences in alcohol dependence/abuse rates: prevalence rates of alcoholism are about 5 to 6% for men, about 1 to 2% for women. The prevalence of alcoholism is highest in men ages 18 to 64 and in women ages 18 to 24, with a gradual drop afterwards (Regier et al, 1988).

Substance use is frequently associated with the presence of other psychiatric disorders. Alcohol use is highly correlated with suicide, homicide, and accidents (Goodwin, 1967; Waller, 1966). A major epidemiological study of psychiatric illness, the National Institute of Mental Health Epidemiologic Catchment Area Program, found high associations between alcohol use and anxiety disorders, depression, and schizophrenia (Regier et al, 1990). Other studies have found associations between cocaine use and opioid use and depressive disorders (Mirin, 1988; Kosten and Kleber, 1988) and associations between nicotine use and depression (Glassman et al, 1990). There appears to be a relationship between substance use and eating disorders, especially in women (Krahn, 1991). The co-morbidity of substance use and psychiatric illness is called *dual diagnosis* and is a major complication in the successful treatment of these patients. While an association between disorders does not indicate whether one disorder causes the other, there are cases in which substance use is directly etiologically related to the psychiatric disorder. Chronic alcohol use is associated with the cognitive and memory deficits of *alcoholic dementia* (alcohol-persisting dementia) and the more restrictive memory deficits of *alcohol amnestic disorder.* Patients with alcohol-related amnestic syndrome have the most difficulty with short-term memory (remembering recent events), but deficits may be noted in long-term memory as well. Patients may try to conceal or compensate for their memory loss by confabulation, making up answers, or talking around questions that require them to use memory. This syndrome, previously known as *Korsakoff's psychosis,* is thought to be due to a deficiency of thiamine, which is required as a cofactor for neuronal transketolase. The memory deficits are often permanent, although about 30% of patients will show improvement with abstinence and thiamine repletion over a long period of time.

Alcohol use may also produce *alcoholic hallucinosis* (alcohol psychotic disorder with hallucinations), characterized by auditory and visual hallucinations in a patient with a relatively clear mental status; *alcoholic paranoia* (alcohol psychotic disorder with delusions), characterized by suspiciousness, and single or multiple delusions usually due to alcoholism; and *alcohol delirium* (delirium tremens) (see also Chapter 4).

RECOGNITION OF SUBSTANCE ABUSE

As with other medical disorders, proper treatment can only be implemented after an accurate diagnosis has been assigned. The diagnosis of alcoholism and other substance-use disorders, however, is often complicated by denial of the problems by patients and their families—or efforts to conceal their use because of the fear of legal and other societal consequences. To recognize and treat alcoholism and other types of substance abuse and dependence, physicians must:

1. know the pharmacokinetics and pharmacodynamics of alcohol and other psychoactive substances;
2. be able to identify the presence of substance abuse or dependence despite efforts of the patient to deny or conceal their substance use;
3. know therapies for the acute management of intoxication and withdrawal of specific psychoactive substances;
4. know options for the short-term treatment and long-term rehabilitation of patients; and
5. be aware of their own attitudes and possible negative biases toward patients with substance-abuse problems.

This chapter provides basic information on the etiology and nosology of substance-use disorders and on the identification and treatment of such disorders in medical and psychiatric patients. Management of specific drug intoxications and emergencies is discussed in Chapter 19 by Dr. Dubin.

Clinical Pharmacology of Psychoactive Substances

For a drug to have psychoactive effects, it must be present in a high enough concentration as free drug at its active site in the brain. The drug must enter the body, be transported by the bloodstream to the brain, and enter the brain tissue. Usually, only a small amount of the total administered drug is delivered to the site of action; the rest of the drug may be bound to serum or tissue proteins, metabolized or excreted, or be otherwise unavailable. Because brain capillaries prevent the passage of many polar molecules into the brain (blood-brain barrier), most psychoactive substances are lipid soluble.

Figure 1 illustrates the competing pharmacokinetic processes that determine the availability of active drug. The *potency, duration*, and *mode of administration* of a drug can be predicted by understanding its *pharmacokinetics*. For example, the different potencies of cocaine hydrochloride and freebase cocaine can be explained by the slower absorption of the hydrochloride from the nasal mucosa and the rapid absorption of freebase from the alveolar mucosa. The rapid absorption of alcohol from the gastric mucosa accounts for its preferred oral administration.

To have psychoactive effects, a drug must also affect some neuronal process. The way drugs act at the active site is known as *pharmacodynamics*. Many psychoactive substances, such as stimulants, sedatives, anxiolytics, and hallucinogens, bind to a specific cellular component, such as a receptor. Receptors have now been identified as the site of action of caffeine (adenosine receptors), cannabis (THC receptor), hallucinogens (serotonin and NMDA receptors), nicotine (nicotinic cholinergic receptors), opioids (opioid receptors), phencyclidine (NMDA receptor), and sedatives (benzodiazepine, barbiturate, and other binding sites associated with the chloride channel). Cocaine and other stimulants appear to bind to specific neurotransmitter transporters. However, other substances, such as alcohol or inhalant solvents, may nonspecifically dissolve in cell membranes and disrupt cellular functions and neurotransmitters.

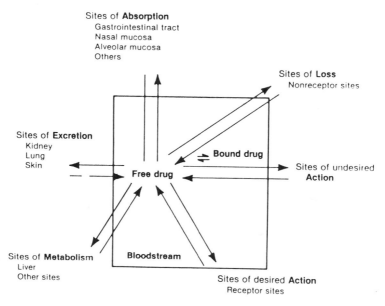

Figure 10–1. *Characteristics of drug movement across membranes. (Morgan JP. Alcohol and drug abuse curriculum for pharmacology faculty. U.S. Department HHS Publication No. (ADM) 85-1368, 1985)*

Ethyl alcohol (ethanol) has been demonstrated to have significant effects on several brain neurotransmitter systems. Acute exposure to ethanol inhibits *excitatory* NMDA receptors, while chronic alcohol exposure causes a *sensitization* of these receptors (Hoffman et al, 1990). Alcohol also may modify the activity of beta-adrenergic and adenosine neurotransmitter receptors linked to adenylate cyclase. Ethanol releases serotonin from neurons and chronic use may lead to depletion of brain serotonin. Alcohol has also been shown to modify the binding of GABA to its receptors and augments the electrophysiologic and behavioral effects of GABA in animals (Hunt, 1983). Alcohol appears to affect the binding of other sedative drugs to the inhibitory chloride channel of cell membranes, which is coupled to the GABA receptor (Seeman, 1972; Skolnick et al, 1981). The existence of a common mechanism for the actions of alcohol and sedative-hypnotics accounts for the cross-tolerance between these substances. (A detailed discussion of neurotransmitters and neurotransmitter receptors may be found in the companion text to this volume; Pedersen et al, in Stoudemire, 1994.)

Identifying Risk Factors for the Development of Substance-Use Disorders

Factors determining an individual's susceptibility to a substance-use disorder are not well understood. Studies of populations at risk for developing substance abuse have identified many factors that foster the development and continuance of substance use, including genetic, familial, environmental, occupational, socioeconomic, cultural, personality, life stress, psychiatric co-morbidity, biologic, social learning, and behavioral conditioning. The relative contributions of these factors vary between individuals, and *no single factor appears to account entirely for the risk.*

The influence of genetic factors has been best studied for alcoholism. It is well established that alcoholism is a familial disorder: children of alcoholics, especially males, are several times more likely to become alcoholic than are children of non-alcoholics (Goodwin, 1985; Cloninger, 1987). *The increased risk of alcoholism exists regardless of whether children are raised by their biologic parents or by non-alcoholic foster parents, suggesting that genetic factors are important.* Children of alcoholics are also more susceptible to other types of drug dependence. A genetic predisposition for alcoholism is also supported by differences in alcoholism rates between identical and fraternal twins. The *concordance* for alcoholism among *identical* twin pairs is *twice* that of fraternal twin pairs (70 vs. 35%). However, environmental influences must also have effects, because 30% of male identical twins of alcoholics do not themselves become alcoholic.

Factors proposed to account for the genetic predisposition for alcoholism include genetic variations in the rate of metabolism of ethanol and acetaldehyde (Thomas et al, 1982); differences in brain electrophysiology (Porjesz and Begleiter, 1982); differential subjective sensitivity to the intoxicating effects of alcohol (Schuckit, 1985); and altered cell membrane properties.

CRITERIA FOR THE DIAGNOSIS OF SUBSTANCE USE

Describing substance-use disorders is complicated by the ambiguity of the language used to describe substance use and by basic questions of whether using psychoactive substances constitutes a medical or a moral condition. In addressing these issues, organizations such as the World Health Organization (WHO) and the American Psychiatric Association (APA) consider the problem use of psychoactive substances to be a medical disorder and have formally defined criteria to determine *when* the use of psychoactive substances constitutes a formal medical disorder.

In a strict pharmacologic sense, *dependence* is often defined as *a state in which a syndrome of drug-specific withdrawal signs and syndromes follows reduction or cessation of drug use* (Table 10–1). *Tolerance* refers to *the state in which the physiologic or behavioral effects of a constant dose of a psychoactive substance decreases over time or when a greater dose of a drug is necessary to achieve the same effect. Withdrawal is a physiologic state that follows cessation or reduction in the amount of drug used.* In general, the behavioral effects of withdrawal are the opposite of those the drug produces (i.e., withdrawal from depressants produces psychomotor activation; withdrawal from stimulants produces psychomotor slowing).

In the *Diagnostic and Statistical Manual of Mental Disorders* (DSM-IV) (APA 1993, in press [1994]), the acute and chronic effects of psychoactive substances are classified under five major categories:

1. **Substance dependence:** A maladaptive pattern of substance use with adverse clinical consequences (see Table 10–1).
2. **Substance abuse:** A residual category that describes patterns of drug use that do not meet the criteria for dependence. Substance *abuse* is defined as a maladaptive pattern of substance use *that causes clinically significant impairment.* This may include impairments in social, family, or occupational functioning; in the presence of a psychological or physical problem; or in situations where use of the substance is physically hazardous, such as driving while intoxicated.
3. **Substance intoxication:** Reversible, substance-specific physiological and behavioral changes due to recent exposure to a psychoactive substance.
4. **Substance withdrawal:** A substance-specific syndrome that develops following cessation of or reduction in dosage of a regularly used substance.
5. **Substance-persisting disorder:** A substance-specific syndrome that persists long after acute intoxication or withdrawal abates (e.g., hallucinogen "flashbacks," memory impairments, or dementia).
6. **Substance-use disorder not otherwise specified:** Includes disorders of mood, thought, cognition, sleep, sexual functioning, etc.,

Table 10–1 **Diagnosing Substance Dependence***

At least *three* of the following occurring over a 12-month period of time:

—*Tolerance;* the need for *increased amounts* of the substance in order to achieve intoxication or other desired effect; or markedly diminished effect with use of the same amount of substance.

—Characteristic *withdrawal* symptoms (may not apply to cannabis, hallucinogens, or PCP); or the use of the substance (or a closely related substitute) to relieve or avoid withdrawal.

—Substance often taken in *larger amounts* or over a *longer period of time* than the person intended.

—Persistent desire or one or more unsuccessful attempts to cut down or to control substance use.

—A great deal of time spent in activities necessary to get the substance (e.g., theft), taking the substance (e.g., chain-smoking), or recovering from its effects.

—Important social, occupational, or recreational activities given up or reduced because of substance use.

—Continued substance use despite knowledge of having a persistent or recurrent social, psychological, or physical problem that is caused by or exacerbated by use of the substance.

* Adapted in part from American Psychiatric Association, DSM-IV (APA 1993, in press [1994])

associated with substance use (e.g., drug-induced anxiety, depression, or psychosis).

While not specifically defined by DSM-IV, the word "addiction" is frequently used in an equivalent sense to dependence but carries a more negative and pejorative connotation.

Eleven distinct classes of psychoactive substances are designated by DSM-IV (Table 10–2): alcohol; amphetamine or related substances; caffeine; cannabis; cocaine; hallucinogens; inhalants; opioids; nicotine; phencyclidine or related substances; and sedatives, hypnotics, and anxiolytics. Under the category of substance-use disorders, all but nicotine and caffeine are associated with both abuse and dependence; dependence *only* is defined for nicotine. Polysubstance dependence is a disorder defined for individuals using three or more categories of substances. "Other substance-use disorders" includes use of other psychoactive agents such as anabolic steroids, nitrate inhalants, anticholinergic agents, and unknown substances.

EVALUATING SUBSTANCE USE

The physician's primary task in evaluating a patient for substance use or dependence is not only to detect and confirm the diagnosis but also to establish an effective therapeutic relationship. In the context of this relationship, the physician should take a detailed alcohol and drug history, conduct a physical and mental status examination, order and interpret necessary laboratory tests, and meet with family or significant others to obtain additional information and to facilitate their involvement in the diagnostic and treatment process.

Assessing and treating patients who have *both* a psychiatric disorder and a substance-use disorder (dual diagnosis) is particularly complex. The physical, psychological, and behavioral effects of psychoactive substances *may be similar to*

Table 10–2 **Classes of Psychoactive Substances***

Alcohol
Amphetamines and related substances
Caffeine
Cannabis
Cocaine
Hallucinogens
Inhalants
Nicotine
Opioids
Phencyclidine and related substances
Sedatives, hypnotics and anxiolytics
Other (steroids, nitrates, etc.)

* Adapted from DSM-IV (APA 1993, in press [1994])

symptoms of a psychiatric disorder or, alternatively, *may mask* the symptoms of a psychiatric disorder. The physical, psychological, and social consequences of substance use may impair treatment of other illnesses as well. An important clinical rule is to generally defer making definitive psychiatric diagnoses until the role of substance use is completely clarified and the patient is completely detoxified. Most authorities would also agree that substance-use disorders must receive *top priority* in the treatment process if more than one Axis I diagnosis is present.

The Interview

As discussed in Chapters 1 and 2, the patient interview remains the *single most important component* of the diagnostic and assessment process. In a well-conducted interview, the physician may not only obtain information relevant to the diagnosis and etiology of a patient's substance-use disorder but may also set the tone for that patient's treatment. The physician should try to obtain a detailed substance-use history and should also inquire about physical or behavioral problems suggesting substance use. Empathy and concern are necessary to instill trust. This may be difficult, as many interviewers have negative feelings about substance users or about their prognosis. Judgmental attitudes and pejorative statements may severely limit the interviewer's ability to gather information and to initiate treatment. The diagnostic interview must almost always include interviews with family members since patients may be exerting denial—or overtly lying—about their pattern of substance use.

In obtaining information about a patient's alcohol and drug use, the *most effective interview strategy* is to focus on whether the patient has experienced *negative consequences* from the use of psychoactive substances, has poor control of use, or has been criticized by others about his or her substance use. Quantity and frequency questions ("How much?" and "How often?") are not especially effective in detecting substance use. The quantity of substance consumed is not the critical factor in making a diagnosis; the major fact to be determined is an assessment of the effects of whatever amount is consumed on the individual's functioning and interpersonal relationships.

Several formalized interviews are well validated in their ability to discriminate alcoholism. The CAGE questionnaire (Ewing, 1984) is a highly sensitive four-item test that uses the letters C, A, G, and E as a mnemonic. A "yes" answer to more than one question is suspicious for alcohol abuse.

> Have you ever felt the need to *C*ut down on drinking?
> Have you ever felt *A*nnoyed by criticisms of drinking?
> Have you ever had *G*uilty feelings about drinking?
> Have you ever taken a morning *E*ye opener?

Another reliable screen for heavy alcohol use is the Michigan Alcohol Screening Test (MAST). This 25-item scale identifies abnormal drinking through its social and behavioral consequences with sensitivity of 90 to 98% (Selzer, 1971). The Brief MAST, a shortened 10-item test, has been shown to have similar efficacy.

Although less documentation exists about the optimal interview to assess the drug-abusing patient, the same considerations apply: *it is more effective to ask about the behavioral and social consequences of drug abuse than about quantity and frequency of use.*

Even under the best interviewing circumstances, many patients who use psychoactive substances are reluctant to report the full extent of their drug and alcohol use and may deny or lie about it. Patients may deny the full extent of their substance use to themselves. In addition, the patient's family, friends, and colleagues collude in the denial of problems with substance use.

The following questions and historical data may help identify occult problem drinking and other types of surreptitious substance abuse:

1. Does the patient have a pattern of unexplained job changes?
2. Is the patient or family vague, evasive, or defensive about alcohol use?
3. Does the patient have convictions for driving under the influence or driving while impaired?
4. Are there multiple unexplained traffic accidents?
5. Does the patient have a history of impulsive behavior, fighting, or unexplained falls and scrapes?
6. Does the patient have any obvious physical stigmata of alcoholism (i.e., spider angiomas or a ruddy nose and face)?
7. Does the patient drink in the morning or find he or she needs an "eye-opener"?
8. Does the patient have a history of blackouts, "lost weekends," binge drinking, "DTs," or "the shakes"?
9. Does the patient relate a history of having to drink to relax or sleep?
10. Is there a history of chronic family chaos and instability?

A "yes" answer to any of these questions may help confirm the likelihood of an alcohol- or substance-related disorder. It should again be emphasized that information from other sources is critical to making the diagnosis—particularly family members who may even obscure the diagnosis by their own denial or attempt to "protect" the patient.

Obviously, patients with an altered mental status due to intoxication or withdrawal from a psychoactive substance may be incapable of providing an accurate history. In these circumstances, it is even more important to interview family members or acquaintances about the assessment. It is also helpful to examine any pill bottles or medications in the patient's possession.

The Physical Examination

The physical examination provides important information about substance use and its medical manifestations. Physical findings of interest include cutaneous abscesses and track marks of intravenous drug abuse, nasal lesions from cocaine abuse, peripheral neuropathy from alcohol use or solvent inhalation, and signs of liver disease from alcoholic or infectious hepatitis. Intravenous drug use should be suspected in any patient who is seropositive for hepatitis B or human immunodeficiency virus (HIV) or who presents with signs and symptoms of acquired immunodeficiency syndrome (AIDS). Substance-use disorders should be considered in all patients who present with accidents or signs of repeated trauma, especially to the head (Skinner et al, 1984).

The physical examination of the severe alcoholic is often marked by telangiectasis of the facial region, facial edema, and parotid gland enlargement. Other aspects of the physical examination that may be pertinent include signs of cirrhosis of the liver, cardiomyopathy, peripheral neuropathy, myopathy, cerebellar dysfunction, and physical signs and symptoms associated with vitamin deficiency, most notably that of thiamine and folate.

In addition to the physical examination, a complete mental status examination should be performed, including tests of memory, concentration, abstract reasoning, affect, mood, and form and content of thought (see Chapter 1).

The effects of alcohol on the central nervous system are dose related and derived from inhibition of the brain stem reticular activating system. As the concentration of alcohol rises in the blood, there is progressive depression of cortical functioning causing drowsiness, incoordination, slurred speech, irritability, and at severely toxic levels stupor, coma, and death. Because tolerance develops to the central nervous system effects of alcohol, some severely addicted individuals can consume large amounts of alcohol without becoming "intoxicated."

Laboratory Testing

Laboratory abnormalities associated with alcoholism are diverse and may be related to end organ damage, vitamin deficiencies, and generalized malnutrition. Abnormalities on hematologic screening including leukopenia, macrocytic anemia, target cells, thrombocytopenia (due to folate deficiency), and evidence of liver disease, and bone marrow suppression. In patients with poor protein intake and liver disease, the blood urea nitrogen level will often be less than 10 mg/dL. Gammaglutamyl transpeptidase (GTT) is considered to be the most sensitive of the laboratory tests in detecting alcoholism but it is nevertheless relatively nonspecific.

Serum and urine toxicologic screens have an important role in assessing and treating patients with substance-use disorders. However, it is important that such tests be properly conducted and that the results be properly interpreted. Informed consent should be obtained for all drug testing. As with all laboratory tests, both false–positive and false–negative results may be obtained; results may be affected by the methods of sample collection and the accuracy of the laboratory (Hansen et al, 1985). To minimize collection errors, all samples for toxicologic analysis should be obtained under direct observation. Both serum and urine samples should be obtained, as substances may be differentially distributed in body fluids. Positive test results should be confirmed by a second test on the same sample using a different analytic method, as closely related compounds in foods or medications may mimic illicit drugs in some drug analyses (for example, eating poppy-seed bagels has been reported to yield a positive urine test for opioids). A positive toxicologic screen may indicate past exposure to a psychoactive substance, but it may not indicate the extent of the exposure, when the exposure occurred, or whether there was behavioral impairment as a result of the exposure. Details regarding laboratory screening for substance use have been discussed in detail elsewhere (Swift, Griffiths, and Camara, 1991).

Abnormal values on diagnostic laboratory testing are widely used to diagnose substance-use disorders, but they are not absolutely reliable or specific. No single laboratory test has been found to discriminate substance users from nonusers. In heavy users of alcohol, laboratory tests such as mean corpuscular volume (MCV) and liver function tests such as aspartate aminotransferase (SGOT) and gamma-glutamyl transferase (GGT) may be abnormal in a high percentage of patients; however, a significant number of heavy drinkers may have normal test values. Opioid users may have abnormal liver function tests and positive serology for hepatitis B or HIV.

Fetal Alcohol Syndrome

Heavy maternal alcohol intake has adverse consequences on the fetus and infant and this disorder is now well defined as the fetal alcohol syndrome. Affected infants are relatively small in length in comparison with weight and most fall below the third percentile for head circumference. They are also notable by the presence of palpebral fissures and epicanthal folds, maxillary hypoplasia, thin vermillion of the upper lip, micrognathia, cleft palate, dislocation of the hips, flexion deformities of the fingers, limited range of motion of other joints, cardiac anomalies (usually septal defects), abnormal external genitalia, and capillary hemangiomata. Infants with this syndrome demonstrate poor sucking and sleeping behavior and are often irritable, hyperactive, and tremulous (Victor and Adams, 1983). Evidence also suggests these infants will have learning disabilities and are prone to a variety of behavioral abnormalities in later childhood.

TREATMENT

General Considerations

To provide optimal treatment of substance use and dependence, the physician must know about therapies for the acute management of intoxicated or withdrawing patients and about options for long-term treatment and rehabilitation. A treatment plan should be practical, economical, and based upon sound principles. The physician's initial task is to establish an effective therapeutic relationship. In the context of this relationship, the physician should engage the patient and if possible the family in short-term and long-term treatment.

There are five objectives of short-term treatment:

1. Relieving subjective symptoms of distress and discomfort due to intoxication or withdrawal;
2. Preventing and/or treating serious complications of intoxication, withdrawal, or dependence;
3. Establishing a drug- or alcohol-free state;

4. Preparing for and referral to longer-term treatment or rehabilitation; and

5. Engaging the family in the treatment process.

The objective of longer-term treatment or rehabilitation is to maintain the alcohol- or drug-free state through ongoing psychological, family, and vocational interventions. Long-term treatment should involve behavioral and psychological interventions to maintain abstinence. Changes in lifestyle, work, or friendships may be necessary to decrease the availability of drugs and to reduce the peer pressure to use drugs. Halfway houses, therapeutic communities, and other residential treatment situations may be useful. Individual and group psychotherapy can help the patient understand the role the drug plays in his or her life, can improve the patient's self-esteem, and can provide alternative methods of relieving psychosocial distress. Treatment of underlying psychiatric or medical illness may reduce the impetus for self-medication. Self-help groups such as Alcoholics Anonymous and Narcotics Anonymous provide education, emotional support, and hope to substance users and their families.

Alcohol Intoxication and Withdrawal: Acute Medical Treatment

Patients presenting for alcohol treatment may show various types of impairment. Many alcoholics have profound social and financial problems that the health-care system is ill-equipped to handle. Particularly frustrating to both physician and patient is an alcoholic with profound social needs who does not require medical treatment or who refuses medical treatment. In this case, referral to social agencies may help the patient, but in many instances no assistance can be obtained.

Acute *alcohol intoxication* results in behaviors ranging from coma to a hyperactive state with affective lability. Ingesting large amounts of alcohol may be fatal. Treatment of alcohol intoxication is essentially supportive and consists of maintaining physiologic homeostasis by supporting vital functions.

Alcohol withdrawal is characterized by tremulousness (the "shakes") and may appear between drinks but is usually most severe after overnight abstinence. Patients may awake with a flushed facies, nausea, anxiety, and tremor, which is relieved by a morning drink eye-opener. The tremor can become severe if alcohol intake is delayed for 12 hours or more. The overt physical tremor is also accompanied by a feeling of internal shakes. The subjective sense of inner shakes may persist for a week or more although the patient's visible tremor will subside within 24 to 48 hours.

Alcohol withdrawal delirium (the DTs) occurs in about 5% of alcoholics (those who are medically untreated for withdrawal) and this syndrome occurs within 3 to 10 days of abstinence. Alcohol withdrawal delirium is characterized by agitation, disorientation, confusion, hallucinations, fever, and hyperactivity of the autonomic nervous system (tachycardia and hypertension). Historically, alcohol withdrawal delirium has been associated with a mortality rate of 5 to 15% (Rogers and Hardison, 1992, p 1840).

Patients presenting with *alcohol withdrawal syndrome* require evaluation of the severity of their withdrawal; they may require behavioral or pharmacologic intervention. The withdrawal syndrome is a complex physiologic process resulting from *increased neuronal activity* in the central and peripheral nervous systems. The consequences of this process may be minimal or may include autonomic hyperactivity seizures, and alcohol withdrawal delirium (Gross, Lewis, and Hastey, 1974). The severity of withdrawal depends on the amount and length of alcohol exposure, the presence of medical complications, and the patient's psychological state. In addition, chronic alcohol ingestion is associated with poor nutrition, poor hygiene, and general debilitation. Current data suggest that less than 5% of patients undergoing detoxification develop severe withdrawal delirium, with a mortality of 1 to 2%.

Physical dependence on alcohol is due to compensatory central nervous system changes that occur in response to a chronically administered depressant substance (ethanol). Historically, the signs and symptoms of the withdrawal syndrome have been reduced by administration of over 100 different pharmacologic agents, including chloral hydrate and similar derivatives, paraldehyde, barbiturates, antihistamines, neuroleptics, antidepressants, lithium, adrenergic blocking agents, and benzodiazepines (Sellers et al, 1983; Sullivan and Sellers, 1986; Liskow and Goodwin, 1987). Today, benzodiazepine derivatives are the treatment of choice, and their efficacy is well established by double-blind controlled studies (Sellers et al, 1983). Benzodiazepines are minimally toxic and have intrinsic anticonvulsant activity.

Thiamine should be administered to all alcohol users as soon as possible (*before* the administration of glucose) to prevent the development of Wernicke's encephalopathy, which is characterized by ataxia, nystagmus, ophthalmoplegia, and mental status changes. The encephalopathic symptoms tend to improve with thiamine repletion. Magnesium and other electrolyte levels should be obtained and deficits replaced. Specific details of detoxification are discussed in Chapter 19.

Recent studies indicate that many alcohol-dependent patients may not require drug-assisted detoxification. Social setting detoxification, a nondrug method, is used with excellent results by many alcohol-treatment facilities. This method, which includes intensive peer and group support in a nonmedical environment, is effective in reducing withdrawal signs and symptoms with no increased incidence of medical complications. Questions have been raised about the possible bias in selecting healthier patients for detoxification in these settings, but Shaw et al (1981) demonstrated that even within a medical setting a significant number of patients respond to supportive care and do not require pharmacologic intervention.

There is an association between alcoholism and anxiety and mood disorders (Von Knorring et al, 1983). Often, mood disturbances are directly related to alcohol and may resolve within 2 or 3 weeks after detoxification. Affective symptoms persisting beyond this time should be treated with antidepressants or electroconvulsive therapy; benzodiazepines or other dependence-producing agents should not be used chronically in patients with alcoholism. In patients with severe mood symptoms or patients previously known to have mood disorders, antidepressant treatment may need to be started during detoxification. For patients who have chronic anxiety (generalized anxiety disorder—see Chapter 8), buspirone (Buspar) should be considered, as this anxiolytic agent is not habit-forming and has no abuse potential.

The Role of the Family in Treatment

Most patients presenting for treatment do so in the context of a family structure that is also dysfunctional. Therefore, *substance dependence should always be considered a disorder involving the entire family*. While family influences may motivate an individual to seek treatment for substance use, more often family members "enable" or facilitate the patient's substance use and may or may not be aware of their contribution to the perpetuation of the identified patient's problem. Substance use by one or more family members may maintain a pathological equilibrium in the family; eliminating the substance use may lead to interpersonal conflicts and loss of family integrity. Therefore, it is important for the physician to be aware of family dynamics and family dysfunction and to recognize the denial, defensiveness, and hostility—as well as the strengths—that may be present in family members.

Spouses and children may experience considerable physical or emotional abuse due to the substance use within the family. The physician should try to involve family members in the patient's treatment as much as possible and should recommend psychological or substance-abuse treatment for other family members when appropriate. Self-help organizations such as Al-Anon, Narc-Anon, Alateen, and groups of adult children of alcoholics (ACOA) may provide valuable emotional support and education for family members. Therapy for the family is as essential as individual treatment for the identified patient.

Confronting the Patient and Family: The Initial Intervention

Effectively confronting patients with their alcohol or drug problem and then getting them into treatment requires special skills and techniques. Some authorities argue that presenting the substance-use problem to the patient and family as a *disease* is most effective. In this model, the patient is told that the use of alcohol or drugs represents a serious threat to his or her health and well-being; the evidence (historical or medical data) is pointed out in an objective and nonjudgmental manner. The physician should emphasize the effects that the alcohol or substance use has had on the patient's health, behavior, or family and should *not* focus on the amount consumed. (The physician should be prepared for denials, excuses, and promises to stop.)

Alcoholism or substance use may be explained as an *addictive disease* with a *genetic basis;* the physician can explain that the alcohol or drug has affected the brain and central nervous system to the extent that the patient can no longer control his or her intake and may have lost sight of the negative effects it is having. Blame for the disease should be placed on the alcohol or drug, *not* on the patient. Lecturing, cajoling, and threatening rarely work and may only heighten the patient's defensiveness, denial, and evasiveness. Most alcoholics or drug abusers have built up a pattern of denial to protect their habit or use denial to avoid embarrassment, shame, guilt, and humiliation. Efforts by the physician to frighten patients into treatment are not usually successful in the long run.

Blaming the alcohol or drug avoids making patients defensive, but the physician should point out that even though the disease may not be the patients' fault, now that they have been advised of the illness, getting effective treatment for managing the illness *is* their responsibility. If this type of presentation is not effective in getting the patient to agree to treatment, then consultation with a specially trained mental health alcohol/addictive disorder specialist is recommended. Even if patients tacitly agree to treatment, the physician should be careful to follow up to see if the recommendations have been followed. The physician should have handy the name and telephone number of a referral for the patient to call; a decision will have to be made as to whether the patient needs initial inpatient treatment. As noted above, it is critical that the family should be involved in this process as well. Alcoholics Anonymous (AA) is a valuable resource for consultations and referral; members of AA will usually visit the prospective patient if the patient initiates the call.

Alcoholism is a family disease: families develop rigid systems of denial to cope with the drinking and maintain the family's equilibrium. The spouse often plays a *codependent* role by enabling the patient to drink, collaborating in the system of denial, and "rescuing" the patient in times of distress. Alcoholism may be the *family secret*, which the family feels would be socially humiliating and embarrassing to acknowledge. *Hence, effective intervention means working with the entire family, not just confronting the alcoholic.* This usually requires careful assessment, planning, and preparation by skilled professionals with a special interest in treating alcoholics and other patients with addictive disorders. The best strategy is to confer with a psychiatrist or other mental-health professional with a special expertise in alcoholism or addiction before direct confrontation, or when an alcohol or substance-abuse problem is suspected. The physician and specialist can then plan a coordinated intervention with clear plans for follow-through and long-term followup.

Long-Term Treatment

The goal of long-term treatment is to maintain abstinence through a comprehensive treatment program that includes psychological, family, and social interventions.

AA is an independent organization founded by a physician alcoholic in 1939. Its only goal is to help individuals maintain total abstinence from alcohol and other addictive substances through group and individual interactions between alcoholics in various stages of recovery. While there is little objective outcome data on the efficacy of self-help groups (Emrick, 1974), they are useful for many individuals. Often, AA groups meet at hospitals, and psychiatric or medical inpatients may easily attend meetings.

Family involvement is extremely important in alcohol treatment. Alcohol use causes many family problems due to the financial and emotional stress the drinking creates. Yet alcoholic family structures often develop a pathological equilibrium that may encourage or maintain alcohol-related behaviors. Spouses and children in alcoholic families adapt to a family member's drinking with their own "wet behaviors." Educating and counseling family members about their role(s) in the patient's alcohol use and treatment is important in avoiding enabling and denial. Often, emotional distress, psychopathology, or substance use by other family members must be treated as well. Valuable emotional support and education for spouses and children may be provided by self-help organizations such as Al-Anon, Alateen, and ACOA (adult children of alcoholics) groups.

Drugs to Reduce Alcohol Consumption/ Pharmacological Prophylaxis

Disulfiram (Antabuse) inhibits the enzyme acetaldehyde dehydrogenase and is used as an adjunctive treatment in selected alcoholics. If alcohol is consumed in the presence of this drug, the toxic metabolite acetaldehyde accumulates, producing tachycardia, skin flushing, dyspnea, nausea, and vomiting. This unpleasant reaction provides a deterrent to the consumption of alcohol (Keventus and Major, 1979). Recently, however, several professional groups have questioned whether disulfiram's toxicity justifies its therapeutic use under any circumstances.

Patients taking disulfiram must be informed about the dangers of even small amounts of alcohol. Alcohol present in foods, shaving lotion, mouthwashes, or over-the-counter medications may produce a disulfiram reaction. The usual dose of disulfiram is 250 to 500 mg once daily. Disulfiram may interact with other medications, notably anticoagulants and phenytoin. It is contraindicated in patients with liver disease.

Naltrexone (Trexan) is a mu-opioid receptor antagonist that *has* been used clinically to treat opioid dependence. Two recent double-blind controlled clinical trials with naltrexone in abstinent alcoholics found that naltrexone-treated subjects had more days of alcohol abstinence, lower rates of relapse to heavy drinking, consumed fewer drinks per drinking day, and had lower dropout than did the placebo group (Volpicelli et al, 1992; O'Malley et al, 1992). Naltrexone treatment had few side effects and was well tolerated by patients. Although the use of naltrexone to treat alcoholism should be considered experimental, the results appear quite promising.

Antidepressants such as imipramine and amitriptyline have been reported effective in reducing alcohol consumption, via an unknown mechanism. Recent studies with serotonin reuptake blocker antidepressants such as fluoxetine and sertraline show the efficacy of these agents in reducing alcohol use in nondepressed heavy drinkers. In several studies, lithium carbonate has also been found to reduce alcohol consumption and to block the intoxicating effects of alcohol but should not be considered a primary treatment intervention.

AMPHETAMINES AND RELATED SUBSTANCES

The amphetamines are a group of drugs structurally related to the catecholamine neurotransmitters norepinephrine, epinephrine, and dopamine. The amphetamines release endogenous catecholamines from nerve endings and are catecholamine agonists at receptors in the peripheral autonomic and central nervous systems. Intoxication with stimulants such as amphetamines, methylphenidate, or other sympathomimetics may produce a clinical picture similar to cocaine intoxication, including sympathetic and behavioral hyperactivity. "Amphetamine psychosis" with manifestations of agitation, paranoia, delusions, and hallucinosis may follow chronic use of these drugs (Ellinwood, 1969), and paranoid states can persist even after detoxification. Antipsychotic medications such as haloperidol are useful in the treatment of stimulant psychoses; however, such patients often require psychiatric hospitalization. Severe hypertension is seen in overdose and may be treated with alpha-adrenergic blockade.

Chronic amphetamine users engage in a pattern of use similar to that of chronic cocaine users: they take escalating doses for a period of several days, then abstain from the drug. Paranoid psychosis diagnostically similar to schizophrenia may occur with chronic use and may persist for some days after cessation of stimulant use. A withdrawal syndrome with physiologic dysfunction does not follow abstinence from amphetamines; however, marked dysphoria, fatigue, and restlessness may occur. Because stimulant users may also suffer from underlying psychiatric illnesses such as affective disorders, a comprehensive psychiatric evaluation is necessary for all patients.

The use of over-the-counter sympathomimetic amines such as ephedrine and phenylpropanolamine as stimulants has increased dramatically in the past decade (Dietz, 1981). These medications are often sold as appetite suppressants, decongestants, or bronchodilators. Signs of intoxication are similar to those for amphetamines, although there tends to be less central nervous system stimulation and greater autonomic effects. Hypertensive crises have resulted from the use of these drugs.

CAFFEINE

Caffeine and the related methylxanthines, theophylline and theobromine, are ubiquitous drugs in our society. More than 80% of the population consumes these agents in coffee, tea, cola, and other carbonated drinks (Dews, 1982). Caffeine is present in chocolate and in a variety of prescription and over-the-counter medications, including stimulants (No-Doz), appetite suppressants (Dexatrim), analgesics (Anacin, APC tablets), and cold and sinus preparations (Dristan, Contac).

Methylxanthines produce physiologic effects through actions at the cellular level. They produce cardiac stimulation, diuresis, bronchodilation, and central nervous system stimulation through several mechanisms. They inhibit the enzyme cyclic AMP phosphodiesterase and increase intracellular levels of this second messenger, thereby augmenting the action of many hormones and neurotransmitters, such as norepinephrine. They also may have a direct stimulatory effect on nerve endings.

Central nervous system effects of caffeine include psychomotor stimulation, increased attention and concentration, and suppression of the need for sleep. Even at low or moderate doses, caffeine can exacerbate the symptoms of anxiety disorders and may increase requirements for neuroleptic or sedative medications (Charney, Henninger, and Jatlow, 1985). At high doses and in sensitive individuals, methylxanthines may produce tolerance and behavioral symptoms of tremor, insomnia, jitteriness, and agitation. Even moderate caffeine users who consume the equivalent of only two cups of coffee per day may develop a significant dependence upon the drug. Abrupt discontinuation of regular caffeine intake resulted in an unpleasant withdrawal syndrome, with headache, lethargy, and irritability (Silverman et al, 1992).

Thus, even low and moderate regular caffeine users to should slowly taper over a period of weeks rather than abruptly stop caffeine.

Treatment of caffeine dependence consists of limiting consumption of caffeine-containing foods, medications, and beverages. In many instances, decaffeinated forms of preferred beverages such as coffee or cola may be substituted. Often, patients are unaware of the extent of their caffeine consumption and of the caffeine content of consumables. They need to be informed about the caffeine content of these substances.

COCAINE

The use of cocaine and "crack" cocaine has undergone an epidemic increase. In 1970, the Haight-Ashbury Clinic reported cocaine use in less than 1% of patients; by 1982, more than 6% were users. Based on the 1985 National Survey of Drug Abuse, 22 million Americans had tried cocaine at least once and 12 million had used it during the preceding year. Along with an increase in use, the manner of cocaine use has changed from intranasal snorting of cocaine powder to smoking or intravenous injection of the more potent form of cocaine, freebase. Freebase cocaine, known as crack, is inexpensive and widely available.

Cocaine is an alkaloid extracted from the leaves of the plant *Erythroxylon coca*, native to South America. It is a local anesthetic that blocks the initiation and propagation of nerve impulses by affecting the sodium conductance of cell membranes. It is a potent sympathomimetic agent that potentiates the actions of catecholamines in the autonomic nervous system, causing tachycardia, hypertension, and vasoconstriction. In addition, cocaine is a central nervous system stimulant, increasing arousal and producing mood elevation and psychomotor activation.

Cocaine intoxication is characterized by elation, euphoria, excitement, pressured speech, restlessness, stereotyped movements, and bruxism. Sympathetic stimulation occurs, including tachycardia, mydriasis, and sweating. Paranoia, suspiciousness, and psychosis may occur with prolonged use. Overdosage produces hyperpyrexia, hyperreflexia, seizures, coma, and respiratory arrest.

Cocaine has a rather short plasma half-life of 1 to 2 hours, which correlates with its behavioral effects (Van Dyke et al, 1978). Along with the decline in plasma levels, most users experience a period of dysphoria known as a *crash*, which often leads to additional cocaine use within a short period. The dysphoria of the crash is intensified and prolonged following repeated use.

Treatment

Optimal treatment for the chronic cocaine user has not been established. While cessation of cocaine use is not followed by a physiologic withdrawal syndrome as severe as that seen with opioids or alcohol, the dysphoria, depression, and drug craving that follow chronic cocaine use are often intense and make abstinence difficult. Psychotherapy, group therapy, and behavior modification have been found to be useful in maintaining abstinence (Rounsaville et al, 1985). Several pharmacologic agents have shown promise as adjunctive treatments. Antidepressants such as imipramine, desipramine, lithium, or trazodone reduce cocaine craving and usage (Rosecan, 1983; Tennant and Rawson, 1983; Gawin and Kleber, 1984). The dopamine agonists bromocriptine and amantadine may block cocaine craving (Dackis and Gold, 1985).

The efficacy of pharmacotherapy for the treatment of cocaine abuse and dependence remains an open question. A statistical analysis of six double-blind studies comparing placebo to desipramine in the treatment of cocaine dependence found that the tricyclic desipramine was no better than placebo in keeping patients in treatment. However, for those who remain in treatment, desipramine is helpful in maintaining abstinence (Levin and Lehman, 1991). Two other recent controlled studies on the use of desipramine in cocaine treatment find no positive effects, except in cocaine patients who are also depressed. A recent review of studies on the pharmacotherapy of cocaine points out that the discrepant results between various cocaine treatment studies may result from poor experimental design and implementation of some of the studies (Meyer, 1992).

Many psychiatric and drug hospitals now offer short-term inpatient treatment of the cocaine user, providing intensive psychological treatment and drug education in a drug-free environment. For recidivists, long-term residential drug-free programs, including therapeutic communities, may be efficacious. Self-help groups such as Narcotics Anonymous may be useful both as a primary treatment modality for cocaine dependence and as an adjunct to other treatment.

Certain psychiatric disorders, such as depression and attention deficit disorder, may be common in cocaine users. Recognizing and treating these underlying disorders may be necessary to stop cocaine use. In addition, many cocaine users also use alcohol or other drugs, particularly sedatives and heroin, and may require treatment for these substances as well.

CANNABIS

Cannabis sativa, also called marijuana, hemp, or "grass," is a plant indigenous to India but now grown worldwide. The leaves, flowers, and seeds of the plant contain many biologically active compounds, the most important of which are the lipophilic cannabinoids, especially δ-9-tetrahydrocannabinol (THC). The biologically active substances are administered by smoking or ingesting dried plant parts (marijuana, bhang, ganja), the resin from the plant (hashish), or extracts of the resin (THC or hash oil). After inhalation or ingestion, THC rapidly enters the central nervous system. It has a biphasic elimination with a short initial half-life (1 to 2 hours), reflecting redistribution and a second half-life of days to weeks. THC is hydroxylated and excreted in bile and urine.

Although it is illegal, a high percentage of the American population has used marijuana. In 1982, 64.1% of young adults (18 to 25) had tried marijuana. Although the use may be declining, millions of individuals continue to use marijuana regularly.

Cannabis intoxication is characterized by tachycardia, muscle relaxation, euphoria, and a sense of well-being. Time sense is altered and emotional lability, particularly inappropriate laughter, may be seen. There is impaired performance on psychomotor tasks, including driving (Klonoff, 1974). Marijuana has antiemetic effects and reduces intraocular pressure; it has been used medically for these effects. Occasionally, with high doses of the drug, depersonalization, paranoia, and anxiety reactions occur. Although tolerance to the effects of cannabis occurs with chronic use, cessation of use does not produce significant withdrawal phenomena. Chronic use of cannabis has been associated with an apathetic, amotivational state that improves upon discontinuation of the drug (Gersten, 1980).

Treatment

Treatment of cannabis dependence is similar to treatment of other drug dependencies. As part of the initial assessment, all patients should undergo complete psychiatric and medical examinations. Short-term goals should focus on reducing or stopping cannabis use and on interventions to ensure compliance. Inpatient treatment may be necessary to achieve abstinence. Because many patients with cannabis dependence are adolescents or young adults, involving the family in assessment and treatment is important.

Long-term treatment should involve behavioral and psychological interventions to maintain abstinence. Often, a change in social situation is necessary to decrease drug availability and reduce peer pressure to use drugs. Individual and group psychotherapy may be useful for helping the patient understand the role marijuana plays in his or her life and may improve self-esteem and provide alternate methods of relieving psychosocial distress. Self-help groups such as Narcotics Anonymous can provide group and individual support.

ANABOLIC STEROIDS

The use of anabolic steroids, once predominantly a problem in fanatical athletes, has now become a relatively common problem in adolescents. A recent study found 6.5% of adolescent boys and 1.9% of girls reported using anabolic steroids without a doctor's prescription (DuRant et al, 1993). The use of anabolic steroids is associated with the use of other substances including cocaine, alcohol, injectable drugs, marijuana, and cigarettes.

Medical complications of the use of anabolic steroids include myocardial infarction, stroke, and hepatic disease. Psychiatric symptoms associated with anabolic steroid use include severe depression, psychotic (paranoid) symptoms, aggressive behavior, homicidal impulses, euphoria, irritability, anxiety, racing thoughts, and hyperactivity. In addition to hypomanic symptoms, a syndrome similar to psychotic depression (severe depression, sleep disturbance, suicidal ideation, anorexia, psychomotor retardation, guilt, delusions of reference, and auditory/visual hallucinations) has been described (Pope and Katz, 1988). While most of these symptoms will gradually abate with drug discontinuation, psychiatric management of these drug-induced syndromes is necessary and, even with discontinuation, a withdrawal syndrome has been noted consisting of depression, fatigue, decreased sex drive, insomnia, anorexia, and dissatisfaction with body image (Brower et al, 1990).

The treatment of anabolic steroid dependency should be within the same general model of other addictions with due consideration to the high likelihood of dependency on other drugs as well (particularly in adolescents). Special narcissistic issues regarding body image are often present in certain types of athletes such as body builders and should be considered in the psychotherapy of such individuals.

Hallucinogens

Many drugs may be used for their hallucinogenic or psychotomimetic effects. These include psychedelics such as lysergic acid diethylamide (LSD), mescaline, psilocybin, and dimethyltryptamine (DMT); hallucinogenic amphetamines such as methylenedioxymethamphetamine (MDMA or Ecstasy) and methylenedioxyamphetamine (MDA); and anticholinergics, such as scopolamine. All can cause a state of intoxication characterized by hallucinosis, affective changes, and delusional states.

The mechanism of action of these substances is thought to involve stimulation of central nervous system dopamine or inhibition of serotonin. Recent studies indicate that administration of hallucinogenic amphetamines to animals produces persistent depletions of brain monoamines, which is consistent with a neurotoxic effect of these substances. Human neurotoxicity has not been established.

Hallucinogens are primarily used by young adults on an intermittent basis. Chronic daily use of hallucinogens is uncommon. In 1982, 21.1% of 18- to 25-year-olds reported using hallucinogens sometime during their life, although more recent statistics report a decrease in use.

The differential diagnosis of hallucinogen-induced psychosis includes schizophrenia, bipolar disorder, delusional disorder, and neurologic disorders such as encephalitis and brain tumor and other toxic ingestions. Psychoses, including those that are drug induced, produce an analgesic state, and medical problems such as pain may be obscured.

Treatment of hallucinogen intoxication includes reducing agitation and psychosis, preventing patients from harming themselves or others, and maintaining vital functions. Agitation and psychosis usually respond to verbal reassurance and decreased sensory stimulation, but sometimes require treatment with benzodiazepines or high-potency neuroleptics. Most hallucinogen intoxications are short-lived (several hours), although prolonged drug-induced psychoses may occur, particularly in patients predisposed to psychiatric illness (Bowers and Swigar, 1983). Some patients experience brief recurrences of the psychotomimetic state (flashbacks) after a drug-free interval.

Inhalants

Inhalants are volatile organic compounds that are inhaled for their psychotropic effects. Substances in this class include organic solvents (such as gasoline, toluene, and ethyl ether), fluorocarbons, and volatile nitrates (including nitrous oxide and butyl nitrate). Inhalants are ubiquitous and readily available in most households and worksites. At low doses, inhalants produce mood changes and ataxia; at high doses, they may produce dissociative states and hallucinosis. Dangers of organic solvent use include suffocation and organ damage, especially hepatotoxicity and neurotoxicity in the central and peripheral nervous systems (Watson, 1982). Cardiac arrhythmias and sudden death may occur. Inhaled nitrates may produce hypotension and methemaglobinemia.

The typical inhalant user is an adolescent male. According to the National Household Survey on Drug Abuse, 9.1% of 12- to 17-year-olds and 12.8% of 18- to 25-year-olds have tried an inhalant at least once.

Optimal treatment of the inhalant user is not well established. Since most users are adolescents, treatment must involve the family. Long-term residential treatment may be helpful in the treatment of heavy users.

Nicotine

Nicotine is an alkaloid drug present in the leaves of the tobacco plant *Nicotiana tabacum*. The plant is indigenous to the New World and has been used for centuries by American Indians in ceremonies and as a medicinal herb. Since its discovery by Europeans, tobacco use has spread worldwide; today nicotine is the most prevalent psychoactive drug. More than 50 million Americans smoke cigarettes daily; another 10 million use another form of tobacco. Nicotine addiction and tobacco use are legally sanctioned forms of substance abuse. Tobacco is clearly the most lethal substance in our society, accounting for over 350,000 premature deaths per year, primarily due to cardiovascular disease and cancer. Since the publication of the Surgeon General's Report on Smoking and Health in 1964, there has fortunately been a gradual decline in the percentage of Americans who smoke. Most of this decline has occurred in men. The numbers of young women who smoke, and the use of other tobacco products such as smokeless tobacco, has increased. Tobacco companies continue their unscrupulous practice of marketing tobacco as either a chic or macho lifestyle-enhancing product; much of their advertising is directed toward young people, from whom most nicotine addicts are recruited.

To maximize the absorption of nicotine, tobacco products are usually smoked in pipes, cigars, or cigarettes or are instilled intranasally or intraorally as snuff or smokeless tobacco. Following absorption from the lungs or buccal mucosa, nicotine levels peak rapidly and then decline, with a half-life of 30 to 60 minutes.

Nicotine has several effects on the peripheral autonomic and central nervous systems. It is an agonist at "nicotinic" cholinergic receptor sites and stimulates autonomic ganglia in the parasympathetic and sympathetic nervous systems, producing salivation, increased gastric motility and acid secretion, and increased catecholamine release. In the central nervous system, nicotine acts as a mild psychomotor stimulant, producing increased alertness, increased attention and concentration, and appetite suppression. The fact that tobacco use can prevent weight gain makes the drug attractive, particularly to young women.

Repeated use of nicotine produces tolerance and dependence. The degree of dependence is considerable: more than 70% of those who quit relapse within a year. Quitting nicotine use produces a withdrawal syndrome characterized by increased irritability, decreased attention and concentration, and an intense craving for and preoccupation with nicotine. Often, there is increased appetite and food consumption and a significant weight gain. Withdrawal symptoms may begin within several hours of cessation and typically last about a week. Craving and weight gain may persist for weeks, however.

The morbidity and mortality resulting from use of nicotine are extensive and include an increase in cardiovascular and respiratory disease and in cancers, particularly of the lung and oropharynx. Many of the deleterious effects of tobacco are due not to nicotine but to other toxic and carcinogenic compounds present in tobacco extract or smoke.

The treatment of the nicotine-dependent patient should follow the principles of treatment common to all psychoactive substances. Short-term goals should consist of reducing and/or quitting tobacco use. Few patients can reduce tobacco use on their own, and a supportive, encouraging relationship of a physician and/or the use of a smoking cessation program is usually necessary to ensure success (Greene, Goldberg, and Ockene, 1988).

Pharmacologic therapy with nicotine gum and absorptive patches has been shown to be safe and at least partially efficacious in the treatment of tobacco dependence. The gum is a sweet, flavored resin containing 2 mg of nicotine, which is released slowly when chewed. The patient chews the gum whenever he or she feels the need, and its use is gradually decreased over time. Proper use of the gum can reduce the craving for tobacco and can decrease the discomfort of withdrawal symptoms (Jarvik et al, 1984; Schneider et al, 1984)). Recently, the alpha$_2$-receptor agonist clonidine has also been reported as partially efficacious in reducing nicotine withdrawal symptoms (Glassman, Stetner, Walsh et al, 1988). The most successful treatment of nicotine dependence combines pharmacologic and behavioral therapies. A detailed discussion of the medical and behavioral treatment of nicotine dependence is found in Chapter 24 of this text.

Opioids

Opioid abuse and dependence remains a significant sociologic and medical problem in the United States, with an estimated 500,000 opioid addicts. These patients are frequent users of medical and surgical services because of the multiple medical sequelae of intravenous drug use and its associated lifestyle. Intravenous opioid users now are the second largest group of persons with AIDS.

The physiologic effects of opiates are due to stimulation of receptors for endogenous hormones, enkephalins, endorphins, and dynorphins. There are at least five distinct opioid receptors, which are designated by the Greek letters mu, kappa, sigma, delta, and epsilon (Jaffe and Martin, 1985). Morphine, heroin, and methadone act primarily through mu-receptors and produce analgesia, euphoria, and respiratory depression. Drugs that appear to be mediated through the kappa-receptor include the so-called mixed agonist-antagonists, butorphanol and pentazocine, which produce analgesia but less respiratory depression. The sigma-receptor appears similar to the receptor for the hallucinogen phencyclidine. The delta-receptor binds endogenous opioid peptides. At high doses, opioid drugs lose their receptor specificity and have agonist or antagonist properties at multiple receptor subtypes.

Treatment

Opioid overdose, a life-threatening emergency, should be suspected in any patient who presents with coma and respiratory suppression. Treatment of suspected overdose includes emergency support of respiration and cardiovascular functions. Parenteral administration of the opioid antagonist naloxone 0.4 to 0.8 mg rapidly reverses coma and respiratory suppression but does not affect depression caused by other sedatives, such as alcohol or barbiturates. Naloxone can precipitate opioid withdrawal, causing the patient whose life has just been saved to be extremely ungrateful.

The opioid withdrawal syndrome is unpleasant but not life-threatening. It is characterized by increased sympathetic nervous system activity, coupled with gastrointestinal symptoms of nausea, vomiting, cramps, and diarrhea. Patients may also report myalgias and arthralgias. There is increased restlessness, increased anxiety, insomnia, and an intense craving for opioids. Treatment for withdrawal consists of minimizing signs and symptoms.

Opioid detoxification is performed by readministering an opioid until withdrawal symptoms cease, then gradually decreasing the dose of opioid over a period of up to 21 days, as specified by federal law (Fultz and Senay, 1975). Although any opioid could be used for detoxification, methadone is most often used due to its long half-life and once-daily oral administration. Initially, patients should be given 10 to 20 mg methadone orally every 2 to 4 hours until withdrawal symptoms are suppressed. The total initial dose is typically 20 to 40 mg for heroin addicts. This dose is then tapered over time.

The alpha$_2$-adrenergic agonist clonidine hydrochloride may also be used to suppress many of the signs and symptoms of opioid withdrawal. Clonidine acts at presynaptic noradrenergic nerve endings in the locus ceruleus of the brain and blocks the adrenergic discharge produced by opioid withdrawal (Aghajanian, 1975; Gold et al, 1979). Clonidine suppresses about 75% of opioid withdrawal signs and symptoms, especially autonomic hyperactivity, anxiety, and gastrointestinal symptoms (Gold et al, 1980; Charney et al, 1981; Washton and Resnick, 1981). Withdrawal symptoms that are not significantly ameliorated by clonidine include drug craving, insomnia, and arthralgias and myalgias. Insomnia may be treated with a short-acting hypnotic such as chloral hydrate, and pain may respond to nonnarcotic analgesics such as ibuprofen or acetaminophen. Clonidine may cause dry mouth, sedation, and orthostatic hypotension. It should be used cautiously in hypotensive patients and those receiving antihypertensives, antidepressants, or antipsychotics (see Chapter 19, Table 19-10).

Methadone Maintenance

Since its introduction in 1965, methadone maintenance has become a major modality of long-term treatment of opioid abuse and dependence (Dole and Nyswander, 1965). Currently, about 100,000 Americans are maintained on methadone. The demand for treatment exceeds the availability, and many programs have long waiting lists, often up to several months. However, a physician can apply to the Drug Enforcement Administration to maintain a patient on methadone outside of an established methadone program.

In a typical methadone program, patients receive a daily dose of oral methadone, coupled with behavioral and psychological therapy. Periodic toxicologic analysis of urine is done to ensure compliance. Patients may receive methadone for various periods of time, often for years.

A recent survey of 172 methadone maintenance programs about treatment practices found wide variations in length of time in treatment and wide differences in upper limits of methadone dosage among the programs (D'Aunno and Vaughn, 1992). Many methadone programs set limits on the highest dose of methadone that could be received and encouraged short periods of methadone maintenance. The authors point out that these practices are in contrast with the evidence on the effectiveness of methadone: the longer clients remain in treatment, the more likely they are to remain abstinent from illicit drugs; treatment with higher doses of methadone is more likely to retain clients in treatment.

Methadone maintenance is clearly effective in reducing illicit drug use and criminality and in improving the social and psychological health of many heroin users. Several theories explain the efficacy of methadone maintenance, including decreasing illicit opioid use by increasing tolerance, treating an endorphin deficiency, and inducing addicts to enter a structured, rehabilitation-oriented treatment.

If hospitalized in a psychiatric or medical facility, patients on a methadone maintenance program can continue to have their daily dose of methadone in the hospital. However, it is important for the physician to keep in touch with the methadone program. If analgesia is needed, patients should receive additional opioids, such as meperidine or oxycodone. This differentiates between the use of opioids for analgesia and for maintenance and does not change the dose of methadone.

Buprenorphine is a semisynthetic opioid used medically as a pain reliever, usually after surgery. Because of its long duration of action, lack of side effects, and relatively mild withdrawal upon cessation of use, buprenorphine maintenance has been proposed as a substitute for methadone maintenance and for the treatment of opioid withdrawal. A recent study comparing buprenorphine with methadone for the treatment of chronic opioid dependence found that buprenorphine at a dose of 8 mg per day is as effective as methadone at a dose of 60 mg per day in preventing withdrawal, retaining clients in treatment, and reducing illicit drug use (Johnson et al, 1992). Several larger-scale clinical trials with buprenorphine in opioid addicts are currently under way.

Opioid Antagonist Therapy

Detoxified opioid users may benefit from opioid antagonist therapy with naltrexone (Trexan R). Naltrexone is a long-acting orally active opioid antagonist that when taken regularly entirely blocks mu-opioid receptors, thus blocking the opioids' euphoric, analgesic, and sedative properties (Resnick et al, 1980). Naltrexone is given either in a daily dose of 50 mg or three times weekly at doses of 100 mg, 100 mg, and 150 mg. The drug appears to be most effective in motivated individuals with good social support and appears less helpful for heroin addicts. Although naltrexone may be prescribed by any physician, it is most effective as part of a comprehensive rehabilitation plan.

Drug-Free Treatment

Drug-free treatment modalities are also useful in treating the opioid abuser (Bale et al, 1984). Such programs emphasize total abstinence from opioids, alcohol, and other drugs, as well as social and psychological rehabilitation. Programs differ widely in their intensity and their theoretical orientation. Therapeutic community programs usually require a long-term treatment commitment of at least several months, during which the addict is taken out of his or her usual environment and involved in intensive psychological and behavioral individual and group therapy. Long-term residential treatment may be most useful for the chronic opioid abuser who requires a change in lifestyle.

Self-help groups such as Narcotics Anonymous (NA) may be useful either as a primary treatment modality for opioid dependence or as an adjunct to other treatment. NA, like AA, uses the 12-step philosophy and stresses total abstinence. Because NA groups often have their own orientations, patients should be encouraged to visit several groups to increase the chances that they will find a group in which they feel comfortable.

Phencyclidine and Related Substances

Phencyclidine (PCP) and similarly acting arylcyclohexylamines, such as ketamine, are used as anesthetics in veterinary medicine and in pediatrics (ketamine). Their mechanism of action is not well understood, although recently this class of drugs has been shown to bind to the so-called sigma opioid receptor in the brain.

PCP intoxication has several definitive features. The agents produce an amnesic, euphoric, hallucinatory state, although the effects may be unpredictable and a prolonged, agitated psychosis with impulsive violence directed at self or others may occur (Petersen and Stillman, 1979; Walker et al, 1981). Vertical and horizontal nystagmus, myoclonus, ataxia, and autonomic instability are common.

As with the hallucinogens, treatment of PCP or similarly acting arylcyclohexylamine intoxication includes supportive measures to prevent patients from harming themselves or others, to maintain cardiovascular and respiratory functions, and to ameliorate psychotic symptoms. Both haloperidol and benzodiazepines have been described as useful for decreasing agitation and psychosis. Psychiatric hospitalization may be necessary in prolonged psychosis.

Sedatives, Hypnotics, and Anxiolytics

Sedatives are among the most prescribed medications and are routinely used for their anxiolytic and hypnotic effects. However, they are also a major source of drug overdoses and of adverse drug reactions. Medications in this group include barbiturates such as secobarbital, butalbital, and phenobarbital; benzodiazepines such as alprazolam and diazepam; and nonbarbiturate sedative-hypnotics such as chloral derivatives, ethchlorvynol, glutethimide, meprobamate, and methaqualone. A patient who becomes dependent on sedative and anxiolytic medications often obtains them by prescription from physicians who are unaware of the patient's abuse or dependence problem.

The effects of sedative-hypnotic and anxiolytic drugs may be mediated through interactions with the GABA–chloride channel receptor complex. In the case of benzodiazepines, there is a neuronal binding site linked to the GABA receptor in both location and function. Binding of benzodiazepines to nerve cell membranes facilitates binding of GABA to its receptors and augments GABA inhibition of nerve cells (Hunt, 1983). Barbiturates, anticonvulsants, and other sedative-hypnotic drugs also have discrete binding sites closely associated with the chloride channel and affect the transport of chloride and inhibition of neurons (Seeman, 1972).

The assessment of the sedative user begins with the history, which should include drug and alcohol use, psychiatric illness, and medical history. Toxicologic screens may be useful in assessing the type of medications used.

Treatment

Treatment of the sedative abuser occurs in two stages, detoxification and long-term rehabilitation. Pharmacologic detoxification is usually necessary, as the withdrawal syndrome following cessation of drug use may be severe and may include seizures, cardiac arrhythmias, and death. The *pentobarbital challenge test* (Wesson and Smith, 1975; Wikler, 1968) is useful for predicting the need for pharmacologic-assisted detoxification to prevent severe withdrawal in heavy users. Pentobarbital 200 mg is administered orally and the patient is observed 1 hour later. The patient's condition after the test dose will range from no effect to sleep. If the patient develops drowsiness or nystagmus on a 200-mg dose, he or she is not dependent on barbiturates. If 200 mg has no effect, the dose should be repeated hourly until nystagmus or drowsiness develop. The total dose administered approximates the patient's daily sedative habit. The barbiturate dose should be tapered over 10 days, with about a 10% reduction each day.

Flumazenil (Mazicon) is the first benzodiazepine *antagonist* to be approved by the Food and Drug Administration. Flumazenil binds competitively and reversibly to the GABA-benzodiazepine receptor complex and inhibits the effects of benzodiazepine. The drug is approved for the treatment of benzodiazepine overdose and/or for the reversal of benzodiazepine oversedation. Recurrence of sedation may occur within 1 hour if the patient is on a long-acting benzodiazepine such as diazepam. It should be noted, however, that flumazenil may reverse the sedative effects of benzodiazepines but *not* fully reverse their effects on the hypoxic respiratory drive, hence respiration monitoring remains essential even though the patient is more alert. Flumazenil may induce seizures particularly when administered to patients who are prone to seizures or who have epilepsy (Fogel and Stoudemire, 1993).

The anticonvulsant carbamazepine has been shown to be effective for ethanol and sedative detoxification (Klein, Uhde, and Post, 1986; Malcolm, Ballenger, Sturgis et al, 1989). The medication is administered until blood levels are in the range for effective anticonvulsant activity, maintained for up to 2 weeks, and then tapered and discontinued.

Long-term treatment should be customized for each patient and may include residential drug-free programs and self-help groups such as AA or NA. Some patients may be found to have an underlying psychiatric disorder, such as an anxiety disorder or depression. If pharmacologic treatment is deemed necessary, antidepressants or nondependence-producing anxiolytics such as buspirone should be used.

SUMMARY

Substance-use disorders are chronic disorders that involve individuals and their families. Identifying and treating such disorders requires the physician to have several skills, including:

1. Knowledge of the biological, psychological, and social substrates of substance use;
2. The ability to interview patients and their families in taking a substance-use history;
3. Knowledge of acute and long-term treatment modalities for intoxication, dependence, and withdrawal; and
4. Knowledge of professionals and special programs in the community for specialized interventions and treatment.

The treatment process involves identifying the problem, making the patient and family aware of the problem, and motivating them to seek help. The process is best conducted in the context of a supportive, empathic, and ongoing physician–patient relationship.

CLINICAL PEARLS

- In diagnosing alcoholism, fully expect the patient and family to deny that a problem exists.
- Alcoholism is a family disease. Usually the entire family uses denial to cope with the alcoholic behavior and to maintain the family homeostasis. Spouses are often enablers and may deny the problem as much as the patient does. Interview and assess multiple family members in making your assessment.
- Effective intervention with alcoholic and substance-abusing patients is best carried out by specialists in intervention and treatment. Find out who is available as a resource for consultation and referral.
- In diagnosing alcoholism and substance abuse, the amount and frequency of ingestion is not the primary issue. Focus on the behavioral, medical, and social *effects* on the individual and family of whatever amount is ingested.

ANNOTATED BIBLIOGRAPHY

Hollister LE: Clinical Pharmacology of Psychotherapeutic Drugs. New York: Churchill Livingstone, 1978.

A well-written, easy-to-understand book on the actions and uses of psychoactive substances used to treat psychiatric disorders. The book also has excellent introductory chapters on basic clinical pharmacology.

Institute of Medicine: Broadening the Basis of Treatment of Alcoholism. Washington, DC, National Academy Press, 1991

An excellent review of the etiology and treatment of alcoholism with an emphasis on social policy aspects.

Jaffe JE: Drug Addiction and Drug Abuse. In Gilman AG, Goodman LS, Gilman A (eds): The Pharmacological Basis of Therapeutics, 6th ed. New York, Macmillan, 1980 .

> An extremely comprehensive and detailed description of the clinical and behavioral pharmacology of psychoactive substances, with emphasis on chemistry and pharmacology. The bible on drugs for medical students.

Lewis DC, Williams CN (eds): Providing Care for Children of Alcoholics: Clinical and Research Perspectives. Pompano Beach, FL, Heath Communications, 1986

> This short, multiauthored monograph of a conference on children of alcoholics provides an excellent review of theoretical, clinical, and policy issues related to the children and families of alcoholics.

Litten RZ, Allen JP: Pharmacotherapies for alcoholism: promising agents and clinical issues. Alcoholism Clin Exp Res 15(4):620–633, 1991

> Discusses potential pharmacological therapies for alcoholism and their uses and limitations.

Nestler EJ: Molecular mechanisms of drug addiction. J Neuroscience 12(7):2439–2450, 1992

> An excellent review of substance dependence, intoxication, and withdrawal from a neurobiological perspective.

Schultes RE, Hofmann A: The Botany and Chemistry of Hallucinogens, 2nd ed. Springfield, IL, Charles C. Thomas, 1980

> A classic text on the chemistry and human uses of hallucinogens.

Senay E: Methadone maintenance treatment. Int J Addictions 20:803–821, 1985

> An excellent review of the principles and practice of the use of methadone to treat opioid dependence.

Stanton MD: Drugs and the family. Marriage Fam Rev 2:1–10, 1979

> A somewhat dated but useful description of the consequences of psychoactive substance use from the perspective of family functioning.

US Department of Health and Human Services: The health consequences of smoking: Nicotine addiction. A report of the Surgeon General. Washington, DC, DHHS Publication No. CDC 88-8406, 1988

> The controversial Surgeon General's report on smoking has excellent sections on the clinical and behavioral pharmacology of nicotine and presents the thesis that nicotine dependence is an addiction.

West LJ: Alcoholism. Ann Int Med 100:405–416, 1984

> A good recent review of the pathogenesis and treatment of alcohol dependence.

Zinberg NE, Harding WM (eds): Control over intoxicant use: Pharmacological, psychological and social considerations. New York, Human Sciences Press, 1982

> Interesting vignettes in this well-written, somewhat controversial book describe the varieties of psychoactive substance use and the way our society deals with such use.

REFERENCES

Aghajanian GK: Tolerance of locus ceruleus neurons to morphine and inhibition of withdrawal response by clonidine. Nature 276:186–188, 1976

American Psychiatric Association: DSM-IV Draft Criteria 3/1/93. Washington, DC. American Psychiatric Association, 1993

American Psychiatric Association: Diagnostic and statistical manual of mental disorders, 4th ed. Washington, DC: American Psychiatric Association, in press [1994]

Bale RN, Zarcone VP, Van Stone WW et al: Three therapeutic communities: A prospective controlled study of narcotic addiction treatment process and follow-up results. Arch Gen Psychiatry 41:185–191, 1984

Bernadt MW, Taylor C, Mumford J et al: Comparison of questionnaire and laboratory tests in the detection of excessive drinking and alcoholism. Lancet 1:325–328, 1982

Bowers MB, Swigar ME: Vulnerability to psychosis associated with hallucinogen use. Psychiatry Res 9:91–97, 1983

Brower KJ, Eliopulos GA, Blow FC et al: Evidence for physical and psychological dependence on anabolic androgenic steroids in eight weight lifters. Am J Psychiatry 147:510–512, 1990

Charney DS, Henninger GR, Jatlow PI: Increased anxiogenic effects of caffeine in panic disorders. Arch Gen Psychiatry 42:233–243, 1985

Charney DS, Sternberg DE, Kleber HD et al: Clinical use of clonidine in abrupt withdrawal from methadone. Arch Gen Psychiatry 38:1273–1278, 1981

Clark WD: Alcoholism: Blocks to diagnosis and treatment. Am J Med 71:275–285, 1981

Cloninger CR: Neurogenetic adaptive mechanisms in alcoholism. Science 236:410–416, 1987

Costa E, Guidotti A: Molecular mechanisms in the receptor action of benzodiazepines. Annu Rev Pharmacol Toxicol 19:231–245, 1981

Dackis CA, Gold M: Bromocriptine as treatment of cocaine abuse. Lancet 1:1151, 1985

D'Aunno T, Vaughn TE: Variations in methadone treatment practices. J Am Med Assoc 267:253–258, 1992

Dews PB: Caffeine. Annu Rev Nutr 2:323–341, 1982

Dietz AJ: Amphetamine-like reactions to phenylpropanolamine. JAMA 245:601–602, 1981

Dole VP, Nyswander M: A medical treatment for diacetylmorphine (heroin) addiction: Clinical trial with methadone hydrochloride. JAMA 193:646–650, 1965

DuRant RH, Rickert VI, Ashworth CS et al: Use of multiple drugs among adolescents who use anabolic steroids. N Engl J Med 328:922–926, 1993

Ellinwood EH: Amphetamine psychosis: A multidimensional process. Semin Psych 1:208–226, 1969

Emrick C: A review of psychologically oriented treatment of alcoholism. Quart J Stud Alcohol 38:1004–1031, 1974

Ewing JA: Detecting alcoholism: The CAGE questionnaire. JAMA 252:1905–1907, 1984

Fogel BS, Stoudemire A: New Psychotropics in Medically Ill Patients. In Stoudemire A, Fogel BS (eds) Medical-Psychiatric Practice, Vol. 2, pp 69–111, ch. 3. Washington, DC, American Psychiatric Press, 1993

Fultz JM Jr, Senay EC: Guidelines for the management of hospitalized narcotics addicts. Ann Intern Med 82:815–818, 1975

Gawin FH, Kleber HD: Cocaine abuse treatment: Open trial with desipramine and lithium carbonate. Arch Gen Psychiatry 41:903–909, 1984

Gay GR: Clinical management of acute and chronic cocaine poisoning. Ann Emerg Med 11:562–572, 1982

Gersten SP: Long-term adverse effects of brief marihuana usage. J Clin Psychiatry 41:60, 1980

Glassman AH, Helzer JE, Covey LS, Cottler LB et al.: Smoking, smoking cessation, and major depression. J Am Med Assoc 264(12):1546–9, 1990

Glassman AH, Stetner F, Walsh BT et al: Heavy smokers, smoking cessation and clonidine: Results of a double-blind, randomized trial. JAMA 259:2863–2866, 1988

Gold MS, Pottash AC, Sweeney DR et al: Opiate withdrawal using clonidine: A safe, effective and rapid non-opiate treatment. JAMA 234:343–346, 1980

Gold MS, Redmond DE Jr, Kleber HD: Noradrenergic hyperactivity in opiate withdrawal suppressed by clonidine. Am J Psychiatry 136:100–102, 1979

Greene HL, Goldberg R, Ockene JK: Cigarette smoking: The physician's role in cessation and maintenance. J Gen Int Med 3:75–87, 1988

Goodwin DW: Alcohol in homicide and suicide. Quart J Stud Alcohol 28:517–528, 1967

Goodwin DW: Alcoholics and genetics: The sins of the fathers. Arch Gen Psychiatry 42:171–174, 1985

Gottschalk L, McGuire F, Heiser J et al: Drug Abuse Deaths in Nine Cities: A Survey Report. NIDA Research Monograph #29. Washington, DC: US Government Printing Office, 1979

Gross M, Lewis E, Hastey J: Acute Alcohol Withdrawal Syndrome. In Kissin B, Begleiter H (eds): The Biology of Alcoholism, Vol. 3. New York, Plenum, 1974

Hansen HJ, Caudhill SP, Boone DJ: Crisis in drug testing: Results of the CDC blind study. JAMA 253:2382–2387, 1985

Harvey SC: Hypnotics and Sedatives. In Gilman AG, Goodman LS, Gilman A (eds): The Pharmacological Basis of Therapeutics, 6th ed. New York, Macmillan, 1980

Hoffman PL, Rabe CS, Grant KA et al.: Ethanol and the NMDA receptor. Alcohol 7:229–231, 1990

Holden C: The neglected disease in medical education. Science 229:741–742, 1985

Hunt WA: The effect of ethanol on GABAergic transmission. Neurosci Biobehav Rev 7:87–95, 1983

Jaffe JH, Martin WR: Opioid Analgesics and Antagonists. In Gilman AG, Goodman LS, Rall TW, et al (eds): The Pharmacological Basis of Therapeutics, 7th ed. New York, Macmillan, 1985

Jarvik ME, Schneider NG: Degree of addiction and the effectiveness of nicotine gum therapy for smoking. Am J Psychiatry 141:790–791, 1984

Johnson RE, Jaffe JJ, Fudala PJ: A controlled trial of buprenorphine treatment for opioid dependence. J Am Med Assoc 267:2750–2755, 1992

Kennedy W: Chemical dependency: A treatable disease. Ohio Med 71:77–79, 1985

Keventus J, Major LF: Disulfiram in the treatment of alcoholism. J Stud Alcohol 40:428–446, 1979

Klein E, Uhde T, Post RM: Preliminary evidence for the utility of carbamazepine in alprazolam withdrawal. Am J Psychiatry 143(2):235–236, 1986

Klonoff H: Marihuana and driving in real-life situations. Science 186:317–324, 1974

Kosten TR, Kleber HD: Differential diagnosis of psychiatric comorbidity in substance abusers. J Subst Abuse Treatment, 5:201–206, 1988

Krahn DD: The relationship of eating disorders and substance abuse. J Subst Abuse 3(2):239–253, 1991

Levin FR, Lehman AF: Meta-analysis of desipramine as an adjunct in the treatment of cocaine addiction. J Clin Psychopharmacol 11(6):374–378, 1991

Lewis DC, Gomolin IH: Emergency treatment of drug and alcohol intoxication and withdrawal. Brown University Program in Alcoholism and Drug Abuse Medical Monograph II, 1982

Lewis D, Gordon A: Alcoholism and the general hospital: The Roger Williams intervention program. Bull NY Acad Med 59:181–197, 1983

Liskow BI, Goodwin DW: Pharmacological treatment of alcohol intoxication, withdrawal and dependence: A critical review. J Stud Alcohol 48:356–370, 1987

Litten RZ, Allen JP: Pharmacotherapies for alcoholism: Promising agents and clinical issues. Alcoholism Clin Exp Res 15(4):620–633, 1991

Malcolm R, Ballenger JC, Sturgis ET, Anton R: Double blind controlled trial comparing carbamazepine to oxazepam treatment of alcohol withdrawal. Am J Psychiatry 146(5):617–621, 1989

Martin WR: Naloxone. Ann Intern Med 85:765–768, 1976

McIntosh I: Alcohol-related disabilities in general hospital patients: A critical assessment of the evidence. Int J Addictions 17:609–639, 1982

Meyer RE: New pharmacotherapies for cocaine dependence ... revisited. Arch Gen Psychiatry 49:900–904, 1992

Mirin SM, Weiss RD, Michael J, Griffin ML: Psychopathology in substance abusers: Diagnosis and treatment. J Drug and Alcohol Abuse, 14:139–157, 1988

National Survey on Drug Abuse. Rockville, MD, Institute of Drug Abuse, 1981

O'Malley SS, Jaffe A, Chang G, Schothenfeld RS, Meyer R, Rounsaville B: Naltrexone and coping skills therapy for alcohol dependence: A controlled study. Arch Gen Psychiatry 49:881–887, 1992

Palestine ML, Alatorre E: Control of acute alcoholic withdrawal symptoms: A comparative study of haloperidol and chlordiazepoxide. Curr Ther Res 20:289–299, 1976

Pederson CA, Golden RN, Petitto JM, et al: Neurobiologic Aspects of Behavior. In Stoudemire A (ed): Human Behavior: An Introduction for Medical Students, 2nd ed, Chapter 12. Philadelphia, J B Lippincott, 1994

Petersen RC, Stillman RC (eds): PCP (Phencyclidine) Abuse: An Appraisal. NIDA Research Monograph 21, DHEW. Washington, DC, US Government Printing Office, 1979

Pope HG, Katz DA: Affective and psychotic symptoms associated with anabolic steroid use. Am J Psychiatry 145:487–490, 1988

Porjesz B, Begleiter H: Evoked brain potential deficits in alcoholism and aging. Alcoholism: Clin & Exp Res 6:53–63, 1982

Rappolt RT, Gay GR, Inaba D: Propranolol: A specific antagonist to cocaine. Clin Toxicol 10:265–271, 1977

Regier DA, Boyd JH, Burke JD et al: One-month prevalence of mental disorders in the United States. Arch Gen Psychiatry 45:977–986, 1988

Regier DA, Farmer ME, Rae DS et al. Comorbidity of mental disorders with alcohol and other drug abuse. J Am Med Assoc 264:2511–2518, 1990

Resnick RB, Schuyten-Resnick E, Washton AM: Assessment of narcotic antagonists in the treatment of opioid dependence. Ann Rev Pharmacol Toxicol 20:463–474, 1980

Rice DP, Kelman S, Miller LS: Estimates of economic costs of alcohol and drug abuse and mental illness, 1985 and 1988. Public Health Rep 106(3):280–292, 1991

Rogers CM, Hardison JE: Alcohol: Tolerance, Addiction, and Withdrawal. In Hurst JW (ed): Medicine for the Practicing Physician, 3rd ed, Chapter 25-1, pp 1840–1842. Boston, Butterworth-Heinemann, 1992

Rosecan JS: The Psychopharmacologic Treatment of Cocaine Addiction (abstract). Vienna, Seventh World Congress of Psychiatry, 1983

Rounsaville BJ, Gawin FH, Kleber HD: Interpersonal psychotherapy adapted for ambulatory cocaine users. Am J Drug Alc Abuse 11:171, 1985

Schneider NG, Jarvik ME, Forsythe AB: Nicotine vs. placebo gum in the alleviation of withdrawal during smoking cessation. Addic Behav 9:149–156, 1984

Schuckit MA: Genetics and the risk for alcoholism. JAMA 254:2614–2617, 1985

Schulz DW, Macdonald RL: Barbiturate enhancement of GABA-mediated inhibition and activation of chloride channel conductance: Correlation with anticonvulsant and anesthetic actions. Brain Res 209:177–188, 1981

Seeman P: Membrane effects of anesthetics and tranquilizers. Pharmacol Rev 24:583–655, 1972

Sellers EM, Cooper SD, Zilm DH et al: Lithium treatment during alcoholic withdrawal. Clin Pharm Ther 20:199–206, 1976

Sellers EM, Kalant H: Drug therapy: Alcohol intoxication and withdrawal. N Eng J Med 294:757–752, 1976

Sellers EM, Narango CA, Harrison M et al: Diazepam loading: Simplified treatment for alcohol withdrawal. Clin Pharm Ther 6:822, 1983

Selzer ML: The Michigan alcoholism screening test: The quest for a new diagnostic instrument. Am J Psychiatry 127:1653–1658, 1971

Shaw JM, Kolesar GS, Sellers EM et al: Development of optimal treatment tactics for alcohol withdrawal: Assessment and effectiveness of supportive care. J Clin Psychopharmacol 1:382–387, 1981

Silverman K, Evans SM, Strain EC, Griffiths RR: Withdrawal syndrome after the double-blind cessation of caffeine consumption. N Engl J Med 327(16):1109–1114, 1992

Skinner HA, Holt S, Schuller R et al: Identification of alcohol abuse using laboratory tests and a history of trauma. Ann Intern Med 101:847–851, 1984

Skolnick P, Moncada V, Barker J, Paul SM: Pentobarbital: Dual action to increase brain benzodiazepine receptor affinity. Science 211:1448–1150, 1981

Stoudemire A (ed): Human Behavior: An Introduction for Medical Students, 2nd ed. Philadelphia, J B Lippincott, 1994

Sullivan JJ, Sellers EM: Treating alcohol, barbituate and benzodiazepine withdrawl. Rational Drug Therapy 20:1–8, 1986

Swift RM, Griffiths W, Camara P: Special Technical Considerations in Laboratory Testing for Illicit Drugs. In Stoudemire A, Fogel BS (eds) Medical-Psychiatric Practice, Vol. 1, Chapter 4, pp 145–163. Washington, DC, American Psychiatric Press, 1991

Tennant FS, Rawson RA: Cocaine and Amphetamine Dependence Treated with Desipramine. In Harris L (ed): Problems of Drug Dependence, pp 351–355. NIDA Monograph Series 43. Rockville, MD, National Institute of Drug Abuse, 1983

Thomas M, Halsall S, Peters TJ et al: Role of hepatic acetaldehyde dehydrogenase in alcoholism. Lancet 2:1057, 1982

Van Dyke C, Jatlow P, Ungerer J et al: Oral cocaine: Plasma concentration and central effects. Science 200:211–213, 1978

Victor M, Adams RD: Alcohol. In Petersdorf RG, Adams RD, Braunwald E et al (eds): Harrison's Principles of Internal Medicine, 10th ed, Chapter 42, pp 1285–1295. New York, McGraw-Hill, 1983

Volpicelli JR, Alterman AI, Hayashida M, O'Brien CP: Naltrexone in the treatment of alcohol dependence. Arch Gen Psychiatry 49:876–880, 1992

Von Knorring A, Cloninger CR, Bohman M et al: An adoption study of depressive disorders and substance abuse. Arch Gen Psychiatry 20:943–950, 1983

Walker S, Yesavage JA, Tinklenberg JR: Acute phencyclidine (PCP) intoxication. Quantitative urine levels and clinical management. Am J Psychiatry 138:674–675, 1981

Waller JA, Turkel HW: Alcoholism in traffic deaths. N Engl J Med 275:532–536, 1966

Washton AM, Resnick RB: Clonidine for opiate detoxification: Outpatient clinical trials. J Clin Psychiatry 43:39–41, 1981

Watson JM: Solvent abuse: Presentation and clinical diagnosis. Hum Toxicol 1:249–256, 1982

Wesson DR, Smith DE: A new method for the treatment of barbiturate dependence. JAMA 231:294–295, 1975

Whitfield CL, Thompson G, Lamb A et al: Detoxification of 1024 alcoholic patients without psychoactive drugs. JAMA 239:1409–1410, 1978

Wikler A: Diagnosis and treatment of drug dependence of the barbiturate type. Am J Psychiatr 125:758–765, 1968

Willow M, Johnston GAR: Dual action of pentobarbitone on GABA binding: Role of binding site integrity. J Neurochem 37:1291–1294, 1981

Alan Stoudemire (ed). *Clinical Psychiatry for Medical Students,* Second
Edition. Copyright © 1994, 1990 by J. B. Lippincott Company.

11 *Geriatric Psychiatry*

David Bienenfeld and
Randon Welton

In 1990 approximately 12% of Americans (over 28 million) were over the age of
65. By the turn of the century it is estimated that one in five Americans will be over 55
years of age and 13% will be over 65 years of age. Estimates reaching to the year 2050
place 22% of Americans over the age of 65 and 5% over 85 years of age. The elderly are
also at increased risk for social stressors including retirement, widowhood, and
physical infirmity.

Aging individuals thus bring to their physicians problems that occur in a
multilayered context. The features of clinical syndromes are often different in
older patients, and therapy frequently requires modification. The examination of
geriatric psychopathology and its treatment begins best with a perspective on
normal aging.

AGING AND THE LIFECYCLE

Most early developmental theorists felt that psychological development stopped
at an early age. According to them, the basic psychologic structure formed during
childhood and was refined during adolescence. This structure determined how the
adult would perceive, interpret, and react to internal drives and the external circumstances of life. Erik Erickson proposed that psychological development continued
throughout life in a series of predictable life crises (see Table 11–1). In his outline,
young adulthood is the time when people confront their ability to maintain intimate

Table 11–1 **Erikson's Stages of Human Development**

STAGE	LIFE CRISIS	AGE	DEVELOPMENTAL TASK
I	Basic trust versus basic mistrust	First year	Knowledge that world and self are trustworthy
II	Autonomy versus shame and doubt	1–3 years	Confidence in own physical and mental capacities
III	Initiative versus guilt	4–6 years	Socially appropriate curiosity and strivings
IV	Industry versus inferiority	6–12 years	Healthy competition with peers
V	Identity versus identity diffusion	Adolescence	Self-definition and differentiation from parents
VI	Intimacy versus isolation	Young adulthood	Sexual, emotional, and spiritual maturity and social responsibility
VII	Generativity versus self-absorption	Middle age	Establishment, guiding, and nurturing of subsequent generations
VIII	Integrity versus despair	Late life	Acceptance of mortality and satisfaction with one's meaning in the world

emotional relationships while in the crisis of *intimacy vs. isolation.* Middle-aged adults struggle with *generativity vs. self-absorption,* trying on the one hand to raise and nurture future generations, and on the other to satisfy self-centered goals. Finally, elderly adults have to deal with *integrity vs. despair.* Their struggle is to reevaluate their lives and accept their roles during life and the meaning of their relationships with others. They learn to own responsibility for their actions and to accept the things that might not be pleasant but that cannot be changed. If they cannot do so they are left with the despair of knowing that the unacceptable aspects of their lives cannot be undone (Erikson, 1959).

The range of life stressors confronting the aging individual is broad. Friends and relatives become ill and die, children grow up and move away, retirement is often mandatory, and physical health may fail. To deal with such a wide array of stressors, one must mobilize a multitude of coping strategies. These strategies, known in psychodynamic terminology as "defense mechanisms," are the ways that people process the data from the environment so as to maintain emotional stability. Such mechanisms may include taking control of and mastering a situation, retreating into fantasy in the face of overwhelming stress, or allowing oneself to ask for and receive necessary help. The individual whose earlier life has allowed him or her to adopt many kinds of defense mechanisms is better able to weather these stressors without psychological symptoms than one who has come to use only a narrow range of coping skills. In dealing with the death of a spouse, for example, some degree of denial and retreat into fantasy may be adaptive if elements of mastery and control are also utilized (Bienenfeld, 1990).   .

COGNITION AND AGING

Cognitive functioning can be divided into learning, memory, and intelligence. Age affects each of these areas differently. Learning is the ability to gain new skills and information. The elderly can continue to learn throughout their life; however, it appears that they tend to learn at a slower rate than younger individuals. This slowing becomes particularly evident in verbal learning. The total amount that can be learned is probably unchanged but this learning takes longer.

Memory can be divided into immediate, short- and long-term memory. Immediate memory, such as repeating words within seconds of hearing them, appears to be largely unaffected by healthy aging. Short-term memory—repeating those same words five minutes later—is also largely undiminished in the healthy elderly person. However, short-term memory is related to attention, and aging individuals are more prone to distraction than younger ones.

Long-term memory, in which information is stored for anywhere from minutes to decades, seems to be the area most seriously affected by aging. While the total amount of stored information is probably unchanged, the retrieval of this information appears to be less efficient. The elderly often require more cues to remember learned objects. Frequently patients or family members will comment that the elderly seem to remember distant events quite well but have considerable difficulty with more recent happenings. This phenomenon is probably more apparent than real. The elderly will tend to remember those events that are emotionally charged or in other ways significant. As they have lived longer they are more likely to have experienced these in the more distant past, so they will tend to remember these events preferentially over more recent but less significant events.

The third major component of cognition is intelligence, which can be defined as the ability to use information in an adaptive way or to apply knowledge to specific circumstances. Intelligence can be further divided into crystallized and fluid intelligence. Crystallized intelligence includes areas such as vocabulary, verbal skills, and general information. With proper intellectual stimulation crystallized intelligence can continue to increase throughout life. Fluid intelligence consists of recognizing new patterns and creative problem solving. This form of intelligence tends to peak in adolescence and declines gradually throughout the rest of life. The decline of fluid intelligence leads people to attempt to maintain constancy so as to minimize the necessity for major cognitive or attitudinal adjustments. This effort to maintain constancy is often perceived as intellectual "rigidity" on the part of elders.

Older individuals often complain about cognitive decline, but the correlation of these subjective complaints with objective measures has repeatedly been found to be weak. On the other hand, aging is associated with certain cognitive difficulties that do not pose a substantial interference with daily functioning. These problems include forgetting names, misplacing items, and experiencing difficulty with complex problem solving. This cluster of complaints has been proposed as a nonpathological entity called "aging-associated cognitive decline."

EVALUATION

While much of the psychiatric evaluation of the elderly is similar to any psychiatric evaluation, there are some features of dealing with the geriatric population that require special consideration. The evaluation needs to take place in a private area that is quiet, well lit, and free from distractions. The physician should ensure that he or she will have the time to perform a complete evaluation. Because of the breadth of the evaluation and the slower response time of some elderly patients, it may often last over an hour. The physician must also be flexible enough to conduct the interview in stages if it becomes clear that the patient cannot tolerate an extended interview.

Because geriatric patients are often referred to physicians by family members or other health professionals, collateral information is essential. This information should be obtained in a timely, efficient manner and include facts about the patient's recent functional baseline and any changes in behavior, cognition, or personality. Family members can often detail changes in behavior that are not otherwise available. This history should include known information about the patient's medical and psychiatric history as well as current medications.

Because geriatric patients have had a different exposure to mental health from that of the (usually) younger examining clinicians, it is useful to ask older patients for their ideas about what the psychiatric examination might be like. Where history and experience have bred misperceptions, examiners can correct them and explain that they are medical specialists who deal with emotional difficulties such as those the patient has described. Reassurance of ongoing communication and cooperation with the patient's primary physician is often helpful. The patient's wishes concerning family involvement in the therapy must also be determined early in the evaluation.

To understand current problems in a developmental context, it is beneficial to conduct a historical review. Not only do examiners ask the patient about past psychiatric symptoms, they also inquire about expectable life stressors and transitions, e.g., marriage, departure of children from the home, and retirement. Knowing the types of coping skills mobilized in these transitions allows the clinician to assess the potential coping skills brought by the patient to the current situation.

It is a principle in all of medicine that diagnosis is only the first step in evaluating a patient. Assessment must follow. Knowing that a patient meets criteria for a major depressive episode does not by itself dictate the appropriate therapy. It is further essential to determine the effect that the illness has had on the patient's life and the resources that can be brought to bear in the service of treatment.

Finally, the clinician should present a formulation to the patient for the latter's comment, correction, or endorsement. The clinician recaps the presenting symptoms, the relevant stressors, the social environment that surrounds the patient, and the historical context of the current distress. The physician then presents a clinical opinion of the syndrome diagnosis in terms comprehensible to the patient, as well as a dynamic formulation explaining the relationship of the chief complaint to this individual's past and present. Once there is concurrence with the patient about the target of the therapy and its meaning to the patient, the physician outlines a treatment plan that follows logically from the biopsychosocial formulation that has been shared.

PSYCHIATRIC DISORDERS IN THE ELDERLY

While the diagnostic criteria for adult mental disorders do not rely on age, clinical diagnosis in geriatric psychiatry entails some particular features. The physician who deals with the elderly confronts presentations of common disorders that change over the course of life as well as disorders that increase in incidence with age.

Dementia and Other Cognitive Disorders

Dementia is a common problem among the elderly. An international review confirmed that the rate of dementia increases with increasing age. The prevalence of dementia in the population between ages 60 and 64 was 0.7%. Between ages 70 and 74, it was 2.8%, and reached 10.5% between the ages of 80 and 84. In the very old this rate can be even higher. Among those elderly who were between 90 and 95, 38.6% had a diagnosable dementia (Jorm, Korton, and Henderson, 1987). Although Alzheimer's disease may be the most common single entity causing dementia, it would be a mistake to dismiss all dementia in the elderly as Alzheimer's disease.

A review that looked at nearly 3,000 elderly with dementia (with a mean age of 72.3 years), found that 57% suffered from Alzheimer's disease, 13% from multiinfarct dementia, and 4% from alcoholism. Drug use and depression were also found to be commonly listed as causes of the dementia (Clarfield, 1988). In a study that looked exclusively at individuals who were 85 years of age, 29.8% had diagnosable dementia. Of those with dementia, only 43.5% were felt to be suffering from Alzheimer's disease. Nearly 47% were felt to have their dementia as a result of either multiple cerebral infarcts or diffuse hypoperfusion of the brain. The remaining 10% of cases were caused by a wide variety of diagnoses including alcoholism, normal pressure hydrocephalus, and vitamin B_{12} deficiency (Skoog et al, 1993). The specific causes and diagnostic criteria for dementia are discussed in Chapter 4 by Dr. Stoudemire. The elderly are also quite susceptible to numerous central nervous system insults that can lead to delirium.

Mood Disorders

Depression

Depressive symptoms and disorders are endemic in the elderly. They account for 50% of all admissions of older adults to acute psychiatric hospitals. Prominent depressive symptoms may exist in 30% of adults over age 60 although some studies put that figure as high as 60%. Ten to 15% of the geriatric population may require treatment for their depressive symptoms and 2 to 3% will meet criteria for either major depression or dysthymia. Beside the discomfort caused by the depressive symptoms alone, the risk of suicide also increases greatly in those with depression.

In 1983 the suicide rate for all Americans was 12.1 suicides per 100,000 people. For those above age 65 the rate increased to 19.2 suicides per 100,000 people. The rate for suicide in males peaks between the ages of 80 and 90 and for women it peaks between 50 and 65 years of age. Part of this increase is attributable to the increased lethality of the elderly person's suicide attempt. Before the age of 50 only one in eight who attempt suicide actually kill themselves with the attempt. After age 65 that completion rate approaches one in two. The elderly suicide tends to use more lethal means, communicates the intent less frequently, and less often uses suicide threats and gestures as tools for manipulating others (Bienenfeld, 1990).

Depressive disorders, including major depression and dysthymic disorder, are not always obvious in the elderly because the clinical presentations may change with age. It is fairly rare, for example, that an elderly patient will give as a chief complaint, "I'm depressed." Much more commonly the patient will describe vague somatic complaints, decreased energy, sleep difficulties, memory disturbances, anxiety, or "nerves." Somatic complaints, in fact, may be the predominant way in which elderly patients present their depression or anxiety. Pain, weakness, and gastrointestinal disturbances are the most frequent avenues of presentation. Often there will be complaints by the patient or others that the elderly individual is becoming regressed and more dependent or is not eating properly. Even someone with numerous neuro-vegetative complaints may deny depression or sadness but admit to feeling "down" or "blue."

A wide variety of cardiovascular, pulmonary, endocrine, and neurologic diseases, most of which increase in prevalence with aging, can present with depressive symptoms such as fatigue, anorexia, and decreased functioning. Depression can also be induced or mimicked by numerous medications commonly used in the elderly, including antihypertensives, benzodiazepines, corticosteroids, and cimetidine. It is equally hazardous to attribute problems in appetite, energy, sleep, or concentration to either depression or to medical causes alone. Appropriate evaluation should be conducted to assess accurately the physical status of the depressed patient with medical illness, including relevant aspects of the history, physical examination, laboratory tests, and radiological procedures.

Prognosis of Depression in the Elderly

The prognosis for elderly patients diagnosed with depression may not be as good as for their younger counterparts. Whereas 20% of a mixed population will remain depressed for more than 18 months, upwards of 30% of elderly patients will remain depressed for that long (Alexopoupolis and Chester, 1992). A study of 124 elderly patients with depression who were followed for one year found that 35% experienced a complete resolution of their depression by the end of the year; 19% had recovered but relapsed within the year, 29% were continuously ill, and 14% died by the end of that first year (Murphy, 1983). Another later study showed slightly more optimistic results with 58% of elderly patients recovered by the end of the year, 15% having recovered and relapsed within the year, 18% continuously ill throughout the year, and 8% dead. This study also followed patients for upward of two years following their depressive episode and found that 22% had a lasting recovery, 38.5% had a recovery with relapses from which they recovered, 32% were made invalids by their depression, and 7% were continuously ill throughout the study (Baldwin and Jolley, 1986).

A significant number of geriatric patients with major depression will also develop delusions. These delusions are most often persecutory or hypochondriacal in nature and can occur in 3% of community-dwelling depressed patients and in 20 to 45% of those elderly depressed patients who require hospitalization. Patients with delusions tend to be less responsive to traditional antidepressant therapy—less than 40% of such patients responded to amitriptyline or imipramine alone. The addition of an antipsychotic or the use of electroconvulsive therapy greatly increases the patient's response. At least one study has indicated a very poor prognosis in psychotic depression with only 10% of elderly patients recovered and well one year after the onset of their depression. Other studies (Baldwin and Jolley, 1986; Murphy, 1983) found no significant difference between the outcomes of depressed patients with or without delusions.

Bereavement

While uncomplicated bereavement (normal grieving) is not a psychopathological condition, it can display many of the features of depressive disorders and it is important to recognize for the purposes of differential diagnosis. Grieving individuals may experience, transiently, such symptoms as anorexia and insomnia in the context of their situational sadness. Normal grieving generally starts with a period of *shock* that lasts a few weeks or less, characterized by emotional numbing and even brief episodes of denial. Next comes a period of *preoccupation* with thoughts of the lost loved one; symptoms including crying, fatigue, and withdrawal. This phase may easily last a year in older widows and widowers, and may recur on the lost person's birthday, the wedding anniversary, or the anniversary of the death. Finally, preoccupation gives way to *resolution*, as somatic and depressive symptoms diminish and the survivor regains interest in social and individual activities (see Chapter 20). These phases are similar at all ages, but in aging somatic symptoms are often predominant expressions of the emotional distress and the phases may take much longer to progress and resolve than at younger ages.

Mania

While bipolar disorder usually begins in the third or fourth decade of life, episodes usually persist into old age. Additionally, first onset of mania in the sixth or even seventh decade is not unusual. Compared with younger manic patients, older individuals are more likely to be *irritable* than euphoric and *paranoid* rather than grandiose. Older patients are more likely than younger ones to present with *dysphoric mania* ("miserable mania") a constellation in which there is pressure of speech, flight of ideas, and hyperactivity, but thought content is as morbid and pessimistic as that of a patient with typical major depression.

Psychotic Disorders

Schizophrenia

Most elderly schizophrenics developed their illness between ages 20 and 40. Only 7% of schizophrenias are first diagnosed after age 60, and only 3% after age 70 (Harris and Jeste, 1988). Aging affects the clinical appearance of schizophrenia, particularly producing a blunting of the "positive" symptoms such as delusions and hallucinations. Residual delusions and hallucinations become less bizarre and more monotonous. The "negative" symptoms, including social withdrawal, apathy, and blunted affect, become more apparent.

Although the numbers are small, some individuals do develop schizophrenia after their 50s and into their 60s, a condition formerly labeled *paraphrenia*. These individuals are more likely to be women than men. The clinical presentation usually centers on persecutory delusions and generally does not include a formal thought disorder. Treated with antipsychotic agents, up to 48% of late-onset schizophrenic patients experience a resolution of symptoms (Pearlson et al, 1989).

Delusional Disorders

Delusional disorders generally present in mid- to late life. These patients are generally brought in by concerned family members as the patients themselves see nothing wrong with their ideas. In the elderly, the delusions most often involve persecutory or somatic themes. Delusions appear to be more common in immigrants and are more common in those with a sensory deficit since sensory deficits are also correlated with delusional disorders. In a community-based study, 78% of elders with persecutory ideation had visual impairment and 58% had hearing deficits, compared with 51 and 37% of age-matched controls without paranoia (Christenson and Blazer, 1984). Medications are only marginally successful at stopping the delusions but do tend to decrease their intensity and lessen the chance of the patient's acting on them. Psychotherapy generally does not produce good results, since the beliefs are unshakably true to the patient, who sees little motivation for therapy.

Anxiety and Somatoform Disorders

Anxiety

As a symptom and diagnosis, anxiety is common in the elderly. Ten to 20% of the elderly complain of anxiety severe enough to warrant a visit to a physician. On self-rating scales, 27% of individuals in their 60s and 29% above the age of 70 report significant anxiety symptoms. Individuals over 65 years of age are five times more likely to be regular users of anxiolytics than are younger individuals. Fifteen percent of those individuals who chronically use anxiolytics are over the age of 65 (Bienenfeld, 1990).

There is a broad differential for anxiety in the elderly. One of the first diagnoses that must be considered is depression. Upward of 70% of elderly individuals with major depression will also experience considerable anxiety. Situational anxiety originating from any one of the many psychosocial changes experienced by the elderly can manifest itself as an adjustment disorder with predominant anxiety symptoms. Numerous medical illnesses can also cause anxiety symptoms (see Table 11–2).

Although anxiety is a common complaint in the elderly, new-onset anxiety disorders are not frequently diagnosed. A caveat to this statement comes with diseases such as obsessive–compulsive disorder, which may have been present for many years but was not discovered by others until later in life.

Disorders such as generalized anxiety disorder (GAD), obsessive–compulsive disorder, and panic disorder—while not uncommon in the elderly (up to 7% of the elderly may have GAD)—rarely begin in old age. Most patients begin to develop their

Table 11–2 **Medical Causes of Anxiety Symptoms in the Elderly**

CARDIOPULMONARY	NEUROLOGICAL
Anemia	Encephalopathies (infectious, metabolic, toxic)
Angina pectoris	Delirium
Arrhythmias	**SUBSTANCE-RELATED**
Chronic obstructive lung disease	Stimulants
Pulmonary infections	Caffeine
Pulmonary embolus	Nicotine
Valvular heart disease	Prescription and over-the-counter drugs
ENDOCRINE AND METABOLIC	Antihypertensives
Hyperthyroidism	Decongestants
Hypocalcemia	Digitalis
Hypoglycemia	Theophylline
Hypoparathyroidism	Withdrawal syndromes
Vitamin deficiencies (B_{12}, folate)	Alcohol
	Narcotics
	Sedative hypnotics

symptoms within the first three or four decades of life. Posttraumatic stress disorder (PTSD) can be common in specific cohorts such as concentration-camp survivors and might develop de novo following the traumatic death of a spouse. The exception to this rule may be specific phobias, which may be experienced by 7% of men and 14% of women above the age of 65 within a six-month period of time. The most common phobia in the elderly who seek psychiatric help is agoraphobia, which can often worsen the social isolation to which the elderly are prone.

Somatoform Disorders

Like those with primary anxiety disorders, most patients with somatoform disorders begin to experience them well before late life. While somatizing behavior, including the expression of anxious and depressive symptoms as somatic complaints, may increase with aging, new-onset somatoform disorders are uncommon in old age. Delusional disorders with predominately somatic symptoms occur in the elderly, but in these conditions the complaints are more bizarre and lack the initial plausibility of those voiced in somatoform disorders. In those individuals with persistent somatoform disorders that started earlier in life, the particular complaints, especially in somatization disorder and hypochondriasis, may change over the course of middle age and late life. Elderly patients with somatization disorder will focus less on sexual function and more on gastrointestinal distress. Elderly hypochondriacs may voice the unfounded conviction that they have a dementia. (See also Chapter 9).

Substance Abuse

Alcoholism

Although alcoholism has no clear definition in any age group, it is clear that alcohol abuse is a common problem in the elderly. Five percent of the elderly population in the community may meet the criteria for alcohol dependence and twice as many drink alcohol in an abusive fashion. According to self reports, 10 to 20% of the elderly drink daily, up to 25% have five to seven drinks a week, and 7 to 8% drink between 12 and 21 drinks a week. One-fifth of elderly medical and psychiatric patients may be problem drinkers, as are as many as 45% of patients admitted to acute geriatric psychiatric units (Liberto et al, 1992).

Despite this evidence of continued problem drinking throughout life, the actual incidence in cross-sectional studies sharply declines after the age of 70. Possible reasons for this decrease include an increased mortality in problem drinkers at ages younger than 70 or a cohort effect as many of those who are in their 70s and 80s currently grew up during the Prohibition era and may have always had a lower prevalence of problem drinking.

Because of the alterations in ethanol metabolism that accompany aging, a given amount of alcohol will produce a higher blood alcohol level in an older person than in a younger one. Additionally, the brain and other organs become increasingly sensitive to the effects of alcohol. As a result, it is fairly common for a person to maintain a constant level of alcohol consumption over many years and only begin to have problems such as confusion, depression, or hepatic dysfunction after age 60.

Confounding the recognition of alcoholism in the elderly is the fact that many of the diagnostic criteria for alcohol abuse and dependence involve features that may not apply to aging individuals. Largely because of retirement the elderly are not likely to suffer occupational problems because of their drinking. They are also less likely to suffer legal consequences. Changes in their behavior such as confusion, self-neglect, malnutrition, and depression may be improperly dismissed as "normal" aging (Bienenfeld, 1990). Using standardized screening tests may also be ineffective. Tests that identify 60% of subjects under the age of 60 who have alcohol abuse identify only 37% of those over the age of 60 who abuse alcohol (Liberto et al, 1992).

There are nonetheless serious medical, social, and psychiatric complications from alcohol abuse in the elderly. Compared to elderly subjects who do not abuse alcohol, those who do are more likely to commit suicide, live alone, and have serious health problems such as hepatic, pulmonary, and cardiovascular diseases. Fifteen percent of those elderly who present to emergency rooms with depression or confusion develop these conditions as a result of alcohol use. Four out of five geriatric patients who abuse alcohol and have evidence of depression are experiencing a depression due to their alcohol use. Up to 60% of older alcoholics will fit the criteria for dementia. They suffer difficulty because of the direct toxic effects of alcohol on the central nervous system or exacerbations of other causes of dementia. Alcohol can exacerbate the changes in sleep and sexual function that normally accompany aging. It can also interact with over 150 prescribed medications including anticoagulants, phenytoin, sedatives, and antidepressants (Bienenfeld, 1990).

Treatment of elderly alcoholics is similar to the treatment of their younger counterparts with only slight differences. Detoxification will more frequently require hospitalization because of concern for autonomic and cardiovascular instability. Because of the particular risk of delirium, it is also generally recommended that they not receive prophylactic benzodiazepines unless they have a history of complicated alcohol withdrawal. If these agents are required, lorazepam and oxazepam are generally preferred because of their rapid hepatic oxidation. Disulfiram, which can be used to discourage alcohol consumption in younger patients, is not recommended in the elderly because it may react with numerous drugs besides alcohol and the elderly can experience severe and even life-threatening reactions.

Abuse of Other Substances

The use of illicit drugs such as narcotics and hallucinogens is not generally a significant problem in the elderly. Much more common is the abuse of prescription and over-the-counter medications. The average American senior citizen receives 3.6 prescriptions per year for psychotropic medications alone. Sixty-two percent of the elderly use at least one prescription medication daily. The elderly often will have multiple providers who are not fully aware of what other medications are being prescribed. Since some elderly individuals tend to hoard pills, trade medications, and take their medications in a nonprescribed manner, the situation is ripe for abuse.

Over-the-counter medications also represent a problem for the elderly. Sixty-nine percent of people over 65 take at least one over-the-counter medication per day. Many of these can interact with alcohol or other medications that the patient is taking. Since these medications are not prescribed, many people do not consider them drugs and will not volunteer them when asked about medications. Over-the-counter cold remedies often include ingredients that can induce delirium, as can nonsteroidal anti-inflammatory drugs. Laxatives, which are taken weekly by one-third of the population over 65, can result in diarrhea, malabsorption, and even hypokalemia. The practitioner is thus well advised to inquire about over-the-counter medications in evaluating the elderly patient (Bienenfeld, 1990).

Personality Disorders

The basic characteristics of individuals with personality disorders are evident early in adult life and are manifest in long-standing patterns of maladaptive perception, communication, and behavior. People do not develop personality disorders in late life, but the characteristic features of these disorders do change over time within individuals. In general, the behavior of individuals with narcissistic, borderline, and histrionic personality disorders becomes less intense with age. Some belated maturation may occur, impulsive actions may become incompatible with the geriatric lifestyle, and early mortality from hazardous behaviors may eliminate those with the most severe personality pathology.

Before making a new diagnosis of a personality disorder in an older patient, one should assess carefully and treat aggressively Axis I disorders, particularly depressive disorders and substance abuse. The influence of a hostile environment in which the patient may really live may temper the clinician's interpretation of ideas that sound unusually suspicious. Psychotherapy (see below) is optimal treatment for personality disorders at any age; in late life it is particularly important to make sure the therapeutic goals of the therapy are matched to the patient's resources and life circumstances.

TREATMENT

Pharmacotherapy

While caution must be used whenever medications are prescribed, there are some special considerations in the use of psychotropic medications in the elderly. Because most elderly psychiatric patients will already be receiving some medication for somatic disorders, their drug regimens may become quite confusing and the clinician must carefully consider the possible drug interactions and additive side effects of any proposed new medication. Additionally, noncompliance becomes a problem when the reason for the medication and the prescribed dosing schedule are poorly understood. Cognitive impairment may mandate that a third party set up or administer the medications.

Certain alterations in metabolism and sensitivity occur with aging. There is a decrease in the lean body mass and total body water along with an increase in body fat. These changes decrease the volume of distribution of hydrophilic drugs such as alcohol and increase the volume of distribution of lipophilic drugs such as benzodiazepines, accounting for the relative increase in blood alcohol content and the decreased clearance of benzodiazepines in the elderly user. Hepatic metabolism decreases in general with age as does the production of albumin. The former effect results in a generalized slowing of hepatic clearance, and the latter effect can cause a relative increase in the free fraction of drugs such as tricyclic antidepressants, which are largely protein-bound. Receptor sensitivity seems to change with age, causing older patients to be more sensitive to the therapeutic and adverse effects of medications.

Drugs for Psychosis

Antipsychotics such as the phenothiazines remain the drugs of choice for psychosis of virtually any etiology. As no one class of antipsychotics appears more effective than the others they are generally selected on the basis of their side effect profile. The high-potency drugs such as haloperidol are widely used in aged patients because of their relatively low anticholinergic and antiadrenergic effects. Antipsychotics seem to be equally effective throughout life, but the risks of extrapyramidal symptoms such as akathisia and parkinsonism increase with age. Lower potency agents, such as thioridazine, minimize the risk of extrapyramidal effects but are potently anticholinergic, producing constipation, postural hypotension, and cognitive impairment. Medium-potency agents, such as perphenazine, provide a reasonable compromise, allowing the clinician to modify the regimen according to observed effects, moving to a higher potency drug if anticholinergic or sedative effects predominate or to a lower potency drug if parkinsonian symptoms appear.

Drugs for Mood Disorders

For depression in the elderly the tricyclic antidepressants are the traditional choices. Secondary amines such as desipramine and nortriptyline are equally effective and have fewer toxic side effects than the older tertiary amines such as imipramine and amitriptyline. The latter category of antidepressants produces sedation and anticholinergic effects that may outweigh their therapeutic benefit. While average therapeutic doses of antidepressants decrease with age, the range of therapeutic plasma levels does not. Once therapeutic plasma levels are attained, therapy may need to be maintained for four to five weeks before maximum clinical benefit is observed.

Of the many tricyclic antidepressant side effects that occur in the elderly, two of the more troubling are confusion, which often is related to the anticholinergic effect, and hypotension due to antiadrenergic effects, which can result in dangerous and even life-threatening falls. Cognitive impairment can develop in up to 35% of patients over the age of 40 who are placed on tertiary amines. In comparison, a study that looked at nortriptyline in the elderly over a seven-week trial found no cognitive changes. In general the tertiary amines are the most likely to cause orthostatic hypotension while nortriptyline is the least likely. Even nortriptyline, however, caused an average decrease of systolic blood pressure of 9 mm/Hg in elderly patients. This orthostasis seems to develop within the first week of therapy and does not correlate well with plasma levels of medication or symptomatic complaints. Tricyclic blood levels can also be altered by many medications. Concurrent use of antipsychotics, fluoxetine, paroxetine, cimetidine, methylphenidate, thiazide diuretics, estrogen, and erythromycin tend to increase serum levels; anticonvulsants, barbiturates, vitamin C, and doxycycline tend to decrease levels. For all of these reasons tricyclic antidepressants and their side effects need to be closely monitored in the elderly (McCue, 1992).

Because of the side effects of the tricyclic antidepressants, many physicians prefer to use the newer antidepressants with their geriatric patients. Trazodone has little anticholinergic effect, moderate antiadrenergic effect, and significant sedation. It can be useful in the depressed patient with significant agitation, anxiety, or insomnia. The selective serotonin reuptake inhibitors (SSRIs) fluoxetine, sertraline, and paroxetine appear to be as effective as the tricyclics and, with the exception of paroxetine, have almost no anti-cholinergic, orthostatic or quinidine-like side effects. In general they are well tolerated by the elderly. Fluoxetine may produce agitation and anorexia and has an active metabolite with a half-life of 10–14 days but its stimulating effects may be desirable in the patient with a retarded depression. Sertraline and paroxetine have half-lives of 24 hours or less and produce little or no sedation.

Monoamine oxidase inhibitors (MAOIs) are used with elderly patients upon occasion and appear to be particularly effective in those who complain of decreased energy or motivation or who are less severely depressed. Caution must be exercised in their use, however, as they can agitate demented patients and can cause autonomic instability. Patients will often have difficulty with orthostatic hypotension while on MAOIs. Compliance with the tyramine-restricted diet required for MAOI therapy may be difficult for the cognitively impaired elder or for someone who depends on others to provide meals.

Psychostimulants such as dextroamphetamine and methylphenidate are used by some physicians in the treatment of their elderly depressed patients. These medications can be used to treat those patients who have prominent medical illnesses and cannot tolerate tricyclic antidepressants or who display prominent lethargy and apathy. One of the great benefits of these medicines is the rapidity of their therapeutic activity. While stimulants improve depressive symptoms quickly in many individuals, their effect on the core depressive illness has never been demonstrated and their long-term usefulness is controversial. The antidepressant bupropion, which has stimulant properties, should be used first if psychostimulants are being considered for long term treatment (see Chapter 18).

Aging bipolar patients continue to require treatment as they can experience both manic and depressive episodes throughout their life. Lithium remains a drug of choice for acute manic episodes and prophylaxis. The elderly are more sensitive to the effects of lithium but can often be managed with serum levels of 0.4 to 0.7 mEq/L. The decrease in renal functioning that occurs with aging slows the elimination of lithium, increasing its half-life from 18 hours at age 20 to 36 hours by age 70 (Jenike, 1989). As a result, the serum lithium levels of an elderly patient can be two or even three times higher than a younger patient's after taking equal doses of the medication. The elderly also seem to be more sensitive to the toxic effects of lithium and can experience difficulty with doses that are considered routine in younger patients. Patients should be periodically assessed for tremor, nausea, diarrhea, and memory deficits. Numerous drugs that the elderly commonly use such as nonsteroidal anti-inflammatory drugs and thiazide diuretics can also raise the serum lithium level and induce lithium toxicity.

Since lithium can be so problematic to use in the elderly, and since the likelihood of symptomatic breakthrough increases with the duration of bipolar illness, there has been some interest in the use of anticonvulsants for mania in the elderly. Agents such as carbamazepine and valproic acid have been shown to be safe and efficacious in younger adults, but investigations in the elderly are still rare. Available information suggests that anticonvulsants, particularly valproate, may be useful in those elderly patients who cannot tolerate lithium or for whom lithium has lost some of its prophylactic benefit.

Drugs for Anxiety

Benzodiazepines have traditionally been overprescribed for the elderly and care needs to be taken that these medications are prescribed only when truly indicated. For adjustment disorders that manifest with anxiety, they should typically be prescribed for only one to two months and then tapered off and discontinued. Long-term therapy with benzodiazepines is indicated only when there are clear chronic symptoms. Drugs with long half-lives and active metabolites such as diazepam and chlordiazepoxide should be used with care. These medications tend to accumulate and cause oversedation and confusion, which is very slow to clear. The very high potency, short half-life drugs such as alprazolam and triazolam also need to be used with care as their use has been related to cognitive impairment. The shorter half-life of these drugs also leaves the elderly patient prone to experience withdrawal when discontinuation is attempted. Drugs such as lorazepam and oxazepam, which are more rapidly and simply metabolized, are generally the drugs of choice in the elderly. Even with these agents, the elderly are more prone to side effects such as sedation, confusion, and memory disturbance.

Buspirone is a nonbenzodiazepine anxiolytic that has demonstrated safety and efficacy in the elderly. It differs from the benzodiazepines clinically in that it may take three to six weeks of therapy before the patient's anxiety diminishes. Elderly patients appear to require the same dosages of buspirone as younger patients—approximately 15 to 40 mg per day given in divided doses.

Psychotherapy

For much of the early history of psychiatry, elderly patients were not considered appropriate candidates for psychotherapy. During that time psychoanalysis was essentially the only method available and individuals over the age of 40 were seen as too close to death and too rigid in their personality structure to benefit. As the scope of psychotherapy has broadened the prospect of treating elderly patients has been reexamined. In fact, the aging process brings about a number of challenges and issues that could be best dealt with by psychotherapy.

The aging person needs to deal with the changing environment around her or him and shifting societal expectations. Retirement, changes in financial status, the loss of loved ones, and decreased social support can threaten the elderly person. The patient may also experience changes in the family role as parent, grandparent, and spouse or widow/widower. Those who obtained self-esteem from their work roles or their roles as parents must begin to find other sources for this esteem. Dependency issues begin to surface as aging individuals find themselves less able to control the environment. Failing health and approaching death are also universal issues that will need to be dealt with in some way. Advancing age can also bring an increased awareness of abilities that were not utilized, goals that were not actively pursued, or personality features that were left underdeveloped.

Grief and loss are central issues in much of the psychotherapy of older persons. From a psychodynamic perspective, the therapeutic task is to identify the particular meaning of the loss to the individual and to find less distressing ways to cope. For example, a man who is embittered in his retirement may come to discover through therapy that he had tied his entire sense of self-worth to his business accomplishments. He can then use the psychotherapy as a forum for exploring other sources of self-esteem. From a more behavioral perspective, the objective is to redirect energy and activity to pursuits more likely to foster emotional recovery, so that the same retiree might be encouraged to participate in church activities or engage regularly with his grandchildren.

Group therapy directly lessens the elder's sense of isolation. The patient is encouraged to practice social and communicative skills in a nonthreatening environment. Feedback concerning communication and behavior is received from peers and not just from the therapist, who might be significantly younger than the patient. The group environment also tends to increase self-esteem by allowing the patient to help others with their problems. To be an appropriate member the patient must be able to make meaningful relationships, be motivated to participate in the group, and be cognitively able to follow the conversation and group interactions.

Despite the increased mobility of our society, families continue to play a pivotal role in the life of the elderly. Almost 10% of American homes contain family members from three generations, and 82% of geriatric Americans live within 30 minutes of one of their children. Over half of elderly Americans have contact with their families more than twice a week and families provide more than 80% of social support services for their elderly members. Families can thus be a part of the therapy and more than just sources of information. The clinician helps the family identify and clarify the problems and frame them into manageable terms. A statement such as, "My children don't care for me," may be reformulated as, "I wish you would visit me more often." Solutions are then crafted in measurable dimensions to address the mutually identified problem.

Typically, too, children overcome the loss of parents more quickly than elders recover from the loss of spouses. There may come a period months after a death when the adult children avoid contact with the still-grieving parent or make comments such as, "You should be over that by now." Education to families about the time course of grieving in later life can prevent the mourning from becoming complicated by guilt and isolation from family.

CLINICAL PEARLS

- Any acute or subacute change in cognition is pathological and needs to be evaluated carefully and not dismissed as just "normal aging."
- Major depression and anxiety in the elderly are frequently secondary to physical illness, drug effects, and alcoholism. These disorders must be sought carefully when evaluating an elderly individual with depression or anxiety.
- While the new onset of schizophrenia in the elderly is uncommon, persistence of schizophrenic signs and symptoms is very common.
- The elderly with sensory impairment are more prone to experience delusional disorders.
- Because of alterations in metabolism and increased sensitivity to the therapeutic and side effects of medication, the elderly generally require less medication for the same symptoms but dosage must be judged on an individual basis.
- A person who has not changed a lifelong pattern of alcohol use may first begin to have alcohol-related problems, including depression and cognitive impairment, in later life.

The opinions expressed herein are solely those of the authors and do not reflect the positions of the Department of Defense, the Department of the Air Force, or any other federal agency.

ANNOTATED BIBLIOGRAPHY

Bienenfeld D (ed): Verwoerdt's Clinical Geropsychiatry, 3rd ed. Baltimore, Williams & Wilkins, 1990

> This book provides comprehensive and readable chapters on most of the major areas in geriatric psychiatry. In particular the chapters on the psychology of aging, the evaluation of the elderly patient, psychopharmacology, and substance abuse in the elderly are of particular interest for those who will deal with the elderly on a regular basis, regardless of specialty.

Blazer D: Depression in late life: An update. Ann Rvw Gerontology Geriatrics 9:197–215, 1989

> This review provides a broad and comprehensive look at this most common of complaints, with a particular emphasis on the psychobiology of depression.

McCue RE: Using tricyclic antidepressants in the elderly. Clin Geriatric Med 8:323–334, 1992

> A thorough examination of the benefits and side-effects that are encountered with the use of these common drugs.

Sadavoy J, Lazarus LW, Jarvik LF (eds): Comprehensive Review of Geriatric Psychiatry. Washington, DC, American Psychiatric Press, 1991

This volume is a useful reference book, featuring 34 chapters on the most important aspects of the field, presented in a factual style by the nation's leading authorities.

Tran-Johnson TK, Krull AJ, Jeste DV: Late life schizophrenia and its treatment: Pharmacologic issues in older schizophrenic patients. Clin Geriatric Med 8:401–410, 1992

A useful overview of schizophrenia in older patients, including late-onset schizophrenia, which also discusses some of the pharmacokinetic and pharmacodynamic changes that accompany aging.

REFERENCES

Alexopoulos GS, Chester JG: Outcomes of geriatric depression. Clin Geriatric Med 8:363–376, 1992
Baldwin R, Jolley D: The prognosis of depression in old age. Br J Psychiatry 149:574–583, 1986
Bienenfeld D (ed): Verwoerdt's Clinical Geropsychiatry, 3rd ed. Baltimore, Williams & Wilkins, 1990
Blazer D: Depression in late life: An update. Ann Rvw Gerontology Geriatrics 9:197–215, 1989
Christenson R, Blazer D: Epidemiology of persecutory ideation in an elderly population in the community. Am J Psychiatry 141:1088–1091, 1984
Clarfield AM: The reversible dementias: Do they reverse? Ann Int Med 109:476–486, 1988
Cohen CI: Outcome of schizophrenia into later life: An overview. Gerontologist 30:790–797, 1990
Erikson EH: Identity and the Life Cycle. New York, International Universities Press, 1959
Finch EJL, Ramsay R, Kalona CLE: Depression and physical illness in the elderly. Clin Geriatric Med 8:275–287, 1992
Harper CM, Newton PA, Walsh JR: Drug-induced illness in the elderly. Postgrad Med 86:245–256, 1989
Harris MJ, Jeste DV: Late onset schizophrenia: An overview. Schizophrenia Bull 14:39–55, 1988
Jenike MA: Geriatric Psychiatry and Psychopharmacology: A Clinical Approach. Chicago, Year Book Medical Publisher, 1989
Jorm A, Korton A, Henderson A: The prevalence of dementia: A quantitative integration of the literature. Acta Psychiatrica Scand 76:465–479, 1987
Lazarus LW (ed): Essentials of Geriatric Psychiatry. New York, Springer Publishing Company, 1988
Liberto JG, Oslin DW, Ruskin PE: Alcoholism in older persons: A review of the literature. Hosp Comm Psychiatry 43:975–984, 1992
McCue RE: Using tricyclic antidepressants in the elderly. Clin Geriatric Med 8:323–334, 1992
Meyers BS: Geriatric delusional depression. Clin Geriatric Med 8:299–308, 1992
Murphy E: The prognosis of depression in old age. Br J Psychiatry 142:111–119, 1983
Pearlson GD, Kreger L, Rabins PV, Chase GA, Cohen B, Wirth JB, Schlaepfer TB, Tune LE: A chart review study of late-onset and early-onset schizophrenia. Am J Psychiatry 146:1568–1574, 1989
Skoog I, Nilsson L, Palmertz B, Andreasson L, Svanborg A: A population-based study of dementia in 85-year-olds. N Eng J Med 328:153–158, 1993
Steiner D, Marcopulos B: Depression in the elderly. Nursing Clin N Am 26:585–600, 1991
Tran-Johnson TK, Krull AJ, Jeste DV: Late life schizophrenia and its treatment: Pharmacologic issues in older schizophrenic patients. Clin Geriatric Med 8:401–410, 1992
Winstead DK, Mielke DH, O'Neill PT: Diagnosis and treatment of depression in the elderly: A review. Psychiatric Med 8:85–98, 1990
Young RC: Geriatric mania. Clin Geriatric Med 8:387–399, 1992

Alan Stoudemire (ed). *Clinical Psychiatry for Medical Students,* Second Edition. Copyright © 1994, 1990 by J. B. Lippincott Company.

12 *Eating Disorders*

Joel Yager

Cases of women who starved themselves have been reported for hundreds of years, including cases of *anorexia mirabilis* in sainted women of the Middle Ages and of notorious "fasting girls" of the sixteenth through nineteenth centuries. Anorexia nervosa as we now recognize it was first described in the late 1870s and interest in the eating disorders has grown considerably over the past two decades. The death of the popular singer Karen Carpenter from anorexia nervosa in 1983 resulted in a flood of television programs and magazine articles that brought considerable attention to the eating disorders. After popular magazines featured articles suggesting that several female idols including Jane Fonda, Olympic gymnast Cathy Rigby, Sally Field, Ally Sheedy, Gilda Radner, Tracey Gold, and even Princess Diana of England may have suffered from anorexia nervosa and/or bulimia nervosa, virtually every female in the United States became aware of the existence of these disorders and their attendant dangers.

EPIDEMIOLOGY

Current studies suggest that among adolescent and young adult women in certain high school and college settings, the prevalence of clinically significant eating disorders is about 4% and for more broadly defined syndromes may be as high as 8% (Kendler et al, 1991). Individual symptoms of eating disorders—body image distortion; extreme fear of being fat out of line with health concerns; the desire to reduce body fat to levels below those ordinarily considered healthy; restrictive and fad dieting; amphetamine and cocaine use for anorectic effects; purging by means of vomiting, laxative abuse, diuretic abuse; and excessive or compulsive exercise among normal-weight and even underweight individuals—are relatively common (Drewnowski et al, 1988). Some of these general symptoms may even be seen in the majority of certain subgroups of the female population, as in select college sororities or among female dance majors.

Males with anorexia nervosa and bulimia form the minority of cases and 90 to 95% of cases are female. The age of onset is most typically in the teenage and early adult years, but cases with prepubertal onset and with onset in the 40s and older have been reported. Although these disorders were previously associated primarily with the upper and upper-middle social classes and almost exclusively with Caucasians, more recent data suggest that these disorders are now well represented among middle and lower-middle class women including nonwhites.

DESCRIPTION, DIAGNOSTIC CRITERIA, AND DIFFERENTIAL DIAGNOSIS

Diagnostic criteria for the eating disorders have been the subject of much discussion and are shown in Table 12–1. Primary symptoms for both *anorexia nervosa* and *bulimia nervosa* are a preoccupation with weight and the desire to be thinner. The two disorders are *not* mutually exclusive, and there appears to be a continuum among patients of the two symptom complexes of self-starvation and the binge-purge cycle: about 50% of patients with anorexia nervosa will also have bulimia nervosa, and many patients with bulimia nervosa may have previously have had at least a subclinical form of anorexia nervosa.

Anorexia Nervosa

Although the diagnosis of anorexia nervosa requires a loss of weight of at least 15% below normal, many patients have lost considerably more by the time they come to medical attention. Patients engage in a variety of behaviors designed to lose weight. In addition to markedly reduced caloric intake—usually in the range of 300 to 600 KCalories/day—strange dietary rituals include the refusal to eat in front of others, avoidance of entire classes of food, and unusual spice and flavoring practices (such as putting huge quantities of pepper or lemon juice on all foods). Some exercise compulsively for hours each day; noneating-related compulsions such as cleaning and counting rituals are not uncommon. Although patients may initially seem cheerful and energetic, about half will develop an accompanying major depression, and all will become moody and irritable. A lifetime prevalence of obsessive–compulsive disorder of 25% has been reported in anorexia nervosa (Halmi et al, 1991). Many complain of having no real sense of themselves apart from the anorexia nervosa. Weight losses of 30 to 40% below normal are not unusual. Accompanying these losses are signs and symptoms indicative of the physical complications of starvation: depletion of fat, muscle wasting (including cardiac muscle loss in severe cases), bradycardia and other arrhythmias, constipation, abdominal pains, leukopenia, hypercortisolemia, osteo-

Table 12–1 **Symptoms of Anorexia Nervosa and Bulimia Nervosa***

Anorexia Nervosa

- The patient refuses to maintain her body weight at a minimal normal weight for age and height, leading to maintenance of body weight 15% below expected; or fails to gain weight as expected during growth, leading to body weight 15% below expected.
- Even though underweight, the patient intensely fears gaining weight or becoming fat.
- The patient experiences her body weight, size, or shape in a disturbed fashion, e.g., claiming to "feel fat" even when clearly underweight.
- In female patients, at least three consecutive missed menstrual cycles that should otherwise be expected to occur (primary or secondary amenorrhea). (Women are considered to have amenorrhea if periods occur only following hormone administration).

Two subtypes are specified:

Restricting Type: Restricters don't usually engage in binge eating, self-induced vomiting, or misuse of laxatives or diuretics for weight loss purposes.

Binge Eating/Purging Type: These patients regularly engage in binge eating and/or self-induced vomiting, misuse of laxatives or diuretics during the course of anorexia nervosa.

Bulimia Nervosa

- Repeated episodes of rapidly binge eating much larger amounts of food in brief periods of time, e.g., two hours, than most people would eat under similar circumstances. Furthermore, during these binges the patient feels that the eating is out of control.
- The patient regularly engages in severe compensatory behaviors to prevent weight gain, e.g., self-induces vomiting, misuse of large amounts of laxatives or diuretics, diet pills, fasts, very strict diets, and/or very vigorous exercise.
- At least two binge eating and purging/severe compensatory behavior episodes per week for a minimum of three months.
- Unrelenting overconcern with weight and body shape.
- These episodes do not occur only during a course of anorexia nervosa.

Two subtypes are specified:

Purging Type: These patients regularly engage in self-induced vomiting and/or misuse of laxatives or diuretics.

Nonpurging Type: These patients don't usually self-induce vomiting or misuse laxatives or diuretics to lose weight. Instead, they engage in other severe compensatory behaviors such as fasting or excessive exercise.

* Adapted from DSM-IV (APA 1993, in press [1994])

porosis, and in extreme cases the development of cachexia and lanugo (fine baby-like hair over the body). Metabolic alterations that conserve energy are seen in thyroid function (low T3 syndrome) and reproductive function, with a marked drop or halt in LH and FSH secretion. All female patients stop menstruating; up to a third stop menstruating even before losing sufficient body fat to account for the onset of amenorrhea.

Anorexia nervosa appears in two general varieties, the *restricting* and *binge eating/purging* subtypes, although these may occasionally alternate in the same patient. The *restricter* tends to exert maximal self-control regarding food intake and tends to be socially avoidant, withdrawn, and isolated, with an obsessional thinking style and ritualistic behavior in nonfood areas. In contrast, the *bulimic* subtype is unable to restrain herself from frequent food binges and then purges by means of vomiting or ingesting extremely large quantities of laxatives and/or diuretics to further weight loss; the bulimic subtype is also commonly depressed and self-destructive; often displays the emotional, dramatic, and erratic personality cluster; and not infrequently abuses alcohol and drugs.

Full recovery within a few years is seen in 30 to 50% of patients. Younger-onset patients and those with the restricter rather than bulimic subtype appear to have a better prognosis. Death from starvation, sudden cardiac arrhythmias, and suicide occurs in 5 to 10% of patients within 10 years and in almost 20% of patients within 20 years of onset (Steinhausen et al, 1991; Hsu, 1987).

A CASE STUDY

A 24-year-old graduate student was brought in by her husband at a weight of 76 pounds because she was fainting repeatedly and would not permit herself to eat in spite of his pleas and concerns for her safety. With a height of 5 feet 4 inches, she had never weighed more than 90 pounds over the past four years and she had not had a menstrual period since age 16. She permitted herself to eat only tiny bits of white colored food and only from someone else's plate. Her exercise pattern included 200 push-ups and sit-ups each morning; if she lost count she was obliged to start at the beginning. In addition, she swam 32 laps each day in the university's pool. On days when she permitted herself an extra morsel and thereby considered herself to have been "bad" with respect to eating, she would force herself to swim an additional even number of laps in multiples of four or she would take handfuls of laxatives to induce severe cramps and diarrhea, both as a punishment and to assure that she lost additional weight. In spite of these limitations she was able to carry out complex and demanding intellectual assignments in her courses. Under duress she finally agreed to gain weight, but could do so only by means of an extremely ritualistic diet of carefully measured amounts of cheese and ice cream.

Bulimia Nervosa

This disorder occurs predominantly in weight-preoccupied females (90 to 95%) who engage in marked eating binges and purging episodes at least twice per week for three consecutive months. According to the DSM-IV (APA 1993a, in press [1994]), two subtypes can be distinguished: the *purging type* uses self-induced vomiting or misuses laxatives or diuretics, and the *nonpurging type* uses other inappropriate compensatory behaviors, such as excessive exercise or fasting, but does not ordinarily self-induce vomiting or misuse laxatives or diuretics. Although the majority of patients with bulimia nervosa appear never to have had frank anorexia nervosa, a past history of the disorder or many of its individual features is not uncommon. Patients frequently consume between 5,000 and 10,000 calories per binge, and binge-purge cycles may occur as frequently as several times per day. The patients always feel as if their eating is out of control, feel so ashamed that they're often secretive about their problem, and have a concurrent major depression or anxiety disorder in up to 75% of cases (Johnson and Connors, 1987). Substantially increased rates of anxiety disorders, chemical dependency disorders, and personality disorders have also been reported among bulimia nervosa patients (APA, 1993b).

All patients with a known or suspected eating disorder need a thorough medical evaluation as well as an assessment of other medical disorders that may cause gastrointestinal symptoms (Table 12–2).

Physical complications of binge-purge cycles include fluid and electrolyte abnormalities with hypochloremic hypokalemic alkalosis, esophageal and gastric irritation and bleeding, large bowel abnormalities due to laxative abuse, marked erosion of dental enamel with accompanying decay, and parotid and salivary gland hypertrophy (squirrel face) with hyperamylasemia of about 25 to 40% over normal values (Mitchell et al, 1987) The medical complications of eating disorders are summarized in Table 12–3.

The disorder is often chronic when untreated, lasting years to decades, but may tend toward slight spontaneous improvement in symptoms (Yager et al, 1988b). Other aspects of outcome are discussed in the treatment section.

A CASE STUDY

An 18-year-old athletically built college freshman had been bulimic since the age of 15, gorging an estimated 5,000 to 20,000 calories of junk food each evening after her family went to bed and vomiting repeatedly when she felt painfully full. The disorder began at a time when her mother became seriously depressed about the deteriorating health of her own alcoholic mother. In addition to feeling out of control and despondent about her eating, the patient had been sexually promiscuous since the age of 16, and since starting college had been drinking heavily and using cocaine whenever it was available. Treatment ultimately required programs that addressed her substance-abuse problems as well as the eating and mood disorders.

Table 12–2 **Differential Diagnosis of Binge Eating and Vomiting**

Binge Eating

** Bulimia Nervosa.
** Binge eating in obesity.
** CNS lesions (e.g., Kleine-Levin syndrome, seizures, and rarely tumors).
** Appetite increases due to metabolic conditions or drugs.
** Other psychiatric disorders such as schizophrenia, mania, and atypical depression.

Vomiting

** CNS causes (e.g., increased intracranial pressure, tumor, and seizure disorder).
** Gastrointestinal causes (e.g., mechanical obstruction, infections, toxins, metabolic, allergic, "functional").
** Migraine.
** Instrumental (goal directed) vomiting (e.g., wrestlers before a match to reduce weight).
** Psychogenic vomiting (other psychiatric disorders such as anxiety, conversion disorders).

Table 12–3 **Medical Complications of Eating Disorders**

A. Related to weight loss:

** Cachexia: loss of fat, muscle mass, reduced thyroid metabolism (low T3 syndrome), cold intolerance, and difficulty maintaining core body temperature.

** Cardiac: Loss of cardiac muscle, small heart, cardiac arrhythmias including atrial and ventricular premature contractions, prolonged His bundle transmission (prolonged Q-T interval), bradycardia, ventricular tachycardia, sudden death.

** Digestive/gastrointestinal: Delayed gastric emptying, bloating, constipation, abdominal pain.

** Reproductive: Amenorrhea, infertility, low levels of lutenizing hormone (LH) and follicle-stimulating hormone (FSH).

** Dermatologic: Lanugo (fine baby-like hair over body), edema.

** Hematologic: Leukopenia.

** Neuropsychiatric: Abnormal taste sensation (zinc deficiency?), apathetic depression, irritability, obsessional thinking, compulsive behaviors, mild organic mental symptoms.

** Skeletal: Osteoporosis.

B. Related to purging (vomiting and laxative abuse):

** Metabolic: Electrolyte abnormalities, particularly hypokalemic, hypochloremic alkalosis; hypomagnesemia.

** Digestive/gastrointestinal: Salivary gland and pancreatic inflammation and enlargement with increase in serum amylase, esophageal and gastric erosion, dysfunctional bowel with haustral dilitation.

** Dental: Erosion of dental enamel (perimyolysis), particularly of front teeth, with corresponding decay.

** Neuropsychiatric: Seizures (related to large fluid shifts and electrolyte disturbances), mild neuropathies, fatigue and weakness, mild degrees of cognitive dysfunction.

ETIOLOGY AND PATHOGENESIS

Theories regarding the etiology and pathogenesis of the eating disorders have implicated virtually every level of biopsychosocial organization.

Biological Theories

Several biological causes have been proposed. One popular theory posits the presence of a hypothalamic or suprahypothalamic abnormality to account for the profound disturbances seen in eating-disorder patients in the secretion of lutenizing hormone (LH), follicle-stimulating hormone (FSH), cortisol, and arginine-vasopressin, among other hormones and peptides, and for abnormalities in opioid and catecholamine metabolism (Fava et al, 1989). Although this possibility may ultimately prove to be at least partly valid, the theory suffers from being based exclusively on data obtained from patients who are already starving or nutritionally unbalanced; no firm support for this theory is as yet available from potentially predisposed but unaffected patients such as unaffected twins or younger sisters of affected patients. Biological data obtained from patients who have recovered and who have been allowed to stabilize for long enough periods of time virtually always show a return to normal values.

Another theory suggests that some eating disorders, particularly bulimic syndromes, may be variants of mood disorders. Supporting arguments include the frequent co-morbidity of affective disturbance with eating disorders, an increased prevalence of mood disturbance in first-degree relatives of bulimic patients, and responses of bulimic patients to antidepressant medications.

Genetically transmitted vulnerability cannot be ruled out, although exactly what the vulnerability might be is obscure. Eating disorders have a familial pattern of transmission, but such patterns do not necessarily suggest genetic as opposed to environmental influences (Yager, 1982). However, the largest series of twins for both anorexia nervosa and bulimia nervosa show much higher concordance for both monozygotic (about 50%) than dizygotic (about 14%) twins (Crisp et al, 1985; Kendler et al, 1991), suggesting that some genetic influences may be important.

Still another theory suggests that the process of dieting and exercise produces an "autointoxication" with endogenous opioids, essentially an altered state of consciousness as a consequence of the starvation state, and that at a certain point this autointoxication creates an autoaddiction to internally generated opioids. According to this theory, the subsequent starvation and exercise are maintained in the effort to continue to generate adequate amounts of endogenous opioid to sustain the good feelings initially produced (Marrazzi and Luby, 1986).

Aside from these speculative theories, the primary biological influences in the pathogenesis of eating-disorder symptoms are those related to starvation and malnutrition per se. Studies with starving normal volunteers have demonstrated that many of the psychopathological as well as physical signs and symptoms of eating disorders are attributable to starvation. Of course, starvation produces all the organ wasting and laboratory findings described above (Garfinkel and Garner, 1982). More interesting from the point of view of the pathogenesis of psychopathology is the observation that starved normal volunteers become food preoccupied, depressed, irritable, hoard food, develop abnormal taste preferences, and binge-eat when food is readily available. Furthermore, in one study in which previously normal volunteers who were starved over a period of several months to 25% below their usual, healthy weights, full psychological recovery didn't occur until six months to a year *after* the subjects had regained all their lost weight. In other words, many of the strange and bizarre psychological symptoms including compulsive rituals and markedly disturbed personality traits may *result* from rather than cause the severe starvation. Many other psychopathological features of patients with severe anorexia nervosa such as immature cognitive capacity as evidenced by decreases in the ability to verbalize feelings, the complexity of cognition, and the use of fantasy also appear related to weight loss rather than to premorbid immaturity; these symptoms improve with weight gain unrelated to psychotherapy. Of course, there do seem to be psychopathological features that antedate the severe weight loss as well.

Psychological Theories

Hypotheses regarding possible psychological factors in etiology and pathogenesis have been derived from classical, operant, cognitive, and social learning theories; psychodynamic schools including classical psychoanalysis, ego psychology, object relations, and self-psychology theories; existential psychology; and several schools of family theory (Garfinkel and Garner, 1985). Accordingly, it is thought that eating disorders may result from the following (not necessarily mutually exclusive) processes:

1. Maladaptive learned responses, based on classical or operant conditioning principles, that reduce anxiety. In the patient with anorexia nervosa these responses may take the form of food and/or weight phobias. In the patient with bulimia nervosa, inner tension states may be relieved by excessive eating. (In many families children at a very young age learn, and may be actively taught, to use food for stress reduction.) Immediately thereafter, the anxiety generated by the shame, guilt, and loss of self-control brought about by the eating binge is in turn relieved by purging.

2. Cognitive distortions that develop in efforts to reduce and manage anxiety in socially awkward and sensitive adolescents (as well as in others). These misguided and erroneous self-statements tend to confound self-worth with physical appearance. The self-statements are constantly repeated as preconscious inner thoughts, cycled over and over again in a ruminative fashion, and have a self-reinforcing quality, so that they become overlearned shibboleths. The thinking distortions include tendencies to overgeneralize, to magnify horrible things (making a mountain out of a molehill), to think in "all or none" and black-and-white terms, to take everything personally, and to think superstitiously. Examples include such self statements as "If I gain one pound everyone will notice how fat and ugly I am"; "If I only had thinner thighs I'd be much more popular and attractive"; "Any bite I take will immediately turn to fat"; "I am special only if I'm thin"; and "I just can't control myself. If I eat one chip I'll never be able to stop and I'll eat the whole bag."

3. Distortions of perceptions and interoceptions. Experiments with photographs, distorting mirrors, and videotape recordings, while not all in agreement, generally tend to support the idea that patients with eating disorders have a greater tendency to distort and misperceive their body widths, seeing themselves as much wider than they are. Although many women without eating disorders also have this tendency, the extent and degree of this distortion is much greater among women with the disorders. Patients with eating disorders also have greater difficulty than others in clearly identifying inner states such as hunger and satiety (interocepts) and in clearly identifying some of their own emotional states as well.

4. Several authorities have suggested that children who will be predisposed to eating disorders suffer developmentally from a weak sense of self and from low self-worth. As patients, they display a

pervasive sense of ineffectiveness (Bruch, 1973). According to one view, these weaknesses may stem from the failure of the parents to treat the child as a legitimate and authentic person in her own right. Instead, such parents are thought to take their child for granted and to value the child primarily for behaving well (so that the parents don't have to be bothered) and for satisfying the parents' own needs to feel valuable and to show off; the child satisfied the parents' needs by means of various achievements and accomplishments (which may have little intrinsic satisfaction for the child); hence, some pre-anorexia nervosa children have been characterized as "the best little girl in the world." Sometimes the inner weakness in the sense of self is very evident, as in the overly timid and anxious child who always clings to the mother and who has a hard time advancing and emancipating at each step of psychosocial development; this character structure may result from constitutional factors as well as from parenting style. Sometimes the weakness is well hidden, at least superficially, by a defensive superficial personality shell and an outer facade that may appear to be strong, willful, and determined, but which lacks the adaptive flexibility of a truly strong personality structure.

5. Conflicts over adolescent development and the tasks of psychosexual maturity. Since anorexia nervosa resembles both psychological and physiological regression from the healthy adolescent state to prepubertal structures, the idea that patients may develop the disorder as a way of putting off the tasks of adolescence has had considerable appeal. In this view patients may avoid the difficult tasks of establishing a separate identity, value system and life plan, separating from their families, and contending with heterosexual urges and peer pressures.

6. Family factors. To start, we must stress that a family cause for eating disorders has not been proven; that a reasonable number of patients seem to come from families that are, for all intents and purposes, "normal"; and that many normal adults grow up in families that manifest the presumed pathogenetic patterns to be described. Therefore, indiscriminate "parent-bashing", i.e., the practice of laying excessive, often undue blame on parents for their childrens' psychiatric disorders—an all too common practice among health workers—is insupportable. Even when family problems are evident, it is far too easy to erroneously attribute the eating disorders to the family's problems; even in such instances the disorders may result from entirely different factors (Yager, 1982).

With this caveat in mind, it can be said that some families are thought to be more likely than others to produce a child with an eating disorder. Several of the hypothesized and observed parental characteristics were described above. These family patterns are not idiosyncratic for eating disorders; they are also believed to produce other types of problems and to possibly exacerbate the course of illness for children with other diseases that may have "psychosomatic components," such as asthma and juvenile diabetes mellitus.

Families believed more likely to produce children with eating disorders include those in which a parent is enmeshed with a child (i.e., overinvolved to the point of being unable to distinguish the parent's needs and wishes from the child's), overt conflict between the parents or between parent and child is studiously avoided, and rules about how family members communicate with one another are so rigid that it may be impermissible to address the sources and even the existence of tensions in the family (Minuchin et al, 1978). Patterns of childhood physical and sexual abuse and other forms of parental "boundary violations" have been cited as contributing factors. A family pattern characterized by "negative expressed emotion" has been empirically linked to poorer outcome for anorexia nervosa (and other psychiatric disorders such as schizophrenia and mood disorders). In this pattern a family member, usually a parent, is highly emotional and unrelentingly critical of the patient, often blaming her for bringing on the disorder and for using it to harm everyone else in the family.

Social and Cultural Factors

Several factors suggest strong social and cultural influences in the appearance of eating disorders. First, *the prevalence of these disorders seems to have increased dramatically over the past several decades.* The prevalence of eating disorders parallels society's attitudes about beauty and fashion. A previous increase in eating disorders was observed in the mid-1920s at the height of the "flapper" era when women's fashion promoted a slim boyish look. The current increase in the prevalence of eating disorders has also occurred concurrent with changing cultural standards of beauty as documented by steadily decreasing weights for height over the past two decades among fashion models, Playboy magazine centerfolds, and Miss America beauty pageant winners. Of note, from the beginning of the 1960s until Barbara Bush, the first ladies of America have also been much slimmer than they were previously.

Social-feminist theorists have suggested that anorexia nervosa may signify the unconscious hunger strikes of women who have been demeaned by society, and the highly skewed sex distribution, with a roughly nine to one preponderance of females to males, has also been interpreted as due to cultural influences. Other factors may be at work, however, including the fact that psychosexual maturation occurs about two years earlier in females than in males, forcing them to face the associated urges and peer pressures at a younger age and perhaps rendering females more vulnerable to maturational conflicts than males. Also, males who develop anorexia nervosa may have more conflicts over sexual identity and even a higher prevalence of homosexual behavior than others. Homosexual male college students' attitudes toward their bodies and food fall midway between those of other college student males and females (Yager et al, 1988a). Once again, such a finding may be due to cultural and/or biological influences.

Given the complexity and diversity of human nature, upbringing, and family life, suffice it to say that although no one theory seems to be universally true, many of the theories of etiology and pathogenesis described above find some support in clinical observations and each has been the basis of some form of intervention.

TREATMENT

Treatment planning for eating disorders must be based on a comprehensive assessment that includes attention to physical status; psychological and behavioral aspects of the eating disorders; associated psychological problems such as substance abuse and mood and personality disturbances; and the family (APA, 1993b). Each patient's problem list will have unique aspects, and treatment components should be targeted to each specific problem. Treatment usually includes attention to weight normalization; symptom reduction through cognitive and behavioral therapy programs, supportive nursing care, dietary management and counseling; individual and family psychological problems through individual, group, and family psychotherapies; and some mood disturbances and some eating-disorder symptoms through psychopharmacological interventions. As is true for many types of disorders, some self-help programs may be useful. At the present time the best treatment approach combines elements pragmatically. The following discussion is organized around the management of specific eating-disorder related problems.

Anorexia Nervosa

Low Weight
Most controlled studies have dealt with short-term weight restoration rather than with long-term treatment and, in current practice, initial attention to weight restoration is followed closely by individual and family psychotherapies (Agras, 1987).

There is general, but not universal, agreement that weight restoration should be a central and early goal of treatment of the emaciated patient. Weight restoration per se may bring about many psychological benefits, including a reduction in obsessional thinking and mood and personality disturbance. Although some underweight patients may be successfully treated outside of the hospital—up to 50% in some series (Garfinkel and Garner, 1982)—such a program usually requires a highly motivated patient, a cooperative family, and good prognostic features such as younger age and brief duration of symptoms. The large majority of severely emaciated patients (25 to 50% below recommended weight) require inpatient treatment in a psychiatric unit, a competently staffed general hospital unit, or a specialized eating-disorder unit. The problem is how to encourage, persuade, or, in the case of the preterminal recalcitrant patient, benevolently coerce the patient into gaining weight.

Carefully designed studies have demonstrated that behavioral programs can reliably encourage weight gain (Agras, 1987). Programs that combine informational feedback regarding weight gain and caloric intake, large meals, and a behavioral program that includes both positive reinforcers (such as praise and desired visits) and negative reinforcers (such as bed rest, room and activity restrictions, and prolonged hospital stays) have the best therapeutic effects on eating and weight gain. Such programs usually require a minimum of several weeks and sometimes several months in the hospital or possibly in a suitable alternative such as an intensive outpatient day hospital.

Compared to programs that use medications or psychotherapy as the principal forms of therapy, programs including behavior therapy programs are at least more efficient, in that lengths of hospital stays are generally shorter for those treated with behavior therapy. However, they have not yet been shown to necessarily be any more effective in the long run. Nasogastric tube feeding and total parenteral nutrition programs are rarely necessary but may sometimes be lifesaving.

Psychotherapies. The role of individual and family psychotherapy in bringing about weight gain per se is difficult to evaluate. To the extent that a patient's motivation to change may be increased through such therapies, they may be valuable. Families can benefit from family therapy and counseling as soon as the problems are identified. In any event, patients often appear to make the best use of these therapies to deal with their own and their families' long-standing psychological problems after they've regained some weight and are better able to think more clearly.

Psychopharmacological Approaches. Many authorities avoid medications in severely malnourished patients with anorexia nervosa because such patients may be especially prone to serious side effects and because no one has yet demonstrated that medication approaches to gaining and sustaining weight have any convincing long-term advantages over nonmedication programs. In one controlled study cyproheptadine in doses of up to 32 mg/day showed some, although by no means striking, benefit for lower weight nonbulimic patients (Halmi et al, 1986). The drug's mechanism of action in this situation is uncertain, but it does seem to increase hunger; paradoxically, this makes it unacceptable to many patients. Low doses of neuroleptics or of antianxiety drugs are sometimes prescribed, but existing studies do not support their general use. Open trials of fluoxetine have been helpful in maintaining weight gain for a year following initial weight gain (Kaye et al, 1991). Thus far, aside from small case series, the value of antidepressant medications for weight gain per se is unproven (Garfinkel and Garner, 1987). Medical regimens are sometimes required for patients with laxative abuse, severe constipation and other abdominal symptoms, and for associated problems.

Psychological Problems

Psychotherapeutic Approaches. For anorexia nervosa, most authorities suggest that individual psychotherapy using a highly empathic and nurturant reality-based perspective is most useful in helping the patient to examine and confront the many psychological distortions and developmental issues described above. Sessions are frequently scheduled weekly or twice weekly. The value of family therapy following hospital discharge has also been demonstrated in controlled studies for younger patients with anorexia nervosa (Russell et al, 1987).

Psychopharmacological Approaches. Antidepressant medication is often used for depression that persists following weight gain and sometimes for depression in the still-underweight patient. However, the efficacy of this approach in the still seriously underweight patient is questionable, and such patients may be more prone to cardiotoxic side effects. Low-dose neuroleptics or antianxiety drugs are sometimes used for specific target symptoms such as psychotic thinking and severe anxiety in patients with anorexia nervosa, but their use in this fashion is based solely on clinical impressions of their occasional value (Garfinkel and Garner, 1987).

Bulimia Nervosa

Binge Eating and Purging

Although with few exceptions psychotherapeutic and psychopharmacological interventions have thus far been evaluated separately from each other, in practice the various approaches are frequently combined, depending on the individual's needs.

Psychotherapeutic Approaches. Many controlled studies have shown the value of individual and group cognitive-behavioral psychotherapies in particular (Fairburn et al, 1991), although other approaches including focal psychodynamic psychotherapy may be of value as well (Hartmann et al, 1992).

A *cognitive-behavioral* approach includes several stages, each consisting of several weeks or more of weekly or biweekly individual and/or group sessions. The *first* stage emphasizes the establishment of control over eating using behavioral techniques such as self-monitoring (e.g., keeping a detailed symptom-relevant diary) and response prevention (e.g., eating until satiated without being allowed to vomit), the prescription of a pattern of regular eating, and stimulus-control measures (e.g., avoidance of situations most likely to stimulate an eating binge). Patients are actively educated about weight regulation, dieting, and the adverse consequences of bulimia. The *second* stage focuses on attempts to restructure the patient's unrealistic cognitions (e.g., assumptions and expectations) and instill more effective modes of problem solving. The *third* stage emphasizes maintaining the gains and preventing relapse, and often provides six months to a year of weekly sessions to provide close follow-up during the time that patients are most likely to relapse (Fairburn, 1981; Johnson and Connors, 1987). Intensive outpatient programs for bulimia have also been employed in which patients start their programs by attending various group programs several hours each day for several weeks. The overall success rate of these methods varies considerably. For those completing the programs, about 50 to 90% experience a substantial reduction in binging and purging rates, averaging about 70%, and about one-third of patients stop these symptoms entirely (the dropout problem is considerable, however, in many groups). Available follow-up reports, generally for less than three years, indicate that many of the gains are maintained, although some recidivism is seen, particularly at times of severe stress.

Psychodynamic Psychotherapy. Although long-term psychodynamic psychotherapy has often been employed in the treatment of bulimia, no controlled studies of its effectiveness in comparison to other modalities are available. Most cognitive-behavioral programs utilize important psychodynamically derived therapy principles, and most psychodynamically oriented therapists who treat patients with bulimia nervosa often effectively employ cognitive-behavioral strategies or work concurrently with other therapists who do.

Psychopharmacological Approaches. Controlled studies indicate that tricyclic antidepressants (particularly imipramine and desipramine), fluoxetine, monoamine oxidase inhibitors (MAOIs) and particularly phenelzine, as well as other antidepressants are useful in reducing binge eating and purging in bulimia nervosa (Agras et al, 1992; Walsh et al, 1991; Levine et al, 1992), although they are not by themselves an adequate treatment program and often more than one type will have to be tried before the best one for the patient is found. Common problems include medication compliance and maintaining good blood levels in the face of persistent vomiting. Fluoxetine and the tricyclics have been best studied and are used most frequently; they are effective in patients with or without concurrent major depression. In the case of MAOIs, patients are very prone to side effects and may have a hard time following a tyramine-free diet. Results of medication treatment are similar to those with cognitive-behavioral psychotherapies, and many patients who do not respond to psychological treatment alone benefit from medication; symptoms are reduced in 70 to 90% of patients, and about one-third are reported to become abstinent (Garfinkel and Garner, 1987). Some evidence suggests that combining medication and cognitive-behavioral psychotherapy is better than either treatment alone (Agras et al, 1992).

Hospitalization. Hospitalization is rarely indicated for uncomplicated bulimia nervosa. Indications include failure to respond to adequate outpatient treatment trials, worrisome medical complications not manageable in the outpatient setting, and a severe mood disorder with suicidality.

ROLE OF THE NONPSYCHIATRIC PHYSICIAN IN PATIENT MANAGEMENT

The nonpsychiatric physician should play a major role in the prevention, detection, and management of patients with eating disorders. Pediatricians and family physicians should be alert to excessive concerns about dieting and appearance in preteens and their families and educate them about healthy nutrition and the dangers of unrealistic appearance-oriented dieting and eating disorders. Because the prevalence of subclinical and full-blown forms of these disorders is so high, physicians should routinely question young female patients about what they desire to weigh; their dietary, dieting, and exercise practices; and their use of laxatives. Psychological problems in young women should stimulate attention to eating-disorder symptoms as well as to problems with mood, substance abuse, sexual behavior, etc. Gynecologists, internists, gastroenterologists, and dentists are also likely to encounter large numbers of eating-disorder patients in their practices.

Once an eating disorder is detected, patients merit a full physical exam; screening laboratory tests including electrolytes, complete blood count, thyroid, calcium, magnesium, and amylase studies; and, for the very thin patient, an electrocardiogram or rhythm strip. The physician should work together with a registered dietician and mental health worker knowledgeable about eating disorders to see if the problems can be ameliorated in outpatient care. With motivated patients this multidisciplinary team approach can be highly successful. The physician's role is to educate and monitor the patient's weight and laboratory tests. For the anorexia nervosa patient, monitoring should include weekly or twice weekly visits to the office for stripped postvoiding weights (with care taken that the patient has not imbibed large quantities of fluid just prior to being weighed) and for ongoing monitoring of any physiological abnormalities of concern.

For young adults, the physician should also be able to prescribe and monitor a course of antidepressant medication for patients with bulimia nervosa and mood or anxiety disorders associated with an eating disorder. The extent to which the physician is willing and/or able to assume a more intense involvement with the psychological and family issues varies considerably.

INDICATIONS FOR PSYCHIATRIC CONSULTATION AND REFERRAL

Every patient with a serious eating disorder warrants consultation with a psychiatrist knowledgeable about eating disorders for guidance to the patient, family, and referring physician about the nature, severity, and prognosis of the disorder, and regarding what treatment options are available. The physician can expect specific guidelines for psychosocial and medical management.

Specific indications for mandatory consultation include failure of the patient to respond to attempts at management in the physician's setting with deteriorating status, severe depression with suicidality, or marked family problems.

CLINICAL PEARLS

A high index of suspicion is warranted with all female adolescents and young adults. Most want to weigh too little.

- Alerting signs include menstrual irregularities, infertility, desires to weigh 10 to 15 pounds less than reasonable for habitus, overconcern with weight or physical appearance, vague gastrointestinal complaints, overuse of laxatives or diuretics, and mood disturbance.
- Signs of self-induced vomiting include puffy cheeks, scars on the knuckles, and decay of the front teeth.
- Alerting laboratory signs include mild disturbances in serum electrolytes, magnesium, and amylase.
- Patients with anorexia nervosa are often devious in providing information and in getting weighed (e.g., drinking large quantities of fluids or putting weights in their clothing). Alternative informants such as family members are always required.

ANNOTATED BIBLIOGRAPHY

Agras WS: Eating Disorders: Management of Obesity, Bulimia and Anorexia Nervosa. Oxford, Pergamon, 1987

Succinct review with special strengths in behavioral approaches to treatment.

American Psychiatric Association Practice Guidelines for Eating Disorders, Am J Psychiatry 150:207–228, 1993

A thorough review with authoritative treatment guidelines.

Garner DM, Garfinkel PE (eds): Handbook of Psychotherapy for Anorexia Nervosa and Bulimia. New York, Guilford Press, 1985

A major collection of authoritative articles describing the rationale and methods for diverse psychotherapeutic approaches including cognitive, behavioral, psychoeducational, and psychodynamic approaches to individual, group, and family therapy in the outpatient and inpatient setting.

Johnson C, Connors ME: The Etiology and Treatment of Bulimia Nervosa. New York, Basic Books, 1987

A complete review of all aspects of bulimia nervosa.

Hsu LKG: Eating Disorders. New York, Guilford Press, 1990

A concise and comprehensive textbook dealing with all aspects from phenomenology through treatment and prognosis.

Mitchell JE, Seim HC, Colon E et al: Medical complications and medical management of bulimia. Ann Int Med 107:71–77, 1987

A thorough review of the physiological problems found in this disorder with guidelines for the primary physician.

Rock CL, Yager J: Nutrition and eating disorders: A primer for clinicians. Int J Eating Disorders 6:267–280, 1987

A review of basic nutritional contributions to the pathogenesis of eating disorders, with corresponding nutrition-related treatment recommendations.

Russell GFM, Szmukler GI, Dare C, Eisler I: An evaluation of family therapy in anorexia nervosa and bulimia nervosa. Arch Gen Psychiatry 44:1047–1056, 1987

A sophisticated research study of 80 patients.

Yager, J. Family issues in the pathogenesis of anorexia nervosa. Psychosomatic Med 44:43–60, 1982

A review of theoretical and clinical aspects of the relationship of the appearance and course of anorexia nervosa to biological and interpersonal factors in families.

REFERENCES

Agras WS: Eating Disorders: Management of Obesity, Bulimia and Anorexia Nervosa. Oxford, Pergamon, 1987

Agras WS, Rossiter EM, Arnow B, Schneider JA, Telch CF, Raeburn SD, Bruce B, Perl M, Koran LM: Pharmacologic and cognitive-behavioral treatment for bulimia nervosa: A controlled comparison. Am J Psychiatry 149:82–87, 1992

American Psychiatric Association: DSM-IV Draft Criteria 3/1/93. Washington DC, American Psychiatric Association, 1993a

American Psychiatric Association: Diagnostic and Statistical Manual, 4th ed. Washington DC, American Psychiatric Association, in press [1994]

American Psychiatric Association: Practice guideline for eating disorders. Am J Psychiatry 150: 207–228, 1993b

Bruch H: Eating Disorders: Obesity, Anorexia Nervosa and the Person Within. New York, Basic Books, 1973

Crisp AH, Hall A, Holland AJ: Nature and nurture in anorexia nervosa: A study of 34 pairs of twins, one pair of triplets and an adoptive family. Int J Eating Disorders 4:5–29, 1985

Drewnowski A, Hopkins SA, Kessler RC: The prevalence of bulimia nervosa in the US college student population. Am J Public Health 78:1322–1325, 1988

Fairburn CG, Jones R, Peveler RK, Carr SJ, Solomon RA, O'Connor ME, Burtin J, Hope RA: Three psychological treatments for bulimia nervosa: A comparative trial. Arch Gen Psychiatry 48:463–469, 1991

Fairburn CG: A cognitive behavioral approach to the treatment of bulimia Psychological Med 11:707–711, 1981

Fava M, Copeland P, Schweiger U, Herzog D: Neurochemical abnormalities of anorexia nervosa and bulimia nervosa. Am J Psychiatry 146:963–971, 1989

Garfinkel PE, Garner DM: Anorexia Nervosa: A Multidimensional Perspective. New York, Brunner/Mazel, 1982

Garfinkel PE, Garner DM (eds): The Role of Drug Treatments for Eating Disorders. New York, Brunner/Mazel, 1987

Halmi KA, Eckert E, LaDu TJ et al: Anorexia nervosa: Treatment efficacy of cyproheptadine and amitriptyline. Arch Gen Psychiatry 43:177–181, 1986

Halmi KA, Eckert E, Marchi P, Sampugnaro V, Apple R, Cohen J: Comorbidity of psychiatric diagnosis in anorexia nervosa. Arch Gen Psychiatry 48:712–718, 1991

Hartmann A, Herzog T, Drinkmann A: Psychotherapy of bulimia nervosa: What is effective? A meta-analysis. J Psychosomatic Res 36:159–167, 1992

Hsu LKG: Outcome and Treatment Effects. In Beumont PJV, Burrows BD, Casper RC (eds): Handbook of Eating Disorders, Part I. Amsterdam, Elsevier, 1987

Johnson C, Connors ME: The Etiology and Treatment of Bulimia Nervosa. New York, Basic Books, 1987

Kaye WH, Weltzin TW, Hsu LKG, Bulick C: An open trial of fluoxetine in patients with anorexia nervosa. J Clin Psychiatry 52:464–471, 1991

Kendler KS, MacLean C, Neale M, Kessler R, Heath A, Eaves L: The genetic epidemiology of bulimia nervosa. Am J Psychiatry 148:1627–1637, 1991

Levine L et al (Fluoxetine Bulimia Nervosa Collaborative Study Group): Fluoxetine in the treatment of bulimia nervosa: A multicenter, placebo-controlled, double-blind trial. Arch Gen Psychiatry 49:139–147, 1992

Marrazzi MA, Luby ED: An auto-addiction opioid model of chronic anorexia nervosa. Int J Eating Disorders 5:191–208, 1986

Minuchin S, Rosman BL, Baker L: Psychosomatic Families: Anorexia Nervosa in Context. Cambridge, Harvard University Press, 1978

Mitchell JE, Seim HC, Colon E et al: Medical complications and medical management of bulimia. Ann Int Med 107:71–77, 1987

Oesterheld JR, McKenna MS, Gould NB: Group psychotherapy of bulimia: A critical review. Int J Group Psychotherapy 37:163–184, 1987

Russell GFM, Szmukler GI, Dare C et al: An evaluation of family therapy in anorexia nervosa and bulimia nervosal. Arch Gen Psychiatry 44:1047–1056, 1987

Steinhausen H-Ch, Rauss-Mason C, Seidel R: Follow-up studies of anorexia nervosa: A review of four decades of outcome research. Psychol Med 21:447–454, 1991

Walsh BT, Hadigan CM, Devlin MJ, Gladis M, Roose SP: Long-term outcome of antidepressant treatment for bulimia nervosa. Am J Psychiatry 148:1206–1212, 1991

Yager J: Family issues in the pathogenesis of anorexia nervosa. Psychosomatic Med 44:43–60, 1982

Yager J, Kurtsman F, Landsverk J et al: Behaviors and attitudes related to eating disorders in homosexual male college students. Am J Psychiatry 145:495–497, 1988a

Yager J, Landsverk J, Edelstein CK: A 20-month follow-up study of 628 women with eating disorders, Part I: Course and severity. Am J Psychiatry 144:1172–1177, 1988b

13 *Dissociative Disorders*

Mark E. James and Steven T. Levy

The diagnostic grouping "dissociative disorders" refers to a group of clinical conditions with the common feature of a disturbance of the integration of consciousness, memory, or identity. The disorders in the category are listed in Table 13–1. These disturbances may be sudden or gradual, transient or chronic. If memory for a significant period of time is lost in the absence of a neurologic disorder, a diagnosis of *dissociative amnesia* is made. If an individual loses memory for his or her entire previous identity and a new identity is assumed along with travel to a new location, the diagnosis is *dissociative fugue*. If more than one distinct personality dominates consciousness at different times in any individual, a diagnosis of *dissociative identity disorder* (or multiple personality disorder) is made. If an individual experiences him- or herself as unreal, strange, or changed in some way, yet remains in contact with reality in the absence of any gross change in identity, the diagnosis is *depersonalization disorder* as long as these symptoms are not part of any other known psychiatric disorder.

This grouping of psychiatric disorders is based both on the similarity of clinical manifestations seen in each, as well as by a presumed underlying psychological process: the phenomenon of *dissociation*. Dissociation is an activity of the mind that results in a "separation of mental structures or content that were previously connected or associatively linked" (Counts, 1990). All individuals are capable of experiencing variable degrees of dissociative alterations of consciousness, information processing, and memory storage and retrieval. Such dissociative experiences of everyday life include "spacing off" during a conversation or lecture; daydreaming; becoming immersed in a movie; or doing something automatically, such as driving a car "on

Table 13–1 **Dissociative Disorders**

Dissociative Amnesia
Dissociative Fugue
Dissociative Identity Disorder (Multiple Personality Disorder)
Depersonalization Disorder
Dissociative Disorder Not Otherwise Specified

autopilot" with little memory of part of the trip. Other phenomena in which dissociative processes play a role include hypnosis, meditation, and other trance phenomena; states of religious fervor and ecstasy; and, in some cultures, states of spirit possession. When dissociation becomes extreme and causes significant distress or impairment of functioning, psychiatric diagnosis and intervention become warranted.

By virtue of their dramatic character, the dissociative disorders have long been of interest to psychiatrists. Explanations of dissociation play an important role in the history of modern psychiatry. Early attempts to explore the process of dissociation did not link it exclusively with those disorders now grouped together in DSM-IV (APA 1993, in press [1994]) as the dissociative disorders. Early investigators thought that a variety of other clinical entities, including hysteria and somnambulism, involved dissociative mechanisms.

Pierre Janet is usually given credit for first using the term "dissociation" in relation to mental disorders. He viewed dissociation as a pathological process in which traumatic memories could not be integrated into preexisting cognitive structures and were instead split off to form "subconscious fixed ideas" that existed outside of an individual's usual conscious experience and continued to exert an effect on behavior (van der Kolk and van der Hart, 1989). According to Janet, dissociation might occur when an individual's mind was weakened, either because of constitutional factors or due to acute states of fatigue, illness, intoxication, or extreme emotional arousal. Josef Breuer (Breuer and Freud, 1893–1895) agreed that pathogenic ideas may be split off from normal conscious awareness in the context of extreme emotional arousal, but added that this may also occur in individuals who enter into abnormal "hypnoid states." Sigmund Freud came to understand the process of the splitting of consciousness differently. In his work with patients, he noticed that certain thoughts were actively kept outside conscious awareness by defensive processes designed to ward off painful feelings resulting from conflict between wishful and prohibited thoughts. This idea that certain mental content can be banned from consciousness (repression) by being unacceptable to the individual became a cornerstone of dynamic psychiatry.

As a part of our modern diagnostic system, dissociative disorders are distinguished by both their clinical manifestations and a presumed common underlying psychological mechanism. This is a departure from diagnostic criteria used in other DSM-IV syndromes, which are diagnosed only on the basis of observable signs and symptoms or known neurologic factors.

Since these early explorations of dissociative processes, various other explanations have been hypothesized. For example, neurobiological investigators have suggested that the disturbances of cognitive integration and memory function seen in dissociative disorders may reflect an underlying pathology of temporal lobe functioning. Patients in dissociated states may demonstrate alterations of brain physiology (electroencephalogram patterns, visual evoked responses, cerebral blood flow), autonomic functioning, dominant-handedness, allergic sensitivities, visual acuity and visual fields, and different responses to medications; how these differences come about remains unclear and speculative. Because these disorders are relatively rare, it has been difficult to study them in a systematic and longitudinal manner.

The capacity for gross alterations in conscious experience, such as is present in patients with dissociative disorders, represents a profound disturbance in mental life available to few individuals. When it does occur, it is usually in the face of overwhelmingly traumatic experiences or memories. Clinical manifestations vary from the mild disturbances seen in many patients with transient depersonalization experiences to episodic and short-lived dramatic episodes of amnesia and fugue to lifelong patterns of disturbance of the greatest severity in certain patients with multiple personality disorder. The various dissociative disorders will be discussed individually in terms of description, etiology, and treatment, with common or linking trends emphasized where appropriate.

DISSOCIATIVE AMNESIA

The following often-cited case of dissociative amnesia in colonial America was described by Benjamin Rush, "the father of American psychiatry," in his lectures (Carlson, 1981). A man named William Tenent, who was preparing for an examination for the Presbyterian ministry, developed an illness with chest pain, intermittent fever, and severe emaciation. He eventually collapsed and was believed dead. Funeral preparations were forestalled by his physician, who believed he felt a slight warmth in Tenent's body. After three days, the presumed corpse "opened its eyes, gave a dreadful groan, and sunk again into apparent death." This occurred again two more times, but after the last he regained consciousness.

He gradually recovered fully during the next year but was completely amnestic for his entire life before the deathlike state. Because he also lost his ability to read or write, his brother began teaching him these skills. One day during a Latin lesson, he suddenly felt a shock in his head. He remembered reading the book before. More recollections occurred and he eventually recovered all memories of his life. He also described an experience during a three-day coma in which he was "transported by a superior being to a place of ineffable glory." He remained healthy for the next 45 years. He became a minister, married, and had three sons.

Description

Dissociative amnesia is characterized by an inability to recall significant personal information beyond what could be explained by ordinary forgetfulness. The most common presentation of dissociative amnesia is a *localized* or circumscribed disturbance of recall; that is, the patient cannot recall any events that occurred during a certain time period, usually the first few hours after a severely upsetting event of a stressful or traumatic nature (Fig. 13–1). Less common is *selective* amnesia, in which certain but not all events within a specified time period are not remembered. On rare occasions a patient may develop *generalized* amnesia (in which the patient cannot recall any information about his or her entire preceding life) or *continuous* amnesia (in which the patient cannot remember anything following a specific event and continuing to the immediate present). In the case above, William Tenent's amnesia was most likely the generalized type. Whether it was psychogenic or caused by his illness is open to speculation.

An episode of dissociative amnesia is usually precipitated by a particularly intense psychological trauma or stressor, either some threat of harm or death, an intolerable and/or inescapable life situation, or a morally unacceptable impulse or act. In some individuals, the amnesia may be preceded by a headache or some alteration of consciousness experienced as sleepiness or dizziness. Occasionally, an amnestic patient may wander aimlessly until the police eventually bring her or him to an emergency room. Some affected individuals may be unaware of their memory disturbance until confronted by another person. Some feel distressed by the

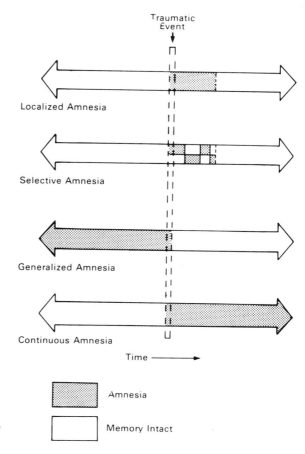

Figure 13–1 *Types of dissociative amnesia.*

amnesia, others seem indifferent, and some may make up information to fill in what is missing.

Epidemiology

The epidemiology of dissociative amnesia is poorly understood. It is believed to be most common in adolescent and young adult females and is most rare in the elderly. There is no information on familial transmission. During war, dissociative amnesia may occur in as many as 5 to 8% of combat soldiers. The incidence is believed to rise during disasters.

Etiology

The precise psychological and/or neurological mechanisms of dissociative amnesia are unknown. One hypothetical model suggests that, in the face of overwhelming psychological trauma, mental mechanisms are activated in susceptible individuals that interfere with the normal retrieval of stored, anxiety-provoking information. The person can then function relatively adaptively compared to the cognitive disequilibrium that might result if the trauma continued to be experienced consciously (as occurs in patients with acute posttraumatic stress disorders). Obviously, the amnesia itself can become disabling or maladaptive.

How memories are sequestered outside of awareness is unclear. One possibility is that a neurologically based retrieval deficit or faulty encoding and storage of information may cause dissociative amnesia since these dysfunctions also cause other types of amnesia. Yet memories can often be recovered using hypnosis or a sodium amobarbital interview, so some capacity for storage and retrieval must remain intact on some level. The psychoanalytic model describes amnesia as unconsciously motivated. If a memory or thought is sufficiently conflict laden or traumatic so that conscious awareness of it is accompanied by significant anxiety, the mind will activate defense mechanisms such as repression to keep the memory or thought outside conscious awareness. The state-dependent learning model suggests that information storage and retrieval depends on the person's state of consciousness. If memories are stored under extreme emotional turmoil, they may not be accessible in other emotional states, resulting in amnesia.

Differential Diagnosis

Any of several neurologic etiologies of amnesia should be ruled out by careful medical-neurological evaluation, particularly central nervous system disease, intoxication, and metabolic derangement (Table 13–2). The classic substance-induced amnesia is the "alcoholic blackout." Chronic alcohol use also may result in anterograde memory disturbances. Postconcussion amnesia may occur after head trauma. Epileptic seizures usually are accompanied by a period of amnesia. If a patient in legal trouble stands to gain by forgetting a period of time, malingering or feigned amnesia should be considered. The short acting benzodiazepine triazolem may cause anterograde amnesia.

Table 13–2 **Medical and Neurological Disorders Causing Dissociative Symptoms**

Alcohol Intoxication—Blackout
Alcohol Amnestic Disorder
Postconcussion Amnesia
Complex Partial Seizures
Migraine Syndromes
Transient Global Amnesia
Carbon Monoxide Poisoning
Hypoglycemia
Hallucinogen Intoxication
Hallucinogen Persisting Perception Disorder (flashback)

Diagnostic Evaluation

For all dissociative syndromes, evaluation should begin with a thorough, comprehensive history. Physical examination should include a complete neurological examination, looking especially for evidence of head injury, intoxication, or focal neurological deficits. Findings on the mental status examination that would point toward a neurologic cause of dissociative syndromes would include clouding of consciousness, impaired attention, disorientation, slurred speech, blunted or labile affect, disorganized flow of thought associations, difficulty with complex mental tasks, impaired cognition beyond specific memory losses, inability to learn new things, and confabulation.

Laboratory evaluation should include assessment of glucose, electrolytes, CO_2, renal and hepatic functioning, blood-alcohol level, and a urine drug screen. Additionally, an electroencephalogram, computed tomography or magnetic resonance imaging of the brain, and neuropsychological testing may be performed. (See Chapters 3 and 4).

Treatment

Therapy involves two general principles: first, to remove the patient from the threatening circumstances, often by hospitalization; second, to explore their distress through psychotherapy. Some recommend an approach designed to retrieve the repressed memories as rapidly as possible, either through free association, hypnosis, or amobarbital interviews. Others believe this approach may be deleterious and advise instead exploring the patient's life situation and any psychological conflicts that may have resulted in the onset of amnesia under the given circumstances in a more circumspect manner.

Psychotropic medications (except for amobarbital interviews) are rarely helpful in treating dissociative amnesia. During therapy, the amnesia often clears rapidly, sometimes completely.

DISSOCIATIVE FUGUE

William James described a famous case of dissociative fugue in *Principles of Psychology* (1918):

Ansel Bourne, a 60-year-old evangelist, disappeared from Providence, Rhode Island. About two weeks thereafter, a man named A.J. Brown opened a small shop in Norristown, Pennsylvania. He conducted business in a quiet and orderly fashion. Six weeks later, he woke up in a frightened state. He said his name was Ansel Bourne, asked to know where he was, and said he had no knowledge of Norristown or shopkeeping. His last memory was of conducting some personal business in Providence, and he could not believe two months had passed. He returned home and maintained complete amnesia for the interval. James later examined Bourne under hypnosis; in this state he evoked the personality of A.J. Brown, who recounted the events in Norristown. James could never facilitate Bourne's recall of any of Brown's memories.

Description

During a classic dissociative fugue a person suddenly and unexpectedly travels away from their home or work place; are unable to recall their past; and are confused about their identity or assume a new identity. During a fugue state, a person may appear perplexed or disoriented. After recovery from the fugue, there is no recall of events that took place during the episode. Patients typically present for help after the fugue, wanting to recall what happened.

Only occasionally will a fugue manifest the more dramatic and classical presentation in which a quiet, ordinary person suddenly assumes a more gregarious, uninhibited manner, travels thousands of miles, and carries on a new, complex social existence for months with a different name and a well-integrated new identity before ultimately shifting back into the former identity with no memory of the interval. More typically, the episode is less elaborate. The affected person engages in brief and apparently purposeful travel, but the new identity is less complete and socialization with others may be minimal. Most episodes of dissociative fugue last several hours to a few days.

Occurrence

As with dissociative amnesia, the occurrence of dissociative fugue increases during wartime or natural disasters. Many cases reported are of soldiers in combat who wandered away from duty. The age of onset is variable. Little information exists about sex ratio or familial incidence.

Etiology

The pathological cause of fugue states is unknown. The same dissociative mental mechanisms discussed under dissociative amnesia apply to dissociative fugue, but in fugue states a different identity is created. This phenomenon is precipitated by severe psychological stress.

Differential Diagnosis and Treatment

As mentioned, evaluation and treatment is usually sought after the fugue has resolved. As with amnesia, the differential diagnosis must include the same list of disorders. Multiple personality disorder should also be ruled out. Treatment of dissociative fugue involves the same principles discussed under dissociative amnesia.

DISSOCIATIVE IDENTITY DISORDER (MULTIPLE PERSONALITY DISORDER)

Description

Multiple personality disorder (newly termed Dissociative Identity Disorder in DSM-IV) is a condition in which there are two or more identities or personalities with each having a distinct pattern of perception, thought, and relating to the environment, and which recurrently take control of the person's behavior. The personality who presents for treatment is usually unaware of the existence of the other personalities. He or she may instead report time lapses, blackouts, or "spells," or may have been told by others about unusual episodes of behavior during which the patient referred to himself or herself by another name (the patient has amnesia for the occurrence). The patient may report hearing voices inside his or her head and may feel controlled by them. Affected individuals also often experience depression, nightmares, suicide attempts, phobias, rapid mood shifts, severe anxiety, depersonalization or derealization, and headaches (Bliss, 1984).

As diagnostic evaluation and treatment proceed, particularly if hypnosis or a sodium amobarbital interview is used, the various personalities manifest themselves. Transition from one to another may also be brought about by severe life stress. The personalities are often quite different: they may appear normal or severely pathological (for example, psychotic or self-mutilating); they may vary in age, sex, race, and habits; and they may prefer different social circles. Each personality may have different mannerisms, speech, cognitive styles, patterns of affect, and behavior, even differing in dominant-handedness. Some personalities may be aware of the presence of the other personalities, while others may not.

There are often significant differences in psychological test profiles and psychophysiological characteristics between personalities. Many studies over the years have replicated the finding of differential skin conductance (galvanic skin response) between personalities. Other measures of autonomic nervous system activity also differ, such as heart rate and muscle tone (Putnam et al, 1990). Optical differences have also been found, including altered visual acuity, visual fields, color vision, and measures of ocular physiology and eye muscle balance across personalities (Miller et al, 1991). Allergic sensitivities and response to medication may vary. Studies of brain physiology suggest different EEG patterns, evoked responses, and regional cerebral blood flow between personalities, but larger studies are needed to verify these findings.

Illustrative Case

One of the most famous cases of multiple personality disorder was Sally Beauchamp, described by Morton Prince in *The Dissociation of a Personality* (1906). Her different personalities had "different trains of thought,... different views, beliefs, ideals, and temperament, and... different acquisitions, tastes, habits, experiences, and memories." She presented for treatment as a conscientious, well-educated young woman who appeared to be an "extreme neurasthenic." She was easily fatigued and had numerous physical complaints. Additionally she was impressionable and emotional, suggesting the diagnosis of hysteria.

Her developmental history indicated that her parents had an unhappy marriage. Her father had a violent temper, and she felt disliked by her mother, who either ignored her or reprimanded her. Miss Beauchamp tended to idealize her mother and blamed herself. She kept feelings to herself and withdrew into fantasy. When she was 7, a brother was born but died soon after. When she was 13 her mother died of a postpartum infection. During the next three years with her father she suffered "continual mental shocks and strains." She had frequent headaches, nightmares, and fatigue. She had "attacks of somnambulism" and would go into trancelike states. At age 16 she ran away from home. Five years prior to seeking treatment she became increasingly agitated and nervous and underwent a gradual change of character.

Dr. Prince began treatment using hypnotherapy. Soon thereafter, during a hypnotic trance, a second personality emerged, which the doctor and patient eventually named "Sally." This personality was physically healthy with considerable stamina. She was lively, bold, amoral, and adventurous. She played mischievous pranks on Miss Beauchamp, such as causing automatisms, telling lies, or going on long walks that caused Miss Beauchamp to feel very fatigued.

Over a year into the treatment a third personality emerged. She had more "womanly" traits and was vivacious, stubborn, ambitious, confident, and self-centered. She had more self-control, courage, and less reserve than Miss Beauchamp and was more "normal" in many respects. This personality remained unnamed, although the patient sometimes referred to her as "the idiot." Dr. Prince came to think of the three personalities as "the saint, the woman, and the devil." He eventually concluded that the patient's original "true" personality had dissociated into her presenting (Miss Beauchamp) personality and the third (unnamed) personality. Sally represented a dissociated state that would come and go. During the six years of treatment the first and third personalities were reintegrated, and the patient felt healthier and functioned better. Sally persisted and continued to "act up."

Occurrence

Multiple personality disorder was previously believed to be rare, with only about 200 reported cases in the literature, but within the past decade there has been an explosion of reports (over 3,000 cases). Investigators who actively look for dissociative disorders report a prevalence of multiple personality in approximately 2 to 5% of individuals screened. There is controversy in this area, however. At one end are investigators who believe dissociation and multiple personality are common and have been historically underdiagnosed or misdiagnosed (Kluft, 1987; Ross et al, 1991). At the other end are investigators who believe that the spontaneous occurrence of multiple personality is rare and that it may be produced iatrogenically in the clinical setting by suggestion (hypnotic or otherwise) or by behavioral shaping in suggestible hysterical patients who are eager to please the doctor (Merskey, 1992). More research is necessary to resolve this debate. Multiple personality disorder almost always begins in childhood, but individuals often do not come to clinical attention until adolescence or adulthood. It is more common in women than men and is more common in first-degree relatives of probands than in the general population.

Etiology

Almost all cases are preceded by physical, sexual, or emotional abuse or exposure to extreme, overwhelming trauma during childhood. Affected individuals seem to have an increased tendency or ability to enter dissociative states or autohypnotic states. Hypothetically, during extreme childhood abuse or trauma, this mechanism may protect the patient from being overwhelmed or incapacitated. However, if the dissociation is acquired through learning or conditioning as a coping strategy, information processed during different states of consciousness may be encoded and stored in different "circuits" inaccessible to one another, which eventually results in the development of different state-dependent personalities. On a biological level, repeated experiences of traumatization may induce an alteration in temporal-limbic circuits analogous to the phenomenon of kindling seen in epilepsy. This may have the result of permanent alterations in the integration of sensory inputs, affects, memories, and cognition. These etiologic explanations remain speculative and will require further study to validate.

Some have noted a similarity between multiple personality disorder and borderline personality disorder (see Chapter 5 by Drs. Ninan and Mance). Patients with either disorder often suffer from depression, anxiety, emotional instability, interpersonal turmoil, and self-destructive behavior. Both groups use "primitive" defense mechanisms, including splitting, denial, dissociation, and projection. Both typically have a history of abuse during childhood. Whether or not the two groups have any etiologic connection is uncertain.

Differential Diagnosis

These patients may be diagnosed as having other psychiatric disorders, particularly schizophrenia, because of the possible history of hearing voices, believing themselves to be influenced by some unknown force, expressing strange ideas, and shifting patterns of identity. As mentioned, co-morbidity may include anxiety disorders, depression, and personality disorders. Dissociative amnesia and dissociative fugue also should be considered. As with amnesia and fugue, any medical or neurological conditions that cause alterations of consciousness, such as drug or alcohol intoxication or withdrawal, metabolic disturbances, and complex partial seizures, should be ruled out. Malingering and factitious disorder with psychological symptoms presenting as multiple personality disorder should also be included in the differential diagnosis.

The diagnosis of multiple personality disorder often brings with it something verging on celebrity status to the patient among psychiatrists and other mental health workers, who may be fascinated by the patient's symptoms. The physician must maintain a high index of suspicion for malingering or elaboration of symptoms in a patient with symptoms of multiple personality disorder who is involved in a criminal justice proceeding and may be seeking a psychiatric defense.

Treatment

Various psychotropic medications may be indicated for relief of symptoms if a patient with multiple personality disorder shows evidence of severe depression, psychosis, or anxiety. If such symptoms pertain to only one or a subgroup of the alter personalities, however, the patient as a whole may not respond particularly well to medication. If EEG findings are suggestive of temporal lobe pathology, an anticonvulsant such as carbamazepine may be of benefit to the patient (Fichtner et al, 1990). Psychotherapy can be used in an attempt to examine and ideally to change the use of dissociation and other pathological defense mechanisms by these patients. Some clinicians advocate using hypnosis to elicit the various personalities and eventually to reintegrate therapeutically the dissociated or split-off aspects of experience. Others believe this technique may reinforce the use of autohypnotic dissociation by patients. In therapy, the patient's past traumas and current stressors and conflicts should be explored supportively to facilitate insight and improve adaptation.

DEPERSONALIZATION DISORDER

Description

Depersonalization is an alteration of experience in which a person feels detached from, or like an outside observer of, his or her body or mental processes. It often is accompanied by a dreamlike state. During a depersonalization episode, the person maintains intact reality testing and is generally distressed by the experience.

The symptom of depersonalization occurs in a number of disorders, including posttraumatic stress disorder, panic disorder, agoraphobia, anxiety disorders due to substances and general medical conditions, hallucinogen intoxication or hallucinogen persisting perception disorder (e.g., LSD flashbacks), severe depression, and schizophrenia (Table 13–3). Patients with seizure disorders, particularly complex partial seizures (especially those of temporal lobe origin) and other brain diseases, may experience depersonalization. Finally, depersonalization can occur in normal people as a result of stress, fatigue, or sleep deprivation. When depersonalization occurs recurrently or persistently in the absence of any of the disorders listed, a diagnosis of depersonalization disorder is made.

Depersonalization may be accompanied by derealization, which involves a sense of the unreality of objects in the external world (as opposed to the alteration of perception of one's self that occurs in depersonalization). Patients with depersonalization disorder may also complain of depression, anxiety, dizziness, obsessional thoughts, somatic worries, and a fear of going insane.

Table 13–3 Other Psychiatric Disorders Presenting with Symptoms of Dissociation

Drug Intoxication or Withdrawal
Schizophrenia and other Psychotic Disorders
Depression
Panic Disorder
Agoraphobia
Anxiety Disorder due to General Medical Conditions or Substances
Posttraumatic Stress Disorder
Borderline Personality Disorder
Factitious Disorder
Malingering

This condition is usually chronic with exacerbations and remissions. Patient impairment is widely variable, and some may develop secondary alcohol or drug dependence or hypochondriasis.

Occurrence

Although single episodes of depersonalization occur in the majority of the population, the prevalence, sex ratio, and familial occurrence of depersonalization disorder are unknown.

Etiology

As with the other dissociative disorders, the etiology of depersonalization disorder is unclear. Intensely traumatic events such as military combat or physical assault may contribute to onset of the disorder. Psychoanalytic theories have viewed depersonalization as a defense against forbidden impulses, as a symptom of defective ego functioning, as a consequence of violation of one's ideals or conscience under abnormal circumstances, and as a response to interpersonal invalidation by significant others. The induction of depersonalization by hallucinogens indicates some neurologic substrate for the symptoms of this disorder.

Treatment

Psychopharmacologic interventions may be used for accompanying symptoms such as anxiety, depression, or obsessions, but the value of medication for depersonalization itself is unknown. Antipsychotics seem to make the condition worse.

The value of psychotherapy is also unknown, but a useful approach would generically include providing support, exploring ongoing stressors, examining the events and thoughts related to the onset of depersonalization experiences, and working to modify psychological defenses and intrapsychic conflicts.

DISSOCIATIVE DISORDER NOT OTHERWISE SPECIFIED

This category includes any disorders in which a dissociative symptom predominates but does not meet criteria for a particular specific dissociative disorder. Examples include cases resembling multiple personality disorder in which other personality states are indistinct or amnesia does not occur; derealization experiences without depersonalization; dissociative states occurring in individuals subjected to "brainwashing" or indoctrination while held captive by cultists or terrorists; stupor, coma, or loss of consciousness not due to a general medical condition; and trance or possession states occurring in particular cultures. In many of the world's societies and cultures, dissociative phenomena manifest most often as states of possession by a spirit, demon, power, or another person, or as experiences of entering trance states beyond one's control, so a separate diagnostic classification is under consideration to account for this, termed dissociative trance disorder.

ROLE OF THE NONPSYCHIATRIC PHYSICIAN AND INDICATIONS FOR PSYCHIATRIC CONSULTATION AND REFERRAL

Most patients with dissociative disorders will present for medical evaluation or treatment with complaints of amnesia, alteration of consciousness, or deteriorating psychosocial functioning. The nonpsychiatrist should be able to recognize these disorders clinically and formulate a differential diagnosis, including both neuropsychiatric and medical diagnoses. All patients with dissociative disorders should be referred for psychiatric intervention since these conditions are complex and require specialized management. The nonpsychiatrist should not leap to the conclusion that patients with dissociative symptoms should be referred elsewhere without first conducting a thorough medical-neurological evaluation to rule out the various illnesses that cause dissociative symptoms.

The dissociative disorders are dramatic clinical entities. They stirred the interest of early psychodynamic investigators, leading to the formulation of concepts such as intrapsychic conflict, altered states of consciousness, mechanisms of defense, and unconscious mental content, which all play a role in the process described as dissociation. These dynamic mental phenomena have become part of our understanding of mental life in general and of various kinds of psychopathology. The dissociative disorders remain poorly understood manifestations of the complexity of mental life.

Patients with such disorders come to the attention of psychiatrists less often than those with more familiar clinical entities. By virtue of their dramatic presentation, such patients are often thought to be feigning their symptoms and are regularly treated with suspicion, mistrust, and even derision. Clinicians are challenged to maintain a professionally appropriate, unbiased, and technically neutral stance in attempting to understand the distress of these perplexing patients. Treatment planning must be flexible and innovative. When confronted with bizarre and somewhat theatrical behaviors, the clinician must persistently strive to be empathic, supportive, and vigorously objective. Many patients are the victims of severe past and present traumas and are reluctant to engage in any self-exploration. A negative attitude by the clinician further alienates the patient and makes a collaborative exploratory effort even less likely.

Dissociative mechanisms are particularly anxiety-provoking for physicians because, despite their bizarre appearance, they occur in patients who appear in other respects in touch with reality, and thus not radically different from those providing them with psychiatric care. Such mechanisms represent extreme instances of psychological processes that are constantly active in all individuals. Therefore, they continue to hold our scientific interest. Ideally, more systematic investigation will lead to a better understanding of them and subsequent improved responsiveness to treatment interventions.

CLINICAL PEARLS

The dissociative disorders should be considered in the differential diagnosis of any patient presenting with alteration of consciousness, amnesia, "spells," disturbance of identity, or alteration of feelings of reality.

- A complete medical-neurological evaluation should be conducted on these patients to rule out the multiple neurologic causes of dissociative symptoms.
- The etiology of dissociative disorders is still poorly understood. Modern theories reflect the thinking of the early pioneers including Janet, James, Prince, Breuer, and Freud. All include the theory that some pathogenic mental content is split off from conscious awareness but continues to exert an influence on emotions, thought, and behavior. This splitting of the mind is thought to arise from state-dependent memory storage (Janet), autohypnotic phenomena (Breuer), and from repression and other defense mechanisms occurring in the context of conflicting forces in the mind (Freud). Neurobiological theory also suggests a role of pathological temporal-limbic functioning that causes a disordered integration of the storage and retrieval of memories.
- Psychological trauma plays a large pathogenic role in the development of dissociative disorders. Multiple personality disorder in particular may arise out of severe childhood physical and sexual abuse.
- Although certain medications may help with symptoms of anxiety, depression, or violent behavior in some patients with dissociative disorders, the treatment of choice continues to be psychotherapy.

ANNOTATED BIBLIOGRAPHY

Bliss EL: Multiple Personality, Allied Disorders, and Hypnosis. New York, Oxford University Press, 1986
> This book discusses the theory and practice of hypnosis and goes on to describe multiple personality and other dissociative disorders and their relationship to autohypnotic phenomena.

Bloch JP: Assessment and Treatment of Multiple Personality and Dissociative Disorders. Sarasota, FL, Professional Resource Press, 1991

The author discusses the identification, diagnosis, assessment, and treatment of dissociative disorders. He defines dissociation as a "defense against the disabling effects of severe and ongoing traumatization during childhood and later development."

Braun BG: Treatment of Multiple Personality Disorder. Washington, DC, American Psychiatric Press, 1986

The chapters of this book discuss different therapeutic approaches including psychotherapy, medication, group therapy, psychoanalysis, and social interventions.

Braun BG (ed): Symposium on multiple personality. Psychiat Clin Am 7:1–198, 1984

This issue contains review articles on various topics related to multiple personality disorder.

Breuer J, Freud S: Studies on Hysteria. In The Standard Edition of the Complete Psychological Works of Sigmund Freud, Vol. 2, 1893–1895. London, Hogarth Press, 1955

This monumental work depicts Breuer and Freud's differing conceptions of the pathogenesis of hysterical phenomena, including both conversion and dissociative mechanisms. Freud goes on to describe the psychological treatment of hysteria.

Fisher C: Amnesic states in war neuroses: The psychogenesis of fugues. Psychoanal Q 14:437–468, 1945

This classic paper discusses the psychodynamic processes involved in dissociation, with emphasis on amnesia and fugue.

Kenny MG: The Passion of Ansel Bourne: Multiple Personality in American Culture. Washington, DC, Smithsonian Institution Press, 1986

This book describes the work of pioneering investigators—including William James and Morton Prince in America and Charcot, Janet, and Freud in Europe—and elaborates on many of the famous cases described by the Americans. It provides a rich historical perspective on the theories of dissociation.

Kluft RP (ed): Childhood antecedents of multiple personality. Washington, DC, American Psychiatric Press, 1985

The chapters of this book describe how severe abuse during childhood can lead to the use of dissociative mechanisms and may result in the development of multiple personality.

Lowenstein RJ (ed): Multiple personality disorder. Psychiat Clin N Am 14:489–791, 1991

This issue of the quarterly publication is devoted to reviews of a variety of aspects of multiple personality disorder.

Nemiah JC: Dissociative disorders (Hysterical Neurosis, Dissociative Type). In Kaplan HI, Sadock BJ (eds): Comprehensive Textbook of Psychiatry/V, 5th ed. Baltimore, Williams & Wilkins, 1989

This textbook chapter by an eminent psychiatrist offers an excellent review of the concepts of hysteria, dissociation, and the dissociative disorders.

Putnam FW: Diagnosis and Treatment of Multiple Personality Disorder. New York, Guilford Press, 1989

The author describes his views of multiple personality disorder and discusses approaches to diagnosis and treatment.

Ross CA: Multiple Personality Disorder: Diagnosis, Clinical Features, and Treatment. New York, John Wiley and Sons, 1989

This book covers the history of the concept of multiple personality, diagnostic and clinical considerations including the use of structured interviews and self-report measures, and discusses principles of treatment.

REFERENCES

Abse DW: Hysterical Conversion and Dissociative Syndromes and the Hysterical Character. In Arieti S, Brody EB (eds): American Handbook of Psychiatry, 2nd ed, Vol. 3. New York, Basic Books, 1974

American Psychiatric Association: DSM-IV Draft Criteria 3/1/93. Washington, DC, American Psychiatric Association, 1993

American Psychiatric Association, Diagnostic and Statistical Manual of Mental Disorders, 4th ed. Washington, DC, in press [1994]

Bliss EL: A symptom profile of patients with multiple personalities, including MMPI results. J Nerv Ment Dis, 172:197–201, 1984

Braun BG (ed): Symposium on multiple personality. Psychiatr Clin N Am 7:1–198, 1984

Breuer J, Freud S: Studies on Hysteria. In The Standard Edition of the Complete Psychological Works of Sigmund Freud, Vol. 2, 1893–1895. London, Hogarth Press, 1955

Carlson ET: The history of multiple personality in the United States: I. The beginnings. Am J Psychiatry 138:666–668, 1981

Counts RM: The concept of dissociation. J Am Acad Psychoanal 18:460–479, 1990

Fichtner CG, Kuhlman DT, Gruenfeld MJ et al: Decreased episodic violence and increased control of dissociation in a carbamazepine-treated case of multiple personality. Biol Psychiatry 27:1045–1052, 1990

Gilmore MM, Kaufman C: Dissociative Disorders. In Michels R, Cavenar JO, Brodie HKH et al (eds): Psychiatry. Philadelphia, JB Lippincott, 1985

James W: The Principles of Psychology. New York, Dover, 1918

Kluft RP: An update on multiple personality disorder. Hosp Comm Psychiatry 38:363–373, 1987

Kopelman MD: Amnesia: Organic and psychogenic. Br J Psychiatry, 150:428–442, 1987

Lowenstein RJ (ed): Multiple personality disorder. Psychiatr Clin N Am 14:489–791, 1991

Merskey H: The manufacture of personalities: The production of multiple personality disorder. Br J Psychiatry 160:327–340, 1992

Miller SD, Blackburn T, Scholes G et al: Optical differences in multiple personality disorder: A second look. J Nerv Ment Dis 179:132–135, 1991

Nemiah JC: Dissociative Disorders (Hysterical Neurosis, Dissociative Type). In Kaplan HI, Sadock BJ (eds): Comprehensive Textbook of Psychiatry/V, 5th ed. Baltimore, Williams & Wilkins, 1989

Prince M: The Dissociation of a Personality. New York, Longmans Green, 1906

Putnam FW, Zahn TP, Post RM: Differential autonomic nervous system activity in multiple personality disorder. Psychiatr Res 31:251–260, 1990

Riether AM, Stoudemire A: Psychogenic fugue states: A review. South Med J 81:568–571, 1988

Ross CA, Joshi S, Currie R: Dissociative experiences in the general population: A factor analysis. Hosp Comm Psychiatry 42:297–301, 1991

van der Kolk BA, van der Hart O: Pierre Janet and the breakdown of adaptation in psychological trauma. Am J Psychiatry 146:1530–1540, 1989

Alan Stoudemire (ed). *Clinical Psychiatry for Medical Students,* Second Edition. Copyright © 1994, 1990 by J. B. Lippincott Company.

14 *Psychosexual Disorders*

Peter J. Fagan and
Chester W. Schmidt, Jr.

Sexual dysfunction is a subclass of sexual disorders in which the essential feature is inhibition in sexual interest or in psychophysiologic disturbances in the sexual response cycle. Sexual dysfunction is distinguished from the other sexual disorder group, paraphilias, in which there is generally no impairment in sexual function. A third category of disorders closely related to sexuality is disorders of gender identity. Readers who wish to learn more about this diagnostic group might consult Blanchard and Steiner (1990) or Stoller (1985).

Sexual dysfunction is not a life-threatening condition, but the negative effects it can have on a patient's self-esteem or relationship should not be underestimated. Given the multiple biological, psychological, and social aspects of human sexual behavior, sexual dysfunctions require a careful and thorough diagnostic evaluation. Because sexuality is so central to self-esteem and the ability to relate to others, a person with a sexual dysfunction deserves skillful and sensitive therapy.

EPIDEMIOLOGY

There is no one adequate demographic survey of the incidence and prevalence of sexual dysfunction in the general population of the United States. The most recent review of the literature on these data was conducted by Spector and Carey (1990) and their general results are seen in Table 14–1. A similar review by Nathan (1986) suggests that the prevalence of arousal and pain disorders among women is less than 5%.

Table 14–1 **Estimated Prevalence of Sexual Dysfunction among the General Population (Spector and Carey, 1990)**

SEXUAL DYSFUNCTION	MEN	WOMEN
Hypoactive desire	16%	34%
Erectile disorder	4–9%	—
Orgasmic disorder	4–10%	4–9%
Premature ejaculation	36–38%	—
Female arousal, dyspareunia, vaginismus	—	n/a

Among those with medical illnesses or postsurgical conditions, the prevalence of sexual dysfunction due to contributing psychogenic factors has been understandably difficult to establish because of the covarying effects of the medical illness. While sample sizes of studies of specific medical conditions are generally too small for epidemiological purposes and specific psychogenic factors are usually not identified, sexual dysfunction is in general clearly highly prevalent among the medically ill (Schover and Jensen, 1988; Kolodny, Masters, and Johnson, 1979; Wise and Schmidt, 1985). There is an increase in orgasmic and erectile dysfunction among the medically ill and a decrease in the incidence of premature ejaculation (Spector and Carey, 1990).

About 30% of sexually dysfunctional individuals also have an additional (Axis I) psychiatric disorder that is not a primary etiological agent in the sexual dysfunction (e.g., major depression) (Maurice and Guze, 1970; Fagan, Schmidt, Wise et al, 1988).

DESCRIPTION

Sexual dysfunctions have traditionally been understood as deviations from the normal human sexual response cycle as described by Masters and Johnson (1966). This has been adapted and amplified in Figure 14–1 to display both the normal physiological arousal pattern (increased heart rate and blood pressure, myotonia) and the particular sexual disorders that may appear in each particular phase.

One of the problems with accepting the Masters and Johnson model of human sexual response uncritically is the possible denial of the cultural factors that are developed and expressed in this model. Since the 1960s this model has been the dominant paradigm of sexual response in Western cultures. There is growing criticism of total reliance on such a physiological model to describe human sexual functioning. The social constructionist school argues that the meaning of sexual behavior (what makes it "unnatural" or "dysfunctional" or "pathological") is constructed from the dominant culture beliefs (Tiefer, 1991). Social constructionists hold that individual deviations from this response pattern might be viewed not as dysfunction but as cultural or experienced-learned differences, e.g., multiorgasmic men (Dunn and Trost, 1989) and women (Darling, Davidson, and Jennings, 1991). Uncritical dependence on traditional sex therapy (based on the Masters and Johnson sensate focus model)

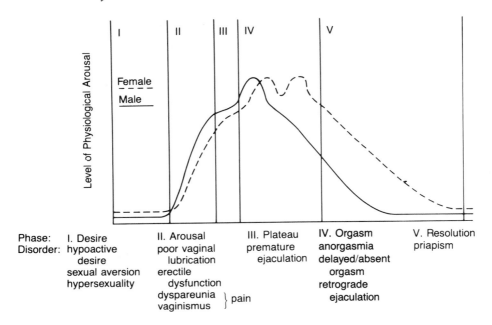

Figure 14–1. *Levels of physiological arousal and sexual disorders in men and women according to phases of sexual response. (Adapted from Masters and Johnson, 1966 and Fagan and Schmidt, 1987)*

might pose obstacles for successful treatment of individuals from non-Western cultures (Lavee, 1991).

However, with this caveat in mind, the human sexual response cycle provides the clinicians with a relative norm with which they can obtain a clear phenomenology of the specific nature of the sexual dysfunction. This can be done during an elaboration of the presenting problem by asking patients to describe their last attempt at sexual intercourse or sexual activity. Particular attention should be paid to quantifying both time (e.g., in foreplay) and physiological response (e.g., vaginal lubrication). These data should then be compared to the human sexual response cycle described by Masters and Johnson (1966) and further elaborated in DSM-IV (APA 1993, in press [1994]). When there appears to be more than one sexual dysfunction, the clinician must determine which disorder was historically first and therefore may be etiologically connected to the secondary condition. For example, a man distressed by premature ejaculation may develop secondary erectile dysfunction.

The DSM-IV groupings of the psychosexual dysfunctions are disorders of desire, arousal, orgasm, and pain. Categories for dysfunctions due to general medical conditions or induced by a substance (drug or medicine) have been added to DSM-IV. A diagnostic category, "sexual dysfunction not otherwise specified," provides for patients whose symptoms elude existing diagnostic taxonomy.

Disorders of Desire

DSM-IV lists two disorders of sexual desire: "hypoactive sexual desire disorder" and "sexual aversion disorder." Hypoactive sexual desire is a condition in which the patient reports usually a global lack of cognitive, emotional, and physiologic readiness to initiate or take part in sexual activity. Compared to others of the same age, sex, health status, and availability of a sexual partner, a person with hypoactive sexual desire has fewer sexual fantasies and lower orgasmic frequency (through masturbation or intercourse). If the condition is acquired, the distress shown by the patient about the low sexual desire may range from preoccupation (e.g., in the "macho" male) to indifference (e.g., in the mother of multiple preschool children). In situations of long-standing hypoactive sexual desire, the condition may be quite ego-syntonic (i.e., not troublesome to the patient).

This disorder does not imply an inability to function sexually. Once activity is initiated, usually by the partner, the person becomes aroused and, unless there is a separate dysfunction, is orgasmic. The hallmark of this disorder is that the baseline of sexual desire (libido) remains significantly low.

Sexual aversion disorder was a new diagnostic category in DSM-III-R. Conceptualized by Helen Singer Kaplan (1987), the disorder is the aversion to and avoidance of sexual activity with a partner. Sexual desire may be normal with fantasy and masturbation frequencies appropriate for age and sex. The patient may avoid intercourse completely or may participate only infrequently out of a sense of duty to the partner. Central to the disorder is a pattern of avoidance that results in infrequent intercourse. When experienced, intercourse is merely tolerated. A sense of enjoyment, satisfaction, and collaboration is usually minimal or absent. Poor body image, especially regarding breasts and genitals, is common; nudity is avoided (Ponticas, 1992; Katz, Gipson, and Turner, 1992).

While disorders of desire may cause marked distress in the individual with hypoactive desire or sexual aversion, it is far more likely that the reason for seeking treatment is the distress of the partner and the resultant interpersonal difficulties.

Disorders of Arousal

Disorders of arousal pertain to an inability to achieve sufficient physiological or cognitive/emotional arousal during sexual activity. In women the disorder is called "female sexual arousal disorder"; in men the disorder is "male erectile disorder." Insufficient physiological arousal for women consists of failure to attain or maintain adequate lubrication-swelling response of the vagina and labia for the completion of sexual activity. Intercourse may be performed, but vaginal dryness will cause pain on initial penetration or throughout coitus. In men the failure to attain or maintain erection until the completion of sexual activity is the criteria for arousal disorder. In most cases it makes intravaginal penetration and ejaculation rare. In others, ejaculation is purposefully rushed after penetration to precede penile detumescence.

In addition to the insufficient peripheral response of the genitals, a disorder of arousal exists when the disturbance causes marked distress or interpersonal difficulty (DSM-IV).

Orgasm Disorders

Female orgasmic disorder is marked by the persistent or recurrent delay in, or absence of, orgasm following a normal sexual excitement phase (DSM-IV). The clinician judges that an orgasm disorder is present in a woman when there is less orgasmic capacity "than would be reasonable for her age, sexual experience, and the adequacy of sexual stimulation she receives" (DSM-IV). Many women do not experience vaginal (as distinct from clitoral) orgasm. During intercourse there may generally be less clitoral stimulation than is necessary for them to achieve orgasm. For them, orgasm is achieved during the sexual experience by manual or oral stimulation of the clitoris. This is a variant of the normal female sexual response cycle and should not be considered a sexual dysfunction. The coital anorgasmia may be etiologically related to constitutional sensory thresholds rather than psychosexual conflicts (Derogatis et al, 1986).

Male orgasmic disorder is likewise the persistent or recurrent delay in, or absence of, orgasm following a normal excitement phase during sexual activity that is adequate in focus, intensity, and duration (DSM-IV). It is important to specify whether the orgasm disorder is present in all sexually stimulating situations (very rare) or only in specific situations, e.g., interpersonal sex.

When evaluating a male patient with an orgasm disorder, the clinician should bear in mind the following clinical conditions. Men may ejaculate without a sense of orgasmic pleasure; this should be designated as "sexual dysfunction, NOS" (not otherwise specified). Others may have orgasm without the emission of ejaculate (e.g., retrograde ejaculation following surgery disrupting innervation of the bladder sphincter muscle); this is not an orgasm disorder. Finally, orgasm and ejaculation may occur without full penile tumescence. This is a disorder of arousal if maximum tumescence has been obtained after sufficient stimulation.

Premature ejaculation occurs persistently with "minimal sexual stimulation or before, upon, or shortly after penetration and before the person wishes it." Premature ejaculation may occur with partial or full tumescence and is usually a condition that has been present since the male was sexually active with a partner. While no reduction in orgasmic pleasure is reported, a man with premature ejaculation is usually distressed that he cannot last long enough for his female partner to have a satisfying sexual experience. As anorgasmia in women may be related to constitutional sensory thresholds, similarly, a relatively low threshold to physical sexual stimuli may be in some men a constitutional "vulnerability" to premature ejaculation (Strassberg et al, 1990). It is classified as a dysfunction only because of the effects of the behavior during interpersonal sexual activity.

Sexual Pain Disorders

There are two sexual pain disorders, "dyspareunia" and "vaginismus." Dyspareunia in a man or woman is "recurrent or persistent genital pain . . . before, during or after sexual intercourse." To assign this diagnosis in women, the dyspareunia should not be caused by a lack of lubrication ("female sexual arousal disorder") or be secondary to vaginismus. In both men and women, the pain is not caused by a medical condition or drugs.

Vaginismus is "recurrent or persistent involuntary spasm of the musculature of the outer third of the vagina that interferes with coitus." Although frequently secondary to genital or sexual trauma, the disorder is not caused *exclusively* by a physical disorder. It should not be more adequately explained by a somatization disorder. The spasms of vaginismus are reflex spasms and are not voluntary responses on the woman's part; her male partner often does not appreciate this fact and feels that his sexual advances are being willfully ejected. The condition is frequently generalized to interfere with a pelvic examination or, in rare cases, the insertion of a tampon.

ETIOLOGY

Human sexual behavior is motivated behavior in which physiological drives are expressed bodily, are experienced by a sentient person, and, if only in fantasy, are nearly always in an erotic relationship with another person (or object surrogate such as a fetish). When sexual behavior fails to achieve the desired end (e.g., intercourse), then sexual dysfunction has occurred. The etiology of the dysfunction can be biogenic or psychogenic or a combination of the two.

Biogenic Causes

Biogenic sexual dysfunction is determined by a careful review of systems as well as by physical examination (Table 14–2) (Buvat et al, 1990). A family history of chronic diseases should also be obtained. Symptomatology or history of endocrine, vascular, or neurologic diseases deserves special attention. Table 14–3 elaborates some of the more common medical and surgical causes of sexual dysfunction in men and women.

Drugs are commonly a principal agent in sexual dysfunction and often contribute to the disorder in a patient whose body has already been compromised by disease. Table 14–4 lists many drugs reported to affect sexual response. Alcohol and drug abuse, beta-adrenergic blockers, centrally acting antihypertensives, and anti-androgens are the most commonly reported drugs implicated in sexual dysfunction (Fagan and Schmidt, 1993).

Referrals to allied medical specialties can be used to determine biogenic factors of sexual dysfunction. A urological examination for erectile dysfunction includes Doppler studies of penile blood flow and measurement of the penile-brachial index (PBI), the ratio of penile systolic pressure to brachial systolic pressure. A PBI less than 0.75 suggests possible vascular etiology for erectile dysfunction (Gerwertz and Zarins, 1985).

Endocrine studies of patients with suspected hormonal etiology should include measurement of fasting blood sugar and assays of follicle-stimulating hormone (FSH), luteinizing hormone (LH), testosterone, and prolactin as well as a general survey (e.g., SMA-18) for liver and renal disease. The level of free (bioavailable) testosterone may be more predictive of endocrine deficiency in male sexual response than the level of serum testosterone (Carani et al, 1990).

(text continues on page 397)

Table 14–2 **Components of Physical Examination of Sexually Dysfunctional Patients**

ORGAN SYSTEM	PHYSICAL EXAMINATION
Endocrine system	
	hair distribution
	gynecomastia
	testes
	thyroid gland
Vascular system	
	peripheral pulses
Gastrointestinal	
	hepatomegaly, or atrophic liver with peripheral neuropathy due to alcoholism
Genitourinary system	
	prostate (in male)
	pelvic examination (in female)
Nervous system	
Sacral innervation	
S1-S2	mobility of small muscles of the foot
S2-S4	internal, external anal sphincter tone bulbocavernosus reflex (in male)
S2-S5	perianal sensation
Peripheral sensation	
Deep Tendon reflexes	
Long tract signs	

Wise TN, Schmidt CW: Diagnostic Approaches to Sexuality in the Medically Ill. In Hall RC, Beresford TP (eds): Handbook of Psychiatric Diagnostic Procedures, Vol 2. New York, Spectrum, 1985

Table 14–3 **Medical Factors That May Affect Sexual Response in Men and Women**

MEN	WOMEN	BOTH
• Peyronie's disease	• Atrophic vaginitis	• Chronic systemic disease
• Urethral infections	• Infections of the vagina	• Chronic pain
• Testicular disease	• Cystitis, urethritis	• Diabetes mellitus
• Hypogonadal androgen-deficient states	• Endometriosis	• Angina pectoris
	• Episiotomy scars, tears	• Hypertension
• Hydrocele	• Uterine prolapse	• Multiple sclerosis
• Lumbar sympathectomy	• Infections of external genitalia	• Hyperprolactinemia
• Radical perineal prostatectomy		• Spinal cord lesions
		• Alcoholism
		• Substance abuse

Reprinted with permission from Schmidt: Sexual disorders. In Harvey AM, Owens A Jr, McKusick A (eds): Principles and Practice of Medicine, p 1149, 16.10–1. E. Norwalk, CT: Appleton and Lange, 1988

Table 14-4 **Medications that May Affect Sexual Response**

DRUG	SEXUAL RESPONSES
Antihypertensives	
1. Diuretics	
Bendroflumethazide (10 mg/day)	Libido, erectile, ejaculation problems
Chlorothiazide (100 mg/day)	Libido, erectile, ejaculation problems
Indapamide (2.5 mg/day)	No reports of impotence
Spironolactone (400 mg/day)	Erectile and libido problems
2. Adrenergic inhibitors—beta-adrenergic blockers	
Atenolol (50–100 mg/day)	Few reports of dysfunction
Bisopropol (5 mg/day)	No sexual dysfunction reported
Metoprolol (200 mg/day)	Few reports of dysfunction
Nadolol (40–240 mg/day)	Few reports of dysfunction
Pindolol (15 mg/day)	Few reports of dysfunction
Propranolol (dose related)	Libido, erectile problems
Timolol (ocular)	Libido, erectile, low ejaculate problems
3. Central-acting adrenergic inhibitors	
Clonidine (0.2–4.8 mg/day)	Libido, erectile problems
Guanabenz (4–64 mg/day)	<1% libido, erectile problems
Methyldopa (1–3 Gm/day)	Libido, erectile, ejaculation problems
4. Peripheral-acting adrenergic antagonists	
Guanadrel + hydrochlorothiazide	Libido, erectile, ejaculation problems
Guanadrel + chlorothiazide	Libido, erectile, ejaculation problems
Guanethidine (>25 mg/day)	Libido, erectile, emission/ejaculation problems
Reserpine (0.1 mg/day)	Libido, erectile problems
5. Alpha-adrenergic blockers	
Prazosin (3–20 mg/day)	Low incidence of sexual dysfunction
Terazosin (1–40 mg/day)	Low incidence of sexual dysfunction
Phenoxybenzamine (5–70 mg/day)	Emission problems
6. Combined alpha- and beta-adrenergic blockers	
Labetalol (200–1000 mg/day)	Erection, ejaculation, delayed detumescence problems
7. Vasodilators	
Hydralazine (35–50 mg/day)	No sexual dysfunction
Minoxidil	No sexual dysfunction
8. Angiotensin-converting enzyme inhibitors	
Captopril (100 mg/day)	19% had worsening of sexual dysfunction
9. Slow channel calcium-entry blocking agents	
Verapamil	No reports when used alone
Psychotherapeutic Agents	
1. Antidepressants	
Amitriptyline (50–200 mg/day)	Libido, arousal, and orgasm problems
Amoxapine (126–210 mg/day)	Libido, arousal, and orgasm problems
Desipramine (75–300 mg/day)	Libido, arousal, and orgasm problems
Imipramine (25–225 mg/day)	Libido, arousal, and orgasm problems
Maprotiline (150 mg/day)	Libido, arousal, and orgasm problems
Nortriptyline (125–200 mg/day)	Libido, arousal, and orgasm problems
Protriptyline (20–60 mg/day)	Libido, arousal, and orgasm problems
Trimipramine	Libido, arousal, and orgasm problems

(continued)

Table 14–4 *(continued)*

DRUG	SEXUAL RESPONSES
Psychotherapeutic Agents	
Clomipramine (25–75 mg/day)	Libido, arousal, and orgasm problems
Fluoxetine (20–80 mg/day)	Anorgasmia, delayed ejaculation
Buproprion (300–600 mg/day)	No reports of sexual dysfunction
Trazodone (50–600 mg/day)	Priapism
Sertraline	15% male, 2% female sexual dysfunction (anorgasmia and delayed ejaculation)
2. Monoamine oxidase inhibitors	
Phenelzine (30–90 mg/day)	Arousal and orgasm problems
Tranylcypromine (20 mg/day)	Arousal and orgasm problems
3. Mood stabilizers	
Lithium	Libido and erectile problems
Carbamazepine	13% had decreased libido or had erectile problems
4. Antipsychotics	
Butaperazine (40–160 mg/day)	Libido, erectile, ejaculation problems
Chlopromazine (1200 mg/day)	Libido, erectile, ejaculation problems, priapism
Chlorprothixine (300 mg/day)	Libido, erectile, ejaculation problems
Haloperidol (5 mg/day)	Libido, erectile, ejaculation problems
Mesoridazine (300–400 mg/day)	Libido, erectile, ejaculation problems, priapism
Perphenazine (24 mg/day)	Libido, erectile, ejaculation problems
Pimozide (16 mg/day)	Libido, erectile, ejaculation problems
Trifluoperazine (20 mg/day)	Libido, erectile, ejaculation problems
Thiothixene (20 mg/day)	Libido, erectile, ejaculation problems
Fluphenazine	Arousal, ejaculation, (painful) orgasm problems
Thioridazine (30–600 mg/day)	Arousal, ejaculation, (painful) orgasm problems, priapism
5. Anxiolytics	
Alprazolam (3–10 mg/day)	Libido, erectile, ejaculation problems, anorgasmia
Diazepam (15–40 mg/day)	Libido, erectile, ejaculation problems in males No negative impact on female sexual function
Lorazepam (1–3 mg/day)	Libido, ejaculation problems
Buspirone	No reported sexual dysfunction
Exogenous Hormones	
1. Androgens	
Testosterone	No negative effect on sexual function
Anabolic steroids	Libido decrease, impotence, testicular atrophy, azoospermia
2. Estrogens	Decreased vaginal atrophy; decreased libido in males
Cancer Chemotherapy Agents	
1. Alkylating agents	Gonadal dysfunction in males and females
Clorambucil	
Cyclophosphamide	
Busulphan	
Melphelan	

(continued)

Table 14–4 *(continued)*

DRUG	SEXUAL RESPONSES
Cancer Chemotherapy Agents	
2. Other agents	
Procarbazine	Gonadal dysfunction in males and females
Vinblastine	Gonadal dysfunction in males and females
Cytosine arabinoside	Gonadal dysfunction in males and females
Ketoconazole (400 mg tid)	Supresses testicular and adrenal androgen synthesis
Carbonic Anhydrase Inhibitors	
Acetazolamide (1 gm/day)	Libido, erectile problems
Methazolamide (100–200 mg/day)	Libido, erectile problems
Dichlorophenamide (100–200 mg/day)	Libido, erectile problems
Antiepileptic Drugs	
Phenytoin	11% males libido or erectile problems
Carbamazepine	13% decreased libido or erectile problems
Phenobarbital	16% decreased libido or erectile problems
Primadone	22% decreased libido or erectile problems

Source: Buffum J: Prescription drugs and sexual function. Psychiatric Med 10:181–198, 1992.

Neurological assessment of the motor, sensory, and autonomic nervous system should pay special attention to the lumbosacral spinal pathways (see Table 14–2 and Fig. 14–2). A cystometrogram or urinary flow studies can grossly define autonomic function in this area. The nerve-sparing technique for retropubic prostatectomy means that such patients should not be considered a priori surgically impotent (Walsh, Lepor, and Eggleston, 1983).

Nocturnal penile tumescence (NPT) studies (Karacan, 1982) monitor the duration, frequency, and amount of penile tumescence during REM sleep. NPT studies can also determine the relationship between penile blood flow and bulbocavernosus and ischiocavernosus muscle activity. In many centers there is also a rigidity challenge in which the buckling force of the erection is measured by a technician with a handheld mercury strain gauge. While NPT is the most complete evaluation of nocturnal erections, recent research (Schiavi, 1990) invites further exploration of the relationship between nocturnal erections and those sought or attained while awake.

When a sexual dysfunction has been linked with a medical illness or treatment, DSM-IV provides for the diagnoses of sexual dysfunction due to general medical conditions, e.g., painful intercourse with vestibular adenitis, or sexual dysfunction induced by either drugs or medications. These two diagnostic categories are new to the DSM series and should be entered on Axis I with the medical condition noted on Axis III and the drug/medication specified in the diagnostic code on Axis I.

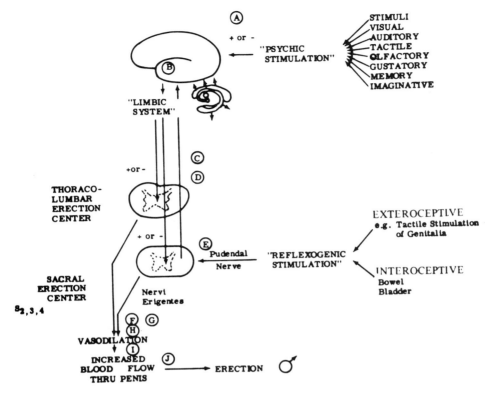

Figure 14–2. *Neurological pathways involved in human penile erection. A—J, sites where lesions could cause sexual dysfunction. (Reproduced with permission from Weiss HD: The physiology of human erection. Ann Intern Med 16:793, 1972)*

Psychogenic Causes

To ascertain the psychogenic causes of sexual dysfunction, a complete psychosocial and psychosexual history should be taken. Table 14–5 lists the data particularly important for the sexual development and behavior of an individual. To obtain the sexual data, the clinician should establish an atmosphere of candor and relative comfort. The physician should ask every and any question that may be relevant to the diagnosis and treatment of the sexual dysfunction. If the clinician is confident that the information being obtained is important, then this attitude will be conveyed to the patient and a condition of relative comfort will exist between them.

Watching experienced clinicians take histories of both sexes will help the novice clinician learn the art of taking a sexual history. It is normal to be somewhat embarrassed in the initial stages of taking sexual histories, especially in patients of the opposite sex. In obtaining a sexual history, the clinician must be aware of and able to confront issues of sexuality in his or her own life. The discomfort or embarrassment should diminish fairly rapidly with experience. If it persists, the clinician should

Table 14–5 **Data Covered for Sexual History**

Childhood

First sex play with peers
Family sleeping arrangements
Sex play with siblings
Sexual abuse, incest, or molestation
Parental attitudes toward sex
Sources of sexual knowledge

Pubertal

Menarche or first ejaculation: subjective reaction
Secondary sex characteristics: subjective reaction
Body image
Masturbation fantasies and frequency
Homoerotic fantasies and behavior
Dating experiences (physical intimacies)
Intercourse
  Age at first occurrence
  Reaction to first intercourse

Young adult

Lengthy or live-in relationships
Pattern of sexual activities with others
Paraphilic behaviors
Previous marriages
  Courtship
  Parental attitudes toward spouse
  Sexual activity (dysfunction?)
  Reasons for termination of marriage
Venereal disease

Adult

Present primary sexual relationship
Development of relationship
Significant nonsexual problems (e.g., money, alcohol, in-laws)
Infertility; contraceptive practices
Children (problems?)

Sexual behaviors
Extramarital affairs
Intercourse frequency during relationship
Variety of sexual behaviors (e.g., oral-genital, masturbation)
Previous dysfunction (in either partner)
Elaboration of onset and history of present problem (without partner
  present)
Perception of partner's reaction to problem
Homosexual activity
Possible exposure to HIV

Reprinted with permission from Fagan PJ, Schmidt CW Jr: Sexual Dysfunction in the Medically Ill. In Stoudemire A, Fogel BS (eds): Psychiatric Care of the Medical Patient, p 311. New York, Oxford University Press, 1993 consult her or his clinical supervisor for assistance. Conversely, if the clinician feels absolutely no twinge of discomfort when initially taking sexual histories, he or she may lack sufficient sensitivity to the emotional issues connected with sexuality. This absence of affect should also be discussed with a supervisor.

If the sexual history follows the lifeline and developmental stages (as suggested in Table 14–5), the patient has a schema of what to expect. This helps to reduce the anxiety that would be generated if the patient felt that a set of completely random questions were being asked about his or her sexual behavior in symptom checklist fashion.

To learn about the phenomenology of the sexual dysfunction, it is helpful to ask patients to describe their most recent attempt at sexual experience. Questions should focus on the person's mental/emotional reactions to the sexual experience (e.g., "Did you think about what you were doing or were you thinking about something or someone else?") as well as on the patient's physiological responses (e.g., "Were you lubricated when penetration was attempted?"). Thoughts and feelings about self and partner convey the emotional reactions. The human sexual response cycle serves as the framework for appreciating the physiological response of the patient. Even with a complete history, however, the multiple determinants of the dysfunction may not become apparent until the person or couple has been in psychotherapy for several sessions. For example, the role of imagery and positive sexual fantasy may be a sufficient component for sexual response in some individuals but the nature and quality of such may not emerge until several therapy sessions have established adequate trust (Whipple et al, 1992).

Psychogenic causes of sexual dysfunction are cognitions or emotions that either ignore (repress) nearly all sexual stimuli in disorders of sexual desire or, in the other sexual disorders, lead to a "fight-or-flight" physiological reaction in which adrenergic effects inhibit the normal human sexual response cycle. The most common example is performance anxiety, in which (usually) the man is so concerned about his sexual functioning that the anxiety itself becomes a self-fulfilling prophecy.

The etiology of these cognitions or emotions that cause sexual dysfunction can be understood from a variety of theoretical frameworks, but none totally explains the etiology of all sexual dysfunction. The major systems that have addressed sexual behavior (and by extension, sexual dysfunction) are psychoanalytic theory, behaviorism, cognitive theory, and social learning theory. What follows is a brief statement about each theory, with a clinical example of the etiology of a sexual dysfunction as explained by that theory.

A *psychoanalytic* approach to sexuality (Person, 1987) and to sexual dysfunction (Meyer, Schmidt, and Wise, 1986) most often explains the disorder as a symptom of an underlying psychological conflict. As such, the dysfunction serves as a psychosomatic symbol of an unconscious conflict and a protection (defense) against consciously experiencing the anxiety of that primary conflict (e.g., separation from a loved object). For example, most sexual dysfunction promotes sexual estrangement, in which physical intimacy is reduced. One with an arousal disorder, therefore, reduces her or his exposure to the possibility of rejection by a lover. A psychoanalytic therapist might also suspect that this fear of rejection is rooted in an infantile experience of rejection by the mother or father.

Behaviorism explains sexual behavior as it does all behavior: as a response to environmental stimuli. In classical conditioning, an object becomes paired with a stimulus so that it can provoke the same response in the organism. In operant conditioning, the organism learns to interact with the environment so that a favorable reward is obtained or a negative result avoided. Sexual pleasure is a reward; sexual pain is a negative result. If sexual intercourse has become paired with pain, including emotional pain, then any approach to it will be avoided. This is commonly seen in sexual aversion disorder. In more extreme cases, the trauma of rape or incest results in aversion disorder or vaginismus.

Social learning theory stresses the role of learning by imitating others (McConaghy, 1987). A person learns how to be sexual with others by observing how others, especially those of the same sex, act sexually. The importance of parental and familial role models in sexual development is crucial. The attitude toward sexuality, the expression of affection, and communication skills in the family of origin are precursors to later adult attitudes and the manner of expressing affection and sexuality. Conflicts about sex role (e.g., insecurity about being able to act like a "real" man or woman) or sex stereotyping can result in sexual dysfunction.

If the parents believe that sex is bad and must be controlled at all costs, then the child as an adult is likely to find it difficult to accept sexual pleasure without emotional conflict. If one "learns" early that sex can be a controlling or manipulating force over others, then sexual activity as an adult will be colored by tones of a power struggle. Sex that is used mainly as an instrument of power usually results in sexual dysfunction in one of the partners unless a primarily sadomasochistic sexual relationship has been established.

Cognitive theory stresses the importance of cognitions or beliefs that determine emotional responses and behaviors in sexual activity (Walen and Roth, 1987). In many ways it is similar to social learning theory, except that it places less stress on early childhood experiences. It is more concerned with the cognitions that are held here and now, and less with their etiology. If an individual believes, for example, that the opposite sex seeks to control, emotionally engulf, or dominate others, then those beliefs (often unrecognized) will influence the emotions the person has during sexual intimacy. Examples are a woman who is anorgasmic because she fears loss of control or a man who gets in and out of a "dangerous" situation with premature ejaculation.

Allied to cognitive etiology of sexual dysfunction are those cases in which a lack of sexual information causes dysfunction. Examples are an older man who expects to achieve an erection (as he did as a youth) without any direct penile stimulation or a menopausal woman who does not realize she may need a vaginal lubricant.

In conclusion, sexual dysfunctions that are psychogenic cannot be directly and universally related to any one specific etiologic event or psychodynamic structure. It is never a case of, "This is premature ejaculation; therefore, X must have caused it." Taking a careful history, further elaborating the patient's psychological constitution in therapy, and testing etiological hypotheses in therapeutic approaches are necessary to confirm the psychogenic factors for a particular patient.

TREATMENT

General Principles

Because patients often have difficulty discussing sexual problems, their presentation of the chief complaint and the history of the present illness may be imprecise. It is therefore necessary to set aside enough time to evaluate the problem; more than one session may be necessary to complete the task. With a patient whose sexual dysfunction involves a partner or a spouse, the evaluation ideally should include the partner's view of the problem. Finally, asking patients about their notions concerning the etiology of their sexual disorder and their expectations for treatment are helpful in understanding patient biases.

The eventual development of a treatment plan depends on the specifics of each case, including several important favorable prognostic factors. Those factors include recent onset of symptoms, mild to moderate severity of dysfunction, prior history of good sexual function, identifiable situational stress factors, good mental health, absence of paraphilia, and a spouse or partner who is cooperative with the evaluation and willing to participate in treatment. Although evaluation often reveals that sexual dysfunctions may be secondary to marital or relational discord, the sexual complaint is the ticket of entry into the care system, and treatment should be provided on the basis of the presenting complaint. Once treatment has begun, relational issues may obtain priority and redirect the goals of treatment.

When patients do not require referral, the PLISSIT model developed by Annon and Robinson (1978) is very useful for evaluation and office counseling. The clinician gives permission (P) to the patient to discuss his or her sexual concerns and apprehensions by initiating discussion with appropriate questions. In response to the questions the patient may have about the sexual problem, the clinician provides limited information (LI) (i.e., enough information to enable informed decisions), without overloading the patient with accurate but excessive detail. As rapport is established between the clinician and patient, the clinician gives specific suggestions (SS) about how to maximize sexual function, taking into account the circumstances of the current relationship and other psychological stressors. Patients that do not respond are referred for intensive therapy (IT).

MEDICAL DISORDERS

Sexual disorders that are secondary to chronic illness, chronic pain, or the side effects of medications may be reversed by medical interventions. Improvement of the patient's overall physical condition and relief of pain may restore sexual function. Drug holidays, a change of medication, or discontinuance of medication may reverse dysfunctions. Dysfunction secondary to the acute side effects of substance abuse or alcoholism will often remit once the abuse is controlled. Prolactin-secreting microadenomas (which cause loss of desire and arousal disorders) may be treated by surgical resection or medically by administering bromocriptine. Inhibited desire in men and/or male arousal disorders secondary to hypogonadism are responsive to intramuscular administration of exogenous testosterone, providing there is no evidence of prostatic carcinoma.

Sexual dysfunction irreversibly impaired by trauma, disease, or the sequelae of surgery is treatable by using the principles of rehabilitation medicine: quantify the loss of function, establish realistic rehabilitative goals, and develop training techniques to maximize residual functional capacities. Patients who suffer irreversible damage can be taught sexual techniques that enable them to maintain sexual relationships, a great psychological benefit to both the patient and the partner. Patients should also be referred to self-help associations (e.g., multiple sclerosis groups, ostomy and cardiac support groups), which hold group meetings and provide literature on sexual function. Dysfunctions secondary to estrogen deficiency are responsive to estrogen replacement (providing no medical contraindications exist), largely by effecting an improved sense of well-being and by increasing the ability to lubricate vaginally.

Postmenopausal women may experience problems with adequate vaginal lubrication due to reduced circulating estrogens. Hormonal replacement of estrogens will reduce vaginal atrophy and improve lubrication during sexual stimulation (Walling, Andersen, and Johnson, 1990). There is also indication that among younger surgically menopausal women the administration of androgens may improve general sexual functioning (Sherwin, 1991).

There are several methods of treatment for medically based erectile dysfunction or dysfunction that is recalcitrant to psychotherapy. The noninvasive method is an external vacuum device that utilizes an elastic band to contain blood in the engorged penis. This method has had a fairly high satisfaction and continued utilization rate (Turner et al, 1991; Witherington, 1991). The main disincentives of the vacuum device are the mastery of the mechanics of the pump and the likelihood of ejaculation not occurring intravaginally if conception is desired.

Yohimbine is an oral medication that acts as a likely alpha-1 and alpha-2 adrenergic antagonist with antidopaminergic properties. While it is widely employed as a first-line medical treatment of erectile dysfunction, it has yet to prove itself as a robust treatment of the impotence (Sonda, Mazo, and Chancellor, 1990).

Intracavernosal injections are an alternative medical treatment for erectile dysfunction and require intact tissue responsive to vasodilating substances (papaverine, phentolamine, prostaglandin E1). The treatment involves injecting small amounts of the vasodilators into the corpora of the penis. Within minutes and with some stimulation, an erection is produced that may last for 60 to 90 minutes. Contraindications are priapism, fibrotic plaque from repeated needle sticks, and some abnormal liver function values (Turner et al, 1989; Althof et al, 1991).

In men for whom the above interventions are not successful, penile prostheses may be implanted. These are either silastic rods or inflatable devices. It is recommended that the man's partner be involved in the choice of this or the other medical and mechanical treatments of erectile failure.

Lastly, both for the well as for the ill, appropriate exercise programs that improve individual fitness will likely have a beneficial effect upon overall sexual functioning (White et al, 1990).

PSYCHOSEXUAL DISORDERS

Desire Disorders

Loss of sexual desire is often associated with depressive disorders, which should be treated with antidepressants, psychotherapy, or both. Marital discord is a common psychogenic cause of loss of desire. Chronic discord leads to anger, and although the partners may be aware of their anger, they fail to connect their loss of sexual interest in each other with their anger toward each other.

Physicians and patients (through self-medication) sometimes try to treat loss of sexual desire with medications such as testosterone, alcohol, antianxiety compounds, or stimulants. Except for confirmed male hypogonadal states, when testosterone is useful, and for the treatment of hyperprolactinemia with bromocriptine, these strategies are rarely successful.

Patients suffering from sexual aversion disorders usually have experienced their dysfunction since beginning adult sexual activity. Aversion disorders exist on a spectrum: at one end is the patient who simply lacks desire to initiate sexual activity but can engage in it with reasonable gratification, and on the other end is the patient who experiences panic attacks when faced with a sexual opportunity. This reaction is clearly a more severe form of the disorder and requires aggressive treatment with chemotherapy and psychotherapy. Panic attacks are responsive to antidepressants including the cyclic antidepressants, the MAO inhibitors, and benzodiazepines. Counseling patients with the less severe form of aversion disorder is directed toward helping the unaffected partner to be more assertive in initiating sexual experiences so that the affected partner is drawn into more frequent participation in sexual relations.

Sexual Arousal Disorder

In both sexes, the inability to develop and maintain levels of sexual excitement may be the result of internal psychological events that interfere with the ability to focus on the stimuli causing sexual excitement. A common psychological distraction is preoccupation with sexual performance. This can become a powerful distraction: as concern about performance becomes more and more absorbing, the psychological activity of worrying about performance crowds out the capacity to attend to sexual stimuli, eventually resulting in the loss of arousal. What occurs is performance anxiety and spectatoring. Other common psychological interferences are worry about stressful life situations and marital discord.

Office counseling is effective for patients who present with the already described prognostic factors. The goal of counseling is to eliminate the distracting psychological event(s) so that the patient can focus on sexual stimuli. This is accomplished by first illustrating the process (i.e., spectatoring) to the patient and then teaching him or her to focus on sexual stimuli by practicing touching exercises in private. The sensate focus exercises are described by Masters and Johnson (Masters and Johnson, 1970). Prescribing small amounts of alcohol or antianxiety medications has not proven to be a successful method of chemically inducing relaxation in order to block the process of spectatoring.

ORGASM DISORDERS

Men who experience delay or absence of orgasm are usually found to have personality traits that require referral for evaluation and treatment. As noted earlier, inhibited orgasm must be differentiated from retrograde ejaculation. Retrograde ejaculation has been reported as a side effect of some medications, including thioridazine (Mellaril).

Women experiencing delay or absence of orgasm who give evidence of the favorable prognostic factors described above, including a past history of orgasmic response, are candidates for office counseling. A recent loss of orgasmic response may often be traced to recent sexual experiences during which the patient could not experience orgasm because of a psychological distraction (the process described above). Counseling is used to resolve the stress and then to shift the patient's focus of attention from her concern about orgasm to enjoyment of the total sexual experience. Again, the touching exercises (sensate focus) are prescribed to the patient and her partner. Single patients should be instructed to practice focusing on sexual stimuli during masturbation, with the expectation that a positive response (i.e., orgasm) will generalize to sexual experiences with a partner. Many women may enjoy sex completely without achieving orgasm and derive sufficient pleasure during the plateau stage. Concern about orgasm varies among women as does the need for specific treatment (McCabe and Delaney, 1992)

PREMATURE EJACULATION

Typically, the patient presents with a history of reaching orgasm as he is attempting to penetrate, just as he has penetrated, or within several pelvic thrusts after penetration. He often reports experiencing premature ejaculation since he became sexually active during late adolescence or early adulthood. Men with this dysfunction usually seek help only when their partners become exasperated with the chronic sexual frustration associated with the disorder. Single patients seek assistance when relationships fail as a result of the dysfunction.

There are two behavioral methods for treating premature ejaculation that effectively teach the patient an awareness of his progression through the sexual response cycle and help him control the timing of that progression. These goals are readily achieved when the patient has a regular sexual partner who will participate in the treatment program. Both the "squeeze" and the "stop-and-go" techniques have been used successfully. With the squeeze technique, the female partner places her thumb and first two fingers around the coronal ridge of the penis and presses firmly for 10 seconds. The pressure results in a 10 to 25% loss of erection and a decrease in the subjective sense of arousal. The stop-and-go technique is practiced by alternately stimulating the penis and resting without touching. Either technique is introduced as an exercise following initial practice with the sensate focus exercises. Control over the pacing of the sexual experience is achieved by practicing the exercises and by using one of these techniques throughout all phases of the response cycle.

Behavioral counseling of this sort can be done in an office setting, but it requires therapist training and experience. Treatment is often complicated by the anger typically experienced and expressed by the female partner and repressed by the patient, necessitating marital therapy in addition to sexually focused treatment.

SEXUAL PAIN DISORDERS

Dyspareunia

Psychogenic dyspareunia is rare, and the diagnosis should be made only after all possible medical causes of pain have been ruled out. Patients subject to psychogenic dyspareunia are likely to have personality traits that support the disorder (e.g., the tendency to somaticize conflict). Depending on the outcome of the evaluation, the type of treatment may be individual, group, or behavioral. For some patients, it may incorporate treatment principles associated with the management of chronic pain.

Vaginismus

The diagnosis of functional vaginismus is often made when a physician attempting a pelvic examination cannot pass a finger or the smallest speculum into the vagina because of contraction of the musculature around the vaginal outlet. Successful treatment is based on behavioral methods that desensitize the patient to the experience of penetration. For some women, the desensitization process must begin with individual behavioral exercises. When she is comfortable with vaginal touching and penetration by herself, the transition is then made to couple exercises. The couple is instructed to create a relaxing milieu by taking a bath together, followed by touching exercises (sensate focus). Next, they are asked to repeat the general touching but to include the genitals, avoiding touching that is overtly sexually stimulating. Having mastered the two sets of exercises, they are asked to repeat the bath, the general body touching, and genital touching, and then to pass a small dilator into the vagina. On subsequent days, the size of the dilators is increased until the dilator approximates the circumference of a penis. The penis is then substituted for the dilator. Patients without partners can be treated in a similar manner with the dilators self-applied. However, it is important to note that the acceptance of the dilators may not generalize to a shared sexual experience. Should this be the case, treatment should be delayed until the patient is in a relationship of sufficient commitment to permit including the partner in the treatment program.

THE ROLE OF THE NONPSYCHIATRIC PHYSICIAN IN PATIENT MANAGEMENT

Physicians in all specialities can expect to be approached by patients about sexual problems. Internists, obstetricians, gynecologists, and pediatricians are frequently questioned by patients about sexual issues. However, regardless of specialty, each physician must decide whether to evaluate the patient's complaint or make a referral. When the choice is to do an evaluation, the physician should schedule at least 30 minutes to complete an initial evaluation. Additional sessions may be necessary to complete the evaluation, to develop a diagnostic formulation, and to design a treatment strategy. Counseling methods and techniques have been described in each subsection for those physicians interested in the office management of psychosexual dysfunction. The physician should contract with the patient or the couple for a specific number of sessions (about five), for a defined amount of time per session (30 to 60 minutes), and a regular meeting date (i.e., Thursday, 2 p.m.). The scheduling details are important components of the therapeutic framework. Patients who do not respond to office counseling should be referred for further treatment.

Once the decision to refer has been made, there are several issues to consider. Should a patient be referred to a general psychiatrist or psychologist, or to someone specializing in the treatment of sexual disorders? How can a physician evaluate the credentials of therapists who state they are expert in evaluating and treating sexual disorders?

Patients with sexual complaints that are secondary to major psychiatric disorders (i.e., schizophrenia, bipolar disorder, major depression) should be referred to a general psychiatrist for the necessary psychotropic medication as well as psychotherapy. When a patient with a sexual dysfunction has a co-morbid anxiety disorder or substance-use disorder, the latter conditions should receive prompt attention from a psychiatrist or psychologist who specializes in the treatment of such disorders. In some cases, the sexual dysfunction can be treated concurrently, but generally the anxiety disorder or substance abuse must be treated first.

Individuals or couples whose major problem is their inability to relate to others (in other words, sex is just one of several issues) need couple/marital therapy provided they are willing to work on general relationship issues rather than narrowly focused sexual problems. Patients whose Axis I diagnosis is a psychosexual disorder are the best candidates for sexually focused treatment. Because sexually focused treatment methods ultimately include relational issues, most therapists expert in the techniques of sexual therapy are also experienced in marital therapies and the relational issues associated with personality disorders. This combination of skills is important and useful because patients often need a course of treatment that includes several methods used in sequence.

The question of credentials may be approached in several ways. The certified generalist with the more advanced degree is likely to be better trained (for psychiatrists, board certified; for psychologists, Ph.D, or Psy.D. and licensed). Since most states do not license or certify sexual therapists, the professional should have trained for at least a year in a sexual disorders program; the best such programs are associated with medical schools. If the referring physician has difficulty identifying a source for referral, the closest medical school is usually a good resource about sexual disorder programs and therapists. Several national organizations (such as the Society for Sex Therapy and Research) keep a list of members, listed geographically.

Sexual dysfunctions are moderately prevalent among medical patients and, to a lesser extent, in the general population. Whether the etiology is psychogenic, biogenic, or both, the physician should take time to ascertain the nature of the disorder and the extent to which the patient is distressed. For some dysfunctions, the physician can make effective office interventions; other patients require additional evaluation and treatment. In either instance, therapeutic attention should be given to the person with sexual dysfunction.

CLINICAL PEARLS

- Most patients have not been trained to talk about sexual problems, and the terms used in most medical situations are not amenable for discussing sexual issues. It is incumbent on the physician to create an atmosphere of comfort and trust that allows the patient to explore his or her sexual difficulties. To do this, the physician must be comfortable with issues concerning human sexuality.
- When a patient is in a committed relationship, it is very helpful to have the partner's view of the problem to understand the whole story. Occasionally, a sexually functional partner will seek help to gain support for obtaining the evaluation of a dysfunctional partner; it is unusual for both partners to present with sexual dysfunctions. However, once treatment has begun, in at least 30% of the cases a sexual dysfunction will be discovered in the partner who supposedly is sexually functional.
- When evaluating or treating couples with sexual problems, extramarital relationships are sometimes uncovered. It is the responsibility of the involved partner to decide whether to reveal such a relationship. The physician should not automatically view the extramarital relationship as a threat to the primary relationship; numerous relationships have survived extramarital affairs. Until the dynamics of the relationships are well understood by the physician, it is prudent to withhold recommendations about such affairs or to defer such decisions to a psychiatrist or psychologist.

ANNOTATED BIBLIOGRAPHY

Friedman RC: Normal Sexuality and Introduction to Sexual Disorders. In Michels R et al (eds): Psychiatry. Philadelphia, JB Lippincott, 1991.

> This chapter provides basic information about biopsychosocial aspects of human sexuality and contains information with which the reader of this chapter is presumed to be familiar. There is also a lengthy treatment of the history of homosexuality as a diagnostic category and of present clinical issues regarding sexual orientation.

Kaplan HS: Psychosexual Dysfunctions. In Michels R et al (eds): Psychiatry. Philadelphia, JB Lippincott, 1991

> Dr. Kaplan provides rich clinical descriptions of sexual dysfunctions and stresses an integrated treatment of them, combining behavioral, psychodynamic, and psychopharmacological modalities and interventions.

Saddock VA: Normal Human Sexuality and Sexual Disorders. In Kaplan HI, Saddock BJ (eds): Comprehensive Textbook of Psychiatry V, vol. 1. Baltimore, Williams & Wilkins, 1989

> This chapter contains a detailed table of the physiological changes that occur during the sexual response cycle as described and documented by Masters and Johnson.

Schover LR, Jensen SB: Sexuality and Chronic Illness. New York, Guilford, 1988

> This book provides clinicians with a comprehensive approach to the evaluation and treatment of sexual problems among individuals with chronic illnesses and disabilities. It is a

practical text that draws its usefulness from abundant case discussions; it should be on a physician's bookshelf.

REFERENCES

Althof SE, Turner LA, Levine SB et al: Sexual, psychological and marital impact of self-injection of papaverine and phentolamine: A long-term prospective study. J Sex Marital Ther 17:101–112, 1991

American Psychiatric Association: DSM-IV Draft Criteria 3/1/93. Washington, DC, American Psychiatric Association, 1993

American Psychiatric Association: Diagnostic and Statistical Manual, 4th ed. Washington, DC, American Psychiatric Association, in press [1994]

Annon JS, Robinson CH: The Use of Vicarious Learning in the Treatment of Sexual Concerns. In LoPiccolo J, LoPiccolo L (eds): Handbook of Sex Therapy. New York, Plenum Press, 1978

Blanchard R, Steiner BW (eds): Clinical management of gender identity disorders in children and adults. Washington, DC, American Psychiatric Press, 1990

Buffum J: Prescription drugs and sexual function. Psychiatr Med 10:181–198, 1992

Buvat J, Buvat-Herbaut A, Lemaire A et al: Recent developments in the clinical assessment and diagnosis of erectile dysfunction. Ann Rvw Sex Res 1:265–308, 1990

Carani C, Zini D, Baldini A et al: Effects of androgen treatment in impotent men with normal and low levels of free testosterone. Arch Sex Behav 19:223–234, 1990

Darling CA, Davidson JK, Jennings DA: The female sexual response revisited: Understanding the multiorgasmic experience in women. Arch Sex Behav 20:527–540, 1991

Derogatis LR, Fagan PJ, Schmidt CW et al: Psychological subtypes of anorgasmia: A marker variable approach. J Sex Marital Ther, 12:197–210, 1986

Dunn ME, Trost JE: Male multiple orgasms: A descriptive study. Arch Sex Behav 18:377–387, 1989

Fagan PJ, Schmidt CW Jr: Sexual dysfunction in the medically ill. In Stoudemire A, Fogel BS (eds): Psychiatric Care of the Medical Patient, chapter 15, pp 307–322. New York, Oxford University Press, 1993

Fagan PJ, Schmidt CW Jr, Wise TN et al: Sexual dysfunction and dual psychiatric diagnoses. Compr Psychiatry 29:278–284, 1988

Gerwertz BL, Zarins CK: Vasculogenic Impotence. In Segraves RT, Schoenberg HW (eds): Diagnosis and Treatment of Erectile Disturbances. New York, Plenum Press, 1985

Kaplan HS: Sexual Aversion, Sexual Phobias and Panic Disorder. New York, Brunner/Mazel, 1987

Karacan I: Nocturnal penile tumescence as a biological marker in assessing erectile dysfunction. Psychosomatics, 23:349–360, 1982

Katz RC, Gipson M, Turner S: Brief report: Recent findings on the Sexual Aversion Scale. J Sex Marital Ther 18:141–146, 1992

Kolodny RC, Masters WH, Johnson VE: Textbook of Sexual Medicine. Boston, Little, Brown, 1979

Lavee Y: Western and non-Western human sexuality: Implications for clinical practice. J Sex Marital Ther 17:203–213, 1991

Masters WH, Johnson VE: Human Sexual Response. Boston, Little, Brown, 1966

Masters WH, Johnson VE: Human Sexual Inadequacy. Boston, Little, Brown, 1970

Maurice WL, Guze SB: Sexual dysfunction and associated psychiatric disorder. Compr Psychiatry 11:539–543, 1970

McCabe MP, Delaney SM: An evaluation of therapeutic programs for the treatment of secondary inorgasmia in women. Arch Sex Behav 21:69–89, 1992

McConaghy N: A Learning Approach. In Geer JH, O'Donohue WT (eds): Theories of Human Sexuality. New York, Plenum Press, 1987

Meyer JK, Schmidt CW Jr, Wise TN (eds): Clinical Management of Sexual Disorders, 2nd ed. Washington, DC, American Psychiatric Press, 1986

Nathan SG: The epidemiology of the DSM-III psychosexual dysfunctions. J Sex Marital Ther 12:267–281, 1986

Person ES: A Psychoanalytical Approach. In Geer JH, O'Donohue WT (eds): Theories of Human Sexuality. New York, Plenum Press, 1987

Ponticas, Y: Sexual aversion versus hypoactive sexual desire: A diagnostic challenge. Psychiatr Med 10:273–281, 1992

Price J, Grunhaus LJ: Treatment of clomipramine-induced anorgasmia with yohimbine: A case report. J Clin Psychiatry, 51:32–33, 1990

Schiavi RC: Sexuality and aging in men. Ann Rvw Sex Res 1:227–249, 1990

Schmidt CW Jr: Sexual Disorders. In Harvey AM, Owens AH Jr, McKusick VA et al (eds): Principles and Practice of Medicine. Norwalk, CT, Appleton and Lange, 1988

Schmidt CW: Changes in terminology for sexual disorders. Psychiatr Med 10:247–255, 1992

Schover LR, Jensen SB: Sexuality and Chronic Illness. New York, Guilford, 1988

Sherwin BB: The psychoendocrinology of aging and female sexuality. Ann Rvw Sex Res 2:181–198, 1991

Sonda LP, Mazo R, Chancellor MB: The role of yohimbine for the treatment of erectile impotence. J Sex Marital Ther 16:15–21, 1990

Spector HP, Carey MP: Incidence and prevalence of the sexual dysfunctions: A critical review of the empirical literature. Arch Sex Behav 19:389–408, 1990

Stoller RJ: Gender Identity Disorders of Childhood and Adults. In Kaplan HI, Saddock BJ (eds): Comprehensive Textbook of Psychiatry/IV, Vol. 1. Baltimore, Williams & Wilkins, 1985

Strassberg DS, Mahoney JM, Schaugaard, M et al: The role of anxiety in premature ejaculation: A psychophysiological model. Arch Sex Behav 19:251–257, 1990

Tiefer L: Historical, scientific, clinical and feminist criticisms of "the human sexual response cycle" model. Ann Rvw Sex Res 2:1–23, 1991

Turner LA, Althof SE, Levine SB et al: Self-injection of papaverine and phentolamine in the treatment of psychogenic impotence. J Sex Marital Ther 15:163–176, 1989

Turner LA, Althof SE, Levine SB et al: External vacuum devices in the treatment of erectile dysfunction: A one-year study of sexual and psychosocial impact. J Sex Marital Ther 17:81–93, 1991

Walen SR, Roth D: A Cognitive Approach. In Geer JH, O'Donohue WT (eds): Theories of Human Sexuality. New York, Plenum Press, 1987

Walling M, Andersen BL, Johnson SR: Hormonal replacement therapy for postmenopausal women: A review of sexual outcomes and related gynecologic effects. Arch Sex Behav 19:119–137, 1990

Walsh PC, Lepor H, Eggleston JC: Radical prostatectomy with preservation of sexual function: Anatomical and pathological considerations. Prostate, 4:473–485, 1983

Weiss HD: The physiology of human erection. Ann Intern Med, 76:793–799, 1972

Whipple B, Ogden G, Komisaruk BR: Physiological correlates of imagery-induced orgasm in women. Arch Sex Behav 21:121–13, 1992

White JR, Case DA, McWhirter D, Mattison AM: Enhanced sexual behavior in exercising men. Arch Sex Behav 19:193–209, 1990

Wise TN, Schmidt CW Jr: Diagnostic approaches to sexuality in the medically ill. In Hall RC, Beresford TP (eds): Handbook of Diagnostic Procedures, Vol. 2. New York, Spectrum, 1985

Witherington R: Vacuum devices for the impotent. J Sex Marital Ther 17:69–80, 1991

Alan Stoudemire (ed). *Clinical Psychiatry for Medical Students*, Second Edition. Copyright © 1994, 1990 by J. B. Lippincott Company.

15 *Paraphilias*

William D. Murphy and Elizabeth D. Schwarz

Paraphilias, or sexual deviations, have provoked both curiosity and abhorrence in laypersons and professionals alike. The paraphilias as described in the DSM-IV (APA 1993, in press [1994]) are a group of disorders whose essential features are recurrent, intense sexual urges and sexually arousing fantasies generally involving either nonhuman objects, suffering or humiliation of one's self or partner (not merely simulated), or children or other nonconsenting persons.

Unlike many disorders described in this text, paraphilias represent not only psychiatric or psychological problems: many are illegal and can cause significant emotional and sometimes physical damage to victims (Finkelhor, 1986). Therefore, in many instances the physician must be concerned not only about the presenting problem of the patient but also about past victims and future danger. For example, in almost every state a physician must report to the local child protection agency any incident of known or suspected child sexual abuse. Many times, the clinician who elects to treat a paraphiliac patient who is involved in illegal acts assumes responsibility not only for the patient's behavior, but also for the protection of society.

Although most nonpsychiatric physicians will not provide direct psychological treatment to such patients, this chapter will serve to increase the physicians' awareness of the extent of these disorders; to improve the physicians' understanding of the characteristics of paraphilias, thus allowing them to better serve victims and family members of paraphiliacs and to allow the physicians to make appropriate referrals. Because knowledge in this area is based largely on paraphiliacs whose behavior is illegal and causes harm to others, this chapter will focus most heavily on this particular group of patients.

EPIDEMIOLOGY

Little is known about the true prevalence of various paraphiliac disorders or other demographic factors, although there is increasing knowledge, at least in the area of the victimization of children. Finkelhor (1986) has extensively reviewed studies surveying college students and adults regarding their sexual contacts with adults before puberty or when under the age of 18. Results vary widely: studies have found prevalence rates ranging from 6 to 62% for females and from 3 to 30% for males. For females, the average rates reported are in the 20 to 25% range, while for males they are in the 8 to 10% range. The variation in rates can be partly explained by three factors: the definition of sexual abuse used (offenses involving touching versus offenses involving hands-off experiences such as exhibitionism); the sample used; and the data collection method used (trained interviewers asking multiple questions provided higher rates than self-administered questionnaires with only one or two questions about sexual abuse). Although there is clear evidence that reporting rates of child sexual abuse have increased (Murram and Weatherford, 1988; Peters, Wyatt, and Finkelhor, 1986), an interesting finding of more recent reviews is that the prevalence rates are similar to those published in the 1940s and 1950s.

Although not as extensive, survey data exist for women who have been the victims of exhibitionists. Rates range from 32% in a female college sample (Cox and McMahon, 1978) to 44% of a group of British nurses (Gittleson, Eacott, and Mehta, 1978). Moser and Levitt (1987) have reviewed similar survey studies for individuals engaging in sadomasochistic fantasies and behavior. As an example, Hunt (1974) found in a sample of 2,026 respondents that 4.8% of men and 2.1% of women reported having obtained pleasure from inflicting pain; 2.5% of men and 4.6% of women reported pleasure from receiving pain. However, it is highly likely that a much smaller percentage of these individuals would meet diagnostic criteria for sexual sadism or sexual masochism.

While the above data cause concern and clearly indicate the extent of the problem of child sexual abuse, they do not provide us with clear evidence of the number of individuals who perpetrate such abuse and how many would actually meet the criteria for a paraphiliac diagnosis. For example, Abel et al (1987) found that pedophiles with male targets averaged about 150 victims, while those with female targets averaged about 20 victims. Exhibitionism and voyeurism averaged 513 and 429 victims, respectively.

Little else is known about the characteristics of paraphiliacs. The disorder is seldom diagnosed in females, except in the area of sexual masochism. Although there is evidence that a small percentage of children are sexually abused by females (Finkelhor and Russell, 1984), it seems evident that the paraphilias are primarily male disorders. There is no clear evidence to suggest that the rates of paraphilias differ between ethnic groups or between geographical areas; however, increasing evidence shows that in many paraphiliacs, the onset of the disorder is in adolescence. Abel and Rouleau (1990), in a study of 561 male paraphiliacs, found that approximately 53% had the onset of their interest prior to age 18. The need for early intervention, before the pattern becomes fixed, is becoming increasingly recognized.

DESCRIPTION

Table 15–1 lists the major paraphilias and their general diagnostic criteria. Proposed diagnostic criteria for the DSM-IV (APA 1993, in press [1994]) are basically unchanged with the exception that telephone scatalogia is listed as a separate disorder rather than combined in the "paraphilia not otherwise specified" category. All the paraphilias require at least that the patient (1) has recurrent, intense sexual urges and sexual fantasies regarding the specific paraphilia and (2) has acted on these urges or is markedly disturbed by them. Additional criteria are listed in Table 15–1.

Much of our knowledge is based on subject populations who are either apprehended for a sexual crime or have sought treatment. The extent to which characteristics of this population parallel other paraphiliacs who have not been caught or who have not sought treatment is unknown. Paraphiliacs are heterogeneous; many people have multiple paraphilias and no one characteristic will apply to all individuals. In the

Table 15–1 **Major Paraphilias***

Exhibitionism: Has had over the last 6 months recurrent sexual urges and sexually arousing fantasies to expose one's genitals to strangers and has either acted on these urges or is distressed by them.

Fetishism: Has had over the last 6 months recurrent sexual urges and/or arousing fantasies that involve the use of nonliving objects as sexual stimuli (e.g., female underwear) and has either acted on these or is distressed by them. The diagnosis should not be made if the fetish objects are only female clothing used in cross-dressing or devices designed specifically for sexual arousal (e.g., vibrators).

Frotteurism: Has had over the last 6 months recurrent sexual urges that involve rubbing against or touching a nonconsenting person and has either acted on these urges or is distressed by them. The touching and rubbing itself is sexually exciting, not the aggressive nature of the act.

Pedophilia: Has had over the last 6 months recurrent sexual urges and arousing fantasies that involve sexual interactions with a prepubescent child (generally younger than 13) and has either acted on these urges or is distressed by them. In addition, the patient should be at least 16 years old and at least 5 years older than the victim.

Sexual masochism: Has had over the last 6 months recurrent sexual urges and arousing fantasies that involve the act (not a simulation of the act) of being made to suffer, being humiliated, beaten, or bound and has either acted on these or is markedly distressed by them.

Sexual sadism: Has had over the last 6 months recurrent sexual urges and arousing fantasies that involve acts (not simulated acts) in which suffering, either physical or psychological, that includes humiliation is found to be sexually arousing by the person and the person has either acted on these or is distressed by them.

Transvestic fetishism: A heterosexual male who over the last 6 months has had recurrent sexual urges and arousing fantasies that involve cross-dressing, which the person has acted on or is markedly distressed by them. The individual should not meet the criteria for gender identity disorder of adolescence or adulthood nontranssexual type or transsexualism.

Voyeurism: Has had over the last 6 months recurrent sexual urges and arousing fantasies that involve observing an unsuspecting person who is either naked, disrobing, or engaged in sexual behavior, and has acted on these or is distressed by them.

Paraphilia not otherwise specified: Includes paraphilias that do not fit any of the above specific categories, such as telephone scatalogia (lewdness), necrophilia (corpses), etc.

* Adapted from DSM-IV (APA 1993, in press [1994])

literature, paraphiliacs are many times described as shy, inhibited, nonassertive individuals who have difficulty managing anger. When these characteristics are evaluated objectively, they are found to only apply to a certain percentage of paraphiliacs; no one personality profile would characterize any one paraphilia.

Exhibitionists obtain sexual pleasure from exposing their genitals to unsuspecting strangers. However, at times an exhibitionist may also expose himself to neighbors or to children he knows. During the act, he may or may not have an erection and may or may not masturbate. Some exhibitionists leave the exhibitionistic situation and masturbate to the fantasy of exposing themselves. The vast majority of exhibitionists expose themselves to females, although we have seen some cases of exposure to males. Targets can be adults, adolescents, or children, and generally the exhibitionist does not attempt any further contact with the victim. However, for those individuals who expose to prepubescent children, the physician should rule out that the exposure is not a prelude to more active sexual involvement with the child. In general, the exhibitionist is looking for some reaction from the victim, such as shock or surprise; some may perceive, at least in fantasy, that their victim is sexually aroused by the behavior. We have also seen some exhibitionists whose arousal is increased when the victim shows fear.

The *voyeur's* behavior involves looking at individuals either undressing, nude, or engaging in sexual activities. In voyeurism, the behavior involves people who are *unaware* that they are being watched; the diagnosis is *not* made for individuals who may watch filmed or live pornography, since in such cases the individuals are aware that they are being seen. Clinicians should also be aware that a history of voyeurism is sometimes seen in rapists, and it is important to rule out that the voyeur does not have an aggressive sexual arousal pattern. At times, an individual may be arrested for voyeurism while, in actuality, he was peeping in a window with the intent of raping the victim.

The *fetishist* obtains sexual arousal from a nonliving object, commonly women's underwear, shoes, boots, or other apparel. The individual will usually masturbate while rubbing, holding, or smelling the object. The person may engage in this behavior alone or ask a partner to wear the object. At times, an individual will steal the fetish object, such as underwear, or both steal and destroy it. In such cases, it is important to consider whether there is a sadistic component to the person's arousal pattern.

If a fetish object is limited to female clothes used in cross-dressing, the appropriate diagnosis is *transvestic fetishism*. Cross-dressing in woman's clothes may be limited to single articles, such as underwear, or may involve total cross-dressing, including a wig and makeup. The transvestite may engage in this behavior alone or with a partner. Many transvestites are heterosexual, and cross-dressing is often part of sadomasochistic activity.

Frotteurs' sexual arousal arises from rubbing against or touching nonconsenting individuals. This behavior usually occurs in crowded places, such as on public transportation, and may involve such things as rubbing their genitals against the buttocks of an unsuspecting woman, grabbing the woman's breasts, or grabbing the woman's genital area.

Pedophiles have sexual attraction to children and, along with exhibitionists, are probably the *most frequent* paraphilias seen by mental health professionals. In diagnosing pedophilia, it is important to state whether the attraction is to the same sex, opposite sex, or both; whether it is limited to incest; and whether it is exclusive (only attracted to children) or nonexclusive. These factors appear to relate to the risk of recidivism since, in general, it has been found that males who molest young males have a high recidivism rate, while incest cases have the lowest recidivism rate.

Pedophiles may report sexual attraction to only one sex and to a limited age range (6 to 8 years old), although some may show attraction to all prepubescent children and either sex. Also, the age of the victim may not reflect the pedophile's true age preference, but may reflect merely the victim's availability. The behavior may be limited to fondling or may include other sexual behaviors such as oral-genital contact, digital penetration, insertion of objects in the vagina or anus, and intercourse. Pedophiles may use force, although many are quite adept at manipulating children into sexual activity. They may be very attentive to children's needs and may be involved in social activities or occupations that give them ready access to children (such as becoming the leader of youth groups). Pedophiles use numerous excuses to justify their behavior, such as it was educational for the child, the child initiated the activity, and the child got pleasure from the activity.

Sadists gain sexual pleasure from causing psychological or physical pain to their victims. In addition to pain, however, an integral part of the sadistic arousal pattern is the humiliation, degradation, and domination of the victim. The sadist may force nonconsenting victims or may engage in sadistic behavior with a consenting partner (a sexual masochist). In consenting relationships, unwritten rules usually govern how far the behavior is allowed to progress. Some sadists show progressive behavior (that is, an escalation in the degree of violence and force used). Behaviors may range from those meant to humiliate and degrade the victim (i.e., bonding, verbal abuse, locking in a cage, dressing the victim in diapers or in women's clothes, or urinating and defecating on the victim) to behaviors geared to elicit pain (spanking, pinching, burning, strangling, piercing with pins or needles, torture, mutilation, and murder).

Sexual masochism is seen as the opposite of sexual sadism, although at times sadism and masochism occur in the same individual, who may engage in both roles in sadomasochistic activity. The person may engage in the behavior alone or with a partner. Again, with a partner limits are many times agreed upon as to how far the behavior is allowed to progress. A dangerous form of this behavior is autoerotic asphyxiation or hypoxiphilia (increasing sexual arousal by oxygen deprivation, obtained through such methods as placing a plastic bag over the head, strangling with a noose, or using chemicals such as nitrates). A number of deaths have been reported in the literature as a result of this behavior.

Differential Diagnosis

In diagnosing paraphilias, there are several factors to keep in mind. First, many paraphilias may meet the criteria for a number of the paraphiliac disorders (Abel et al, 1987). If a patient presents complaining of one paraphilia, it is important to ask specifically about each other possible paraphilia in language understandable to the patient. Patients do not always volunteer this information spontaneously. Second, the paraphiliac fantasies, urges, and behaviors may be continuous or episodic. In some patients, the paraphiliac urges, fantasies, and behaviors may occur only during periods of stress or interpersonal conflict, while in other patients the paraphiliac fantasies or behaviors are always necessary for sexual arousal.

Differential diagnosis is less complicated by an overlap in symptomatology between disorders than by the patient's failure to provide honest details of his history. At times, paraphiliac behavior is seen in other diagnostic categories (such as schizophrenia, mania, neuropsychiatric disorders, and mental retardation), but clinical experience suggests it is unlikely that another disorder is primarily responsible for the aberrant behavior. However, in transvestism and fetishism it is important to rule out temporal lobe complex partial seizures (Blumer, 1969); numerous reports have suggested a relationship of these paraphilias to temporal lobe disorders and more recently a relationship between pedophilia and temporal lobe dysfunction has been reported (Langevin, 1990). However, most patients with temporal lobe disorders are not paraphiliacs, and probably most paraphiliacs do not have temporal lobe disorders. It is important that these diagnoses be assessed for and appropriate treatment given if another disorder is diagnosed.

It is important to continue assessing for the presence of paraphilia, even in cases where acute psychotic episodes or other disorders have been resolved. For example, our group saw one patient with clear evidence of paranoid schizophrenia. Following appropriate and reasonably successful pharmacologic treatment, this patient continued with recurrent and intense pedophiliac urges that required specific treatment in and of themselves. Similar observations have been made in patients with mental retardation and substance-abuse disorders.

Criteria for the diagnosis of paraphilia are based largely on the patient's self-report. Paraphiliacs (especially those whose behavior is illegal) often provide very unreliable histories; specialists in the area have turned to other sources to assist in adequate treatment formulation and diagnosis. As part of the evaluation, extensive use is made of victims' statements, police reports, and interviews with significant others to get a clearer picture of the extent and nature of the patient's problem. Many clinical and research facilities use penile plethysmography as a means of direct assessment of sexual arousal to assist in diagnosis of sexual preference (Murphy, Haynes, and Worley, 1991).

ETIOLOGY

Data are extremely limited about the etiology of the development of paraphilias. Therefore, the information reviewed in this area should be considered speculative. Traditional theories regarding etiology follow standard psychiatric theorizing (that is, from psychoanalytic, behavioral, biological, or family systems perspectives). Some descriptive factors, however, warrant special attention.

The first is clinical reports that pedophiles appear to have been victimized themselves sexually as children at a higher rate than one would expect in normals (Groth, Hobson, and Gary, 1982). More recent data suggest, however, this rate is not as high as previously thought. Hanson and Slater (1988), in reviewing a large number of studies, found that with large sample studies the rate of sexual abuse in offenders was approximately 30%. In addition, given the large number of males who appear to have been abused in the general population, it would appear that most young males who are sexually abused do not become sex offenders. Although being sexually abused may be a risk factor for the development of pedophilia, it would appear that there are other, unidentified factors that lead to the development of pedophilia. A number of factors could be proposed, such as whether the abuse had ever been disclosed, whether the young victim ever received treatment, adult reaction to disclosure of the abuse, and the general family stability. To date, few of these factors have been investigated, although such knowledge would allow more appropriate early interventions in individuals at risk for sexual abuse.

A second factor about paraphiliacs is that the vast majority are male. Although this might raise both biological and genetic explanations, it also brings into question the role of male enculturation in the development of paraphiliac behavior. Feminist writers (Brownmiller, 1975) and some researchers (Murphy, Coleman, and Haynes, 1986) have clearly described various aspects of male social learning that may relate to sexual aggression against adult women. Such factors include males' need for dominance, perceptions of women as objects, society's reinforcement of rape myths, and various sex role stereotypes that, at least in the past, were culturally accepted. For pedophiles, such factors might include the masculine requirement to be dominant and powerful in sexual relationships, erotic portrayal of children in advertising, male tendencies to sexualize all emotional needs, and repressive norms about sexuality (Finkelhor, 1984).

Psychoanalytic theories predominated early thinking regarding paraphilias (Karpman, 1954). Many of the early writings in this area tended to follow directly Freud's theories of infantile sexuality, in which all humans are born with primitive, reflectively unformed, instinctual sex drives. Most individuals reach adult heterosexual orientation by progressing through psychosexual levels of development, including adequate resolution of the oedipal complex. In contrast, other individuals may develop neurotic behaviors and symptoms as a result of aberrant patterns of psychosexual development. The paraphiliac, however, because of extreme castration or mutilation anxiety, expresses these infantile sexual desires directly through paraphiliac fantasies or acts. Hammer and Glueck (1957), in a study of incarcerated offenders, found that paraphiliacs feared sexual contact with adult females as a result of their failure to resolve the oedipal complex. All were found to suffer from forms of unconscious castration anxiety. The authors proposed that the various paraphilias allow the individual to resolve in unconscious ways his castration anxiety and fears of adult women. The pedophile tends to choose children, who are less threatening than mature adult women; the exhibitionist displays his genitals, therefore provoking reactions from females and proving the existence of his penis; and the transvestic fetishist may use his cross-dressing to identify with the mother figure as a defense against his castration anxiety (Blair and Lanyon, 1981; Hammer and Glueck, 1957; Wise, 1985).

Early behaviorist writers, rather than focusing on early relationship with parental figures, have instead focused on early sexual experiences and the integration of such experiences into masturbatory fantasies. The basic tenet is that paraphiliac arousal patterns are conditioned by the pairing of masturbatory fantasies with the paraphiliac stimuli (McGuire, Carlisle, and Young, 1965; Rachman, 1966; Rachman and Hodgson, 1968).

Later behavioral theories included other factors that at least might maintain or assist in the development of paraphiliac behavior. For example, a lack of social skills or significant heterosexual anxiety might make it difficult for the individual to develop sexual relationships with appropriate sexual partners, leaving the paraphiliac outlet as the only means of sexual gratification (Barlow and Abel, 1976; Murphy and Stalgaitis, 1987). A number of cognitive-oriented behavior therapists have focused on the role of what are called cognitive distortions (that is, the justifications paraphiliacs use to legitimize their behavior) in the maintenance of deviant sexual behavior (Conte, 1986; Murphy, 1990).

Throughout the literature on paraphilias, various case reports have associated the onset of paraphiliac behaviors with neurological or other biological abnormalities. For example, Regestein and Reich (1978) described four cases of the onset of pedophilia after illness that led to substantial cognitive impairment. Also, Berlin (1983) reports 34 cases of paraphilias (the majority pedophilic) with a variety of associated biological abnormalities, including elevated testosterone levels, schizophrenia, childhood dyslexia, Klinefelter's syndrome, and cortical atrophy. Also, as noted, temporal lobe epilepsy has been associated with fetishism and transvestite fetishism (Blumer, 1969) and more recently temporal lobe disorders have been noted among some pedophiles (Langevin, 1990).

None of these studies were based on random samples of either paraphiliacs or individuals suffering from the various biological abnormalities. Therefore, it is unclear what percentage of patients with such neurological or biological findings develop paraphilias and what percentage of paraphiliacs show such abnormalities. It cannot be assumed from studies that a biological abnormality is the factor leading to the development of paraphilia. At the clinical level, however, these case reports do suggest that the clinician needs to consider that individual paraphiliacs may have additional neurologic disorders; the clinician should try to determine whether the neurologic disorder has any relationship to the paraphilia. Because of the well-documented role that the temporal lobe and associated limbic structures play in regulating sexual behavior, further studies of temporal lobe disorders in paraphilias seem warranted.

Family interactions have also been implicated, at least within the subset of pedophiles involved in incest (Alexander, 1985; Larson and Maddock, 1986). Such theories have focused on factors such as the family's isolation, role confusion in the family, daughters who assume the mother's role, and a general emotional enmeshment among family members. Although it is clear to any clinician working with these families that many are quite dysfunctional, it is not clear whether this is causative or secondary to the abusive behavior (Conte, 1986).

Although a number of factors have been implicated as etiological in the paraphilias, none have produced sufficient evidence to be considered predominant. Like many psychiatric disorders, it is likely that we will find that paraphilias are multiply determined by an interaction of biological, psychological, and social/cultural variables. It is also likely that as our diagnostic abilities improve, we will be able to develop more clearly subtypes of paraphiliacs and will be better able to determine the role and importance of the various etiological factors in these subtypes.

TREATMENT

In this section, we will attempt to review the current general framework that paraphiliac treatment takes and treatment issues that are addressed in sex offender–specific programs. In addition, recent biological approaches will be integrated into this general treatment framework. There has been an increased use of the antiandrogen drug Depo-Provera (medroxyprogesterone acetate, MPA) and recent clinical reports of the use of serotonin reuptake blockers such as fluoxetine with this population.

Treatment in general focuses heavily on the specific paraphiliac behavior or sex offense and the factors surrounding the offense, usually from a cognitive-behavioral framework. Less attention is given to early childhood experiences; therefore, psychodynamic or traditional psychotherapy approaches are usually not considered primary treatment modalities (Knopp, 1984). Most specialized programs use group therapy approaches with other paraphiliacs as the primary treatment modality and use male/female cotherapy teams.

In treating sex offenders, the therapist needs to be more directive and to set limits more clearly on patients' behaviors (such as having no contact with children) than in a traditional therapeutic setting. This includes having patients waive confidentiality so that treatment failure and noncompliance can be reported to appropriate agencies. Most programs work closely with the courts, parole, probation, and child protection agencies; these systems are considered active members of the treatment team rather than agencies that interfere with the therapeutic relationship. Finally, offenders are clearly told that there is no "cure" and the techniques learned in treatment should be employed on a lifelong basis.

The rest of this section will focus on specific components of treatment found in a number of treatment programs (Conte, 1985; Murphy and Stalgaitis, 1987).

Reducing Denial

Until an offender admits to the paraphiliac behavior and provides specific details of the behaviors and factors surrounding the behaviors, it is difficult for treatment to progress. Therefore, one of the initial goals of treatment is to challenge the patient's denial. Denial is sometimes total ("I didn't do it") or partial ("I didn't do everything he/she said I did"). Therapeutic approaches to reduce denial rely heavily on group confrontation, including the use of victims' statements and results of psychophysiological assessment of sexual arousal (Abel, Cunningham-Rathner, Becker et al, 1983).

Sexual Arousal

By definition, paraphiliacs experience fantasies of and recurrent urges to engage in paraphiliac behaviors. Therefore, most programs use some specific behavioral procedure to reduce such urges or to at least give the patient methods for controlling such urges. Although using mild electrical stimulation aversive techniques were frequently used in early treatment studies (Quinsey, 1977), a number of alternative procedures have been more recently developed.

In *covert sensitization* (Cautela and Wisocki, 1971), the patient is taught to imagine a graphic picture of his paraphiliac behavior and to link it with an equally graphic description of an aversive consequence, such as going to jail or losing his family (Barlow, Leitenberg, and Agras, 1969; Brownell and Barlow, 1976; Brownell, Hayes, and Barlow, 1977). In another technique that is used either in conjunction with covert sensitization (Maletzky, 1980) or alone (Laws and Osborne, 1983), the paraphiliac stimulus or fantasy is linked with a noxious odor, such as spirits of ammonia or valeric acid. Also, many programs use some form of masturbatory satiation or verbal satiation that requires patients to verbalize their deviant fantasies for long periods of time (30 to 45 minutes) without ejaculating (Laws and Osborne, 1983; Marshall, 1979; Marshall and Lippens, 1977). This leads to a reduction in the reinforcing value of the fantasies.

A number of biologically oriented approaches have also been used to reduce sexual arousal, although these are not specific to deviant sexual arousal and are geared to reducing libido in general (Berlin, 1983; Bradford, 1985; Freund, 1980). Two antiandrogen drugs that are receiving increased attention are cyproterone acetate (CPA), which is available only in Canada and Europe, and medroxyprogesterone acetate (MPA, Depo-Provera), which has been used in the United States (Berlin, 1983; Bradford, 1985). Although CPA has been used on a larger number of sex offenders, because it is unavailable in the United States we will focus on MPA.

According to Bradford (1985), MPA reduces testosterone through a number of mechanisms, primarily by inducing A-ring reductase inhibition in the liver, therefore increasing testosterone metabolism. Berlin (1983) recommends a starting dose of 500 mg per week of the 100 mg/ml solution, with no more than 250 ml given in a single injection site. Using periodic blood levels to assess whether testosterone levels have been suppressed, the drug is then titrated so as not to cause total impotence and so the drug is not feminizing. Optimal drug levels have not yet been determined. Common side effects of MPA include weight gain, mild lethargy, cold sweats, nightmares, hot flashes, and hypertension.

Berlin (1983) reported a series of 20 chronic paraphiliacs treated with MPA. While on the drug, only three relapsed (or only three were known to relapse); however, nine subjects dropped out of treatment and eight of the nine recidivated while off the drug. Similar dropout problems have been reported by Meyer, Cole, and Emory (1992) and Hucker, Langevin, and Bain (1988). Quinsey and Marshall (1983) have been critical of MPA because of these large dropout rates ranging from 30 to 100% across studies. Further studies are needed on increasing the acceptability of this drug to patients and on ways of increasing compliance. At the current time, Depo-Provera should be seen as a potential component of a comprehensive treatment program but should not be viewed as a treatment that can stand alone.

In addition to Depo-Provera, there have been recent clinical reports of the use of other pharmacological agents in the treatment of paraphiliac and other compulsive sexual behaviors, such as compulsive masturbation. Because of the clinical observation that some individuals with paraphilias are quite compulsive in the behavior, there has been a specific interest in serotonin reuptake blockers, such as clomipramine and fluoxetine. Kafka (1991) reported significant results in a group of ten individuals who showed a mixture of paraphiliac behavior and nonparaphiliac sexual compulsions with co-morbid affective disorders. Seven of the 10 patients were treated with fluoxetine. Stein, Hollander, Anthony et al (1992) report a second series of 13 patients, again the patients being mixed, some with paraphiliac and others with compulsive sexual behaviors, and many with co-morbid obsessive–compulsive disorders. All the patients in the series were treated with either fluoxetine or clomipramine and the results were much more mixed; none of the patients with paraphilias showed any significant changes. Finally, Kruesi, Fine, and Valladares (1992) report a double-blind cross-over comparison of clomipramine versus desipramine with an initial placebo phase. Although only eight subjects were included, there were no differences between clomipramine and desipramine, although both were superior to placebo. At the current time, no firm conclusions can be drawn regarding the efficacy of serotonin reuptake blockers because of the small sample sizes, heterogeneity of populations studied, and variety of co-morbid disorders within the studies to date. However, even the moderate improvements observed warrant further investigations of these agents, which have much fewer side effects than Depo-Provera.

Identifying Antecedents to Sexual Abuse and Increasing Social Competence

Paraphiliac behavior is at times influenced by certain environmental stimuli or certain emotional events (Pithers, Marques, Gibat et al, 1983). Many paraphiliacs have trouble managing various emotional states and have difficulty with appropriate assertiveness and social skills. Therefore, programs provide a variety of structured social competency programs as part of treatment, such as stress management, anger management, interpersonal skills training, and assertiveness training.

Cognitive Distortions and Victim Empathy

Paraphiliacs whose behavior harms others tend to show limited empathy for their victims. We have hypothesized (Murphy, 1990) that one reason for the lack of empathy is that patients engage in a number of distortions that they use to reduce the guilt they feel about the behavior. These include blaming the victim ("she asked for it"), denying the impact on the victim ("she/he liked it," "I didn't hurt her"), or attempting to make the behavior socially acceptable ("I was only providing sex education to the child"). Methods to challenge such belief systems involve educating the patient regarding victim impact, directly confronting the distortions, and teaching patients to identify the distortions themselves. Treatment programs commonly use books or articles written by victims or movies presented from a victim's standpoint; some programs use actual confrontations between the offender and the victim's therapist or the actual victim.

Other Treatment Issues

Several other issues need to be addressed with paraphiliac patients. For example, offenders with alcohol and drug problems or with other concurrent psychiatric problems may need treatment for those problems. Alcohol and drug issues must be addressed, and appropriate medication is warranted for patients with major affective disorders or schizophrenic disorders. Similarly, marital therapy, family therapy, or sexual dysfunction therapy may be required for paraphiliacs with partners and for incest families that plan on reuniting.

ROLE OF THE NONPSYCHIATRIC PHYSICIAN IN PATIENT MANAGEMENT AND INDICATIONS FOR PSYCHIATRIC CONSULTATION AND REFERRAL

The vast majority of patients who present to physicians, victims or perpetrators, will require referral to an appropriate mental health professional. In almost all states, professionals are required by law to report to the proper authorities reasonable suspicion or evidence of child abuse, sexual or otherwise.

Physicians may encounter individuals who engage in paraphiliac behavior or who have paraphiliac urges that are not likely to harm others, the patient, or society (fetishism and transvestism, for example), and whose urges do not distress the patient. In such cases, depending on the physician's own moral beliefs and ethical standards, the physician might feel comfortable counseling the patient about the wide variety of sexual behaviors people engage in and letting the patient decide whether he needs to consult a specialist. Whenever a patient's fantasies and/or behavior involve either harming others or infringing on others' rights, more specialized services are required. The physician should remember that many paraphiliacs are not forthcoming with all their fantasy material or urges. In addition, as we have noted previously, many paraphiliacs have multiple paraphilias, and even though the one being presented may not seem to be of serious harm to others, there may be other issues the patient has not addressed. Even when the paraphilia is a hands-off offense, such as exhibitionism or voyeurism, many such patients also have other paraphilias that might be more directly harmful. Also, these paraphilias in and of themselves do infringe on the privacy of others. The physician faced with such a patient should maintain a nonjudgmental stance regarding the patient and should encourage the patient to disclose further material.

In making referrals, the physician should realize that not all mental health professionals (psychiatrists, psychologists, and social workers) have specialized training in treating paraphiliac patients; in fact, they may have very little experience with this specific diagnostic category. Many times, district attorneys, parole and probation officers, and child protection workers may have the best knowledge of individuals who specialize in the treatment of paraphiliacs in the community.

Physicians can play an important role in prevention. Most primary-care physicians who provide medical care to children on a regular basis can provide their patients with information on child sexual abuse the same way they provide them with pamphlets and brochures on a variety of medical problems. Also, the physician, regardless of specialty, should continually be aware of the high frequency of sexual abuse in the population. Many patients being treated by physicians for a variety of disorders may have been sexually abused, and sometimes the physical complaints can be directly tied to the abuse. The physician should keep this in mind and should not be afraid to ask patients routinely about past or present traumatic sexual experiences as part of their diagnostic workup.

CLINICAL PEARLS

- Many paraphiliac behaviors are both a psychiatric disorder and a crime. The patient's risk to society must always be considered.
- Patients may have multiple paraphilias, and these should always be considered when evaluating the patient.
- When evaluating a paraphiliac, especially those whose behavior harms others, the clinician should never rely solely on the patient's self-report and should seek collaborative information.
- Treatment of paraphilias is specialized. Not all mental health professionals have adequate training with this diagnostic group. Where possible, referrals should be to individuals with training in this area.
- Physicians should remember that victimization occurs frequently in our society. Physicians can play a key role in identifying victims and in prevention.

ANNOTATED BIBLIOGRAPHY

Blair CD, Lanyon RI: Exhibitionism: Etiology and treatment. Psychol Bull 89:439–463, 1981

  A good overall review of exhibitionism both clinically and theoretically. Provides excellent description of the theoretical approach to understanding exhibitionism and common treatment techniques.

Bradford JMW: Organic treatments for the male sexual offender. Behav Sci Law 3:355–375, 1985

  Reviews biological approaches to treatment of sex offenders, provides a good literature review, and discusses in some detail the pharmacology and application of antiandrogen drugs.

Finkelhor D: A Sourcebook on Child Sexual Abuse. Beverly Hills, Sage, 1986

  Probably the best single source for a general presentation of the whole area of child sexual abuse with discussion of victim, offender, and prevention.

Gelder M, Gath D, Mayou R: Oxford Textbook of Psychiatry. Oxford, Oxford University Press, 1983

  Includes a brief description of the major paraphilias, with some attention to etiology and a cursory outline of treatment.

Kaplan HI, Saddock B: Comprehensive Textbook of Psychiatry, 4th ed. Baltimore, Williams & Wilkins, 1985

  Contains a good overview of paraphilias and their proposed etiologies including environmental, biological, and analytic formulations, and highlighting clinical features, differential diagnosis, and a very brief discussion of treatment.

Marshall WL, Laws DR, Barbaree HE: Handbook of Sexual Assault: Issues, Theories, and Treatment of the Offender. New York, Plenum Press, 1990

  A most comprehensive review of sexual aggression against women and children. Includes information on the psychological, sociological, and biological aspects of this disorder plus clinical approaches.

REFERENCES

Abel GG, Becker JV, Mittelman M et al: Self-reported sex crimes of nonincarcerated paraphiliacs. J Interpers Viol 2:3–25, 1987

Abel GG, Cunningham-Rathner J, Becker JV McHugh J: Motivating sex offenders for treatment with feedback of their psychophysiologic assessment. Paper presented at the World Congress of Behavior Therapy, Washington, DC, December 1983.

Abel GG, Rouleau JL: The Nature and Extent of Sexual Assault. In Marshall WL, Laws DR, Barbaree HE (eds): Handbook of Sexual Assault: Issues, Theories, and Treatment of the Offender. New York, Plenum Press, 1990

Alexander PC: A systems theory conceptualization of incest. Fam Process 24:79–88, 1985

American Psychiatric Association: DSM-IV Draft Criteria 3/1/93. Washington, DC, American Psychiatric Association, 1993

American Psychiatric Association: Diagnostic and Statistical Manual of the Mental Disorders, 4th ed. Washington, DC, in press [1994]

Barlow DH, Abel GG: Recent Developments in Assessment and Treatment of Sexual Deviation. In Craighead WE, Kazdin AE, Mahoney MJ (eds): Behavior Modification: Principles, Issues, and Applications. Boston, Houghton Mifflin, 1976

Barlow DH, Leitenberg H, Agras WD: The experimental control of sexual deviation through manipulation of the noxious scene in covert sensitization. J Abnorm Psychol 74:596–601, 1969

Berlin FS: Sex Offenders: A Biomedical Perspective and a Status Report on Biomedical Treatment. In Greer JG, Stuart IR (eds): The Sexual Aggressor: Current Perspectives on Treatment. New York, Van Nostrand Reinhold, 1983

Blair CD, Lanyon RI: Exhibitionism: Etiology and treatment. Psychol Bull 89:439–463, 1981

Blumer D: Transsexualism, Sexual Dysfunction, and Temporal Lobe Disorder. In Green R, Money J (eds): Transsexualism and Sex Reassignment. Baltimore, Johns Hopkins, 1969

Bradford JMW: Organic treatment for the male sexual offender. Behav Sci Law 3:355–375, 1985

Brownell KD, Barlow DH: Measurement and treatment of two sexual deviations in one person. J Behav Ther Exp Psychiatry 7:349–354, 1976

Brownell KD, Hayes SC, Barlow DH: Patterns of appropriate and deviant sexual arousal: The behavioral treatment of multiple sexual deviations. J Consul Clin Psychol 45:1144–1155, 1977

Brownmiller S: Against Our Will: Men, Women and Rape. New York, Simon and Schuster, 1975

Cautela JR, Wisocki PA: Covert sensitization for the treatment of sexual deviations. Psychologic Rec 21:37–48, 1971

Conte JR: Sexual Abuse and the Family: A Critical Analysis. In Trepper TS, Barrett MJ (eds): Treating Incest: A Multimodal Systems Perspective. New York, Haworth, 1986

Conte JR: Clinical dimensions of adult sexual abuse of children. Behav Sci Law 3:341–354, 1985

Cox DJ, McMahon B: Incidence of male exhibitionism in the United States as reported by victimized female college students. Int J Law Psychiatry 1:453–457, 1978

Finkelhor D: A Sourcebook on Child Sexual Abuse. Beverly Hills, Sage, 1986

Finkelhor D: Child Sexual Abuse: New Theory and Research. New York, Free Press, 1984

Finkelhor D, Russell D: Women as Perpetrators: Review of the Evidence. In Finkelhor D (ed): Child Sexual Abuse: New Theory and Research. New York, Free Press, 1984

Freund K: Therapeutic sex drive reduction. Acta Psychiatr Scand 62:(suppl 287)5–38, 1980

Gittleson NL, Eacott ST, Mehta BM: Victims of indecent exposure. Br J Psychiatry 132:61–66, 1978

Groth AN, Hobson WF, Gary TS: The child molester: Clinical observations. Soc Work Hum Sexuality 1:129–144, 1982

Hammer RF, Glueck BC Jr: Psychodynamic patterns in sex offenders: A four-factor theory. Psychiatr Q 31:325–345, 1957

Hanson RK, Slater S: Sexual victimization in the history of sexual abusers: A review. Ann Sex Res 1:485–499, 1988

Hunt M: Sexual Behavior in the 1970s. Chicago, Playboy Press, 1974

Hucker S, Langevin R, Bain J: A double-blind trial of sex drive reducing medication in pedophiles. Ann Sex Res 1:227–242, 1988

Kafka MP: Successful antidepressant treatment of nonparaphilic sexual addictions and paraphilias in men. J Clin Psychiatry 52:60–65, 1991

Karpman B: The Sexual Offender and His Offenses: Etiology, Pathology, Psychodynamics and Treatment. New York, Julian Press, 1954

Knopp FH: Retraining Adult Sex Offenders: Methods and Models. Syracuse, NY, Safer Society Press, 1984

Kruesi MJP, Fine S, Valladares L et al: Paraphilias: A double-blind cross-over comparison of clomipramine versus desipramine. Arch Sex Behav 21:587–593, 1992

Langevin R: Sexual Anomalies and the Brain. In Marshall WL, Laws DR, Barbaree HE: Handbook of Sexual Assault: Issues, Theories, and Treatment of the Offender. New York, Plenum Press, 1990

Larson NR, Maddock JW: Structural and Functional Variables in Incest Family Systems: Implications for Assessment and Treatment. In Trepper TS, Barrett MJ (eds): Treating Incest: A Multimodal Systems Perspective. New York, Haworth Press, 1986

Laws DR, Osborne CA: How to Build and Operate a Behavioral Laboratory to Evaluate and Treat Sexual Deviates. In Greer JG, Stuart IR (eds): The Sexual Aggressor: Current Perspectives on Treatment. New York, Van Nostrand Reinhold, 1983

Maletzky BM. Assisted Covert Sensitization. In Cox DJ, Daitzman RJ (eds): Exhibitionism: Description, Assessment and Treatment. New York, Garland Press, 1980

Marshall WL: Satiation therapy: A procedure for reducing sexual arousal. J Appl Behav Anal 12:10–22, 1979

Marshall W, Lippens BA: The clinical value of boredom: A procedure for reducing inappropriate sexual interests. J Nerv Ment Dis 165:283–287, 1977

McGuire RJ, Carlisle JM, Young BG: Sexual deviations as conditioned behavior: A hypothesis. Behav Res Ther 2:185–190, 1965

Meyer WJ, Cole C, Emory E: Depo-Provera treatment for sex offending behavior: An evaluation of outcome. Bull Am Acad Psychiatry Law, 20:249–259, 1992

Moser C, Levitt EE: An exploratory-descriptive study of a sadomasochistically oriented sample. J Sex Res 23:322–337, 1987

Murphy WD: Assessment and Modifications of Cognitive Distortions in Sex Offenders. In Marshall WL, Laws DR, Barbaree HE (eds): Handbook of Sexual Assault: Issues, Theories, and Treatment of the Offender. New York, Plenum Press, 1990

Murphy WD, Coleman EM, Haynes MR: Factors related to coercive sexual behavior in a nonclinical sample of males. Violence and Victims 1:255–278, 1986

Murphy WD, Haynes MR, Worley PJ: Assessment of Adult Sexual Interest. In Hollin CR, Howells K (eds): Clinical Approaches to Sex Offenders and Their Victims. West Sussex, England, John Wiley and Sons, 1991

Murphy WD, Stalgaitis SJ: Assessment and Treatment Considerations for Sexual Offenders Against Children: Behavioral and Social Learning Approaches. In McNamara JR, Appel MA (eds): Critical Issues, Developments, and Trends in Professional Psychology, Vol. 3. New York, Praeger, 1987

Murram D, Weatherford T: Child sexual abuse in Shelby County, Tennessee: Two years of experience. Adolesc Pediatr Gynecol 1:114–118, 1988

Peters SD, Wyatt GE, Finkelhor D: Prevalence. In Finkelhor D (ed): A Sourcebook on Child Sexual Abuse. Beverly Hills: Sage, 1986

Pithers WD, Marques JK, Gibat CC et al: Relapse Prevention with Sexual Aggressives: A Self-Control Model of Treatment and Maintenance of Change. In Greer JG, Stuart IR (eds): The Sexual Aggressor: Current Perspectives on Treatment. New York, Van Nostrand Reinhold, 1983

Quinsey VL: The assessment and treatment of child molesters: A review. Can Psych Rev 18:204–220, 1977

Quinsey VL, Marshall WL: Procedures for Reducing Inappropriate Sexual Arousal: An Evaluation Review. In Greer JG, Stuart IR (eds): The Sexual Aggressor: Current Perspectives on Treatment. New York, Van Nostrand Reinhold, 1983

Rachman S: Sexual fetishism: An experimental analogue. Psychol Rec 16:293–296, 1966

Rachman S, Hodgson R: Experimentally induced "sexual fetishism." Replication and development. Psychol Rec 18:25–27, 1968

Regestein QR, Reich P: Pedophilia occurring after onset of cognitive impairment. J Nerv Ment Dis 166:794–798, 1978

Stein DJ, Hollander E, Anthony DT et al: Serotonergic medications for sexual obsessions, sexual addictions, and paraphilias. J Clin Psychiatry 53:267–271, 1992

Wise TN: Fetishism—etiology and treatment: A review from multiple perspectives. Compr Psychiatry 26:249–257, 1985

Alan Stoudemire (ed). *Clinical Psychiatry for Medical Students,* Second
Edition. Copyright © 1994, 1990 by J. B. Lippincott Company.

16 *Psychiatric Disorders of Childhood and Adolescence*

Mina K. Dulcan

This chapter addresses the identification, evaluation, and treatment of psychiatric disorders as they occur in children and adolescents. The most detailed coverage is given to the diagnoses most likely to present in childhood and adolescence (see Table 16–1) and those that are most likely to be encountered in family and pediatric medicine or surgical practices. Although phobias, obsessive–compulsive disorder, posttraumatic stress disorder, mood disorders, schizophrenia, anorexia nervosa, and bulimia nervosa occur in youth, these disorders are covered primarily in the chapters on adult psychopathology. This chapter highlights the *differences* between adult and childhood forms of psychiatric illness in clinical manifestations, evaluation, and treatment.

It should also be noted that children and adolescents may be given any psychiatric diagnosis for which they meet criteria. In general, personality disorder diagnoses are not given to patients younger than 18 years old because personality development is not considered to be completed until adulthood. Space does not allow for detailed specification of diagnostic criteria in this chapter. They are documented in the *Diagnostic and Statistical Manual of Mental Disorders,* 4th Ed (APA 1993, in press [1994]).

The last section of this chapter covers psychological aspects of medical illness in children and adolescents. This topic is of particular importance to students interested in family practice, pediatrics, and surgery. Students who plan a career in internal medicine will find that many of the emotional reactions to physical illness described in children and their families also occur in adults (see also Chapter 20 by Dr. Levenson).

426

Table 16–1 **Disorders Usually First Diagnosed in Infancy, Childhood, or Adolescence***

Attention-deficit Hyperactivity Disorder
Conduct Disorder
Oppositional Defiant Disorder
Separation Anxiety Disorder
Rumination Disorder
Encopresis
Enuresis
Tic Disorders
Mental Retardation
Pervasive Developmental Disorders
Learning Disorders
Communication Disorders

* Adapted from DSM-IV (APA 1993, in press [1994])

PSYCHIATRIC EVALUATION

When evaluating a child or adolescent, a great deal of the history is gathered from the parents or guardians (see Table 16–2). Standardized questionnaires supplement information from interviews. An excellent example is the Child Behavior Checklist (CBCL), which comes in several forms: for parents of children ages 2 to 3 years and 4 to 18 years (Achenbach, 1991a), the Youth Self-Report Form for ages 11 to 18 years (Achenbach, 1991b), and the Teacher's Report Form (Achenbach, 1991c).

The importance of a thorough knowledge of normal development cannot be overemphasized. The symptoms of many psychiatric disorders in childhood and adolescence are characteristic of all normal children at earlier developmental stages (such as bedwetting or tantrums) or appear occasionally in many normal children (for example, lying, stealing, or short attention span). Psychopathology is determined by the pattern of symptoms as well as their severity, intensity, frequency, duration, and by the child's degree of impairment in functioning.

When interviewing the child or adolescent, important information is gathered by direct questioning and by observations of appearance, affect, and behavior. The interview must be adapted for the age and maturity of the patient. Children and adolescents are often better reporters than their parents about feelings of anxiety and depression and about conduct problems such as stealing, truancy, or substance abuse.

A physical examination is usually indicated to search for medical causes of symptoms and to discover and treat any unrelated but coexisting medical disorders. The decision to conduct additional medical evaluations, such as a neurological examination or laboratory tests, is made based on the findings of the medical history and physical examination (see Chapter 1 by Drs. Yates, Kathol, and Carter). Anticipated pharmacologic treatment may require additional studies to establish baseline values and to rule out contraindications to a particular medication.

Table 16–2 **Biopsychosocial History of a Child or Adolescent**

Chief complaint
History of present illness
    Development of the symptoms
    Attitudes toward the symptoms
    Effects on the child and family
    Stressors
    Prior psychiatric treatment and results
        Psychotherapy: type, frequency, duration
        Medication: exact doses, schedule, beneficial effects, side effects
        Environmental changes
Past history
    Medical
    Psychiatric
Medical review of systems
Review of psychological symptoms
Developmental history (milestones)
School history
Family history
    Medical
    Psychiatric
    Developmental

Information from the school is always useful and is essential when there is concern about learning, behavior in school, or functioning with peers. With parental consent, the clinician may interview teachers; obtain records of testing, grades, and attendance; and have school personnel complete a standardized rating form such as the Teacher's Report Form of the Child Behavior Checklist (Achenbach, 1991c). Ideally, a visit to the school is arranged to observe the youngster in the classroom and on the playground.

Psychological testing, including an individually administered intelligence test and achievement tests, is obtained when there is any question about learning or IQ (see Table 16–3 and Chapter 3 by Drs. Kaslow and Farber). Additional testing for specific learning disabilities is conducted as indicated by school reports and the results of initial tests.

In a typical pediatric clinic, 15 to 20% of the children suffer from an emotional or behavioral problem of sufficient severity to warrant mental health care (Costello and Pantino, 1987). Parents and children, however, often do not spontaneously report their concerns about behavior, development, and/or emotional problems because they perceive physicians as "too busy," not interested, or unable to help with "nonmedical" problems (Costello and Pantino, 1987). In medical settings, parents should be asked if they have any worries about the child's development, school performance, emotions, or behavior. Children and adolescents are asked if they have been feeling depressed or sad or worried or nervous. The primary care physician should be prepared to detect physical or sexual abuse or neglect or to provide anticipatory guidance regarding sexuality.

Table 16–3 **Psychoeducational Test Instruments**

Estimated Cognitive Developmental Level in Very Young Children

Bayley Scales of Infant Development
  Age 3 to 30 months

Intelligence

Kaufman Assessment Battery for Children (K-ABC)
  Age 2½ to 12½ years
  Less dependent on culturally based information and schooling
Peabody Picture Vocabulary Test (PPVT-R)
  Brief test of receptive language abilities, often used as a screening test for IQ
Stanford-Binet Intelligence Scale, 4th ed.
  Age 2 years to adulthood
  Heavily language based
Wechsler Preschool and Primary Scale of Intelligence (WPPSI)
  Age 4 to 6½ years
Wechsler Intelligence Scale for Children, 3rd ed. (WISC-III)
  Age 6 to 16 years
Wechsler Adult Intelligence Scale (WAIS)
  Age 16 years and over

Academic Achievement

Peabody Individual Achievement Test (PIAT)
Wide Range Achievement Test (WRAT)
Woodcock Reading Mastery Tests

Developmental Level of Adaptive Functioning

Vineland Adaptive Behavior Scales

Indications for consultation with a child and adolescent psychiatrist after the initial screening assessment include:

Physical symptoms with unexplained etiology or severity
Noncompliance with medical treatment
Developmental delays
Physician observation or child's or parent's report of depression, anxiety, or hyperactive behavior
Impaired school performance
Problems with peer or family relationships
Suspected substance abuse
Parental difficulties with child rearing

GENERAL PRINCIPLES OF TREATMENT PLANNING FOR CHILDREN AND ADOLESCENTS

The initial treatment plan is based on the diagnosis, target symptoms, and strengths and weaknesses of the patient and the family. The child's environment, including school, neighborhood, and social support network, will also influence the choice of treatment strategy. Children and adolescents are usually best served by a combination of treatment modalities. Parents should be included in treatment planning by informing them of the probable course of the disorder if untreated, describing available treatments, and estimating the potential benefits and risks for their child. The child or adolescent patient is included in this discussion as appropriate. With only a few exceptions, all of the treatments used for adults may be used for children and adolescents, with modifications for the patient's developmental status. In most cases, coordination with the parents, school, pediatrician, child welfare agency, courts, or recreation leader will be part of the treatment plan.

Parents of children and adolescents with psychiatric or learning problems need and deserve education in the nature of their child's disorder and in managing difficult behaviors. Parents spend far more time with their children than the therapist does and parents can powerfully assist or impede the process of treatment. Treatment planning is an ongoing process, with reevaluations done as interventions are attempted and as additional information about the child and family comes to light.

Pharmacologic Treatment

When using psychopharmacologic agents with children and adolescents, important general principles include minimizing the use of multiple medications and **virtually never using medication as the only form of treatment.** It is important to educate the family regarding the medication, and resources are now available to assist in this process (see Dulcan, 1992). The physician must consider the potential meaning of medication to the child, family, school, and the child's peer group.

In considering a specific medication treatment for a child or adolescent, the physician has a special responsibility to consider the risk/benefit ratio. Both therapeutic and side effects of the medication must be actively evaluated, seeking information from the child, parent, and other relevant adults such as teachers. There is a need to balance the potential risks of the medication with the prognosis of the untreated disorder and with what is known about the relative efficacy of medication. It is important to note that the U.S. Food and Drug Administration guidelines, as published in the *Physicians Desk Reference* (PDR), are meant to regulate the advertising of pharmaceutical companies—not the clinical practice of physicians. These companies often do not go to the expense and trouble of testing in children and adolescents drugs marketed primarily for adults. This often results in overly conservative doses or lack of "approval" for certain indications. For older drugs, the PDR may recommend indications or doses that are no longer considered appropriate. The clinician should therefore rely on the scientific literature rather than the PDR.

Adjunctive Treatments

Modified school programs are indicated for those children and adolescents who cannot perform satisfactorily in regular classrooms, who need additional structure or specialized teaching techniques to reach their academic potential, or whose behavior requires a small class and specifically trained teachers.

Prior to being placed in a special education class, youngsters must have individually administered psychological tests, including an intelligence test, achievement tests, and an evaluation for learning disabilities. Federal law 94-142 requires that all children who need them receive special services. These must be provided in the least restrictive environment—that is, as much in the "mainstream" with other children and adolescents—as possible.

Learning a sport or hobby may be an especially important adjunct in the treatment of children and adolescents who lack positive relationships with peers or adults. A relationship with an adult such as a Big Brother or Sister or a YMCA counselor, or an opportunity to attend a camp, may improve self-esteem and peer relationships.

Placement in a foster home may be needed when parents are unwilling or unable to care for a child or adolescent. Indications are clearest in cases of physical neglect or physical or sexual abuse. Other families may be unable to provide the appropriate emotional or physical environment.

DISRUPTIVE BEHAVIOR DISORDERS

Attention-Deficit Hyperactivity Disorder

Children who have problems at home and school because they are fidgety, restless, overactive, inattentive, distractible, and impulsive have been described in the past as having minimal brain damage or dysfunction, hyperactivity, hyperkinetic reaction or syndrome of childhood, or attention-deficit disorder (ADD) with or without hyperactivity. The current diagnostic term is attention-deficit hyperactivity disorder (ADHD). There are three subtypes: (a) attention deficits only (inattentive type), (b) hyperactivity and impulsivity, and (c) both groups of symptoms (combined type).

Epidemiology

Between 14 and 20% of preschool and kindergarten boys and approximately a third as many girls have ADHD (Campbell, 1985). In elementary schools, 3 to 10% of students have ADHD symptoms. Many overactive, distractible, and impulsive children can be identified by parents and teachers but have not been diagnosed or treated. A 1987 survey in Baltimore County, Maryland, found 6% of all public elementary school students, 3.7% of middle school students, and 0.4% of high school students to be receiving stimulant treatment for ADHD (Safer and Krager, 1988). Boys outnumber girls in the prevalence of ADHD more dramatically in clinical settings than in school populations.

Description

Diagnostic criteria for ADHD require a pattern of behavior that appeared no later than the age of 7 years, has been present for at least 6 months, and is excessive for age and intelligence. The symptoms are divided into inattention and hyperactivity-impulsivity and must be present often, although not necessarily all of the time or in every situation. Possible symptoms are listed below, but all are not required in a specific child (APA 1993, in press [1994]):

1. Fidgety or restless
2. Difficulty staying seated
3. Easily distracted
4. Difficulty waiting in lines or awaiting his/her turn
5. Impulsive speech
6. Difficulty following instructions
7. Short attention span at work and play
8. Difficulty playing quietly
9. Doesn't seem to listen
10. Loses things
11. Makes careless mistakes
12. Difficulty organizing
13. Avoids engaging in effortful mental activities, particularly when not interested
14. Forgetful
15. Runs about or climbs excessively in situations where these activities are inappropriate

Potentially dangerous impulsive behavior may also occur. Variability of symptoms from time to time and in different situations is a hallmark of ADHD. Many youngsters with ADHD can pay attention for an hour or more to a highly engaging activity of their own choosing, such as television or a computer game.

Teachers complain that children with ADHD are frequently "off task" and disturb others by fidgeting, making noises, or talking. Their written work is often messy and characterized by poor handwriting and impulsive, careless errors. Virtually all youngsters with ADHD have deficits in learning, achievement, or completion of school work by the time the diagnosis is made.

Hyperactive behavior per se is no longer considered the key or even a necessary feature of this disorder, although the term is often used as shorthand for ADHD. Douglas (1983) proposes as primary deficits:

1. Lack of investment, organization, and maintenance of attention and effort in completing tasks
2. Inability to inhibit impulsive action
3. Lack of modulation of arousal levels to meet the demands of the situation
4. Unusually strong inclination to seek immediate reinforcement

Commonly associated features of ADHD are low self-esteem, feelings of depression and demoralization, and lack of ability to take responsibility for one's actions. In social situations, these youngsters tend to be immature, bossy, intrusive, loud, uncooperative, out of synchrony with situational expectations, and irritating to both adults and peers. As a result, they may have few friends, preferring to play with older or younger children.

In a specific child, association between ADHD and neurological soft signs, minor physical anomalies, and EEG abnormalities are not clinically useful because they are not always present in ADHD and because many normal children and those with other psychiatric diagnoses have such findings (Rutter, 1982).

From 50 to 80% of children with ADHD continue to show symptoms of hyperactivity, impulsivity, and inattention during adolescence, which frequently results in academic failure and/or school behavioral problems, depressed mood, low self-esteem, family conflict, and poor peer relationships. *In young adulthood, two-thirds of grown-up hyperactive children continue to show at least some symptoms of restlessness, poor concentration, impulsivity, and/or explosiveness, with resulting impairments in academic, vocational, and social functioning.*

In clinical settings, *at least two-thirds of patients with ADHD also have oppositional defiant disorder (ODD) or conduct disorder.* (These disorders are discussed in detail later.) Youngsters with coexisting attentional and conduct disorders tend to have an earlier age of onset, exhibit a greater total number of antisocial behaviors, and display more physical aggression. Of all children with ADHD, those with co-morbid conduct disorder are virtually the only ones at risk for antisocial behavior and drug use as adults.

Differential Diagnosis

Inexperienced or overly critical parents or teachers may confuse *normal age-appropriate overactivity* with ADHD. Onset of symptoms after age seven or a duration of less than six months may indicate an *adjustment disorder*, especially if there is an identifiable stressor in the child's life. Children who are fidgety and preoccupied may have an *anxiety disorder* instead of (or in addition to) ADHD.

Prepubertal children with *bipolar disorder* may manifest a chronic mixed affective state marked by irritability, overactivity, and difficulty concentrating. Family history may be helpful in differentiating this from ADHD, but long-term follow-up may provide the only conclusive answer.

Children who are restless and inattentive only at school may have *mental retardation* or a *specific developmental disorder* rather than ADHD. ADHD can be diagnosed *in addition to* mental retardation if symptoms are excessive for the child's *mental* age. Delays in specific learning skills, such as reading, math, and language, are commonly associated with ADHD.

Symptoms resembling ADHD can be caused by *drugs* such as phenobarbital (prescribed as an anticonvulsant) or theophylline (for asthma). *Hyperthyroidism* can be differentiated from ADHD by the presence of physical signs and by laboratory measures.

Etiology

Familial factors have been strongly implicated, although teasing out genetic from environmental influences is difficult. Children with ADHD alone have an elevated rate of first-degree relatives with ADHD. Children who have both ADHD and conduct disorder tend to come from families with an increased rate of ADHD, conduct disorder, ODD, and antisocial personality disorder (Biederman et al, 1986).

Neurotransmitter abnormalities in ADHD have been suggested but have not been consistently documented. Recent imaging studies suggest delayed or abnormal maturation of the frontal lobes of the brain. Biological insults associated with some cases of ADHD include complications of pregnancy, maternal alcohol use or smoking, postmaturity, long labor, health problems or malnutrition in infancy, lead poisoning, phenylketonuria, and glucose-6-phosphate dehydrogenase deficiency.

Evaluation

Reports should be obtained from multiple sources, always including the teacher and preferably incorporating rating scales with standardized norms such as the Child Behavior Checklist for parents (Achenbach, 1991a) and the Teacher's Report Form (Achenbach, 1991c). Children often do not demonstrate problem behaviors in the doctor's office but may be overactive, impulsive, and distractible in the waiting room. Psychological testing is nearly always needed to evaluate the IQ and academic achievement and to search for specific developmental disorders. Motor or vocal tics should be sought in both the patient and family, because patients with Tourette's disorder commonly have coexisting ADHD.

Treatment

Psychotherapy. Dynamically oriented individual therapy is not effective as a primary treatment for ADHD. These children have little insight into their behavior and its effect on others and may be genuinely unable to report their problems or to reflect on them. Supportive psychotherapy may be helpful in addressing low self-esteem and demoralization resulting from the parent, teacher, and peer reactions to the ADHD child's behavior, or in resolving the effects of a parental divorce or other stressor. Family therapy can address problems caused by living with a difficult child or other marital or family dynamics that may interfere with consistent management. Group therapy is useful in improving social skills and peer relations.

Behavior Modification. Behavior modification can improve both academic achievement and behavioral compliance if they are specifically targeted. Both *noncorporal* punishment (time out and response cost) and reward components are required. Behavioral techniques, including the teaching of specific social skills, can improve peer interactions. Behavior modification addresses symptoms that stimulants do not, but more cooperation from parents and teachers is required, and generalization and maintenance are elusive. Many youngsters require programs that are intensive and prolonged for months to years. The most effective behavioral treatment programs specify target behaviors at both home and school.

Classroom behavior modification techniques include explicit class rules, token economies, attention to positive behavior, and response cost programs (withdrawal of reinforcers following undesirable behavior) (Abramowitz and O'Leary, 1991). Reinforcers such as praise, stars on a chart, or privileges may be dispensed by the teacher or by parents through the use of daily report cards.

Cognitive Behavioral or Problem-Solving Therapy. This form of treatment combines behavior modification techniques, such as contingent reinforcement and modeling, with instruction in cognitive strategies, such as stepwise problem solving and self-monitoring. It was developed in an attempt to improve the generalization and durability of behavior modification techniques and directly addresses presumed deficits in the control of impulsivity and problem solving (Kendall and Braswell, 1985). Unfortunately, most empirical studies have shown limited efficacy in the treatment of ADHD.

Psychopharmacologic Treatment. The decision to use medication for ADHD is based on symptoms (not due to another treatable cause) of inattention, impulsivity, and often hyperactivity that are persistent and of sufficient severity to cause functional impairment at school and, usually, at home and with peers. Parents must be willing to monitor the medication and to attend appointments. Behavioral and school-related interventions are usually considered first unless severe impulsivity and non-compliance create an urgent situation.

Measures from both home and school of baseline symptoms and progress are essential in monitoring response to treatment. Prior to starting medication, the child, family, and teacher should be educated about the use and possible positive and side effects of the medication. It is helpful to debunk common myths about treatment. The physician should work closely with parents on dose adjustments and obtain frequent reports from teachers and annual academic testing.

It is clear that medication alone is not sufficient treatment. Every study of pharmacologic treatment of hyperactivity that has used more than one outcome measure has shown that even children who respond positively continue to show deficits in some areas.

Stimulants. Stimulants, which include methylphenidate, dextroamphetamine, and magnesium pemoline, are the most commonly used medications in the treatment of ADHD. One theory regarding their mechanism of action suggests that stimulants act by canalizing or reducing the excessive, poorly synchronized variability in the various dimensions of arousal and reactivity seen in ADHD (Evans, Gualtieri, and Hicks, 1986). Contrary to previous belief, normal and hyperactive children, adolescents, and adults have similar cognitive and behavioral responses to comparable doses of stimulants, although children do not report euphoria. Stimulants do *not* have a paradoxical sedative action; they do *not* lead to drug abuse or addiction; and many adolescents with ADHD continue to require and benefit from their use.

Up to 96% of children with ADHD have at least some positive behavioral response to methylphenidate and/or dextroamphetamine, although side effects limit efficacy or require discontinuation of medication in some children (Elia, Borcherding, Rapoport, and Keysor, 1991). Both preschool children and adolescents may require lower weight-adjusted doses than school-aged children, and may have greater likelihood of side effects and somewhat lower therapeutic efficacy. Up to 25% of children who respond poorly to one stimulant medication have a positive response to another. Stimulants reliably decrease physical activity, especially during times when children are expected to be less active (such as during school but not during free play). They decrease vocalization, noise, and disruption in the classroom to the level of normal peers and improve handwriting. Stimulants consistently reduce off task behavior and improve compliance to adult commands.

Stimulants produce improvement on cognitive laboratory tasks measuring sustained attention, distractibility, impulsivity, and short-term memory. Cognitive learning strategies that the child typically uses are enhanced. Stimulants increase productivity and decrease errors in tests of arithmetic, reading comprehension, sight vocabulary, and spelling, and increase the percentage of assigned seat work completed (Pelham and Hoza, 1987).

Methylphenidate and behavior modification at home and school have been shown to be additive in effect on motor, attention, and social measures for many ADHD children (Pelham and Murphy, 1986). Stimulant medication and behavior modification can be synergistic in improving classroom behavior. Behavior modification plus a low dose of medication yields a benefit equivalent to a higher dose of medication alone (Carlson et al, 1992).

Stimulant medication should be initiated with a low dose and titrated weekly according to response and side effects (see Tables 16–4 and 16–5). Weight-corrected doses provide an approximate range. Stimulants should be given after meals to reduce anorexia. The need for medication after school or on weekends is individually determined. In most cases, the presence of motor or vocal tics in the patient or family contraindicates the use of a stimulant medication.

If target symptoms are not too severe, stimulants are discontinued for an annual drug-free trial for at least two weeks in the summer. If school functioning is stable, a trial off the medication in the middle of the school year is useful to assess whether it is still needed.

Tolerance has been reported occasionally, but compliance is often irregular and missed doses should be the first possibility considered when medication appears to lose its effect. It is not wise for children to be responsible for their own medication. Alternate reasons for apparent decreased drug effect are an increase in the patient's weight (prior to puberty only) or a reaction to a change at home or school.

Recent data suggest that the long-acting stimulant formulations—Ritalin Sustained Release (S-R) and Dexedrine Spansule—are more effective than previously thought, although there may be a delay in the onset of action and increased variability from day to day (Pelham, Sturges, Hoza et al, 1987). For some children, Dexedrine Spansule appears to be more consistently efficacious than other stimulant preparations (Pelham et al, 1990). The longer-acting formulations are especially useful when the short-acting forms last only 2.5 to 3 hours or cause severe rebound symptoms or when medication cannot be administered at school. Highly individualized regimens combining short- and long-acting forms may be best for some children. Unpredictably high doses may result if a child chews a long-acting tablet instead of swallowing it.

Magnesium pemoline is a longer-acting, mild central nervous system stimulant structurally dissimilar to methylphenidate and dextroamphetamine. Pemoline may be able to be given once a day although absorption and metabolism vary widely, and some children need twice-daily doses.

Stimulant side effects are listed in Table 16–5. There is no evidence that stimulants produce a decrease in the seizure threshold. The combination of methylphenidate and the tricyclic imipramine has been associated with a syndrome of confusion, affective lability, marked aggression, and severe agitation in children (Grob and Coyle, 1986).

Table 16–4 Clinical Use of Medications to Treat ADHD in Prepubertal Children

	Methylphenidate (Ritalin)	Dextroamphetamine (Dexedrine)	Pemoline (Cylert)	Desipramine (Norpramin)	Clonidine (Catapres)
How Supplied (mg)	5,10,20 Sustained Release 20	5,10 (tablet) Elixer Spansule 5,10,15	18.75,37.5,75	10,25,50,75,100,150	0.1 (scored tablet) 0.1,0.2,0.4 mg/day skin patch
Usual Single Dose Range	0.3–0.8 mg/kg/dose	0.15–0.5 mg/kg/dose	0.5–2.5 mg/kg/dose	10–100 mg/dose	0.05–0.1 mg/dose
Usual Daily Dose (mg/kg/day)	0.6–2	0.3–1.25	0.5–3.0	4–6	0.003–0.006
Range (mg/day)	10–60	5–40	37.5–112.5		0.15–0.30
Usual Starting Dose (mg)	5 daily or BID	2.5–5 daily or BID	18.75–37.5 daily	10–25 daily (0.5 mg/kg)	0.05–0.1 daily
Maintenance					
Number of doses per day	2–4	2–4	1–2	2–3	3–4
Monitor	Pulse Blood pressure Growth Dysphoria Tics	Pulse Blood pressure Growth Dysphoria Tics	Pulse Blood pressure Growth Dysphoria Tics Liver functions	EKG Blood pressure	Blood pressure EKG Fasting glucose Sedation Dysphoria

Table 16–5 **Side Effects of Stimulant Medications**

Common Initial Side Effects (Try dose reduction)

Anorexia
Weight loss
Irritability
Abdominal pain
Headaches
Emotional oversensitivity, easy crying

Less-common Side Effects

Insomnia
Dysphoria
Social withdrawal
Rebound overactivity and irritability (Try adding small afternoon or evening dose or using time-release medication)
Impaired cognitive test performance (especially at very high doses)
Less than expected weight gain
Anxiety
Nervous habits (picking at skin, hair twisting or pulling)
Allergic rash or hives

Rare But Potentially Serious Side Effects

Motor or vocal tics
Tourette's disorder
Depression
Growth retardation (more likely with high doses)
Tachycardia
Hypertension
Psychosis with hallucinations
Compulsions or stereotyped activities

Side Effects More Common in Preschool Children *

Sadness
Irritability
Clinginess
Insomnia
Anorexia

Side Effects Reported with Pemoline Only **

Choreiform movements
Dyskinesias
Night terrors
Lip licking or biting
Chemical hepatitis (very rare)

* Campbell, 1985
** McDaniel, 1986

Tricyclic Antidepressants. Desipramine, a drug with less anticholinergic side effects than other cyclic antidepressants, is useful in the treatment of children and adolescents with ADHD, including some unresponsive to stimulants (Biederman, Baldessarini, Wright, Knee, and Harmatz, 1989). Drawbacks to using tricyclics such as desipramine include potentially serious cardiac side effects, especially in prepubertal children, and the danger of accidental or intentional overdose. When properly monitored, however, desipramine does not appear to be associated with an increased risk of sudden death in children with normal cardiac electrophysiology (J Biederman, personal communication, 1992). *Desipramine is used in patients who do not respond to stimulants, who develop significant depression on stimulants, who have a personal or family history of tics, or who develop tics when on a stimulant.* Desipramine has a longer duration of action than methylphenidate, so a dose at school is not needed and rebound is not generally a problem. Prepubertal children should be given three divided doses to avoid excessive peaks and valleys in blood levels. Desipramine is begun at 10 or 25 mg/day and gradually titrated to a maximum dose of 2 to 5 mg/kg/day. The use of tricyclics in children is discussed further in the section on childhood mood disorders.

Clonidine. This alpha-adrenergic agonist, given in pill or transdermal form, is useful for a subgroup of children with ADHD, including those with tics or a family history of Tourette's disorder or when a stimulant is only partially effective (Hunt, Capper, and O'Connell, 1990). Clonidine is particularly useful in decreasing hyperactivity, impulsivity, defiance, emotional lability, and temper tantrums and in improving frustration tolerance and the ability to fall asleep at night. Maximum therapeutic effect may not be seen for several months. Although clonidine is not helpful in improving attention per se, if a stimulant is not contraindicated, they may be used together. Vital signs, complete blood count, fasting glucose, and urinalysis should be obtained before starting clonidine. Some clinicians recommend an EKG. The most troublesome side effect of clonidine is sedation, although it tends to decrease after several weeks. Hypotension and dizziness may occur at high doses. Dry mouth, photophobia, dysphoria, bradycardia, and abnormal glucose tolerance have been reported. The transdermal form may produce a pruritic skin rash. Clonidine should be tapered rather than stopped suddenly to avoid a withdrawal syndrome consisting of increased blood pressure, elevated pulse, and motor restlessness (Leckman, Ort, Caruso et al, 1986).

Environmental Interventions for ADHD

Academic deficits, learning disabilities, and/or behavior problems may necessitate tutoring, a special class for all or part of the day, or a special school. Recreational or camp programs are often useful.

Many parents ask about special diets to treat childhood behavior problems. At most 5% of hyperactive children show minimal behavioral or cognitive improvement on the so-called Feingold or Kaiser-Permanente diet (Wender, 1986). Inducing the child to comply is extremely difficult. Controlled studies have been unable to demonstrate consistently that ingestion of sugar has any effect on the behavior or cognitive performance of normal or hyperactive children, even those identified by their parents as sugar responsive (Milich, Wolraich, and Lindgren, 1986).

The Role of the Primary Care Physician

The pediatrician or family physician is likely to be the first to be approached by parents concerned about the possibility of ADHD. Milder, uncomplicated cases of ADHD can be managed by the primary care physician in close collaboration with a psychologist to perform testing to identify intellectual deficits and learning disabilities, and a child and adolescent psychiatrist or psychologist to provide psychotherapeutic interventions as needed. Cases with psychiatric co-morbidity or that do not respond to simple stimulant regimens should be referred to a child and adolescent psychiatrist.

Conduct Disorders

The diagnosis of conduct disorder describes children and adolescents with a pattern of disruptive, willfully disobedient behavior.

Epidemiology

The prevalence of conduct disorder in children and adolescents has been estimated at 3 to 7%. Males predominate, especially in aggressive conduct disorders, but the prevalence in females is rising. *Conduct problems are the most common complaint in referrals to child and adolescent psychiatric clinics and hospitals.*

Description

This diagnosis requires a repetitive and persistent pattern of behavior that violates the basic rights of others or age-appropriate rules of society, manifested by at least three of a list of specific behaviors, which include stealing, running away from home, staying out after dark without permission, lying in order to "con" people, deliberate fire-setting, repeated truancy (beginning before age 13), vandalism, cruelty to animals, bullying, physical aggression, and forcing someone into sexual activity (APA 1993, in press [1994]).

Conduct disorder is a purely descriptive label for a heterogeneous group of children and adolescents. Many patients seem to lack appropriate feelings of guilt or remorse, empathy for others, and a feeling of responsibility for their own behavior. Irritability, tantrums, cheating, low frustration tolerance, inability to delay gratification, and provocative behavior are common. Precocious and promiscuous sexual activity is often seen. Social skills are poor with both peers and adults.

This is a potentially serious disorder because a substantial minority of patients will develop antisocial personality disorder or alcoholism in adulthood. The severity of prognosis increases with the number, variety, and frequency of problem behaviors. Among young children, the strongest predictors of adolescent delinquency are aggression, drug use, stealing, truancy, lying, and low educational achievement (Loeber, 1990). The combination of ADHD and conduct disorder results in a high risk of later delinquency.

Differential Diagnosis

Rule-violating behavior may be placed on a continuum. The least severe is the *normal* occasional lying and stealing seen in children less than 6 years old. A single occurrence of serious misconduct would be diagnosed *childhood or adolescent antisocial behavior.* Behavior problems that are not as severe as those seen in conduct disorder and that are less persistent than in *oppositional defiant disorder (ODD)* are diagnosed as *adjustment disorder with disturbance of conduct* if there is an identifiable stressor.

Etiology

A number of causal factors have been implicated, but there is no known single cause and all factors are not present in each case. ADHD and/or oppositional defiant disorder (ODD) often precede the development of conduct disorder. Conduct disorder symptoms may result from depression (Puig-Antich, 1982), mania, or psychosis. Mentally retarded youth may be led into antisocial acts by peers, or their lack of more adaptive coping strategies may result in aggression or stealing.

Conduct disorder appears to result from an interaction among the following factors (selection differs from child to child):

1. *Temperament* characterized by an initial resistance to childrearing, poor adaptability to change, high activity level, intense reactivity, and low threshold of responsiveness.
2. *Parents who provide attention to problem behavior and ignore good behavior,* who tend toward prolonged negative interactions with the child, who do not provide adequate supervision, and whose discipline is inconsistent, ineffective, and either lax or extremely severe and even abusive. One or more generations of parental irritability and explosive discipline lead to the poor socialization of children and inadequate parenting skills as adults. Children develop noncompliant and poorly controlled behaviors and lack social and academic survival skills, leading to rejection by normal peers and school failure (Patterson, DeBaryshe, and Ramsey, 1989).
3. *Association with a delinquent peer group.*
4. *Parental modeling* of impulsivity and rule-breaking behavior.
5. Genetic predisposition.
6. Parental marital conflict.
7. Placement outside of the home as an infant or toddler.
8. Poverty.
9. Low IQ or brain damage (especially in violent delinquents).

Evaluation

Reports from both parent and child, and often community sources, are required to accurately assess the severity of the behavior. A search should be made for the common concurrent diagnoses, especially ADHD, anxiety and mood disorders, substance abuse, specific developmental disorders (especially developmental reading disorder and expressive language disorder), and mental retardation. Because of the high frequency of brain damage in patients with violent conduct disorders, the physician should conduct a careful search for symptoms suggestive of complex partial seizures.

Treatment

Psychotherapy. Dynamically oriented individual therapy is not usually an effective treatment for children and adolescents with conduct disorders, although specific symptoms associated with psychological trauma such as divorce or abuse may benefit from this modality. Conduct disorders are generally treated more effectively in family or group therapy or in a structured milieu such as a residential treatment center. A recently developed model of individual supportive-expressive play psychotherapy, based on object relations theory that is often combined with parent training and/or play group psychotherapy has been demonstrated to be effective in treating children with ODD or mild to moderate conduct disorder, as long as the child has the capability for social bonding and for appropriate degrees of guilt (Kernberg and Chazan, 1991).

Multisystemic therapy (Henggeler and Borduin, 1990) is a comprehensive treatment model of documented efficacy that includes the combination of systemic family therapy with behavior modification techniques, the use of social service agencies, and active outreach to influence the youth's teachers and peer group. Individual psychotherapy based on a supportive therapeutic relationship using cognitive-behavioral, self-control, or social skills training may be included, as may individual or marital therapy with parents.

Behavior Modification. Several effective parent management training programs, based on social learning theory, exist for parents of noncompliant oppositional and aggressive children (Forehand and McMahon, 1981; Patterson, 1975). Parents are taught to use clear and consistent rules, to positively reinforce good behavior, and to use noncorporal discipline (limit setting and consequences other than physical punishment) effectively. One frequently used negative contingency is the "time out," so called because it puts the child in a quiet boring area, where there is a time out from whatever positive reinforcement he or she may be receiving for the problem behavior. Treatment is more effective the earlier it is begun, with adolescents being particularly resistant.

Cognitive behavior modification (CBM) is a technique that combines training in problem-solving skills with behavior modification. Children are taught to delay action and to consider alternative ways of resolving conflict. Both CBM and parent management training in behavior modification have been demonstrated to decrease aggressive and delinquent behavior and increase positive social skills in preadolescent conduct-disordered children. The combination of the two treatments is more effective than either alone in improving child behavior and in reducing parental stress and depression (Kazdin, Siegel, and Bass, 1992).

Psychopharmacologic Treatment. *Lithium* may be considered in the treatment of severe impulsive aggression, especially when accompanied by explosive affect (Campbell et al, 1985). (See section in this chapter on mood disorders for more details on lithium use as well as Chapter 18 by Drs. Silver, Hales, and Yudofsky.)

Carbamazepine may benefit patients with severe impulsive aggression accompanied by emotional lability and irritability and who have an abnormal EEG or a strong clinical suggestion of epileptic phenomena (Evans, Clay, and Gualtieri, 1987). Medical and behavioral side effects of carbamazepine are similar to those seen in adults

(Evans, Clay, and Gualtieri, 1987; Herskowitz, 1987; Pleak et al, 1988) (see Chapter 17 by Drs. Ursano, Silberman, and Diaz).

Propranolol, a beta-adrenergic blocker, may be useful in patients with otherwise uncontrollable rage reactions and impulsive aggression, especially those with evidence of neurologic dysfunction (Williams, Mehl, Yudofsky et al, 1982).

Neuroleptics such as haloperidol and molindone may reduce aggression, hostility, negativism, and explosiveness in severely aggressive children (Campbell et al, 1985; Greenhill et al, 1985). (See the section in this chapter on schizophrenia for more detail on the use of neuroleptics.)

If the conduct disorder is secondary to a major depression, successful treatment with *antidepressants* leads to remission of the conduct symptoms (Puig-Antich, 1982). In cases with coexisting ADHD, *stimulant* treatment may decrease impulsive conduct symptoms and defiance as well as overactivity and inattention.

Environmental Interventions Community-based recreation programs or a Big Brother or Sister may be helpful. A special education placement may be needed to manage behavior, remediate learning disabilities and academic deficits, and provide vocational training. Hospitalization may be required for severely aggressive youth. Effective residential treatment programs use close supervision and a strict token economy, which are combined with instruction in adaptive social and educational skills. Legal sanctions may be necessary to enforce cooperation with treatment. Long-term treatment is necessary to prevent relapse.

The Role of the Primary Care Physician

These children and adolescents are at high risk for injuries and accidents, resulting in frequent hospitalizations and emergency room visits. The primary care physician must be alert to possible medical complications such as venereal disease, pregnancy, and sequelae of drug abuse.

Oppositional Defiant Disorder

This relatively new diagnostic category was intended to describe *milder forms of chronic behavior problems than those seen in conduct disorder.* Children diagnosed with oppositional defiant disorder (ODD) are at risk for developing a conduct disorder.

Epidemiology

From 6 to 10% of youth have ODD, with boys outnumbering girls from two to three to one (Anderson et al, 1987). This disorder is extremely common among children referred to psychiatric services.

Description

Children with ODD display a chronic pattern of stubborn, negativistic, provocative, hostile, and defiant behavior *without* serious violation of the rights of others. They are often irritable, resentful, and quick to take offense. These children are usually most difficult to manage at home, but problems extend to school and peers. They often continue to resist compliance even when cooperation would be in their own best interest. Specific diagnostic criteria include loss of temper, arguments with adults, noncompliance (refusal to follow commands, directions, or minor rules), blaming others, and vindictiveness (APA 1993, in press [1994]).

Differential Diagnosis

Oppositional defiant disorder must be distinguished from milder forms of *stubbornness*. Negativity and tantrums are *normal* prior to three years of age, as are early adolescent arguments with adults and resistance to rules. Intentional and provocative noncompliance characteristic of ODD should be differentiated from the noncompliance resulting from impulsivity and inattention in *ADHD*, although both disorders are often present. In that case, both should be diagnosed. Oppositional behavior that is limited to school may be a result of *mental retardation* or a *specific developmental disorder*.

Etiology

Hypothesized factors include an inherited predisposition (perhaps mediated by difficult temperament), modeling of parental oppositional and defiant behavior, and parental inability to reward positive behavior or to set firm, fair, and consistent limits.

Evaluation

Symptoms are more prominent when the patient is with familiar people. Behavior may not seem abnormal in a diagnostic interview, especially if few demands are placed on the child. Parent and teacher reports are important. Psychological testing may be needed to discover low IQ or learning disabilities.

Treatment

Behavior Modification. An operant approach, using environmental positive and negative contingencies to increase or decrease the frequency of behaviors, is the most useful. A token economy is one type of operant approach, points, stars, or tokens can be earned for desirable behaviors (and lost for problem behaviors) and exchanged for backup reinforcers such as money, food, toys, privileges, or time with an adult in a pleasant activity. Techniques can be taught to parents (see Forehand and McMahon, 1981) and can be used by teachers in classrooms. It is especially helpful if parents and teachers can learn to structure situations to provide the child with appropriate choices and to avoid power struggles (similar to the strategies used with toddlers in the "terrible twos").

Psychopharmacology. In children with coexisting ADHD and ODD, stimulant medication may reduce oppositional behavior and improve compliance as well as address inattention, impulsivity, and hyperactivity.

ANXIETY DISORDERS

The prevalence of anxiety disorders in children and adolescents has been estimated to be from 2 to 15%, depending on severity. There is considerable overlap among anxiety disorders and between anxiety and depressive disorders (Kashani and

Orvaschel, 1990; Last, Strauss, and Francis, 1987). After puberty, anxiety disorders are more common in girls than boys. There is substantial continuity in anxiety disorders, both from generation to generation and in the childhood histories of adult patients with anxiety disorders. In contrast to common notions that anxiety disorders are of minor importance, overanxious disorder and separation anxiety disorder can be chronic, relapsing, and result in considerable social and academic impairment.

Etiology

Familial factors are strongly implicated, although sorting out genetic predisposition from family dynamic factors and imitation of a fearful parent is difficult. In patients with separation anxiety disorder seen in a clinical setting, 83% of the mothers had an anxiety disorder and 63% had a mood disorder (Last, Strauss, and Francis, 1987).

Children identified at age two as extremely inhibited, quiet, and restrained in unfamiliar situations tend to remain shy and socially avoidant at age seven. They have greater sympathetic reactivity than outgoing children, as measured by heart rate acceleration and early morning salivary cortisol levels. Two year olds who are uninhibited tend to remain fearless and outgoing (Kagan, Reznick, and Snidman, 1988). Certain medications, such as propranolol (for headache) and haloperidol (for Tourette's disorder) may produce symptoms of separation anxiety and school refusal.

Evaluation

Techniques of assessment are similar for all of the anxiety disorders in children and adolescents. Children who are anxious about being interviewed or who are having difficulty separating from their parents may be helped by being seen together with the parent initially. The clinical interview with the young person is especially important because parents usually underreport phobic, anxiety, and mood symptoms. A detailed history of school experiences should be taken. Family history should focus particularly on anxiety and mood disorders. A medical history and physical exam will generally rule out a medical cause for somatic complaints such as headaches, abdominal pain, nausea, or vomiting. In *separation anxiety disorder*, somatic symptoms are worst on evenings and mornings before school and absent on weekends and holidays, except the night before school starts. Extensive medical evaluations should be avoided unless there are clear indications for them. Information should be sought regarding any possible advantage or "secondary gain" that results from the patient's symptoms.

Treatment

A variety of treatment techniques are applicable to several of the anxiety disorders in children and adolescents.

Psychotherapy. Individual psychotherapy may be useful, with special attention to the child's relationship to the therapist and to separations that occur in the therapy. Supportive psychotherapy may permit children to deal with their anxiety in a more adaptive way. The goal of insight-oriented psychodynamic individual psychotherapy, using verbal and play techniques, is to resolve the underlying psychological conflicts and promote more functional intrapsychic defenses to deal with anxiety.

Cognitive therapy techniques aim to reduce anxiety and improve coping skills by using specific training to change the patient's maladaptive, self-defeating thoughts to ones that describe the child or adolescent as competent (Ollendick and Francis, 1988).

Family therapy may be valuable to reduce parental modeling or subtle encouragement of fearful behavior.

Behavior Modification. Behavioral techniques used to treat anxiety disorders include relaxation training, systematic desensitization, assertiveness training, shaping, and operant conditioning (Ollendick and Francis, 1988).

Psychopharmacologic Treatment. Although there are few systematic data, benzodiazepines may be used in the short-term treatment of children and adolescents with severe anticipatory anxiety. Infants and children absorb diazepam faster and metabolize it more quickly than adults (Simeon and Ferguson, 1985). Dosage schedule depends on age and the specific drug (Coffey, 1990). Side effects are similar to those seen in adults.

The efficacy of imipramine in patients with school avoidance secondary to separation anxiety is controversial, but it may be tried for children or adolescents who do not respond to psychological treatments such as family therapy, behavior therapy, and modification of the school situation.

Separation Anxiety Disorder

Description

Separation anxiety disorder is characterized by excessive anxiety for the patient's age—lasting for at least four weeks—concerning separation from parents (or others to whom the child is attached). Specific criteria include severe and persistent worries that something terrible will happen to the child or his or her parents that will keep them apart, reluctance or refusal to go to school because of fear of separation, refusal to sleep alone or away from home, avoidance of being alone, nightmares about separation, and excessive distress and/or physical symptoms in anticipation of or during separation from parents (APA 1993, in press [1994]). In the past, this disorder was considered synonymous with "school phobia."

Differential Diagnosis

Normal age-appropriate separation anxiety may transiently worsen under stress, especially in children under six years of age. Avoidance of school may be due to separation anxiety disorder or to a number of other causes. In *truancy*, the child stays away from home and the parents are not usually aware, unless told by the school. Some families may keep a child home from school to help with family tasks. The child may have a *realistic fear* (for example, of a bully), a *simple phobia* of something in the school environment, or a *social phobia*. Anxiety may be precipitated by unreasonable demands for academic performance at school or an undiagnosed *specific developmental disorder*. Social withdrawal and lack of energy secondary to *major depression* may lead to avoidance of school.

The Role of the Primary Care Physician

The primary care physician is in a position to distinguish the temperamentally shy but normal child from the one whose anxiety results in impairment in school or with peers.

Mild cases of school avoidance secondary to separation anxiety disorder can be managed by the primary care physician with encouragement to the child, family, and school. The child should be sent to school unless there are objective signs of illness, such as a fever. If the child stays home, she or he should rest in bed and not be allowed to engage in activities that are fun. If significant school refusal persists for more than a week, immediate referral for psychiatric evaluation and treatment should be made, because the longer the child is out of school, the more difficult treatment becomes.

The primary physician can use a contingency management program for young children whose separation anxiety is manifested primarily by refusal to sleep in their own bed. This includes an explanation to child and parents, supporting the parents in insisting the child stay in his or her own room, helping to devise a schedule of rewards for successful performance, and increasing the child's motivation by the physician's own attention and praise for sleeping alone.

Generalized Anxiety Disorder

The child or adolescent with *generalized anxiety disorder* suffers from and verbalizes excessive or unrealistic worry in multiple areas. Specific characteristics include worry about future events, past behavior, and the child's own competence; somatic complaints; self-consciousness; excessive need for reassurance; and marked feelings of tension. Associated features may include such habits as nail biting, thumb sucking, and hair pulling or twisting. This diagnosis includes the former diagnosis of overanxious disorder.

Phobias

A *phobia* is defined as a persistent, specific fear that is out of proportion to the actual danger and that leads to impairment in social and/or academic functioning because of the need to avoid the feared object or situation.

Normal fears are common in children. Specific fears vary with age. For example, infants react with fear to loss of physical support, loud noises, and rapidly approaching large objects. Fear of strangers develops around seven months of age. Toddlers (age one to three years) are frightened by loud noises, storms, some animals, the dark, and separation from their parents. These fears continue to be prevalent among three to five year olds and are joined by fears of monsters and ghosts. All of these fears tend to decline after age six. Common fears observed in school-age children (six to twelve years) are those relating to bodily injury, burglars, being kidnapped, being sent to the principal, being punished, and failure. Fears of tests in school and of social embarrassment take the lead from puberty through adolescence (Ollendick and Francis, 1988). Girls generally report more fears than boys, although it is not clear whether they actually *have* more fears or are simply more willing to report them.

Traditional Freudian theory proposed that phobias result from unconscious defenses against unacceptable wishes and feelings, as described in the classic case of "Little Hans." Oedipal dynamics were thought to be prominent in childhood phobias.

According to classical conditioning (behavioral) theory, phobias are learned by the generalization of fears to other objects or situations that are similar or that are coincident in time or place. Phobias persist because avoiding the feared object reduces anxiety. This removal of an aversive stimulus strengthens the preceding behavior (the phobic avoidance).

Behavioral treatments are generally the treatment of choice for children with one or two phobias. Symptom substitution (the appearance of a new symptom if the phobia is removed without addressing the presumed underlying conflicts) is not a problem if attention is paid to removal of secondary gain and to ensuring that the child has the skills and the opportunities to deal with the problem situation in other ways.

Children and adolescents with a *social phobia* fear one or more situations in which they will be observed by others and where their actions may lead to humiliation or embarrassment. Answering questions or speaking in front of the class are commonly feared, leading to impaired grades in school despite adequate learning. If severe, the phobia may lead to an avoidance of school altogether or "school phobia."

Obsessive–Compulsive Disorder

This serious and difficult-to-treat illness occasionally begins in childhood or adolescence (see Chapter 8 by Drs. Nagy, Krystal, and Charney). Estimated prevalence is 0.3 to 1% (Flament et al, 1988). Many cases go undetected and untreated until adulthood. Diagnostic criteria are the same as in adults, and the clinical phenomena are remarkably similar at all ages. Frequency, severity, chronicity, bizarre characteristics, and interference with daily life distinguish obsessions and compulsions from typical childhood worries, rituals, and superstitious habits. As in adults, clomipramine and fluoxetine may reduce the force of obsessions and compulsions sufficiently to improve quality of life. Supplemental behavior modification and/or psychotherapy are often necessary.

Panic Disorder

The existence of panic disorder in youth has been controversial, but recent data document its presence in children and adolescents who have a parent with panic disorder and/or depression, suggesting genetic or behavioral modeling etiologic contributions. There are few studies of the treatment of panic in children and adolescents, but preliminary evidence suggests clonazepam may be useful (Reiter, Kutcher, and Gardner, 1992). Supportive individual and family psychotherapy with an educational focus and the encouragement of exposure to feared situations may be helpful (see also Chapter 8).

Posttraumatic Stress Disorder

Description
Posttraumatic stress disorder (PTSD) is characterized by the development of specific, long-lasting emotional and behavioral symptoms precipitated by a shocking,

unexpected event that is outside the range of usual human experience. During the event the individual felt intensely fearful and helpless (see Chapter 8). Trauma may be chronic rather than acute, as in repeated sexual or physical abuse, when the stress is exacerbated by dread of the next episode. Symptoms include reexperiencing the traumatic event, avoidance of reminders of the event, and increased arousal. The precipitant may be experienced directly, by observation (as it occurs to another person), or vicariously after learning about a traumatic event or a severe threat to a close friend or relative.

The clinical phenomena seen in children differ in some ways from those seen in adults (Terr, 1987a). Immediate effects include fear of separation from parent(s), fear of death, and fear of further fear. Children withdraw from new experiences. Perceptual distortions occur, most commonly in time sense and in vision, but auditory, touch, and olfactory misperceptions have been described. Many details of the experience are accurately remembered, but sequencing and/or duration of events is often altered.

In children, reexperiencing the event is likely to occur in the form of nightmares, daydreams, and/or repetitive and potentially dangerous reenactment in symbolic play or in actual behavior. Despite obvious similarities between the reenactments and the original event, most children are unaware of the connection. Even children younger than age three demonstrate through play and/or dreams memories of traumatic events that they cannot describe verbally.

A variety of fears of repetition of the experience and of other situations develop that may involve separation or danger or remind them of the event. Children may experience somatic symptoms, such as headaches and stomachaches. Later, many traumatized children develop a sense of pessimism and hopelessness about the future. As long as four to five years after the event, children remain deeply ashamed of their helplessness in the face of danger. Children with PTSD most often demonstrate increased arousal by sleep disturbances that may add to functional impairment in other areas (Pynoos et al, 1987). Children commonly regress (show behaviors characteristic of a previous developmental stage).

Associated symptoms may include anxiety and/or depression. Impulsivity, difficulty concentrating, and decreased motivation may interfere with school performance. Guilt due to surviving and/or to perceived or actual deficiencies in attempts to save others is common. The normal cognitive egocentricity and magical thinking of children may contribute to a false belief that their thought or action somehow caused the traumatic event.

Etiology

Children with preexisting stressors, anxiety, or depression, or children who have experienced a previous loss, are at risk for more severe and prolonged symptoms. A sufficiently severe stressor, however, may produce the disorder without any predisposition. The degree of exposure to a life-threatening situation is directly related to severity of PTSD (Pynoos et al, 1987). The changes in living circumstance caused by disasters, such as the loss of the family home, isolation from usual social supports, and even the death of parents or other family members, can exacerbate PTSD. Symptoms may be partially ameliorated by a stable, cohesive, supportive family.

Evaluation

PTSD should be suspected in any child or adolescent who has had a significant change in behavior. A clinical interview technique for child and adolescent victims begins with the use of play and fantasy, using a projective drawing and storytelling task. The interviewer then structures a detailed recounting of the traumatic event, including affective responses and fantasies of revenge. The concluding stage includes a review of the child's current life concerns, a reassessment of the traumatic experience, anticipatory guidance regarding reactions that the child may experience, and efforts to support the child's self-esteem (Pynoos and Eth, 1986).

Treatment

Individual insight-oriented play and verbal psychotherapy is the most commonly used modality (Terr, 1987b). Time-limited focal psychotherapy may be effective in some cases (Pynoos and Eth, 1986). Group therapy with victims who have been exposed to the same event organized in schools or in the community may be helpful in decreasing distortions and reducing the spread of posttraumatic fears and symptoms. On the other hand, mixed groups of victims who have experienced different events (such as rape or incest) may actually lead to contagion of fears (Terr, 1987b).

Supportive therapy for parents and siblings can provide information about the child's symptoms and their cause, as well as deal with vicarious trauma experienced by family members and reduce contagion. Anecdotal reports suggest that propranolol may be effective in the treatment of agitated, hyperaroused children and adolescents with PTSD (Famularo, Kinscherff, and Fenton, 1988).

ELIMINATION DISORDERS

One of the most common developmental problems seen by primary care physicians is the child who has not attained or who has lost bladder or bowel control. Although these disorders are called "functional" enuresis and encopresis to differentiate them from medically caused incontinence, they have significant physiologic components.

Enuresis

Epidemiology

Most children achieve urinary control between two and three years of age. Virtually all are dry in the daytime by age four, but nocturnal control may lag behind. On average, boys are slower in achieving continence than girls. Among five year olds, 14% of boys and girls wet at least once a month. Approximately 10% of first graders are still nocturnally enuretic. By age 14, 1% of boys and 0.5% of girls remain enuretic (almost exclusively nocturnal). The spontaneous remission rate is high.

Description

Enuresis is defined as a pattern of involuntary or intentional voiding of urine into bed or clothes after age five years. The diagnostic criteria require a frequency of at least twice a week for at least three consecutive months or marked impairment or distress (APA 1993, in press [1994]). *Diurnal* is used to describe wetting in the daytime and *nocturnal* for wetting only during sleep, by far the more common form. Enuresis may result in family conflict and punitive treatment of shaming of the child, teasing by peers, restriction of social activities due to peer rejection and fear of embarrassment, and low self-esteem.

Differential Diagnosis

Transient loss of urinary control is common in young children when physically or psychologically stressed. Some children are careless in wiping, or leave the toilet before urination is complete, leading to the appearance of enuresis.

Specific medical causes of urinary incontinence include:

Urethritis secondary to use of bubble bath
Urinary tract infections
Diabetes mellitus
Diabetes insipidus
Sickle cell anemia
Seizure disorders
Neurogenic bladder (e.g., secondary to spina bifida)
Genitourinary tract malfunction, malformation, or obstruction
Pelvic masses

Etiology

Enuresis has a strong genetic component. Seventy-five percent of enuretic youth have a first-degree relative with a history of enuresis. Nocturnal enuresis in younger children is largely a consequence of delayed maturation of bladder control mechanisms. General neuromaturational delay, small bladder capacity, and lack of systematic toilet training may contribute to enuresis. Constipation has also been implicated as a causative factor (O'Regan et al, 1986). Common physiologic causes of diurnal enuresis in females are vaginal reflux of urine, bladder spasm when frightened or laughing, and urgency incontinence.

Enuresis is occasionally related to other psychiatric disorders. In young children it may be a symptom of an *adjustment disorder. Anxious* children may experience urinary frequency, resulting in incontinence if toilet facilities are not immediately available. Children with *oppositional defiant disorder* may refuse to use the toilet as part of their battle for control. Many children with *ADHD* wait until the last minute to use the bathroom and may lose control on the way. Avoidance of dirty, dangerous, or insufficiently private toilet facilities in school may also lead to incontinence. Recent research does *not* show a relationship between enuresis and specific sleep stages for children with or without other psychiatric diagnoses.

Evaluation

The history includes details of wetting, including time of occurrence, amount, frequency, precipitants, details of toilet training, and family history of enuresis. A careful medical history, physical and neurological examination, and urinalysis are indicated in all cases. Urine cultures should be obtained in girls. Radiologic studies or instrumentation of the genitourinary tract are not indicated unless there are specific indications of abnormality on the history or physical exam.

Treatment

Environmental Interventions. Nocturnal enuresis in children younger than seven years old should be treated with patience while waiting for the child to mature. Secondary symptoms should be minimized by discouraging the parents from punishing or ridiculing the child. Older children can be taught to change their own beds in order to reduce negative reactions from parents. Measures such as restricting fluids and waking the child during the night to urinate are not notably successful. Exercises to increase bladder capacity may reduce nocturnal enuresis, and start-and-stop exercises may strengthen the bladder sphincter muscles and improve control.

Behavior Modification. If treatment of uncomplicated enuresis is necessary, behavioral methods are the first choice, although parent and child motivation and participation are required. The first step is a simple monitoring and reward procedure using a chart with stars (for dry days or nights) to be exchanged for rewards. For children and adolescents who do not respond to simple interventions, more elaborate behavioral programs or a urine alarm device (available for about $50) may be used.

Children who are secondarily enuretic (having previously been dry) and those who have accompanying psychiatric problems are more difficult to treat. Referral to a child and adolescent psychiatrist for specialized evaluation and treatment may be necessary.

Psychotherapy. Individual or family psychotherapy may be indicated to deal with secondary effects of the enuresis or with coexisting psychiatric disorders that may be exacerbating the problem.

Psychopharmacologic Treatment. Prior to starting medication, baseline frequency of wet and dry days or nights is recorded. Daily charting is then used to monitor the child's progress. If medication is used chronically, the child or adolescent should have a drug-free trial at least every six months to see if medication is still required.

Low doses of the *tricyclic antidepressants* imipramine, amitriptyline, desipramine, and nortriptyline are partially effective in the treatment of nocturnal enuresis. The mechanism remains unclear, but they do not seem to work by altering sleep architecture, treating depression, or increasing peripheral anticholinergic activity. Wetting usually returns when the drug is discontinued. Tolerance to the medication may develop, necessitating a dose increase. In some children, tricyclics lose their effect entirely. Parents must take special precautions to avoid overdoses by the patient or siblings. Imipramine may be useful on a short-term basis or for special occasions (such as camp).

Desmopressin (DDAVP), an analogue of antidiuretic hormone, can be administered as a nasal spray to treat nocturnal enuresis. Onset of action is within several days. Few patients become completely dry, however, and relapse occurs when the medication is stopped (Klauber, 1989). In patients with normal electrolyte regulation, side effects are minimal (headache and rare nasal mucosa dryness or irritation).

Because excessive water intake can result in hyponatremic seizures, fluids should be limited during the evening and night (Beach, Beach, and Smith, 1992). A major drawback of DDAVP is its expense (as high as $240 per month in 1992).

Encopresis

Epidemiology

Bowel control is usually achieved between 30 months and four years of age. The prevalence of encopresis is approximately 1.5% after age five and decreases with age. In late adolescence it is almost nonexistent in the absence of severe mental retardation, psychosis, or conduct disorder. Boys outnumber girls six to one. Encopresis is slightly more common in poor children. Encopresis is less often an isolated symptom than enuresis is. Twenty-five percent of encopretics seen in psychiatric settings are also enuretic.

Description

This disorder is characterized by repeated involuntary (or, rarely, voluntary) passage of feces into clothing or other places other than the toilet (such as the floor or closets) at least once a month for at least three months after the age of four years (APA 1993, in press [1994]). Encopresis rarely occurs during sleep. The older the child, the more resistant to treatment and the more negative the prognosis. Rejection by peers, school, and family increases with age.

Differential Diagnosis

Transient loss of continence may follow a stressor such as hospitalization or parental divorce. Medical causes of fecal incontinence include:

Metabolic
  Hypothyroidism
  Hypercalcemia
Dietary
  Lactase deficiency
  Overeating of fatty foods
Lower gastrointestinal tract
  Congenital aganglionic megacolon (Hirschprung's disease)
  Anal fissure
  Rectal stenosis
Neurologic—e.g., myelodysplasia

Etiology

Children with functional encopresis may be divided into three groups according to etiology. In all cases, predisposing subtle abnormalities in colon motility and sphincter function are likely. Familial factors are suggested by the 15% rate of childhood encopresis in fathers of encopretic children. The first group includes children who have never been systematically toilet trained, who are retarded, or who have neuromaturational delays.

The second group is characterized by chronic severe constipation. This may be involuntary (due to dietary factors or pain on defecation caused by a skin rash or an anal fissure) or a result of a lack of opportunity to use the toilet. Voluntary stool withholding may result from punitive toilet training, improper management of common toilet-related fears, or environmental interference with normal toilet habits (unsafe or dirty bathrooms or lack of privacy). As a result of the constipation, the child develops impaired colon motility and contraction patterns, stretching and thinning of the walls of the colon (functional megacolon), and decreased sensation or perception of the urge to defecate or of actual passage of stool. Impaction results, with leakage of loose stool around the obstruction (overflow incontinence). The child becomes habituated to the smell and often does not know when he or she has soiled (a fact difficult for adults to believe).

In the third group, encopresis is secondary to a psychiatric disorder such as oppositional defiant disorder, attention-deficit hyperactivity disorder, conduct disorder, phobia, or adjustment disorder.

Evaluation

A complete medical history, a physical examination, and routine laboratory tests are indicated. A detailed history is needed to distinguish between passage of full bowel movements (likely to be volitional), overflow of loose stool around an impaction, or staining of underwear due to careless wiping after toileting. A history of toilet training and bathroom environments is needed. An X-ray of the abdomen or a barium enema may be required to assess fecal impaction. Urinalysis will detect an associated urinary tract infection (common in encopretic girls).

Treatment

Psychotherapy. Traditional individual psychotherapy may be used in addition to other treatments. Children with encopresis are often angry and may benefit from improving their ability to express their emotions verbally. Psychotherapy may also be useful in improving self-esteem. Behavioral treatments are essential in most cases. Parents should be helped to avoid hostile or punitive responses to the child's incontinence and should be cautioned that relapses may occur.

The Role of the Primary Care Physician

Medical treatment is essential for children with chronic constipation and resulting functional megacolon. Children and parents are educated in the physiology and anatomy of the lower bowel. Enemas and suppositories are used to evacuate the bowel. A bowel "retraining" program follows, using orally administered mineral oil, a high roughage diet, development of a regular toileting routine, and a mild suppository (such as Dulcolax) if necessary. Routine administration of enemas by parents is contraindicated as that alone does not improve bowel function and is toxic to the parent–child relationship.

Because children with encopresis more commonly have associated psychiatric disorders than those with enuresis, psychiatric consultation is indicated for most encopretic children older than six years of age.

MOOD DISORDERS

Mood disorders in children and adolescents are potentially serious, long-lasting, and recurrent (Kovacs et al, 1984a; Kovacs et al, 1984b). This section will focus on age-related differences from mood disorders in adults which are covered in Chapter 7 by Drs. Risby, Risch, and Stoudemire.

Epidemiology
The incidence of mood disorders has increased in children and adolescents (Ryan et al 1992) as the age of onset of both unipolar depression and bipolar disorder have declined. The prevalence of major depression has been estimated at 2% in prepubertal children and 5% in adolescents. Dysthymic disorder without coexisting major depression is found in 3.3% of adolescents (Kashani et al, 1987). Prior to puberty, depression is more common in boys than girls, with a change to the adult sex ratios (females greater than males) in adolescence. Mania is rare prior to puberty. In late adolescence the incidence approaches 20% of the adult rate.

Description
Diagnostic criteria are essentially the same for children as for adults, except that mood can be irritable instead of depressed, and failure to make expected weight gain can be seen instead of weight loss. The behaviors may be manifested in different ways, appropriate for developmental level. Reduction in school performance and activities with friends or complaints of boredom or aches and pains may be key indicators of depression in young people. Young depressed patients are less likely than adults to show anhedonia, diurnal variation, psychomotor retardation, delusions (Carlson and Kashani, 1988), insomnia, or the classic vegetative signs of depression (Kutcher and Marton, 1989).

Among adolescents with major depression, subsequent bipolarity is predicted by precipitous onset of symptoms, psychomotor retardation, psychotic features, pharmacologically precipitated hypomania, and a family history of bipolar disorder (Strober and Carlson, 1982).

Differential Diagnosis
Adolescent mania is frequently misdiagnosed as *schizophrenia* because of the psychotic manifestations and regression common to both. Because of the lack of cyclical vegetative symptoms in prepubertal children, mania often resembles *ADHD*. Belligerence, poor judgment, and impaired impulse control in mania (stealing, sexual activity) may be confused with *conduct disorder*. Secondary mania may result from prescribed (steroids, carbamazepine, tricyclic antidepressants) or abused (cocaine, amphetamines) *drugs, metabolic abnormalities, neoplasm*, or *epilepsy*.

Children less than four years of age may develop a clinical picture similar to major depression when separated from their parents. Children suffering from *reactive attachment disorder* secondary to parental abuse or neglect who present with lethargy, apathy, and withdrawal may appear depressed. In a subgroup of children with *conduct disorder*, a major depression precedes the development of the conduct problems (Marriage et al, 1986; Puig-Antich, 1982).

Evaluation

Children can be asked direct questions related to depression, although the wording must be adjusted for their level of cognitive and emotional development. Young children have more difficulty recognizing and verbalizing their feelings and may use idiosyncratic words such as "bored" to describe dysphoria or anhedonia. "Cranky" may be more understandable to a child than "irritable." Although some children report their mood states more accurately than their parents can, observation of depressed affect by a trained clinician is often essential. Longitudinal course and family history are important.

It is crucial to assess the degree of suicidality. Children can be questioned regarding ideation, plans, and attempts. This questioning will *not* increase the likelihood of self-destructive behavior. If a child or adolescent is seen following a suicide attempt, a detailed evaluation should be made of the circumstances preceding and following the attempt, history of substance abuse or impulsive behavior, wishes to die or to influence others at the time of the attempt and at the time of evaluation, whether a friend or family member has committed suicide, and coping skills and supports in the patient and family. A careful search should be made for frequent co-morbid conditions, such as anxiety disorders, ADHD, conduct disorders, and alcohol or drug abuse.

Treatment

Psychotherapy. Individual and family psychotherapy are cornerstones of the management of depression in childhood and adolescence. Even after successful treatment with medication, impaired interpersonal relations with peers and family members may require individual, group, or family therapy to address developmental deficits or the sequelae of the depression (Puig-Antich et al, 1985).

Cognitive therapy techniques developed for the treatment of depression in adults are being adapted for use with children and adolescents (Emery, Bedrosian, and Garber, 1983). Behavior therapy techniques such as social skills training or contingency management to reduce withdrawal may be useful adjunctive treatments.

Psychopharmacologic Treatment. The evidence for efficacy is less than in adults, and drugs should be used in conjunction with other treatments. For nonpsychotic depression, psychotherapy should be the first step, with medication added if there is no improvement in four to six weeks.

Tricyclic antidepressant drugs may be useful in the treatment of children and adolescents with major depression. Tricyclic pharmacokinetics differ before and after puberty. As a result, prepubertal children generally need a higher milligram per kilogram dose than adults, and are prone to rapid, dramatic swings in blood levels from toxic to ineffective. Medication should be divided into three daily doses to produce more stable levels (Ryan, 1992). Tricyclics may be given once or twice daily in adolescents.

The starting dose of imipramine, amitriptyline, and desipramine is 1.5 mg/kg/day, which may be increased every four days by 1 mg/kg/day to a maximum dose of 5 mg/kg/day. Nortriptyline may have fewer side effects and a more precise therapeutic window of 75 to 150 ng/ml, usually attained at 0.5 to 2 mg/kg/day (Ryan, 1990). It has a longer half-life than imipramine and can be given twice a day in children. Milligram per kilogram doses are lower than for imipramine and variation in metabolism is greater (Geller et al, 1986).

Parents must be reminded to supervise closely administration of medication and to keep pills in a safe place to prevent intentional overdose or accidental poisoning not only by the patient but by other family members, especially young children.

Tricyclics have a quinidinelike effect. At doses of more than 3 mg/kg/day of imipramine or desipramine, children and adolescents develop small but statistically significant EKG changes (intraventricular conduction defects) (Bartels et al, 1991). A small group of children and adolescents may have a genetic inability to metabolize tricyclics normally, resulting in high risk for cardiotoxicity (Rancurello, 1985). An initial EKG is essential for all patients to establish a baseline and to detect preexisting Wolf-Parkinson-White syndrome or other cardiac conduction abnormalities that could result in fatality because of the quinidinelike effect of tricyclics. In prepubertal children the EKG should be repeated at significant dosage increases and monitored periodically thereafter. Blood pressure and pulse should be taken initially and when the dose is increased. The dose should be decreased if any of the following limits is reached (N Ryan, personal communication, 1992):

Pulse = 130 beats per minute
Sustained resting heart rate = 100 beats per minute
Resting blood pressure = 140/90 mm Hg
EKG
    PR interval = 0.18 (children) or 0.20 sec (adolescents)
    QRS interval = 0.12 sec or 150% of baseline
    QTc interval = 0.48 sec

Plasma levels are recommended in patients who fail to respond to usual doses (possibly low levels) or those who have severe side effects at usual doses (possibly very high levels).

Anticholinergic side effects are similar to adults (Herskowitz, 1987) but less common. Tricyclics may cause lowering of the seizure threshold with worsening of preexisting EEG abnormalities and, rarely, a seizure. Central nervous system toxicity that may be mistaken for a worsening of the original depression is manifested by irritability, psychotic symptoms, agitation, anger, aggression, nightmares, forgetfulness or confusion, especially at plasma levels of imipramine + desipramine > 450 ng/ml (Preskorn, Weller, Hughes, Weller, 1988). Depressed children who are withdrawn and nonverbal may show a transient apparent worsening of sadness, crying, irritability, and aggression as their depression responds to medication.

Sudden withdrawal of moderate or higher doses results in a flulike gastrointestinal syndrome with nausea, cramps, vomiting, headaches, and muscle pains. Other manifestations of tricyclic withdrawal may include social withdrawal, hyperactivity, depression, agitation, and insomnia (Ryan, 1990). Tricyclics should therefore be tapered over a two- to three-week period rather than being abruptly discontinued. The short half-life of tricyclics in prepubertal children may produce daily withdrawal symptoms if medication is given only once a day or if a dose is missed (Ryan, 1992).

Lithium carbonate may be considered in the treatment of children and adolescents with bipolar disorder, whether mixed or manic. Lithium should not be prescribed unless the family is willing and able to comply with regular multiple daily doses and with lithium levels. The medical workup is the same as in adults. Growth and thyroid and kidney function (serum creatinine and morning urine specific gravity) should be monitored every three to six months.

Therapeutic lithium blood levels are the same as for adults, 0.6 to 1.2 mEq/liter, which can usually be attained with 900 to 1200 mg/day, in divided doses, although daily doses of up to 2,000 mg may be required (Campbell et al, 1985).

Since lithium excretion occurs primarily through the kidney and most children have more efficient renal function than adults, they may require higher doses for body weight than adults (Ryan, 1992; Weller, Weller, and Fristad, 1986). Lithium should be taken with food to minimize gastrointestinal distress. Children are at risk for the same side effects as adults but may experience them at lower serum levels (Campbell, Silva, Kafantaris et al, 1991). In growing children, the consequences of hypothyroidism are potentially more severe than in adults. *Because of its teratogenic potential, lithium is contraindicated in sexually active girls.* Lithium's tendency to aggravate acne may also be of particular clinical significance in adolescents.

Adequate salt and fluid intake is necessary to prevent lithium levels from rising into the toxic range. The family should be instructed in the importance of preventing dehydration from heat or exercise and in the need to stop the lithium and contact the physician if the child or adolescent develops an illness with fever, vomiting, diarrhea, and/or decreased fluid intake. Erratic consumption of large amounts of salty snack foods may cause fluctuations in lithium levels (Herskowitz, 1987).

Carbamazepine may be useful in the treatment of mania that is resistant to lithium and neuroleptics or rapidly cycling (see Chapter 18).

SCHIZOPHRENIA

Schizophrenia in adults is covered in Chapter 5 by Drs. Ninan and Mance. The presentation of schizophrenia in adolescence is similar to that in adulthood, but clinical features in children are somewhat different.

Epidemiology
Childhood schizophrenia has been estimated to be present at a rate of 0.5 per 1,000. The prevalence increases after puberty, approaching adult levels in late adolescence.

Description
Diagnostic criteria are the same as for adults, with the exception that failure to reach expected levels of adaptive functioning may be seen instead of regression. Schizophrenic children are characterized by markedly uneven development and the insidious onset of symptoms. Language and social behavior are usually delayed and are qualitatively different from normal children at any developmental stage. Visual hallucinations are more common in children than in adults.

Differential Diagnosis

Acute hallucinations are not uncommon in children and can result from *acute phobic reactions, physical illness* with fever or metabolic aberration, or *medications*. Some schizophrenic children younger than age six years have symptoms characteristic of *autistic disorder* prior to the development of the core symptoms of schizophrenia (delusions, hallucinations, formal thought disorder) (Watkins, Asarnow, and Tanguay, 1988).

Treatment

Psychotherapy. Individual psychotherapy may be useful as a part of a comprehensive treatment plan for schizophrenic children (Cantor and Kestenbaum, 1986). Family psychoeducational treatment (Anderson, Hogarty, and Reiss, 1980) may also prove beneficial. Token economies may be useful in shaping adaptive behavior and reducing inappropriate behaviors.

Psychopharmacologic Treatment. Neuroleptics (also called major tranquilizers) are less likely to be effective in schizophrenic adolescents than in adults and even less so in children. Neuroleptics should be used only as part of a comprehensive treatment program. Target symptoms that may respond include overactivity, aggression, agitation, stereotyped movements, delusions, and hallucinations.

The dose range for haloperidol in children is 0.5 to 16 mg/day (.02 to 0.2 mg/kg/day) (Campbell et al, 1985). An initial trial of about four weeks is needed to assess efficacy. Laboratory studies should be monitored at regular intervals. A drug-free trial after four to six months may be useful in assessing the continued need for medication.

Acute extrapyramidal side effects occur as in adults and may be treated with oral or intramuscular diphenhydramine (25 to 50 mg) depending on age. Chronic extrapyramidal side effects in adolescents can be treated with diphenhydramine or the anticholinergic drug benztropine—1 to 2 mg/day—in divided doses. Adolescent boys seem to be more vulnerable to acute dystonic reactions than adult patients, so prophylactic antiparkinsonian medication may be indicated. In children, reduction of neuroleptic dose is preferable to the use of antiparkinsonian agents (Campbell et al, 1985).

Tardive or withdrawal dyskinesias—some transient, but others irreversible—are seen in 8 to 51% of neuroleptic-treated children and adolescents (Campbell et al, 1985) and are one of the major reasons why these drugs should not be used casually. Tardive dyskinesia has been documented in children and adolescents after as brief a period of treatment as five months (Herskowitz, 1987). A careful examination for abnormal movements using a scale such as the Abnormal Involuntary Movements Scale (AIMS) should be conducted before placing the patient on a neuroleptic and periodically reused thereafter. Parents and patients (as they are able) should receive regular explanations of the risk of movement disorders.

Potentially fatal neuroleptic malignant syndrome has been reported in children and adolescents, with a presentation similar to that seen in adults (Latz and McCracken, 1992). Weight gain may be problematic with the long-term use of the low-potency neuroleptics. Abnormal laboratory findings are less often reported in children than in adults, but the clinician should be alert to the possibility of blood dyscrasias and hepatic dysfunction. If an acute febrile illness occurs, medication should be withheld and a complete blood count (with differential) and liver enzymes should be determined (Campbell et al, 1985).

Abdominal pain may occur, especially early in treatment. Enuresis has been reported (Realmuto et al, 1984). Photosensitivity due to chlorpromazine may be a problem when youngsters play outside.

Of particular concern is behavioral toxicity, manifested as the worsening of preexisting symptoms or development of new symptoms such as hyper- or hypoactivity, irritability, apathy, withdrawal, stereotypies, tics, or hallucinations (Campbell et al, 1985). The so-called low-potency antipsychotic drugs such as chlorpromazine and thioridazine can produce cognitive dulling and sedation, interfering with the ability to benefit from school (Campbell et al, 1985) and are probably best avoided. Children and adolescents are more sensitive to sedation than are adults (Realmuto et al, 1984).

Environmental Interventions The best outcome is obtained with an intensive school-based treatment program that incorporates multiple methods of intervention. Hospitalization or long-term residential treatment may be needed.

EATING DISORDERS

Rumination Disorder of Infancy

This potentially fatal disorder is one of the key differential diagnoses in the evaluation of children seen in pediatric services with failure to thrive (the unexplained failure to gain weight).

Epidemiology
Rumination appears in infants between three months and one year of age and in persons with moderate or severe mental retardation. In both groups, males predominate five to one (Mayes et al, 1988).

Description
This disorder is characterized by repeated voluntary regurgitation and rechewing of food, without apparent nausea or associated gastrointestinal illness, accompanied by weight loss or failure to make expected weight gain. Rumination appears to be an enjoyable source of pleasurable stimulation or a means of tension release. When not ruminating, the child may appear apathetic and withdrawn, irritable and fussy, or quite normal.

Differential Diagnosis
Medical causes of vomiting include gastroesophageal reflux (due to esophageal sphincter dysfunction or hiatal hernia), gastrointestinal infections, congenital malformations (such as pyloric stenosis), or hyperactive gag reflex. Failure to gain weight may result from inadequate feeding, malabsorption syndromes, systemic infection, or inborn errors of metabolism.

Etiology

About one-third of infants with rumination disorder have a history of obstetrical complications; one-fourth have developmental delays attributed to mental retardation or pervasive developmental disorder. Abnormalities in parental caretaking have been implicated, either understimulation with neglect or excessive stimulation out of phase with the infant's needs accompanied by harsh handling. Cases with no apparent abnormalities in the infant or in the mother–child relationship may represent habit disorders that were encouraged by characteristics of the child's gastrointestinal physiology or triggered by a transient medical illness.

Evaluation

Pediatric hospitalization is usually required for evaluation, with a search for possible causes and for sequelae such as dehydration, electrolyte imbalance, and malnutrition. Calorie counts and weight should be recorded. A detailed history is taken of physical and emotional development and of feeding. Upper gastrointestinal contrast and esophageal motility studies may be indicated. The mother–child interaction is observed during times of feeding and playing. It is important not to confuse the anxiety, frustration, and disgust the child's constant vomiting and unrewarding weight gain *induce* in the mother with dysfunctional mothering that may have *caused* the disorder. Some infants are so irregular and unpredictable in their rhythms and labile in their responses that the best parent has a difficult time. The child should be evaluated for developmental delay and the parents for possible primary psychiatric disorders.

Treatment

Psychotherapy. Supportive psychotherapy for the parents, with attention to any psychopathology that may have become apparent in the evaluation, is indicated. Parents and child may be seen together to model feeding techniques and ways of interacting with the baby that will be rewarding to both.

Behavior Modification. Treatment programs using social rewards such as cuddling and playing that are combined with mild noncorporal punishments (brief ignoring, scolding) for rumination may be useful.

Environmental Interventions. Pediatric hospitalization may be necessary to restructure the feeding behavior of both parent and child and to reduce parental anxiety. A visiting nurse or homemaker may be arranged to support a mother who is overwhelmed. Developmentally delayed infants may benefit from an organized stimulation program. If parents refuse to cooperate with treatment, or parenting ability is so impaired that the infant is in danger, laws in all states mandate reporting to a child protective services agency.

The Role of the Primary Care Physician

The pediatrician is the key player in cases of rumination disorder, conducting the medical evaluation and working together with social services and the child psychiatrist on psychosocial evaluation and treatment. These families require close and prolonged pediatric care to monitor progress and mobilize additional resources.

Anorexia Nervosa and Bulimia Nervosa

These disorders are covered in detail in Chapter 12 by Dr. Yager. Anorexia nervosa typically begins at puberty or in early adolescence and bulimia in late adolescence. The immediate and long-term medical sequelae are often more serious in young patients than in adults. Family treatment has a more central role in the care of adolescents compared to adults. The twelve-step programs commonly used in adult treatment are generally not relevant for teenagers with eating disorders, whose dynamics more commonly relate to separation-individuation issues than addictive mechanisms.

Obesity

Obesity virtually always has its onset in childhood. It is not technically a psychiatric disorder, but it has significant psychosocial as well as medical sequelae. (Overeating affecting a patient's medical status can be designated under Psychological Factors Affecting Medical Conditions in DSM-IV.) An estimated 10 to 35% of American children and adolescents are overweight; many suffer from low self-esteem and impaired peer relationships as a result. Obese youngsters are typically physically inactive and spend many hours watching television and snacking. The majority of obese children over the age of ten become persistently obese adults (see Chapter 24 by Drs. Goldstein, Ruggiero, Guise, and Abrams).

The most effective treatment programs actively involve both parents and child and include education, a balanced diet, regular exercise, and peer activities (Epstein et al, 1990). Contingency management programs may be useful for children, while adolescents benefit from cognitive strategies such as those used for adults.

TOURETTE'S DISORDER

Tourette's disorder is the most severe and chronic of the group of tic disorders. The others are chronic or transient vocal or motor tic disorders. Tourette's disorder is defined by chronic and frequent motor and vocal tics that typically change in location, pattern, frequency, and severity. A tic is an involuntary, sudden, rapid, recurrent, nonrhythmic, steroryped motor movement or vocalization (words or sounds) (APA 1993, in press [1994]). Tics may be temporarily suppressed by conscious effort, and typically diminish markedly during sleep. Estimated prevalence of Tourette's disorder is 3 in 10,000, with a male predominance of three to ten to one. Etiology is strongly genetic, but a variety of environmental influences can affect severity. Often far more disabling than the tics themselves are the commonly associated symptoms of hyperactivity, impulsivity, distractibility, defiance, or obsessions and compulsions. It is controversial whether these problems are a part of Tourette's disorder per se or whether they are accounted for by genetic links with ADHD and obsessive–compulsive disorder.

Initial treatment requires education of the child, family, teachers, and peers regarding the nature of the disorder. This often drastically reduces patient distress and school and family disruption. A variety of psychotherapeutic and behavior modification interventions may be helpful in reducing tics or other specific target symptoms as well as secondary depression, anxiety, and low self-esteem. Special education may be useful. Low doses of haloperidol, pimozide, or clonidine may reduce tics and behavioral problems. Obsessions and compulsions may respond to clomipramine or fluoxetine. The use of stimulants to treat symptoms of ADHD in children with Tourette's disorder is highly controversial because of the risk of exacerbating tics. Desipramine or clonidine is generally preferred. Because of Tourette's disorder's chronic waxing and waning course and the high frequency of medication side effects, pharmacologic treatment is best used sparingly.

MENTAL RETARDATION

Epidemiology
The prevalence of mental retardation in the United States has been estimated at 1 to 3%. Males predominate 1.5 to one.

Description
Mental retardation is defined as significantly subaverage general intellectual functioning as demonstrated by an IQ of 70 or below on an individually administered intelligence test, accompanied by deficits in adaptive functioning, with onset before the age of 18. The four degrees of severity of mental retardation are seen in Table 16–6.

Differential Diagnosis
Children who have been severely *neglected* may test in the retarded range. True intellectual capacity can only be assessed after a period of remediation. Children with *specific developmental disorders* have delays in circumscribed areas with normal functioning in other areas. The DSM "V code" *borderline intellectual functioning* is used for children with IQ scores between 71 and 84. These youngsters are impaired primarily in the school setting.

Children with *autistic disorder* have uneven developmental delays and qualitative abnormalities of behavior and emotions. Many have mental retardation *in addi-*

Table 16–6 **Categories of Severity of Mental Retardation**

DESCRIPTION	RANGE OF IQ	PROPORTION OF RETARDED POPULATION
Mild ("educable")	IQ 50–55 to 70	85%
Moderate ("trainable")	IQ 35–40 to 50–55	10%
Severe	IQ 20–25 to 35–40	3–4%
Profound	IQ below 20–25	1–2%

* (APA 1993, in press [1994])

tion to autistic disorder. Some children identified by schools as having *ADHD* are, in fact, mentally retarded. For children with *sensory impairments* such as deafness or blindness or *neurological disorders* such as cerebral palsy, expert psychological evaluation is needed to distinguish mental retardation from interference by the disabilities.

Etiology

Mental retardation is a diverse category with a large number of etiologies. Identifiable single gene or chromosomal abnormalities and metabolic, traumatic, and toxic causes are more common in those with moderate to profound retardation. In mild retardation, etiology is more often attributed to a genetic endowment at the low end of the normal distribution or to psychosocial factors such as poverty and lack of stimulation. Many cases are idiopathic.

Evaluation

Intelligence testing is administered by a psychologist skilled in working with children in a setting that will encourage the child's cooperation. Commonly used tests of intellectual functioning are listed in Table 16–3. Adaptive functioning is evaluated by history, clinical observation, and standardized evaluation using the Vineland Adaptive Behavior Scales. A medical evaluation is indicated to seek causative disorders, sensory handicap, and associated physical problems such as congenital malformations, inborn errors of metabolism, or epilepsy. Genetic evaluation may be important in counseling the parents regarding risk to future children. Psychiatric evaluation may be necessary to define associated psychiatric disorders, which are three to four times as common in the retarded as in the general population.

Treatment

Psychotherapy. Individual psychotherapy or parent counseling may be useful to deal with developmental or situational crises or in the treatment of coexisting psychiatric disorders. Parents may need assistance in dealing with their grief over having a "defective" child. Specific behavioral programs are useful in teaching adaptive behaviors and reducing stereotypic behaviors, aggression, and self-injury.

Psychopharmacologic Treatment. Children and adolescents with mental retardation are at increased risk of psychopathology. The same medications used for youth of normal IQ may be tried. For example, stimulants are effective in treating ADHD target symptoms, although efficacy decreases with decreasing IQ (Gadow, 1985).

Environmental Interventions Mentally retarded children and adolescents require special education programs. Moderate to profoundly retarded youth benefit from comprehensive multidisciplinary habilitation programs. Specialized infant stimulation and preschool programs can reduce intellectual and adaptive deficits. Institutionalization is now indicated only for the most severely affected, usually those with accompanying medical disorders or severe behavior problems. Adolescents and young adults benefit from vocational training programs, sheltered workshops, and group homes in the community.

The Association for Retarded Citizens, a national organization, has state and local chapters that provide assistance to retarded persons and their families.

PERVASIVE DEVELOPMENTAL DISORDERS

This category (abbreviated as PDD) contains *autistic disorder*, formerly known as infantile autism, and a residual category called *pervasive developmental disorder not otherwise specified* for children with similar features who do not meet full criteria for autistic disorder. These patients are characterized by an uneven pattern of development that includes both severe delays and qualitative abnormalities.

Epidemiology
Strictly defined autistic disorder occurs at a rate of 4 per 10,000 persons. Other cases in the pervasive developmental disorder spectrum appear at a rate of 10 to 20 per 10,000. There is a male predominance of three to four to one.

Description
Autistic disorder is characterized by severe and sustained impairment, relative to chronological and mental age, in three areas:

1. Reciprocal social interaction,
2. Communication, and
3. Patterns of behavior, activities, and interests.

The onset is in infancy or early childhood. Autistic persons do not view other people as having thoughts or feelings. They do not seek out adults or peers for emotional gratification, although they may cling mechanically to their parents when frightened. They do not engage in social or imaginative play, preferring stereotyped activities with objects. There is often strong attachment to an inanimate object such as a string or rubber band. Speech and language development are both markedly delayed and abnormal in content, form, and tone. Echolalia, incorrect use of pronouns, and idiosyncratic meanings for words are common. Even when grammatically correct speech and language develop, there is impairment in the ability to initiate or sustain conversation due to an inability to make use of social cues and a lack of an understanding of the other's point of view. Stereotyped body movements, such as hand-flicking or head-banging, are common. Changes in the environment or in routines often produce extreme distress. There is a marked restriction in interests and a preoccupation with parts of objects or a narrow area of knowledge.

Development may be markedly abnormal from early infancy, with indifference or aversion to cuddling. Eye contact may be absent or present but impersonal. Some children may initially appear normal, with symptoms appearing at age two or three years as more complex communication and social interaction are expected.

Differential Diagnosis
Children with pure *mental retardation* have a more even pattern of delays and do not have bizarre behaviors or deficits in social relatedness. Many children with PDD

also have mental retardation, usually in the moderate range. In *aphasia, developmental language disorders*, or *deafness*, the deficits in language are partially compensated by nonverbal gestures; social interest is normal. *Degenerative neurological diseases* may transiently resemble PDD.

History and clinical examination can distinguish PDD from *reactive attachment disorder of infancy* or severe reactions to trauma or separation from parents. In very young or nonverbal children, the symptoms of autism and *schizophrenia* may be difficult to distinguish (Watkins et al, 1988).

Etiology

There is no evidence that child-rearing practices contribute to the development of this disorder. PDD is more common in children with certain chromosomal abnormalities (such as fragile X syndrome) and can follow a wide range of infections (especially maternal rubella during pregnancy) and traumatic insults to the central nervous system. Neuroanatomic imaging findings have been inconsistent. Pedigree studies have indicated a genetic contribution to the spectrum that includes PDD, language disorders, dyslexia, and mental retardation. In some families, autosomal recessive inheritance appears likely.

Evaluation

Medical evaluation is needed to seek sensory deficits, possible treatable metabolic disorders, and degenerative diseases. A genetic evaluation may be useful for counseling family members. The physician should be alert to the possibility of epilepsy; major or minor motor or complex partial seizures develop in 20 to 35% of patients with autism by age 20. In evaluating family dynamics, the reciprocal effects on parents of the child's behavior must be taken into account. Baseline measurements are taken of cognitive level, social communication skills, language function, and additional psychiatric symptoms such as hyperactivity, aggression, severe anxiety, compulsions, depression, or mania.

Treatment

Psychotherapy Group therapy with autistic or normal peers may significantly improve social functioning. Supportive psychotherapy may be of benefit to parents. Behavioral techniques are valuable in increasing learning and reducing maladaptive or injurious behaviors. These management strategies should be taught to parents and incorporated into the school setting.

Psychopharmacologic Treatment. No medications are known to affect the autistic disorder per se, and medication should not be used as the sole treatment.

Neuroleptics. In some hyper- or normoactive autistic children, haloperidol (in doses of 0.5 to 3.0 mg/day) decreases behavioral target symptoms such as hyperactivity, aggression, temper tantrums, withdrawal, and stereotypies. In combination with a structured behavioral/educational program, it may enhance language acquisition. In general, hypoactive autistic children do not respond well to haloperidol (Campbell et al, 1985). (See the section on schizophrenia in this chapter for the use of neuroleptics in children and adolescents.)

Stimulants. Contrary to previous belief, recent reports indicate that methylphenidate in doses similar to those used to treat ADHD may reduce overactivity in autistic children and improve attention span without producing psychosis or increasing stereotyped behaviors (Birmaher, Quintana, and Greenhill, 1988; Strayhorn et al, 1988).

Antidepressants. Clomipramine or fluoxetine may be useful in decreasing the compulsive rituals and perservative behaviors that often appear in persons with autism.

Opiate Antagonists. Naltrexone has been found to be useful in the treatment of some children and adolescents with autistic disorder by decreasing withdrawal and self-injurious behavior and increasing communicative speech and social relatedness (Campbell, Anderson, Small et al, 1990).

Environmental Interventions. The best outcome is obtained with a specialized therapeutic educational program that integrates social, language, and behavioral components, beginning as early as possible (age two to four years). Sufficiently intensive early treatment can avert institutionalization for all but the most handicapped. Adolescents and young adults can benefit from sheltered workshops, vocational training programs, and group homes in the community. Support and advocacy groups for parents (such as a local chapter of the Autism Society of America) are useful.

The Role of the Primary Care Physician
The pediatrician is usually the first to whom parents bring their concerns about a child with PDD, often in the first 18 months of life. It is essential for the physician to take these concerns seriously. If a screening examination indicates delay or deviance in development, immediate arrangements for definitive diagnosis and early intervention are indicated. Whenever possible, referral should be made to a center with experience in this rare disorder where a multidisciplinary team assessment can be conducted. The primary physician will maintain an important role in coordinating medical care for these patients, whose medical disorders may be difficult to diagnose and treat due to the lack of verbal ability and cooperation. The physician must be aware that parents of autistic children, driven to desperation by the severity of the disorder and the absence of curative treatments, are at risk for pursuing unconventional, unproven, and perhaps even harmful interventions that promise miraculous results.

SPECIFIC DEVELOPMENTAL DISORDERS

Description
This group of disorders is characterized by developmental delay in a specific domain (relative to that expected for mental age) that results in functional impairment. The delay must not be due to a diagnosable physical disorder, a visual or hearing impairment, a pervasive developmental disorder, mental retardation, or inadequate

educational opportunities. It is common for a child to have more than one specific developmental disorder (see Table 16–7). Frequent secondary symptoms include low self-esteem, demoralization, refusal to exert effort in school, and behavior problems.

Etiology

Genetic factors are suggested by the clustering of specific developmental disorders in families. Etiology is presumed to relate to delayed or abnormal maturation of or damage to local areas of the cerebral cortex. Substantial genetic contributions to dyslexia (developmental reading disorder) have been demonstrated.

Evaluation

Early diagnosis is crucial in facilitating remediation and reducing secondary emotional and behavioral symptoms. Assessment requires psychological testing (see Table 16–3) to establish IQ followed by academic achievement tests and tests of specific language, speech, and motor functions. Visual and hearing impairment must be ruled out. A careful history should be taken of school attendance and performance and of the quality of teaching. Schools overidentify boys and fail to identify girls with developmental reading disorder (Shaywitz et al, 1990).

Treatment

Children do not simply grow out of learning disabilities but retain some degree of impairment into adulthood.

Psychotherapy. Supportive psychotherapy may be required to deal with low self-esteem, passivity, lack of motivation, anxiety, or depression resulting from the learning

Table 16–7 **Specific Developmental Disorders**

DISORDER	ESTIMATED PREVALENCE* (AGE 5–12)
Academic Skills Disorders	
Developmental Arithmetic Disorder	Unknown
Developmental Expressive Writing Disorder	2–8%
Developmental Reading Disorder (dyslexia)	7–9% **
Language and Speech Disorders	
Developmental Articulation Disorder	5–10%
Developmental Expressive Language Disorder	3–10%
Developmental Receptive Language Disorder	3–10%
Motor Skills Disorder	
Developmental Coordination Disorder	6%
Developmental Disorder Not Otherwise Specified	Unknown

* (APA, 1987)
** (Shaywitz et al, 1990)

difficulties. Family therapy can deal with sequelae of parental criticism and child academic failure. Behavioral techniques may be useful in motivating children to practice and learn skills that are difficult for them.

Educational and Adjunctive Interventions. Most important is specific remediation of the deficits, using teaching techniques tailored to the child's strengths and weaknesses. Special educational programs may be needed, ranging from tutoring to a resource room several periods a week, to full-time special classes. The most severe cases may require a special school or residential treatment program. Articulation or language therapy is indicated for language and speech disorders. Physical or occupational therapy may be needed.

MEDICAL ILLNESS IN CHILDREN AND ADOLESCENTS

Response of Child and Family to Physical Illness

Infancy

When infants less than six months old are hospitalized, they are usually most upset by changes in their usual routine. It is helpful to have the parents do as much of the care as possible and to arrange for consistency of nurses. For the older infant who has formed strong differential attachments, separation is traumatic, especially in the unfamiliar hospital environment and when accompanied by physical discomfort and medical procedures. Stranger anxiety adds to the baby's distress. The infant's immature language development exacerbates the problem since explanations are not useful in understanding the situation.

The constant presence of a parent is extremely important. In the absence of an attachment figure, the baby's thrashing, refusal to eat, and inability to sleep may have serious medical consequences. Fortunately, most pediatric hospital settings not only permit but encourage parents to "live in" while their young child is hospitalized.

Early Childhood

Hospitalized children aged one to three years react primarily to separation from their parents. They may react by rejecting parents when they visit, being aggressive toward physicians and nurses, regressing in bowel and bladder control, and refusing to eat. If parents are absent, children may develop depression, sleep disturbance, diarrhea, or vomiting. Toddlers also have great concern for the intactness of their bodies and may be extremely fearful of minor procedures (such as blood-drawing). Maximizing parental presence and providing the child with familiar items from home are helpful.

For children aged three to five years, separation from parents by hospitalization is still difficult, even for a child who is comfortably able to separate in other circumstances. Anesthesia and surgery are especially frightening because this is a time of normal fears of bodily injury. Children believe that illness and painful treatments are punishment for real or fantasized misbehavior. When possible, preparation by simple explanations and a visit to the hospital may help. Constant presence of a parent is important.

School Age

Children aged six to 12 years usually tolerate acute illness and hospitalization relatively well, especially if they are prepared, parents visit daily for substantial periods, and preceding development was normal. They may still have irrational explanations of illness (that they are being punished or that their parents were unable to protect them). Behavioral regression or oppositional behavior often occurs.

Adolescence

Adolescents have more realistic fears regarding the outcome of illness, especially regarding changes in appearance or inability to continue favorite activities. An injury may make impossible a planned career (such as professional sports or the military). Loss of autonomy and privacy are especially painful, as are differences from peers.

Parents

At the time of diagnosis, the parents of a chronically ill or handicapped child must go through a period of mourning. The stages are similar to those following a death: anger, denial, grief, and resignation. Medical problems in a child may be viewed by the parent (and others) as a negative reflection on the parent. Parents feel guilty, especially for genetic diseases or complications that may be attributed (rightly or wrongly) to maternal behavior. The parents' anger, resentment, guilt, and/or denial may interfere with their ability to work together with the pediatric team. Realistic additional caretaking and financial burdens may stress parents beyond their ability to cope. (Regressive behavior precipitated by physical illness in adults is discussed in Chapter 20.)

Chronic Illness

Sequelae of chronic illness include interference with normal developmental tasks attained through school, peers, sports, and other activities. Autonomy and control of the child's own body is jeopardized. Children and adolescents with chronic illness, but without disability, are twice as likely as controls to have a psychiatric disorder. Those with disability as well as chronic illness are even more likely to have emotional problems, attention-deficit disorders, social isolation, or school performance problems. The majority of chronically ill youngsters do not, however, have psychiatric disorders or major difficulties with social or school adjustment (Cadman et al, 1987).

Compliance

Lack of compliance with medical regimens (e.g., medication, diet, exercise) is a major problem in the care of children and adolescents. Factors that contribute to noncompliance are seen in Table 16–8. Attention to and remediation of specific causes of noncompliance will improve medical management. (General issues in noncompliance are discussed in Chapter 20.)

Table 16–8 **Causative Factors in Noncompliance**

Patient Factors

Denial or lack of acceptance of the disorder
Frustration with the outcome or nature of treatment
Wish to obtain parental attention or special privileges via symptoms
Wish to regain control
Rebellion against parents
Lack of knowledge or skills
Inability to resist peer pressure
Lack of relationship or miscommunication with health care team
Psychopathology
   Depression
   Suicidal intent
   Attention-deficit hyperactivity disorder
   Oppositional defiant disorder
   Anorexia nervosa or bulimia

Family Factors

Unresolved guilt, denial, anger, and/or fear
Lack of knowledge and skills
Inability to encourage adolescent independence
Competition with medical personnel
Lack of support system
Other stressors on family
Family conflict acted out through the child's medical care
Rivalry between patient and healthy siblings

Treatment-related factors

Interference with usual activities
Side effects of drugs (pain, nausea, weight gain, hair loss)
Clarity of connection between noncompliance and sequelae
Disinterested, inconsistent medical personnel

SPECIFIC INTERVENTIONS FOR MEDICALLY ILL CHILDREN AND ADOLESCENTS

A child and adolescent psychiatrist or pediatric psychologist can offer consultation and treatment for emotional and behavioral problems. Coexisting psychiatric disorders are treated as in medically healthy children, although modifications are often needed.

Psychotherapy

Supportive individual, family, and/or group psychotherapy is often valuable for both patient and parents. Instruction in social problem solving and coping skills may also be beneficial.

Behavior Modification

Techniques such as behavioral contracting with contingency management and self-monitoring with self-reinforcement are invaluable in improving medical and behavioral compliance. Children who refuse or are unable to swallow oral medication can be taught to take pills using instruction, modeling, contingent rewards, and shaping pill-swallowing using successively larger candies or placebos (Pelco et al, 1987).

Behavioral medicine techniques have been adapted for the level of the youngster's cognitive or emotional development. Relaxation training has been used in the treatment of pediatric migraine, juvenile rheumatoid arthritis, hemophilia, asthma, and hyperventilation in patients with cystic fibrosis. Hypnosis can be used in the treatment of physical symptoms with a psychological component or to help a child manage severe pain or nausea associated with a physical disorder or its treatment.

Behavioral therapy techniques in the management of chronic pain include operant techniques, self-monitoring, and stress management planning. Emphasis is placed on fostering a sense of control and mastery and on promoting normal functioning in spite of pain (Masek, Spirito, and Fentress, 1984; Varni et al, 1986).

"Stress inoculation" uses education, modeling, systematic desensitization, hypnosis, contingency management, and training and practice in coping skills such as imagery and breathing exercises. It is useful in the prevention of stress and anxiety in children before medical and dental procedures and in chronically ill children for reduction of anxiety, pain, or other discomfort connected to repeated procedures such as spinal taps, bone marrow aspirations, and chemotherapy injections (Melamed, Klingman, and Siegel, 1984; Varni et al, 1986).

Psychopharmacologic Treatment

Tricyclic antidepressants may be used to treat depression. Situational and anticipatory anxiety related to procedures may benefit from hydroxyzine, diazepam, or alprazolam (Pfefferbaum et al, 1987).

Environmental Interventions

Peer activities and school should be normalized as much as possible. Chronically ill children may benefit greatly from special camps and recreation programs with medical supervision. Families may require a variety of concrete assistance to provide for an ill child.

The Role of the Physician

Members of the medical team will be more successful if they are able to deal with their own feelings of guilt, helplessness, inadequacy, and anxiety. Staff support groups may be useful. In dealing with adolescents, efforts to respect and reinforce the patient's competence and autonomy, to give information in a way that permits the adolescent to understand and to save face, and to encourage questions will be rewarded with improved compliance and psychological adjustment. Children and adolescents with potentially fatal illnesses appreciate accurate information, titrated to their ability to understand and emotional readiness to hear.

CLINICAL PEARLS

Emotional and behavioral reactions should be anticipated.

- Explain in advance as much as the child's age, coping style, and medical situation allow.
- Minimize separations from parents, especially for children under eight years old.
- Try to understand the meaning of the illness to the child and correct her or his misconceptions.
- Understand that the child or adolescent needs to control *something* in the environment and arrange the milieu so that this will not interfere with treatment.
- Do not criticize or blame the child or parents for regressive behavior.

ANNOTATED BIBLIOGRAPHY

General

Adams PL, Fras I: Beginning Child Psychiatry. New York, Brunner/Mazel, 1988

> An introductory text.

Dulcan MK, Popper CW: Concise Guide to Child and Adolescent Psychiatry. Washington, DC, American Psychiatric Press, 1991

> A brief paperback handbook.

Garfinkel BD, Carlson GA, Weller EB (eds): Psychiatric Disorders in Children and Adolescents. Philadelphia, Saunders, 1990

> Manageable, comprehensive coverage of the diagnosis and treatment of psychiatric disorders of childhood and adolescence. Available in paperback.

Lewis M, Volkmar F: Clinical Aspects of Child and Adolescent Development, 3rd ed. Philadelphia, Lea and Febiger, 1990

> Good coverage of both normal and pathological development.

Wiener JM (ed): Textbook of Child and Adolescent Psychiatry. Washington, DC, American Psychiatric Press, 1991

> A complete, clinically focused textbook. Chapters on assessment, treatment, all Axis I and II disorders, and special issues such as abuse and suicide.

Evaluation and Treatment

Adams PL: A Primer of Child Psychotherapy, 2nd ed. Boston, Little, Brown, 1982

Dulcan MK: Treatment of Children and Adolescents. In Hales RE, Yudofsky SC, Talbott JA (eds): The American Psychiatric Press Textbook of Psychiatry, 2nd ed. Washington, DC, American Psychiatric Press, 1994

Green WH: Child and Adolescent Clinical Psychopharmacology. Baltimore, Williams & Wilkins, 1991

Simmons JE: Psychiatric Examination of Children, 4th ed. Philadelphia, Lea and Febiger, 1987

Attention-deficit Hyperactivity Disorder

Barkley RA: Attention-deficit Hyperactivity Disorder: A Handbook for Diagnosis and Treatment. New York, Guilford Press, 1990

Oppositional Defiant Disorder

Forehand R, McMahon RJ: Helping the Non-Compliant Child: A Clinician's Guide to Parent Training. New York, Guilford Press, 1981

Anxiety Disorders

Eth S, Pynoos RS (eds): Posttraumatic Stress Disorder in Children. Washington, DC, American Psychiatric Press, 1985

Ollendick TH, Francis G: Behavioral assessment and treatment of childhood phobias. Behavior Modif 12:165–204, 1988

Reiter S, Kutcher S, Gardner D: Anxiety disorders in children and adolescents: Clinical and related issues in pharmacological treatment. Can J Psychiatry 37:432–438, 1992

Wolff RP, Wolff LS: Assessment and treatment of obsessive–compulsive disorder in children. Behavior Modif 15:372–393, 1991

Elimination Disorders

Howe AC, Walker CE: Behavioral management of toilet training, enuresis, and encopresis. Pediatric Clin N Am 39:413–432, 1992

Levine MD: Encopresis. In Levine MD, Carey WB, Crocker AC (eds): Developmental-Behavioral Pediatrics, 2nd ed, pp 389–397. Philadelphia, Saunders, 1992

Rappaport LA: Enuresis. In Levine MD, Carey WB, Crocker AC (eds): Developmental-Behavioral Pediatrics, pp 384–388. Philadelphia, Saunders, 1992

Mood Disorders

Kutcher SP, Marton P: Parameters of adolescent depression: A review. Psychiatric Clin N Am 12:895–918, 1989

Schizophrenia

Cantor S: Childhood Schizophrenia. New York, Guilford Press, 1988

Eating Disorders

Casey PH: Failure to Thrive. In Levine MD, Carey WB, Crocker AC (eds): Developmental-Behavioral Pediatrics, 2nd ed, pp 375–383. Philadelphia, Saunders, 1992

Chatoor I, Kickson L, Einhorn A: Rumination: Etiology and treatment. Pediatr Annals 13:924–929, 1984

Yates A: Current perspectives on the eating disorders, I: History, psychological, and biological aspects. J Am Acad Child Adolesc Psychiatry 28:813–828, 1989

Yates A: Current perspectives on the eating disorders, II: Treatment, outcome, and research directions. J Am Acad Child Adolesc Psychiatry 29:1–9, 1990

Obesity

Neumann CG, Jenks BH: Obesity. In Levine MD, Carey WB, Crocker AC (eds): Developmental-Behavioral Pediatrics, pp 354–363. Philadelphia, Saunders, 1992

Tourette's Disorder

Cohen DJ, Brunn RD, Leckan JF (eds): Tourette's Syndrome and Tic Disorders: Clinical Understanding and Treatment. New York, John Wiley, 1988

Mental Retardation

Bregman JD, Hodapp RM: Current developments in the understanding of mental retardation. Part I: Biological and phenomenological perspectives. J Am Acad Child Adolesc Psychiatry 30:707–719, 1991

Bregman JD: Current developments in the understanding of mental retardation. Part II: Psychopathology. J Am Acad Child Adolesc Psychiatry 30:861–872, 1991

Sparrow SS, Fletcher JM, Cicchetti CV: Psychological Assessment of Children. In Cohen DJ, Schowalter JE (eds): Child Psychiatry. In Cavenar J (ed): Psychiatry, Vol. 2. Philadelphia, Lippincott, 1985

Autistic Disorder/Pervasive Developmental Disorder

Denckla MB, James LS (eds): An update on autism: A developmental disorder. Pediatrics 87:5 (suppl), 1991

Specific Developmental Disorders

Silver L: The Misunderstood Child: A Guide for Parents of Learning Disabled Children. New York, McGraw-Hill, 1984

Medically Ill Children

Van Dongen-Melman JEWM, Sanders-Woudstra JAR: The Chronically Ill Child and His Family. In Cohen DJ, Schowalter JE (eds): Child Psychiatry. In Cavenar J (ed): Psychiatry, Vol. 2. Philadelphia, Lippincott, 1985

Van Dongen-Melman JEWM, Sanders-Woudstra JAR: The Fatally Ill Child and His Family. In Cohen DJ, Schowalter JE (eds): Child Psychiatry. In Cavenar J (ed): Psychiatry, Vol. 2. Philadelphia, Lippincott, 1985

REFERENCES

Abramowitz AJ, O'Leary SG: Behavioral interventions for the classroom: Implications for students with ADHD. School Psychol Rvw 20:220–234, 1991

Achenbach TM: Manual for the Child Behavior Checklist/4–18 and 1991 Profile. Burlington, University of Vermont Department of Psychiatry, 1991a

Achenbach TM: Manual for the Youth Self-Report and 1991 Profile. Burlington, University of Vermont Department of Psychiatry, 1991b

Achenbach TM: Manual for the Teacher's Report Form and 1991 Profile. Burlington, University of Vermont Department of Psychiatry, 1991c

American Psychiatric Association: Diagnostic and Statistical Manual of Mental Disorders, 3rd ed., Rev. Washington, DC, American Psychiatric Press, 1987

American Psychiatric Association: DSM-IV Draft Criteria 3/1/93. Washington, DC, American Psychiatric Association, 1993

American Psychiatric Association: Diagnostic and Statistical Manual of Mental Disorders, 4th ed. Washington, DC, American Psychiatric Press, in press [1994]

Anderson CM, Hogarty GE, Reiss DJ: Family treatment of adult schizophrenic patients: A psycho-educational approach. Schizophr Bull 6:490–505, 1980

Anderson JC, Williams S, McGee R, Silva PA: DSM-III disorders in preadolescent children: Prevalence in a a large sample from the general population. Arch Gen Psychiatry 44:69–76, 1987

Barkley RA: Attention-deficit Hyperactivity Disorder: A Handbook for Diagnosis and Treatment. New York, Guilford Press, 1990

Bartels MG, Varley CK, Mitchell J, Stamm SJ: Pediatric cardiovascular effects of imipramine and desipramine. J Am Acad Child Adolesc Psychiatry 30:100–103, 1991

Beach PS, Beach RE, Smith LR: Hyponatremic seizures in a child treated with desmopressin to control enuresis. Clin Pediatrics 31:566–569, 1992

Biederman J, Baldessarini RJ, Wright V, Knee D, Harmatz JS: A double-blind placebo controlled study of desipramine in the treatment of ADD: I. Efficacy. J Am Acad Child Adolesc Psychiatry 28:777–784, 1989

Biederman J, Munir K, Knee D et al: A family study of patients with attention deficit disorder and normal controls. J Psychiatr Res 20:263–274, 1986

Birmaher B, Quintana H, Greenhill LL: Methylphenidate treatment of hyperactive autistic children. J Am Acad Child Adolesc Psychiatry 27:248–251, 1988

Cadman D, Boyle M, Szatmari P, Offord DR: Chronic illness, disability, and mental and social well-being: Findings of the Ontario Child Health Study. Pediatrics 79:805–813, 1987

Campbell M, Anderson LT, Small AM et al: Naltrexone in autistic children: A double-blind and placebo-controlled study. Psychopharmacol Bull 26:130–135, 1990

Campbell M, Green WH, Deutsch, SI: Child and Adolescent Psychopharmacology. Beverly Hills, Sage Publications, 1985

Campbell M, Silva RR, Kafantaris V et al: Predictors of side effects associated with lithium administration in children. Psychopharmacol Bull 27:373–380, 1991

Campbell SB: Hyperactivity in preschoolers: Correlates and prognostic implications. Clin Psychol Rvw 5:405–428, 1985

Cantor S, Kestenbaum C: Psychotherapy with schizophrenic children. J Am Acad Child Psychiatry 25:623–630, 1986

Carlson CL, Pelham WE, Milich R, Dixon J: Single and combined effects of methylphenidate and behavior therapy on the classroom performance of children with attention-deficit hyperactivity disorder. J Abnormal Child Psychol 20:213–232, 1992

Carlson GA, Kashani JH: Phenomenology of major depression from childhood through adulthood: Analysis of three studies. Am J Psychiatry 145:1222–1225, 1988

Coffey BJ: Anxiolytics for children and adolescents: Traditional and new drugs. J Child Adolesc Psychopharmacology 1:57–83, 1990

Costello EJ, Pantino T: The new morbidity: Who should treat it? Dev Behav Pediatrics 8:288–291, 1987

Dorsett PG: Behavioral and Social Learning Psychology. In Stoudemire A (ed): Human Behavior: An Introduction for Medical Students, 2nd ed. Philadelphia, Lippincott, 1994

Douglas VI: Attentional and Cognitive Problems. In Rutter M (ed) Developmental Neuropsychiatry. New York, Guilford Press, 1983

Dulcan MK: Information for parents and youth on psychotropic medications. J Child Adolesc Psychopharmacology 2:81–101, 1992

Dulcan MK: Childhood and Adolescent Development. In Stoudemire A (ed): Clinical Psychiatry for Medical Students, 2nd ed. Philadelphia, Lippincott, 1994

Elia J, Borcherding BG, Rapoport JL, Keysor CS: Methylphenidate and dextroamphetamine treatments of hyperactivity: Are there true nonresponders? Psychiatry Res 36:141–155, 1991

Emery G, Bedrosian R, Garber J: Cognitive Therapy with Depressed Children and Adolescents. In Cantwell DP, Carlson GA (eds): Affective Disorders in Childhood and Adolescence: An Update. New York, Spectrum Publications, 1983

Epstein LH, Valoski A, Wing RR, McCurley J: Ten-year follow-up of behavioral, family-based treatment for obese children. JAMA 264:2519–2523, 1990

Evans RW, Clay TH, Gualtieri CT: Carbamazepine in pediatric psychiatry. J Am Acad Child Adolesc Psychiatry 26:2–8, 1987

Evans RW, Gualtieri CT, Hicks RE: A neuropathic substrate for stimulant drug effects in hyperactive children. Clin Neuropharmacol 9:264–281, 1986

Famularo R, Kinscherff R, Fenton T: Propranolol treatment for childhood posttraumatic stress disorder, acute type. AJDC 142:1244–1247, 1988

Flament MF, Whitaker A, Rapoport JL et al: Obsessive–compulsive disorder in adolescence: An epidemiological study. J Amer Acad Child Adolesc Psychiatry 27:764–771, 1988

Forehand RL, McMahon RJ: Helping the Noncompliant Child: A Clinician's Guide to Parent Training. New York, Guilford Press, 1981

Gadow KD: Prevalence and efficacy of stimulant drug use with mentally retarded children and youth. Psychopharmacol Bull 21:291–303, 1985

Geller B, Cooper TB, Chestnut BS: Preliminary data on the relationship between nortriptyline plasma level and response in depressed children. Am J Psychiatry 143:1283–1286, 1986

Greenhill LL, Solomon M, Pleak R et al: Molindone hydrochloride treatment of hospitalized children with conduct disorder. J Clin Psychiatry 46:20–25, 1985

Grob CS, Coyle JT: Suspected adverse methylphenidate-imipramine interactions in children. JDBP 7:265–267, 1986

Henggeler SW, Borduin CM: Family Therapy and Beyond: A Multisystemic Approach to Treatment the Behavior Problems of Children and Adolescents. Pacific Grove, CA, Brooks/Cole, 1990

Herskowitz J: Developmental Toxicology. In Popper C (ed): Psychiatric Pharmacosciences of Children and Adolescents. Washington, DC, American Psychiatric Press, 1987

Hunt RD, Capper S, O'Connell P: Clonidine in child and adolescent psychiatry. J Child Adolesc Psychopharmacol 1:87–102, 1990

Kagan J, Reznick JS, Snidman N: Biological bases of childhood shyness. Science 240:167–171, 1988

Kashani JH, Carlson GA, Beck NC et al: Depression, depressive symptoms, and depressed mood among a community sample of adolescents. Am J Psychiatry 144:931–934, 1987

Kashani JH, Orvaschel H: A community study of anxiety in children and adolescents. Am J Psychiatry 147:313–318, 1990

Kazdin AE, Siegel TC, Bass D: Cognitive problem-solving skills training and parent management training in the treatment of antisocial behavior in children. J Consulting Clin Psychol 60:733–747, 1992

Kendall PC, Braswell L: Cognitive-Behavioral Therapy for Impulsive Children. New York, Guilford Press, 1985

Kernberg PF, Chazan SE: Children with Conduct Disorders: A Psychotherapy Manual. New York, Basic Books, 1991

Klauber GT: Clinical efficacy and safety of desmopressin in the treatment of nocturnal enuresis. J Pediatrics 114:719–722, 1989

Kovacs M, Feinberg TL, Crouse-Novak MA et al.: Depressive disorders in childhood: I. A longitudinal prospective study of characteristics and recovery. Arch Gen Psychiatry 41:229–237, 1984a

Kovacs M, Feinberg TL, Crouse-Novak MA et al: Depressive disorders in childhood: II. A longitudinal study of the risk for a subsequent major depression. Arch Gen Psychiatry 41:643–649, 1984b

Kutcher SP, Marton P: Parameters of adolescent depression: A review. Psychiatric Clin N Am 12:895–918, 1989

Last CG, Strauss CC, Francis G: Comorbidity among childhood anxiety disorders. J Nerv Ment Dis 175:726–730, 1987

Latz SR, McCracken JT: Neuroleptic malignant syndrome in children and adolescents: Two case reports and a warning. J Child Adolesc Psychopharmacol 2:123–129, 1992

Leckman JF, Ort S, Caruso et al: Rebound phenomena in Tourette's Syndrome after abrupt withdrawal of clonidine. Arch Gen Psychiatry 43:1168–1176, 1986

Loeber R: Development and risk factors of juvenile antisocial behavior and delinquency. Clin Psychol Rvw 10:1–41, 1990

Lyons JA: Posttraumatic stress disorder in children and adolescents: A review of the literature. Dev Behav Pediatrics 8:349–356, 1987

Marriage K, Fine S, Moretti M, Haley G: Relationship between depression and conduct disorder in children and adolescents. J Am Acad Child Adolesc Psychiatry 25:687–691, 1986

Masek BJ, Spirito A, Fentress DW: Behavioral treatment of symptoms of childhood illness. Clin Psychol Rvw 4:561–570, 1984

Mayes SC, Humphrey FJ, Handford HA, Mitchell JF: Rumination disorder: Differential diagnosis. J Am Acad Child Adolesc Psychiatry 27:300–302, 1988

McDaniel KD: Pharmacologic treatment of psychiatric and neurodevelopmental disorders in children and adolescents (Part 1). Clin Pediatr 25:65–71, 1986

Melamed BG, Klingman A, Siegel LJ: Individualizing Cognitive Behavioral Strategies in the Reduction of Medical and Dental Stress. In Meyers AW, Craighead WE (eds): Cognitive Behavior Therapy with Children. New York, Plenum Press, 1984

Milich R, Wolraich M, Lindgren S: Sugar and hyperactivity: A critical review of empirical findings. Clin Psychol Rvw 6:493–513, 1986

Ollendick TH, Francis G: Behavioral assessment and treatment of childhood phobias. Behavior Modif 12:165–204, 1988

O'Regan S, Yazbeck S, Hamberger B, Schick E: Constipation: A commonly unrecognized cause of enuresis. Am J Diseases Child 140:260–261, 1986

Patterson GR: Families: Applications of Social Learning to Family Life. Champaign, IL, Research Press, 1975

Patterson GR, DeBaryshe BD, Ramsey E: A developmental perspective on antisocial behavior. Am Psychol 44:329–335, 1989

Pelco LE, Kissel RC, Parrish JM, Miltenberger RG: Behavioral management of oral medication administration difficulties among children: A review of literature with case illustrations. Dev Behav Pediatrics 8:90–96, 1987

Pelham WE, Greenslade KE, Vodde-Hamilton M et al: Relative efficacy of long-acting stimulants on children with attention-deficit hyperactivity disorder: A comparison of standard methylphenidate, sustained-release methylphenidate, sustained-release dextroamphetamine, and pemoline. Pediatrics 86:226–237, 1990.

Pelham WE, Hoza J: Behavioral assessment of psychostimulant effects on ADD children in a summer day treatment program. Advances in Behavioral Assessment of Children and Families 3:3–34, 1987

Pelham WE, Murphy HA: Attention Deficit and Conduct Disorders. In Herson M (ed): Pharmacological and Behavioral Treatment: An Integrative Approach. New York, John Wiley, 1986

Pelham WE, Sturges J, Hoza J et al: The effects of Sustained Release 20 and 10 mg Ritalin b.i.d. on cognitive and social behavior in children with Attention Deficit Disorder. Pediatrics 80:491–501, 1987

Pfefferbaum B, Overall JE, Boren HA et al: Alprazolam in the treatment of anticipatory and acute situational anxiety in children with cancer. J Am Acad Child Adolesc Psychiatry 26:532–535, 1987

Pleak RR, Birmaher B, Gavrilescu A et al: Mania and neuropsychiatric excitation following carbamazepine. J Am Acad Child Adolesc Psychiatry 27:500–503, 1988

Preskorn SH, Weller EB, Hughes CW, Weller RA: Relationship of plasma imipramine levels to CNS toxicity in children. Am J Psychiatry 145:897, 1988

Preskorn SH, Weller EB, Hughes CW et al: Depression in prepubertal children: Dexamethasone nonsuppression predicts differential response to imipramine vs. placebo. Psychopharmacol Bull 23:128–133, 1987

Puig-Antich J: Major depression and conduct disorder in prepuberty. J Am Acad Child Adolesc Psychiatry 21:118–128, 1982

Puig-Antich J, Lukens E, Davies M et al: Psychosocial functioning in prepubertal major depressive disorders: II. Interpersonal relationships after sustained recovery from affective episode. Arch Gen Psychiatry 42:511–517, 1985

Pynoos RS, Eth S: Witness to violence: The child interview. J Am Acad Child Adolesc Psychiatry 25:306–319, 1986

Pynoos RS, Frederick C, Nader K et al: Life threat and posttraumatic stress in school-age children. Arch Gen Psychiatry 44:1057–1063, 1987

Rancurello MD: Clinical applications of antidepressant drugs in childhood behavioral and emotional disorders. Psychiatr Annals 15:88–100, 1985

Realmuto GM, Erickson WD, Yellin AM et al: Clinical comparison of thiothixene and thioridazine in schizophrenic adolescents. Am J Psychiatry 141:440–442, 1984

Reiter S, Kutcher S, Gardner D: Anxiety disorders in children and adolescents: Clinical and related issues in pharmacological treatment. Can J Psychiatry 37:432–438, 1992

Rutter M: Syndromes attributed to "Minimal Brain Dysfunction" in childhood. Am J Psychiatry 139:21–33, 1982

Ryan ND: Heterocyclic antidepressants in children and adolescents. J Child Adolesc Psychopharmacology 1:21–31, 1990

Ryan ND: The pharmacologic treatment of child and adolescent depression. Psychiatric Clin N Am 15:29–40, 1992

Ryan ND, Puig-Antich J: Affective illness in adolescence. In Frances AJ, Hales RE (eds): American Psychiatric Association Annual Review, Vol. 5. Washington, DC, American Psychiatric Press, 1986

Ryan ND, Williamson DE, Iyengar S, Orvaschel H, Reich T, Dahl RE, Puig-Antich J: A secular increase in child and adolescent onset affective disorder. J Am Acad Child Adolesc Psychiatry 31:600–605, 1992

Safer DJ, Krager JM: A survey of medication treatment for hyperactive/inattentive students. JAMA 260:2256–2258, 1988

Schuster CR, Lewis M, Seiden LS: Fenfluramine: Neurotoxicity. Psychopharmacol Bull 22:148–151, 1986

Shaywitz SE, Shaywitz BA, Fletcher JM, Escobar MD: Prevalence of reading disability in boys and girls: Results of the Connecticut Longitudinal Study. JAMA 264:998–1002, 1990

Simeon JG, Ferguson HB: Recent developments in the use of antidepressant and anxiolytic medications. Psychiatr Clin N Am 8:893–907, 1985

Strayhorn JM, Rapp N, Donina W, Strain PS: Randomized trial of methylphenidate for an autistic child. J Am Acad Child Adolesc Psychiatry 27:244–247, 1988

Strober M, Carlson G: Bipolar illness in adolescents with major depression: Clinical, genetic, and psychopharmacolgic predictors in a three- to four-year prospective follow-up investigation. Arch Gen Psychiatry 39:549–555, 1982

Terr LC: Chowchilla revisited: The effects of psychic trauma four years after a school-bus kidnapping. Am J Psychiatry 140:1543–1550, 1983

Terr LC: Childhood Psychic Trauma. In Call JD, Cohen RL, Harrison SI, Berlin IN, Stone LA (eds): Basic Handbook of Child Psychiatry, Vol. V. New York, Basic Books, 1987a

Terr LC: Treatment of Psychic Trauma in Children. In Call JD, Cohen RL, Harrison SI, Berlin IN, Stone LA (eds): Basic Handbook of Child Psychiatry, Vol. V. New York, Basic Books, 1987b

Varley CK: Effects of methylphenidate in adolescents with attention deficit disorder. J Am Acad Child Psychiatry 4:351–354, 1983

Varni JW, Jay SM, Masek BJ et al: Cognitive-Behavioral Assessment and Management of Pediatric Pain. In Holvman AD, Turk ED (eds): Handbook of Psychological Treatment Approaches. New York, Pergamon Press, 1986

Watkins JM, Asarnow RF, Tanguay PE: Symptom development in childhood onset schizophrenia. J Child Psychol Psychiatry 29:865–878, 1988

Weller EB, Weller RA, Fristad MA: Lithium dosage guide for prepubertal children: A preliminary report. J Am Acad Child Psychiatry 25:92–95, 1986

Wender EH: The food additive-free diet in the treatment of behavior disorders: A review. JDBP 7:35–42, 1986

Williams DT: Hypnosis as a Psychotherapeutic Adjunct. In Harrison SI (ed): Basic Handbook of Child Psychiatry, Vol. 3. New York, Basic Books, 1979

Williams DT, Mehl R, Yudofsky S et al: The effect of propranolol on uncontrolled rage outbursts in children and adolescents with organic brain dysfunction. J Am Acad Child Psychiatry 21:129–135, 1982

Alan Stoudemire (ed). *Clinical Psychiatry for Medical Students,* Second Edition. Copyright © 1994, 1990 by J. B. Lippincott Company.

17 The Psychotherapies: Basic Theoretical Principles and Techniques

Robert J. Ursano,
Edward K. Silberman, and
Alberto Diaz, Jr.

Psychotherapy is the "talking cure." Through the use of words to create understanding, guidance, and support and lead the patient to new experiences, the psychotherapist aims to eliminate symptoms and increase the patient's productivity and enjoyment of life. The brain itself is the target of psychotherapy. Behavior, thoughts, and emotions derive from brain activity and have a neuroanatomical, neurochemical, and neurophysiologic basis. The psychotherapies aim to alter brain "patterning" and function. Psychopathology frequently limits a patient's ability to see and experience options and choices. The patients' behaviors, thoughts, and feelings are constricted by their psychiatric illness. Through the various psychotherapies, the therapist attempts to increase the patients' range of behavioral options and decrease painful constricting symptoms.

Psychotherapeutic approaches to psychopathology vary widely and reflect different concepts and theories of mental life, personality development, abnormal behavior, and the role of environmental and biological determinants. The increasing understanding of the nature of the interaction of human beings with each other as individuals and as members of social groups has facilitated the application of some of these principles to the psychotherapeutic relationship as a treatment tool. Experience indicates that an integrated approach to treatment is the most successful approach. Different patients benefit from different types of psychotherapy. In addition, patients may substantially benefit from the appropriate combined use of medications and psychotherapy. Because of this, the medically trained psychiatrist can provide the most comprehensive evaluation for combining medication with psychotherapeutic treatment. The psychiatrist can use combined medication and psychotherapeutic treatments and is trained to recognize and manage the potential interactions of these two treatments. The psychiatrist is also alert to changes in the patient's medical status that can be a cause of or a result of psychiatric illness. Patients with significant medical illness as part of their health history (e.g., migraine, ulcers, psychosomatic illnesses, and so forth) are best treated by the psychiatrist who, as a physician, is knowledgeable of these disorders and their effects on feelings, behaviors, and life adjustment and is a skilled psychotherapist. Often the seriously depressed or psychotic patient may also be more comfortable with a psychiatrist who is trained in managing life-and-death issues, chronic illness, and the medical side effects of medication.

In the following pages, the major psychotherapies are reviewed. An understanding of these techniques and their theoretical concepts used in patient selection is important to the treatment armamentarium of inpatient, outpatient, and consultation–liaison psychiatric practices as well as general medical practice.

PSYCHOANALYTIC PSYCHOTHERAPIES

Psychoanalysis

Psychoanalysis was developed by Sigmund Freud in the late 19th century. Freud found that patients' life difficulties were related to unrecognized (unconscious) conflicts that arise in the course of child development and continue into adult life. Such conflicts are typically between libidinal and aggressive wishes and the fear of loss, condemnation retaliation, the constraints of reality, or the opposition of other incompatible wishes. "Libidinal wishes" are longings for both sexual and emotional gratification. Sexual gratification in psychoanalysis refers to the broad concept of bodily pleasure, the state of excitement and pleasure experienced by various bodily sensations beginning in infancy. Aggressive wishes may either be primary destructive impulses or arise in reaction to perceived frustration, deprivation, or attack. Such (neurotic) conflicts may give rise to a variety of manifestations in adulthood, including anxiety, depression, and somatic symptoms, as well as work, social, or sexual inhibitions and maladaptive ways of relating to other people.

The goal of psychoanalysis is to understand the nature of the patient's childhood conflicts (the "infantile neurosis") and their consequences in adult life. This is accomplished through reexperiencing these conflicts in relation to the analyst (the "transference neurosis"). This is a major undertaking that requires a great deal of the patient to sustain the treatment. It requires individuals who are able to access their fantasy lives in an active and experiencing manner and are able to "leave it behind" at the end of a session. Psychoanalysis is frequently criticized for being used to treat reasonably healthy people. However, all medical treatments require certain innate capacities of the patient (e.g., an intact immune system for successful antibiotic therapy). As with a generally healthy person with a relatively focal, yet painful physical disorder that impairs their functioning, a generally healthy person may have painful neurotic conflicts that interfere with both their work and personal life, and therefore require treatment.

Psychoanalysis focuses on the recovery of childhood experiences as they are re-created in the relationship with the analyst (Sandler et al, 1973). This re-creation in the doctor–patient relationship of the conflicted relationship with a childhood figure is called the "transference neurosis" (see Table 17–1). In the therapeutic relationship with the analyst, the emotional conflicts and trauma from the past are relived. The feelings and conflicts toward major figures in the child's development, most frequently the parents, are "transferred" to the analyst. When the transference neurosis is present, the patient emotionally experiences and reacts to the analyst in a very real manner "as if" the analyst was the significant figure from the past. Frequently, this experience is accompanied by other elements of the past being experienced in the patient's life. Countertransference, the analyst's transference response to the patient, is increased by life stress and unresolved conflicts in the analyst. It can appear as either an identification with or a reaction to the patient's conscious and unconscious fantasies, feelings, and behaviors. Understanding their own countertransference reactions can allow analysts to recognize subtle aspects of the transference relationship and better understand the patient's experience.

Psychoanalytic treatment attempts to set up a therapeutic situation in which the patient's observing capacity can be used to analyze the transference neurosis. *Transference reactions occur throughout life in all areas and are a frequent accompaniment of the doctor–patient relationship in the medical setting.* However, psychoanalysis is unique in its efforts to establish a setting in which the transference, when it appears, can be analyzed and worked through in an intense manner to facilitate recovery from psychiatric illness.

Modern psychoanalysis requires four to five sessions per week (45 to 50 minutes per session) continued, on the average, for 3 to 6 years. This extensive amount of sessions is necessary for patients to develop sufficient trust to explore their inner life and their subjective experience. Likewise, given the number of events that occur daily in one's lifetime, the frequent meetings are necessary for the patient to be able to explore fantasies, dreams, and reactions to the analytic situation instead of focusing

Table 17–1 **Psychoanalysis**

Goal	Resolution of symptoms and major reworking of personality structures related to childhood conflicts
Selection Criteria	No psychotic potential
	Able to use understanding
	High ego strength
	Able to experience and observe intense emotional states
	Psychiatric problem derived from childhood conflicts
Technique	Focus on fantasies and the transference
	Free association
	Couch
	Interpretation of defenses and transference
	Frequent meetings
	Neutrality of the analyst
Duration	3–6 years

only on daily reality-based crises and stresses. Individuals who are in severe crisis and, therefore, are focused on the crises in their life are generally not candidates for psychoanalysis. If major crises do occur during analysis, formal analysis may be temporarily suspended for a more supportive psychotherapeutic approach. In general, psychoanalytic patients are encouraged to use a recumbent position on the couch to further facilitate their ability to freely associate and verbalize their thoughts and feelings. In addition, the analyst usually sits out of the patient's view to assist unencumbered the process of *free association.*

Free association, the reporting of all thoughts that come to mind, is a major element in psychoanalytic technique. In point of fact, free association is difficult to attain, and much of the work of psychoanalysis is based on identifying those times when free association breaks down (the occurrence of a defense, clinically experienced by the analyst as "resistance"). When the patient is able to free associate easily, the neurotic conflicts have been largely removed and the termination of treatment is near.

Early in treatment, the analyst establishes a *therapeutic alliance* with the patient that allows for a reality-based consideration of the demands of the treatment and for a working collaboration between analyst and analysand (patient) directed toward understanding the patient. The analyst points out the defenses the patient uses to minimize awareness of conflicts and disturbing feelings. Dreams, slips of the tongue, and symptoms provide avenues to the understanding of unconscious motivations, feelings, and ideas.

The specific treatment effects of psychoanalysis result from the progressive understanding of defensive patterns and, most important, the feelings, cognitions, and behaviors that are "transferred" to the analyst from significant individuals in the patient's past. In the context of the arousal associated with the reexperiencing of these figures from the past and the simultaneous understanding of the experience, behavioral change occurs. Interpretation is an important technical procedure in this process. An interpretation links the patient's current experience with the analyst to an experience with a significant childhood figure during development.

The analyst operates under several rules that facilitate the analysis of the transference. These include the *rule of neutrality,* by which the analyst favors neither the patient's wishes (id) nor the condemnations of these wishes (superego), and the *rule of abstinence,* whereby the analyst does not provide emotional gratification to the patient similar to that of the wished-for childhood figure.

Medications are infrequently used in psychoanalysis, although some analysts are integrating psychoanalytic treatment with medication, particularly for mood disorders. In these cases, psychoanalysis is directed toward aiding the change in behaviors that may have been learned over a long time and may be interfering with the return of good psychosocial functioning. In general, however, the necessity for the use of medication may indicate the patient's need for greater support and structure than can be provided in the psychoanalytic treatment.

The assessment of a patient for psychoanalysis must include diagnostic considerations as well as an assessment of the patient's ability to make use of the psychoanalytic situation for behavior change. A patient's ability to use psychoanalysis depends on the patient's psychological-mindedness, the availability of supports in their real environment to sustain the psychoanalysis (which can be felt as quite depriving), and the patient's ability to experience and simultaneously observe highly charged emotional states. Because of the frequency of the sessions and the duration of the treatment, the cost of psychoanalysis can be prohibitive. However, low-fee training clinics frequently make a substantial amount of treatment available to some patients who could not otherwise afford it. Psychoanalysis has been useful in the treatment of obsessional disorders, conversion disorders, anxiety disorders, dysthymic disorders, and moderately severe personality disorders. Individuals with chaotic life settings and an inability to establish long-term, close relationships are usually not good candidates for psychoanalysis. In the present cost-effective climate, psychoanalysis is more frequently recommended after a course of brief psychotherapy has proved either ineffective or insufficient. Little empirical research is available on the efficacy of psychoanalysis compared with other psychotherapies. In general, those patients who can use understanding, introspection, and self-observation to modify their behavior find the treatment beneficial and productive.

Intensive (Long-Term) Psychoanalytically Oriented Psychotherapy

Psychoanalytically oriented psychotherapy, also known as psychoanalytic psychotherapy, psychodynamic psychotherapy, and explorative psychotherapy, is a psychotherapeutic procedure that recognizes the concepts of transference and resistance in the psychotherapy setting (Bruch, 1974; Reichmann, 1950). Both long-term and brief psychodynamic psychotherapy are possible. (See following section for brief psychodynamic psychotherapy.) Psychoanalytic psychotherapy is usually more focused than is the extensive reworking of personality undertaken in psychoanalysis. In addition, psychoanalytic psychotherapy is somewhat more "here and now" oriented, with less attempt to completely reconstruct the developmental origins of conflicts.

The psychoanalytic techniques of interpretation and clarification are central to psychoanalytic psychotherapy. Psychoanalytic psychotherapy makes more use of supportive techniques—such as suggestion, reality testing, education, and confrontation—than does psychoanalysis. This allows for its application to a broader range of patients, including those with the potential for severe regression.

Patients in long-term psychoanalytic psychotherapy are usually seen two or three times per week, although once per week is also increasingly common. Patient and therapist meet in face-to-face encounters with free association encouraged. Psychoanalytic psychotherapy may extend several months to several years, at times being as long as a psychoanalysis. The length is determined by the number of focal problem areas undertaken in the treatment. Medications can be used in psychoanalytic psychotherapy and provide another means of titrating the level of regression (the experience of feelings, thoughts, and actions from childhood being readily accessed) a patient may experience.

The same patients who are treated in psychoanalysis can be treated in psychoanalytic psychotherapy (see Table 17–2). The psychosocial problems and internal conflicts of patients who cannot be treated in psychoanalysis, such as those with major depression, schizophrenia, and borderline personality disorder, can be ad-

Table 17–2 **Psychoanalytically Oriented Psychotherapy**

Goal	Understanding conflict area and particular defense mechanisms used
	More "here and now" than psychoanalysis
Selection	Similar to psychoanalysis
	Also includes personality disorders with psychotic potential (Borderline, Narcissistic)
	Some major depressions and schizophrenia may be helped when combined with medication during periods of remission for the treatment of psychosocial features
Techniques	Face to face—sitting up
	Free association
	Interpretation and clarification
	Some supportive techniques
	Medication as adjunct
Duration	Months to years

dressed in a long-term psychoanalytic psychotherapy. In long-term psychoanalytic psychotherapy, the regressive tendencies of such patients can be titrated with greater support, medication and reality feedback through the face-to-face encounter with the therapist. Little empirical data are available on the efficacy of psychoanalytically oriented psychotherapy, although it is highly valued by many clinicians and patients. Recent studies tend to support the importance of working with the transference to create behavioral change (Luborsky and Crits-Cristoph, 1990). Interpersonal psychotherapy (IPT) (Klerman et al, 1984) has many psychodynamic principles and has been shown effective in studies using combined psychotherapy and medication interventions.

Brief Psychodynamic Psychotherapy

Following World War II there was a rapid growth in the demand for psychotherapy that considerably increased the pressure upon psychiatrists to develop briefer forms of psychotherapy. In addition, the community mental health movement and, more recently, the increasing cost of mental health care have stimulated efforts to find briefer forms of psychotherapy. At present, brief psychotherapy is a necessary part of the psychiatrist's armamentarium rather than the "second-best" alternative, as it was viewed in the 1950s.

The goals of brief psychotherapy are described by most authors as facilitation of health-seeking behaviors and the mitigation of obstacles to normal growth. From this perspective, brief psychotherapy focuses on the patient's continuous development throughout adult life in the context of conflicts relating to environment, interpersonal relationships, biological health, and developmental stages. This picture of brief psychotherapy supports modest goals and the avoidance of "perfectionism" by the therapist.

While many of the selection criteria emphasized in the literature of brief psychotherapy are common to all kinds of psychodynamic psychotherapy, certain unique selection criteria are required because of the brief duration of treatment (see Table 17–3). Patients in brief psychodynamic psychotherapy must be able to engage quickly with the therapist, and terminate therapy in a short period of time. The necessity of greater independent action by the patient mandates high levels of emotional strength, motivation, and responsiveness to interpretation. The importance of rapidly establishing the therapeutic alliance underlies a substantial number of the selection and exclusion criteria.

Some exclusion criteria for brief psychotherapy were developed by Malan (1975). He excludes patients who have had serious suicidal attempts, drug addiction, long-term hospitalization, more than one course of electroconvulsive therapy (ECT), chronic alcoholism, severe chronic obsessional symptoms, severe chronic phobic symptoms, or gross destructive or self-destructive behavior. Patients who are unavailable for therapeutic contact or those who need prolonged work to generate motivation, penetrate rigid defenses, deal with complex or deep-seated issues, or resolve intense transference reactions are also not likely to benefit from brief psychotherapy and may have negative side effects.

The importance of focusing on a circumscribed area of current conflict in brief psychotherapy is mentioned by most authors (Davanloo, 1980; Malan, 1975; Mann, 1973; Sifneos, 1972). They also emphasize the importance of the evaluation sessions to determine the focus of treatment. The formulation of the focus to the patient may be, for example, in terms of the patient's conscious fears and pain, but it is important for the therapist to construct the psychodynamic focus at a deeper level in order to understand the work being done. Maintaining the focus is the primary task of the therapist. This enables the therapist to deal with complicated personality structures in a brief period of time. Resistance is limited through "benign neglect" of potentially troublesome but nonfocal areas of personality. The elaboration of techniques of establishing and maintaining the focus of treatment is critical to all brief individual psychodynamic psychotherapies.

Table 17–3   **Brief Psychodynamic Psychotherapy**

Goal	Clarify and resolve focal area of conflict that interferes with current functioning
Selection Criteria	High ego strength
	High motivation
	Can Identify focal issue
	Can form strong interpersonal relationships, including with therapist, in a brief time
	Good response to trial interpretations
Techniques	Face to face
	Interpretation of defenses and transference
	Setting of time limit at start of therapy
	Focus on patient reactions to limited duration of treatment
Duration	12–40 sessions; usually 20 sessions or less

Transference interpretations (that is, making comments that link the patient's reactions to the therapist to feelings for significant individuals from the patient's past) are generally accepted as important in brief psychotherapy. However, the manner and rapidity in which transference is dealt with varies considerably.

There is remarkable agreement on the duration of brief psychotherapy. Although the duration ranges from 5 to 40 sessions, authors generally favor 10 to 20 sessions. The duration of treatment is critically related to maintaining the focus within the brief psychotherapy. When treatment extends beyond 20 sessions, therapists frequently find themselves enmeshed in a broad character analysis without a focal conflict. Change after 20 sessions may be quite slow. Clinical experience generally supports the idea that brief individual psychodynamic psychotherapy should be between 10 and 20 sessions unless the therapist is willing to proceed to long-term treatment of greater than 40 or 50 sessions.

COGNITIVE PSYCHOTHERAPY

Cognitive psychotherapy is a method of brief psychotherapy developed over the last two decades by Aaron T. Beck and his colleagues at the University of Pennsylvania primarily for the treatment of mild and moderate depressions and for patients with low self-esteem (Beck, 1976; Rush and Beck, 1988). It is similar to behavior therapy in that it aims at the direct removal of symptoms rather than the resolution of underlying conflicts, as in the psychodynamic psychotherapies. However, unlike traditional behavioral approaches, the subjective experience of the patient is a major focus of the work. Cognitive therapists view the patient's conscious thoughts as central to producing and perpetuating symptoms such as depression, anxiety, phobias, and somatization. Both the content of thoughts and thought processes are seen as disordered in people with such symptoms. Therapy is directed toward identifying and altering these cognitive distortions.

The cognitive therapist sees the interpretations that depressed persons make about life as different from those of nondepressed individuals. Depressed people tend to make negative interpretations of the world, themselves, and the future (the negative cognitive triad). Depressed individuals interpret events as reflecting defeat, deprivation, or disparagement and see their lives as filled with obstacles and burdens. They view themselves as unworthy, deficient, undesirable, or worthless and see the future as bringing a continuation of the miseries of the present. These evaluations are the result of the negative biases inherent in depressive thinking and applied regardless of the objective nature of the individual's circumstances. Other psychiatric conditions have their own characteristic cognitive patterns that determine the nature of the symptoms. The "thinking" distortions in depression include arbitrary inferences about an event, selective use of details to reach a conclusion, overgeneralization, overestimating negative and underestimating positive aspects of a situation, and the tendency to label events according to one's emotional response rather than the facts.

Such cognitions (verbal thoughts) often feel involuntary and automatic. This kind of thinking is so automatic in response to many situations—and the resultant cognitions so fleeting—that people may often be virtually unaware of them. Such automatic thoughts differ from unconscious thoughts in that they can easily be made fully conscious if attention is directed to them. A large portion of the work of cognitive psychotherapy is to train patients to observe and record their automatic thoughts.

Cognitive theory postulates a chronic state of depression-proneness that may precede the actual illness and remain after the symptoms have abated. Depression-prone individuals have relatively permanent depressive cognitive structures ("cognitive schemas") that determine how new stimuli are perceived and conceptualized. Typical schemas of depression include "I am stupid," or "I cannot exist without the love of a strong person." Unlike automatic thoughts, patients are not typically aware and cannot easily become aware of such underlying general assumptions. These must be deduced from many specific examples of distorted thinking. Schemas such as "I am stupid" may lie dormant much of the time only to be reactivated by a specific event, such as difficulty in accomplishing a task. These enduring self-concepts and attitudes are assumed to have been learned in childhood on the basis of the child's experiences and the reactions of important family members. Once formed, such attitudes can be self-perpetuating.

Just as depressive thoughts can be triggered by events, episodes of depressive illness may, from the cognitive perspective, be triggered by sufficient stress. Such stresses may be specific to the individual and her or his particular sensitivities developed in childhood. Alternatively, sufficient degrees of nonspecific stress may precipitate depression in vulnerable individuals. Experiences of loss, a setback in a major goal, a rejection, or an insolvable dilemma are especially common precipitants of depression. The onset of medical illness, with its attendant limitations and associated meanings, is also seen as likely to trigger depression in many people.

Researchers have accumulated considerable evidence that depressed individuals do indeed manifest negative biases in their views of themselves, their experiences, and the future. In addition, they have attitudes (schemas) that distinguish them from nondepressed subjects as well as distortions in logic and information processing. It is less clear whether all depressed people show the thinking distortions that Beck has described. Much of the cognitive depression research has been criticized because the studies have been on nonpatient populations, such as student volunteers, with relatively mild degrees of depression. These individuals may be very different from actual psychiatric patients. Whether cognitive distortions are a predisposing factor to depression is also unclear. Most researchers have found that most distorted thinking disappears when depression is successfully treated, even with antidepressant medication, suggesting that these distortions are a symptom of depression rather than an enduring trait of depression-prone people. Clearly, further research is needed to test the causality of cognitive factors in depression.

Technique of Cognitive Psychotherapy

Cognitive psychotherapy is a directive, time-limited, multidimensional psychological treatment. The patient and therapist together discover the irrational beliefs and illogical thinking patterns associated with the patient's depressive affects (see Table 17–4). They then devise methods by which patients themselves can test the validity of their thinking. The therapist helps patients to become aware of their

Table 17–4 **Cognitive Psychotherapy**

Goal	Identify and alter cognitive distortions
Selection	Unipolar, nonpsychotic depressed outpatients
	Contraindications include delusions, hallucinations, severe depression, severe cognitive impairment, ongoing substance abuse, enmeshed family system
Technique	Behavioral assignments
	Reading material
	Taught to recognize negatively biased automatic thoughts
	Identify patients' schemas, beliefs, attitudes
Duration	Time limited: 15–25 sessions

irrational beliefs and distorted thinking ("automatic thoughts") and to see for themselves whether their ideas are objectively true or logical.

Cognitive psychotherapy was developed for unipolar, nonpsychotic, depressed outpatients. The presence of bipolar illness, delusions or hallucinations, or extremely severe depression is a contraindication for cognitive psychotherapy as the sole or primary treatment modality. Other contraindications include the presence of underlying medical illness or medications that may be causing the depression, the presence of an organic mental disorder, or an ongoing problem of substance abuse. In addition, cognitive psychotherapy may not be indicated as the sole form of treatment for major or "endogenous" depression (which may be accompanied by endocrine, sleep, or other biological abnormalities in which antidepressant medication or ECT is needed) or for patients enmeshed in family systems that maintain a fixed view of themselves as helpless and dependent. Cognitive psychotherapy may be useful in patients who refuse to take, fail to respond to, or are unable to tolerate medication, as well as those who prefer a psychological approach in the hope of greater long-term benefits.

Cognitive psychotherapy is generally conducted over a period of 15 to 25 weeks in once-weekly meetings. With more severely depressed patients, two or three meetings per week are recommended for the first several weeks. While cognitive psychotherapy was developed and is usually administered as an individual treatment, its principles have also been successfully applied to group settings.

A course of cognitive psychotherapy proceeds in a succession of regular stages. The first stage is devoted to introducing the patient to the procedures and rationale of the therapy, setting goals for the treatment, and establishing a therapeutic alliance. The therapist may assign reading material on the cognitive theory of depression. In the next stage, the therapist begins to demonstrate to the patient that cognitions and emotions are connected. Patients are taught to become more aware of their negatively biased automatic thoughts and to recognize, both during and outside of the psychotherapy hours, that negative affects are generally preceded by such thoughts. Behavioral assignments may be used.

In the next phase, which normally comprises the majority of the work, the emphasis shifts to a detailed exploration of the patient's cognitions and their role in perpetuating depressive feelings. In the final stage of psychotherapy, patients will have had a great deal of experience in recognizing their habitual thought patterns, testing their validity, and modifying them when appropriate, with the result of substantial symptomatic relief. Psychotherapy then focuses on the attitudes and assumptions that underlie the patient's negatively biased thinking. For example, the patient might assume that, "If I'm nice, bad things won't happen to me." A logically equivalent assumption would then be, "If bad things happen to me, it is my fault because I am not nice." Target symptoms that might be the focus of a session include intense sadness, pervasive self-criticism, passivity and avoidance, sleep disturbance, or other affective, motivational, or cognitive manifestations of depression. The therapist repeatedly formulates the patient's beliefs and attitudes as testable hypotheses and helps the patient to devise and implement ways of verifying them. The therapist maintains an inquiring attitude toward the patient's reactions to the therapist and the therapeutic procedures. Such reactions are explored for evidence of misunderstanding and distortion, which are then dealt with in the same way as the patient's other cognitions.

A great variety of different techniques are used by cognitive therapists to break the cycle of negative evaluations and dysfunctional behaviors. Behavioral methods are often useful in the beginning of psychotherapy, particularly when the patient is severely depressed. Activity scheduling, mastery and pleasure exercises, graded task assignments, cognitive rehearsal, and role-playing may all be used.

More cognitively oriented methods are applied in the middle and late stages of psychotherapy as psychotherapy progresses. The therapist and patient explore the patient's inner life in a spirit of adventure. Patients become more observant of their peculiar construction of reality and usually focus more on actual events and their meanings. The fundamental cognitive technique is teaching patients to observe, record, and validate their cognitions.

Efficacy of Cognitive Psychotherapy

In contrast to most other psychotherapies, there is a growing literature on the efficacy of cognitive psychotherapy. Although the number is still relatively small, all studies examining the outcome of cognitive psychotherapy have found it to be an effective treatment at least in ambulatory outpatients with mild to moderate degrees of depression. Cognitive psychotherapy has been shown to be more effective than no psychotherapy in treating both depressed volunteers and psychiatric patients with diagnoses of depression.

It should be emphasized that the choice of treatment for a depressed patient should often involve a combination of both psychotherapy and antidepressant medication. To withhold antidepressants from patients who have a clear biological component to their depression, based on their signs and symptoms and family history, because of a "bias" toward one sort of psychotherapy or another is unjustifiable on clinical grounds. Hence, integrated psychotherapeutic *and* pharmacologic treatment is often indicated and should be considered in every patient.

SUPPORTIVE PSYCHOTHERAPY

Supportive psychotherapy aims to help patients maintain or reestablish the best level of functioning given the limitations of their illness, personality, native ability, and life circumstances (see Table 17–5). In general, this goal distinguishes supportive

Table 17–5 **Supportive Psychotherapy**

Goal	Maintain or reestablish best level of functioning
Selection	Very healthy individuals exposed to stressful life circumstances (e.g., Adjustment Disorder)
	Individual with serious illness, ego deficits, e.g., Schizophrenia, Major Depression (psychotic)
	Individuals with medical illness
Techniques	Available, predictable therapist
	No/limited interpretation of transference
	Support intellectualization
	Therapist acts as a guide/mentor
	Medication frequently used
	Supportive techniques: suggestion, reinforcement, advice, teaching, reality testing, cognitive restructuring, reassurance
	Active stance
	Discuss alternative behaviors, social/interpersonal skills
Duration	Brief (days–weeks) to very long term (years)

psychotherapy from the change-oriented psychotherapies that aim to reverse primary disease processes and symptoms or restructure personality.

The line between supportive and change-oriented psychotherapy, however, is frequently not clear. The situation is somewhat analogous to the medical treatment of viral versus bacterial infections. Treatment of the former is basically supportive in that it aims to maintain normal bodily functions (e.g., fever reduction, control of cerebral edema, dietary compensation for liver failure) in the face of infection, while in the latter, the aim is to eliminate the infection. However, in addition to the supportive aspects of treating bacterial infections, antibiotic treatment itself is supportive in the sense that it works as an adjunct to the body's natural immune system, without which it is relatively ineffective. However, there are supportive elements in all effective forms of psychotherapy, and the terms "supportive" and "change-oriented" merely describe the balance of efforts in a particular case.

Patients who are generally very healthy and well adapted but who have become impaired in response to stressful life circumstances, as well as those who have serious illnesses that cannot be cured, can receive supportive psychotherapy. Supportive psychotherapy may be brief or long-term. The "healthy" individual, when faced with overwhelming stress or crises (particularly in the face of traumas or disasters), may seek help and be a candidate for supportive psychotherapy. The relatively healthy candidate for supportive psychotherapy is a well-adapted individual with good social supports and interpersonal relations, flexible defenses, and good reality testing who is in acute crisis. This individual continues to show evidence of well-planned behaviors and a healthy perspective on the crisis, making use of social supports, not withdrawing, and anticipating resolution of the crisis. Although the patient is functioning below his or her usual level, this patient remains hopeful about the future and makes use of resources available for problem solving, respite, and growth. This patient uses supportive psychotherapy to more rapidly reconstitute, to avoid errors in judgment by "talking out loud," to relieve minor symptomatology, and to grow as an individual by learning about the world.

The more typical candidate for supportive psychotherapy has significant deficits in ego functioning, including poor reality testing, impaired impulse control, and difficulties in interpersonal relations. Patients who have less ability to sublimate and are less introspective are frequently treated in supportive psychotherapy, where more directive techniques and environmental manipulation can be used.

Ego strength and the ability to form relationships may be more important than diagnosis in the selection of patients for supportive psychotherapy (Werman, 1984; Rockland, 1989). The ability of the patient to relate to the therapist, a past history of reasonable personal relationships, work history and educational performance, and the use of leisure time for constructive activity and relaxation bear importantly on the treatment recommendation. Almost no information is known regarding which characteristics of the patient may predict a good result from supportive psychotherapy rather than merely a poor response to the change-oriented psychotherapies. Delineation of the minimum level of personal strengths needed to benefit from supportive individual psychotherapy is an important task for future research.

Technique of Supportive Psychotherapy

Psychoanalytic theory provides the major contributions to the theory of the supportive psychotherapy. In-depth psychological understanding of patients in supportive psychotherapy is as necessary as in the change-oriented, explorative psychotherapies (Rockland, 1989; Pine, 1986; Werman, 1984). Understanding unconscious motivation, psychic conflict, the patient–therapist relationship, and the patient's use of defense mechanisms is essential to understanding the patient's strengths and vulnerabilities. This knowledge is critical to providing support as well as insight.

Therapists who are predictably available and safe (i.e., who accepts the patient and puts aside their own needs in the service of the treatment) assume some of the holding functions of the "good parent." In such a therapeutic situation, the patient is able to identify with and incorporate the well-functioning aspects of the therapist, such as the capacity for self-observation and the ability to tolerate ambivalence (Pine, 1986).

The containment of affect and anxiety is an important supportive function. Patients in need of supportive psychotherapy typically fear the destructive power of their rage and envy. They are helped to modulate their emotional reactions by the reliable presence of the therapist and the therapeutic relationship that remains unchanged in the face of emotional onslaughts.

The therapist fosters the supportive relationship by refraining from interpreting positive transference feelings and waiting until the intensity of feelings has abated before commenting about negative transference feelings. Interpretations of the negative transference are limited to those needed to assure that the treatment is not disrupted. While maintaining a friendly stance toward the patient, the therapist respects the patient's need to establish a comfortable degree of distance. The therapist must not push for a more intimate or emotion-laden relationship than the patient can tolerate. The rapport with the patient, which the supportive psychotherapist tries to establish, differs from the "therapeutic alliance" of insight-oriented therapy. The doctor–patient relationship does not require the patient to observe and report on their own feelings and behavior to the same extent as in the change-oriented, explorative psychotherapies. The therapist acts more as a guide and a mentor.

There is virtually unanimous agreement among writers on supportive psychotherapy that fostering a good working relationship with the patient is the first priority. The therapist must be available in a regular and predictable manner. Rather than approach the patient as a "blank screen," the therapist actively demonstrates concern, involvement, sympathy, and a supportive attitude. The therapist serves as an "auxiliary ego" for the patient. The auxiliary ego functions of the therapist can be seen in the therapist's use of suggestion, reinforcement, advice, teaching, reality testing, cognitive restructuring, and reassurance. In taking such an active stance, it is especially important for the therapist to guard against grandiosity and personal biases so as not to "become an omnipotent decision maker." Rather the therapist acts as "a strong, benign individual who is reasonably available when needed." To the extent that patients develops the capacity to observe themselves, the psychotherapy may proceed beyond support and take on features of the explorative and change-oriented psychotherapies.

The defenses of denial and avoidance are handled by encouraging the patient to discuss alternative behaviors, goals, and interpretations of events. Reassurance has a variety of forms in supportive psychotherapy including: supporting an adaptive level of denial (such as a patient may employ in coping with a terminal illness); the patients' experience of the therapist's empathic attitude; or the therapist's reality testing of the patients' negatively biased evaluations of themselves or their situation. Reassuring a patient is not easy. Reassurance requires a clear understanding of what the patient fears. Overt expressions of interest and concern may be reassuring to a patient who fears rejection but threatening to one who fears intrusion. Interpretations in supportive psychotherapy are limited to those that will decrease anxiety and strengthen (rather than loosen) defenses, particularly the defenses of intellectualization and rationalization.

The therapist's expressions of interest, advice giving, and facilitation of ventilation reinforce desired behaviors. Expressions of interest and solicitude are positively reinforcing. Advice can lead to behavioral change if it is specific and applies to frequent behaviors of the patient. Desired behaviors are rewarded by the therapist's approval and by social reinforcement. Ventilation of emotions is useful only if the therapist can help the patient safely contain and limit them, thus extinguishing the anxiety response to emotional expression. Cognitive and behavioral psychotherapeutic interventions that strengthen the adaptive and defensive functions of the ego (e.g., realistic and logical thinking, social skills, containment of affects such as anxiety) contribute to the supportive aspects of the psychotherapy.

Efficacy of Supportive Psychotherapy

Most data on the effectiveness of supportive psychotherapy come from studies in which supportive psychotherapy has been used as a control in testing the efficacy of other treatments. In such studies, the procedures used in supportive psychotherapy tend to be poorly specified, and no attempts are made to correlate individual supportive techniques with outcome. There are no studies in which supportive psychotherapy is compared with no treatment or minimal treatment. However, despite its limitations, the research literature offers some evidence that supportive psychotherapy is an effective treatment, particularly when combined with medication. This appears to be true in the treatment of depression, anxiety disorders, and schizophrenia.

There is a body of research indicating that supportive psychotherapy is an effective component of the treatment of patients with a variety of medical illnesses, including those with ulcerative colitis or myocardial infarction and cancer patients undergoing radiation treatment. In general, patients in supportive psychotherapy improve emotionally and have fewer days in the hospital, fewer complications, and more rapid recovery.

The evidence to date, though preliminary, suggests that supportive psychotherapy can be effective in both psychiatric and medical illnesses and is frequently more cost effective than more intensive psychotherapies for some disorders. More research is needed on the indications, contraindications, and techniques of supportive psychotherapy.

BEHAVIORAL THERAPY

Behavioral therapy (behavior modification) is based on the concept that all symptoms of a psychological nature are learned maladaptive patterns of behavior in response to environmental or internal stimuli. It does not concern itself with the intrapsychic conflicts that are the focus of the psychodynamically oriented psychotherapies. Rather, it uses the concepts of learning theory to eliminate the involuntary, disruptive behavior patterns that constitute the essential features of psychopathology and substitutes these with highly adaptive and situation-appropriate patterns (Lazarus, 1971). Behavioral therapy has been useful in a wide range of disorders when specific behavioral symptoms can be targeted for change and this change is central to recovery. Eating disorders, chronic pain syndromes and illness behavior, phobias, sexual dysfunction, and conduct disorders of childhood are frequently treated with behavioral therapy techniques.

Techniques of Behavioral Therapy

A variety of techniques exist that permit the modification of undesirable and unwanted behaviors when applied by therapists skilled in their use (see Table 17–6). These approaches require careful history taking and behavioral analysis in order to identify the behaviors to be targeted for extinction or modification. Often, adjunctive techniques, such as the use of hypnosis and drugs, are used to facilitate behavior modification but are not requisite for therapeutic success. Present-day behavioral therapists are usually alert to interpersonal and emotional aspects of psychiatric symptoms and the doctor–patient relationship. Psychodynamic, cognitive, and interpersonal techniques are frequently integrated into the therapy but are not seen as

Table 17–6 **Behavioral Therapy (Behavioral Modification)**

Goal	Eliminate involuntary disruptive behavior patterns and substitute appropriate behaviors
Selection	Habit modification
	Targeted symptoms
	Phobias
	Some psychophysiologic responses: headache, migraine, hypertension, Raynaud's phenomena
	Sexual dysfunction
Techniques	Systemic desensitization
	Implosion therapy and flooding
	Aversive therapy
	Biofeedback
Duration	Usually time limited

central to the therapeutic effect. Four of the more common behavioral techniques follow.

Systematic Desensitization

Systematic desensitization refers to a technique whereby individuals suffering primarily from phobic responses are gradually exposed to anxiety-provoking situations or objects in small increments. The therapist first identifies a hierarchy of behaviors directed to approaching the phobic object or situation. Relaxation techniques are used to decrease anxiety at each stage of the hierarchy. The patient moves up to the next level of intensity when the stimulus no longer provokes intense anxiety. This particularly effective technique is useful in an office setting as well, because experience has demonstrated that the patient can confront the anxiety-provoking stimulus in his imagination with very much the same effects. Again, a hierarchy of increasingly anxious imaginary scenes is constructed. The patient visualizes each scene and reexperiences the anxiety associated with it and then uses relaxation techniques to gradually become comfortable with the fantasy. Patients move up the hierarchy of images until they are able to fully visualize the phobic object/situation without undue anxiety. Usually, this in vitro technique will be accompanied by in vivo practice exposures. Hypnotic procedures and the use of anxiolytic drugs are useful adjuncts in certain types of patients. There is some controversy regarding the mechanisms underlying the effect of systematic desensitization. Various explanations have been suggested regarding the underlying mechanisms. It is possible, for example, that the graduated exposure to the anxiety-provoking situation represents nothing more than a sequential or progressive "flooding" technique (see next section). It is also possible that by exposing the individual to only small, and therefore more tolerable, amounts of anxiety, the individual is able to develop more appropriate and successful coping mechanisms. Other authors have suggested that the key to systematic desensitization lies in the suppression of anxiety, which is achieved by evoking a competitive physiological response such as deep muscle relaxation.

Implosion Therapy and Flooding

These two techniques vary only in the presentation of the anxiety-eliciting stimulus. Animal behaviorists discovered early on that avoidant behavior, which by its very nature can be expected to be highly resistant to extinction, could be extinguished rather rapidly by submitting the subject to a prolonged conditioned stimulus while restraining it and making the expression of the avoidant behavior impossible. In the therapeutic situation, the patient is directly exposed to the stressful stimulus until the anxiety subsides. This is in contrast to the graded exposure of systematic desensitization. In theory, each session should result in ever-decreasing intervals between exposure and cessation of anxiety. In implosion therapy the patient uses mental images as substitutes for the actual feared object or situation, whereas in the flooding approach the therapist conducts the procedure in vivo. Results appear to indicate that both approaches are equally effective. Some have questioned the ethics of submitting patients to such painful experiences, especially when other alternatives are available. A risk associated with this technique is the danger that the patient may refuse to submit to such an uncomfortable experience and may terminate the exposure prior to the abatement of the anxiety. This will result in a successful "escape" and will therefore reinforce the phobic response.

Aversive Therapy

This treatment modality has its roots in classical and operant conditioning. Controversial by its very nature, it has nevertheless found acceptance as a potentially useful avenue of therapy for a narrow range of disorders and unwanted habits. Perhaps the most common form of aversive therapy is the use of disulfiram (Antabuse) in alcoholics. This treatment approach is based on the fear of an extremely unpleasant, and indeed sometimes fatal, physiologic response (the unconditioned stimulus) when someone who has been taking Antabuse then imbibes alcohol (which becomes the conditioned stimulus). In theory, the alcoholic patient on Antabuse therapy will avoid alcohol to avoid the alcohol–Antabuse reaction. The use of mild aversive stimuli has also been found to be useful in smoking-cessation programs. Because of safety considerations, and to ensure continued patient participation, aversive stimuli used under these conditions are often mild and may not constitute much more than having to hold the smoke in the oral cavity for a prolonged period of time. Various aversive techniques have also been used in the treatment of sexual offenders and have included the use of such stimuli as mild electric shocks and unpleasant odors. Ethical considerations, understandable patient reluctance to participate in treatment, and pejorative associations by the general public with torture and other forms of maltreatment have resulted in rather limited applications for these techniques. In addition, its effectiveness has been more variable than that of other behavioral techniques.

Biofeedback

Biofeedback is not a type of behavioral therapy per se but rather a tool or technique that can be integrated with other operant procedures for the management of a number of psychophysiological disorders. Some of the conditions in which there is documented short-term efficacy for biofeedback are: hypertension, migraine headaches, tension headaches, some cardiac arrhythmias, and Raynaud's phenomenon. This approach presumes that many pathological psychophysiologic responses could be subject to modification if the individual could become aware of their existence and of positive changes incurred as a result of learned responses (Gaarder and Montgomery, 1977). For the conditioned response to be reinforced and learning to take place, the organism must be aware that a response has taken place. The biofeedback techniques consist of the use of sophisticated instrumentation to detect changes in skin temperature, muscle tension, or heart rate. Biofeedback first burst on the scene amid great publicity and exaggerated claims regarding its efficacy. This was followed by an expected period of disenchantment and skepticism. Nevertheless, for selected patients, especially those suffering from psychophysiologic disorders characterized by measurable vascular and neuromuscular changes, such as chronic tension headaches, this approach may be of some use either by itself or in conjunction with other therapies, including medication and formal psychotherapy. Biofeedback is often administered in clinics by technicians. There is a paucity of evidence, however, that for tension-related syndromes such as chronic headache it is any more effective than simple relaxation exercises.

Effectiveness of Behavioral Therapies

The behavioral approaches have proved to be of considerable value in the treatment of a wide spectrum of disorders, particularly phobias and muscle tension, as well as migraine headaches. They also may be considered as valuable adjunct techniques in the overall management of psychiatric and other medical conditions such as headaches and eating disorders. Often, much time and effort are devoted to discussing the relative merits of the behavioral techniques versus the psychodynamic therapies. Elements from each approach play a significant factor in the other. Even in the most dynamically oriented therapy situation, the achievement of new insights, improvements in the quality of life, and the lessening of anxiety facilitate the progress toward wellness. Similarly, there has been little research into the nature of the relationship between the patient and her or his behavioral therapist. The degree to which conflicts between the behavioral therapist and the patient may re-create past relationships and how this is handled and influences treatment progress are not well known.

GROUP THERAPIES

In its most basic form, group therapy can be described as the attainment of therapeutic goals through the skilled manipulation of group processes or mechanisms. The changes effected can be limited and situation-specific or they can be far-reaching and foster personality development and growth. Family therapy and couples therapy are specific forms of group therapy directed to the family and the couple—usually the marital couple—in special group/interpersonal settings. In contrast to the individual therapies, the group therapies have direct access to the interpersonal processes of the patient with individuals of varying age and sex. Intrapsychic, interpersonal, communication, and system theories, as well as a knowledge of family and couple development and roles, are used to elucidate various aspects of behavior and increase the patient's awareness. In addition, new behaviors can be tried in the group with the therapist present (Yalom, 1986). The different types of group therapy emphasize different theoretical perspectives and may have different group compositions (see Table 17–7). All groups provide members with support, a feeling of belonging, and a safe, secure environment where change can be effected and tried out first. The therapist uses the vast array of processes at work in a group to facilitate interaction among its members and to guide the work of the group toward the desired goal. Skill, training, and a keen understanding of group dynamics are required. Particular awareness of group fantasies, projections, scapegoating, and denial are a part of most group therapy work. Frequently, cotherapists run the group. This often increases the ability to attend to the many processes occurring in the group and aids in the avoidance of countertransference pitfalls.

Group Psychotherapy

Group psychotherapists use a variety of techniques derived from knowledge of the dynamics and behavior of social groups to foster desired change in the individual members (Yalom, 1986). The theoretical framework supporting the various therapeutic modalities, however, varies with the goals and purposes of the group, the type of group, and the composition of the group. A review of the literature reveals widely diverging definitions and classifications. Different approaches achieve a measure of fame and popularity, such as the so-called encounter groups, then recede from the scene. In general, however, groups can be divided into three separate and distinct categories: (1) directive, (2) psychodynamic/interpersonal, and (3) analytic. This classification is based largely on the degree to which the group fosters the exploration and evocation of repressed, unconscious material. As a result, each group type will vary widely in approach, techniques, composition, conceptual model, and defined goals. Group psychotherapy occurs both in inpatient and outpatient settings.

Table 17–7 **Group Therapies**

Goal	Alleviation of symptoms
	Change interpersonal relations
	Alter specific family/couple dynamics
Selection	Varies greatly based on type of group
	Homogeneous groups target specific disorders
	Adolescents and personality disorders may especially benefit
	Families and couples where the system needs change
	Contraindications: substantial suicide risk, sadomasochistic acting out in family/couple
Types	Directive/Supportive Group Psychotherapy
	Psychodynamic/Interpersonal Group Psychotherapy
	Psychoanalytic Group Psychotherapy
	Family Therapy
	Couples Therapy
Duration	Weeks to years; time limited and open-ended

Directive/Supportive Group Psychotherapy

These groups usually have very specific, well-defined, and relatively limited goals. Good examples are the Alcoholics Anonymous (AA) and Overeaters Anonymous groups. The groups function within a very narrow set of guidelines defined by a specific philosophy, set of values, or religious orientation. In the case of AA, for example, the members help each other achieve sobriety and cope with everyday problems of living by adhering to "The Twelve Steps" and entrusting their fate to a "Higher Power." The group leader serves as a role model, stressing commonsense, reality-oriented solutions to problems while using the group to apply peer pressure, enhance self-esteem, foster a feeling of togetherness and belonging, and provide a supportive and nurturing environment. Members usually share at least one major attribute in common (for example, alcoholism), but in many other respects the group is very heterogeneous in composition. There may be a wide divergence in social background, education, personality types, and even the absence or presence of major psychiatric disorders. Behavioral techniques are often applied in similar group situations to treat individuals with phobias while using group support and encouragement to enhance efficacy.

Psychodynamic/Interpersonal Group Psychotherapy

These groups address the individual members' psychopathology, foster the development of insight, promote the development of better interpersonal and social skills, and, in general, promote improved coping skills for the here and now. Defenses are identified and challenged in an atmosphere of support and acceptance. Positive change is encouraged and reinforced. These groups may adhere to any of a wide variety of theoretical models (such as gestalt therapy, psychodrama, and so forth) or may be eclectic in their approach and incorporate aspects of these into the system to fit the needs and characteristics of the group. They tend, however, to focus on the individual's subjective experience and interpersonal behaviors.

Psychoanalytic Group Psychotherapy

This type of group essentially uses the psychoanalytic approach as applied in individual therapy. The therapist remains neutral and nondirective, thus promoting a transference neurosis that can be analyzed. Defenses are identified and resistances interpreted. The group focuses on past experiences and repressed unconscious material as the underlying factors in psychopathology. The therapist attempts to identify individual transferences of the members as well as shared group fantasies or assumptions.

In general, most patients who benefit from individual psychotherapy benefit from group psychotherapy. Empirical data are lacking except for directive/supportive group psychotherapy approaches (e.g., AA, Overeaters Anonymous, type A personality). The differences and similarities in behavior change following group and individual psychotherapy are largely unknown. Although there is no hard evidence for the greater or lesser efficacy of either technique applied to appropriate patients, not all patients will do well in all groups, and some patients should not be considered for inclusion in a treatment group under any circumstances. Specifically, severely depressed and suicidal individuals should not be assigned to outpatient groups. Their emotional state will prevent them from becoming integrated into the group, and the lack of an initial strong therapeutic relationship with a specific therapist may increase the risk of suicide. Such patients should be considered for individual and other more intensely supportive modalities, and inpatient hospitalization when indicated. Manic patients tend to be disruptive to group process, and their impulsivity and lack of control prevent them from obtaining any real benefit from group work. Some types of personality disorders, such as explosive, narcissistic, borderline, and antisocial personalities, may also present insurmountable difficulties for treatment with this modality. Schizophrenics may do well in highly directive groups with emphasis on reality testing and improving interpersonal coping skills. Group therapy can be used as a useful adjunct to either individual psychotherapy or psychotropic medications. Inpatient group psychotherapy is a very common treatment modality and differs from outpatient treatment because of the heterogeneity of the group and its frequent change in membership. Group psychotherapy may be particularly helpful with adolescents who are highly sensitive to peer group support and influence. Groups also provide a powerful arena in which individuals with personality disorders can become increasingly aware of their interpersonal problems.

Family Therapy

In family therapy, psychological symptoms are considered to be the pathological expression of disturbances in the social system of the family. For the purposes of this discussion, the latter can include any members, ranging from the basic couple to children, grandparents, distant relatives and, in some cases, even close friends of the family. The essential feature is the relationship among the various members and how their behavior can affect the group as a whole as well as the individual family members. The theoretical models may run the whole gamut of therapeutic approaches, ranging from the psychoanalytic to the behavioral (Beels, 1988).

Most family therapists agree that family groups are extremely complex and dynamic systems with a definite hierarchical structure that is a result of cultural and societal proscribed roles, repetitive behavior patterns, and ingrained ways in which the family members have interrelated. Family structure can be seen as a self-regulating system with multiple control mechanisms designed to ensure some degree of a homeostatic equilibrium. The family system seeks stability and inherently resists change. When the system is subjected to internal or external stresses, the family may respond by "designating" one of its members as the "patient," and his or her "illness" may act as a safety valve to maintain system integrity. This same resistance to change will of course oppose any therapeutic efforts and may take the form of refusal to explore family issues by the other members of the family, missed appointments, no apparent therapeutic progress, and so forth. Some change does occur in any family as the passage of time thrusts on the system irresistible forces such as maturation of children, illness, death, old age, and, of course, personal growth and maturity. The family system may thus be conceived as three-dimensional: highly structured, homeostatic, but slowly evolving and changing its character over long periods of time.

The clinical indications for family therapy are very broad. Psychopathology in any member of a family will undoubtedly influence family dynamics, and vice versa.

The treatment of children and adolescents frequently requires family therapy to deal with the environment that may be causing or sustaining the symptoms. Recent research indicates the particular value of family therapy in the treatment of schizophrenic patients in reducing rehospitalization rates. Practical considerations such as geographical distance, economic situation, or refusal to participate can rule out family participation. When family members are being extremely destructive to the family unit or important familial relationships, family therapy should not be instituted or should be suspended for a brief time. The treatment of childhood disorders, eating disorders, alcoholism, and substance abuse generally requires a family therapy intervention.

Each clinician brings to the field their own conceptual framework, clinical experience, philosophical orientation, and training background. The orthodox psychoanalyst may conceive of family therapy as the individual treatment of the symptomatic member, while at the other end of the spectrum, the social worker specializing in this form of treatment may include any or all members of the family in the sessions and may use a highly directive approach including didactic presentations and environmental manipulation. The focus of most family therapy is on current issues (the here and now) and achievement of discrete changes toward an identifiable goal. Developmental conflicts, communication patterns, boundary management, flexibility, familial conflict resolution techniques, and roles accepted and proscribed by the system for each member are areas of therapeutic attention. Exploration of individual unconscious material is usually avoided. The use of family (or couples) therapy, when an individual psychotherapy is stalled, can help resolve environmental and family system variables that are inhibiting further individual progress. In such cases, a course of family (or couples) therapy can frequently reestablish the momentum of an individual treatment. Family therapy can be an important adjunct to inpatient treatment to facilitate discharge and psychosocial readjustment.

No single technique or procedure dominates family therapy. Therapists may see one or two members of the family or they may see the entire group. The family may be seen together by a single therapist, individually by different therapists, together by more than one therapist, or more than one family may be seen in special forms of multifamily group therapy. Similarly, the therapeutic techniques can range from inducing change by crisis to focusing on small aspects of how the family functions in order to create positive changes that the system can assimilate and incorporate over varying periods of time.

Couples Therapy

Couples therapy is the treatment of dysfunctional couples. In modern society, this includes both married and unmarried "dyads" as well as homosexual couples. It is very similar to, and, in fact, may be described as a form of, family therapy. The same theoretical concepts and treatment approaches described above apply. If the couple has an extreme sadomasochistic relationship, therapy may be blocked. During times when one partner is being overly destructive to the relationship or the other partner, the therapist may need to directly intervene. If this cannot be limited in the treatment, a brief individual therapy with each partner separately may sufficiently resolve the tension to allow the couples therapy to continue. The goal of treatment may be to resolve conflict and reconstruct the dyadic relationship or to facilitate disengagement in the least painful way possible.

SEXUAL DYSFUNCTION THERAPY

The term "sexual dysfunction therapy" encompasses the entire spectrum of accepted psychotherapies from the purely behavioral techniques to the psychodynamically oriented approaches. Treatment may be restricted to a single form of therapy or may consist of a combination of approaches. The focus, however, is the resolution of a specific sexual dysfunction, such as premature ejaculation, impotence, orgasmic dysfunction, or vaginismus (Masters and Johnson, 1970). Most sex therapists emphasize focusing on symptom relief with the use of behavior modification techniques followed by attempts at resolution of underlying conflicts (which may represent the core of the disorder) by more traditional insight-oriented dynamic methods (see Table 17–8). In general, the brief focused therapies, whether used singly or in combination with other forms, seem to have a greater success rate with specific symptom relief than do the longer-term treatments.

The evaluation of sexual dysfunction should include a complete investigation of possible medical causes (see Chapter 14). A considerable number of physical illnesses, injuries, and congenital malformations can result in symptoms suggestive of a psychosexual disorder and, if not addressed, will render all other therapies useless. Intraabdominal adhesions and masses, for example, can result in pain during intercourse. Endocrine disturbances may affect sexual drive, and spinal injuries can inhibit penile erections. Similarly, a number of medications can result in dysfunctional symptoms causing great distress to the patient. Thioridazine, a commonly used neuroleptic, is often associated with reversible retrograde ejaculation in the otherwise normal male. In this situation, simple counseling and reassurance may suffice to calm the patient. Thus, the role of careful history taking, a complete physical examination, and indicated laboratory testing cannot be overemphasized.

Table 17–8 **Sexual Dysfunction Therapies**

Goal	Resolution of specific sexual dysfunctions
Selection	Couples
	Sexual dysfunction: impotence, premature ejaculation, vaginismus, orgasmic dysfunction
	Rule out medical causes
Types	Behavior modification techniques, including systematic desensitization, homework, education
	Psychodynamic approaches
	Hypnotherapy
	Group therapy
	Couples therapy as needed to deal with the system dynamics
Duration	Weeks to months

The human sexual response cycle may be divided into four distinct phases: (1) appetitive (baseline), (2) excitement, (3) orgasmic, and (4) resolution. For the purposes of our discussion, the last phase bears little relation to disturbances in sexual functioning. The psychosexual disorders may be grouped according to where the dysfunction occurs in the response cycle. Sexual desire disorders are part of the appetitive phase; sexual arousal disorders are part of the excitement phase; and orgasmic disorders are part of the orgasmic phase. Sexual pain disorders are difficult to assign but may directly or indirectly affect the cycle at any level. This classification must be borne in mind when deciding upon the most appropriate therapeutic regimen. Disorders affecting the orgasmic phase are readily treatable by simple behavioral techniques, and the results appear to be dramatic and long lasting. Disorders affecting the appetitive phase, however, reflect deep-seated conflicts and are much more resistant to therapeutic intervention. They often require the use of insight-oriented therapies and the uncovering of repressed material in conjunction with behavioral therapy. The disturbances of the excitement phase fall somewhere between these two in terms of prognosis and choice of treatment.

Choice of Therapeutic Approach for Sexual Dysfunction

Proponents of the various therapeutic approaches can make a case for the efficacy of their methods in the treatment of these disorders. A basic understanding of the more commonly used and successful treatments is essential for appropriate treatment planning or selection of optimal referral sources.

Individual Psychodynamic Therapy

Individual brief-term psychodynamically oriented psychotherapy remains one of the more useful and effective techniques available when dealing with psychosexual disorders that have complex intrapsychic conflicts at their roots with pervasive negative influences over many other aspects of the individuals' lives. In actual practice, individual psychotherapy by itself may not bring about the desired results, but its efficacy may be greatly enhanced by the application of one of the many behavioral therapies in conjunction with the more traditional approach.

Behavioral Therapy

The use of behavioral techniques such as systematic desensitization and, to a lesser degree, implosion or flooding therapy is often extremely useful in treating sexual dysfunctions—particularly those associated with disturbances of the orgasmic phase. The actual techniques differ very little from the tried and true methods used in other disorders amenable to treatment by these methods (see Chapter 14). The therapist performs a detailed behavioral analysis and develops a hierarchical list of anxiety-producing situations during the sexual act that culminate in the pathological response, be it premature ejaculation, retarded ejaculation, or inhibited orgasm. Through gradual exposure to the anxiety-provoking stimulus, the patient eventually learns to cope in a more appropriate fashion and to perform sexually in an enjoyable, rewarding fashion. As noted earlier, these techniques are particularly effective when dealing with disorders of the orgasmic phase, but their primary value when treating disturbances of the appetitive phase is as an adjunctive technique. Specific techniques of behaviorally oriented therapy for specific types of sexual dysfunction are discussed in Chapter 14.

Hypnotherapy

Hypnotic suggestion can be used effectively to convince a patient that he or she does not need to feel pain during intercourse and to relieve disabling anxiety that may impair performance or consummation and enjoyment of the sexual act.

Group Therapy

Group therapy may be of value for selected patients whose perceived inadequacies and concerns about their symptoms may make them feel "different," socially isolated, and unable to share their feelings, fears, and irrational fantasies. Support from other members of the group with whom they can relate and identify may result in decreased anxiety and improvement in symptoms and may make the patient more amenable to participation in other forms of treatment, such as behavioral therapy.

Dual Sex (Couples) Therapy

This variant of behavioral therapy was initially proposed by Masters and Johnson and in its original form approached sexual dysfunction disorders as a "dyad" issue, that is, a patient suffering from a psychosexual disorder did so in the context of his relationship with his sexual partner. The two would be treated together as members of the "dyad" unit by a team consisting of a male and a female therapist. The latter not only directed what was for all intents and purposes a behavioral treatment approach, complete with educational sessions and schedule of assignments (systematic desensitization), but also served as role models for the same-sex member of the "dyad." In recent years, adherence to the male–female team and male–female "dyad" concept has not been as strict, and the makeup of the participants has been tailored to fit individual circumstances. Nevertheless, it remains an extremely effective approach that uses education, behavioral modification, modeling, and couples therapy to effect change in sexual dysfunction.

SUMMARY

The psychotherapies are important components of the treatment plan for nearly all psychiatric illnesses. Both short- and long-term techniques are available. Which psychotherapy for which patient with which therapist is less clear. Psychotherapy provides the patient with new problem-solving techniques. Some patients prefer one type of problem solving or can learn one type and not another.

How the outcomes from the different psychotherapies may differ and what this may mean for long-range health/relapse warrant further research. Increasingly, data indicate the effectiveness of the psychotherapies in reducing hospitalization rates and the use of other medical resources. Studies on the use of psychotherapy as an adjunct in the treatment of various physical illnesses also tend to indicate cost benefits in overall medical care dollars. The ability to use a range of psychotherapies is important in the treatment of psychiatric illness and in obtaining maximum benefit from medical case management and the therapeutic effectiveness of the doctor–patient relationship.

For the nonpsychiatric physician, a referral for psychiatric assessment is essential when psychotherapy may be indicated. The psychiatric consultant can evaluate the interplay of biological, psychological, and social context variables that may be causing or maintaining illness in the patient. A comprehensive treatment plan and goals can then be formulated. Prior to referring a patient, the physician should educate the patient. Many patients will have the belief that psychiatric illness is fake or imaginary. They should be reassured that their distress and pain are real and that there is a wide array of possible treatments. Patients are best prepared when they can understand the role of medication in providing possible relief of symptoms and the role of the psychotherapies in learning new ways to handle the problems that may be precipitating their distress. For instance, the physician refers a patient to physical therapy to learn a new way to walk when the patient has developed a limp to compensate for chronic pain. (The limp may persist even after the pain is relieved by medication.) Similarly, the psychotherapies teach, through various means, new problem-solving techniques to relieve patterns of behaviors, feelings, and thoughts that are causing or maintaining impairment.

Finally, as noted earlier, it should be emphasized that the best form of treatment is often integrated psychotherapy and pharmacotherapy. Psychiatrists or nonpsychiatric clinicians who are polarized one way or the other may offer a narrow range of treatment and overlook a biological or psychological therapy that might potentially be dramatically effective for the patient. Hence, in making a referral for an initial evaluation, it is recommended that one consult a clinician with a balanced, integrated approach. The success of a referral for psychiatric evaluation or psychotherapy is *critically* dependent on the attitude, confidence, and enthusiasm of the referring physician.

CLINICAL PEARLS

- It is important to exhibit confidence and enthusiasm when making a referral for psychiatric evaluation or psychotherapy. Patients will detect ambivalence and skepticism on the physician's part about the need for such treatment. It is usually helpful to recommend a psychiatrist or other health professional who is known *personally* by the physician.
- Always present the psychiatric referral as part of the patient's ongoing medical care. Some patients will view a psychiatric referral as meaning you are "dumping" them onto another doctor and as a "rejection." Patients should be reassured that any psychiatric treatment will be in parallel with their ongoing medical care.
- Have the name and telephone number of your referral source readily available to give to the patient.
- Call the psychiatrist to personally explain the reason and need for the referral and what role you would like to continue to play in the patient's care.

- Make the appointment for the psychiatric evaluation while the patient is still in the office or clinic.
- Be sure to schedule a follow-up appointment after the date of the psychiatric evaluation to check on the patient's reaction to the referral and their response to initial treatment.

ANNOTATED BIBLIOGRAPHY

Balint M, Ornstein P, Balint E: Focal Psychotherapy. Philadelphia, JB Lippincott, 1972

This book is one of the first written in the area of brief psychodynamic pscyodynamic psychotherapy. It is a superb demonstration of a case of brief psychotherapy in an individual with moderately severe psychopathology. The case illustrates the exceptional clinical skill and technical requirements in carrying out a brief psychodynamic psychotherapy.

Bruch H: Learning Psychotherapy. Cambridge, Harvard University Press, 1974

This eloquent and well-written introduction to psychotherapy presents basic principles of psychotherapeutic relations of the management of psychotherapy that are applicable to nearly all psychotherapeutic endeavors. It is based on the author's extensive career as a psychotherapist. An excellent introduction to psychotherapy.

Coleman J: Aims and conduct of psychotherapy. Arch Gen Psychiatry 18:1–6, 1968

This is a clearly written, classic article that articulates without jargon the basic doctor–patient relationship, goals, and orientation maintained by the psychiatrist in conducting psychotherapy.

Novalis PN, Rojcewicz SJ, Peele R: Clinical Manual of Supportive Psychotherapy. Washington, DC, American Psychiatric Press, 1993

Stone L: The Psychoanalytic Situation. New York, International University Press, 1961

This brief book describes the structural elements of psychoanalysis—setting, organization, techniques, and contribution to the treatment. Well written.

Sullivan HS: The Psychiatric Interview. New York, WW Norton, 1954

This excellent introduction to the psychiatric interview is written from the perspective of the interpersonal school of psychiatry. However, its basic presentation is applicable to all of the psychotherapies. It provides a basic science to the application of talk as a curative agent.

Ursano RJ, Hales RE: A review of brief individual therapies. Am J Psychiatry 143(12):1507–1517, 1986

This article is an overview of both individual and group brief psychotherapies. It has a detailed list of references and presents the psychotherapies as medical interventions with substantive technical and selection criteria. In addition, there is a brief overview of the cost-benefit issues in psychotherapy.

Ursano RJ, Silberman EK: Psychodynamic and Supportive Psychotherapy. In Hales RE, Yudofsky SC, Talbot JA (eds): Textbook of Psychiatry. Washington, DC, American Psychiatric Press, 1994

This chapter reviews psychodynamic and supportive psychotherapies. It contains an extensive review of supportive psychotherapy, perhaps the most widely used and understudied of all of the psychotherapies.

Ursano RJ, Sonnenberg SM, Lazar SG: Concise Guide to Psychodynamic Psychotherapy. Washington, DC, American Psychiatric Press, 1991

This book is a concise, highly readable text on the techniques of psychodynamic psychotherapy. It includes a glossary and sections on supportive and brief psychotherapy.

Werman DS: The Practice of Supportive Psychotherapy. New York, Brunner/Mazel, 1984

This book is one of a very few that describe supportive psychotherapy in a technical manner. It is a substantive contribution to the literature and to the clinician's ability to learn supportive psychotherapy as a technique.

Yalom ID: The Theory and Practice of Group Psychotherapy. New York, Basic Books, 1985

This book is the basic text of group psychotherapy. It is a comprehensive review with technical directions for the application of the technique by clinicians.

REFERENCES

Beck AT: Cognitive Theory and the Emotional Disorders. New York, International Universities Press, 1976

Beels CC: Family Therapy. In Talbott JA, Hales RE, Yudofsky SC (eds): Textbook of Psychiatry. Washington, DC, American Psychiatric Press, 1988

Bion WR: Experiences in Groups. New York, Basic Books, 1961

Bruch H: Learning Psychotherapy. Cambridge, Harvard University Press, 1974

Davanloo H (ed): Short-Term Dynamic Psychotherapy. New York, Jason Aronson Press, 1980

Fiore J, Stoudemire A, Kriseman N: The Family in Human Development and Medical Practice. In Stoudemire A (ed): Human Behavior: An Introduction for Medical Students, 2nd ed. Philadelphia, JB Lippincott, 1994

Gaarder K, Montgomery P: Clinical Biofeedback. Baltimore, Williams & Wilkins, 1977

Kaplan HS: The New Sex Therapy. New York, Brunner/Mazel, 1974

Klerman GL, Weissman MM, Rounsaville BJ et al: Interpersonal Psychotherapy of Depression. New York, Basic Books, 1984

Lazarus A: Behavior Therapy and Beyond. New York, McGraw-Hill, 1971

Luborsky L, Crits-Cristoph P: Understanding Transference. New York, Basic Books, 1990

Malan DH: A Study of Brief Psychotherapy. New York, Plenum Press, 1975

Mann J: Time-Limited Psychotherapy. Cambridge, Harvard University Press, 1973

Masters WH, Johnson VE: Human Sexual Inadequacy. Boston, Little, Brown & Co, 1970

Pine F: Supportive psychotherapy: A psychoanalytic perspective. Psychiatr Ann 16:524–534, 1986

Reichmann FF: Principles of Intensive Psychotherapy. Chicago, University of Chicago Press, 1950

Rockland LH: Supportive Therapy: A Psychodynamic Approach. New York, Basic Books, 1989

Rush AJ, Beck AT (eds): Cognitive Therapy. In Frances A, Hales RE (eds): American Psychiatric Press Review of Psychiatry. Washington, DC, American Psychiatric Press, 1988

Sandler J, Dare C, Holder A: The Patient and the Analyst. New York, International Universities Press, 1973

Sifneos PE: Short-Term Psychotherapy and Emotional Crisis. Cambridge, Harvard University Press, 1972

Werman DS: The practice of supportive psychotherapy. New York, Brunner/Mazel, 1984

Yalom I (ed): Group Psychotherapy. In Frances A, Hales RE (eds): American Psychiatric Press Review of Psychiatry. Washington, DC, American Psychiatric Press, 1986

Alan Stoudemire (ed). *Clinical Psychiatry for Medical Students,* Second
Edition. Copyright © 1994, 1990 by J. B. Lippincott Company.

18 *Biological Therapies for Mental Disorders*

Jonathan M. Silver,
Robert E. Hales, and
Stuart C. Yudofsky

GENERAL CONSIDERATIONS IN SELECTING A SOMATIC THERAPY

The use of a somatic treatment for a psychiatric illness is a decision that should be made only after careful consideration of many factors for that individual patient. Medication alone is never *the* treatment for a patient; rather, medications may be important components of a larger overall treatment plan. All psychiatric patients require a skilled and thorough psychiatric, neurologic, and physical evaluation. A key component of a well-considered decision to use a somatic treatment is the specification of *target symptoms*. One should list those specific symptoms that are designated for treatment and monitor response of these symptoms to treatment. However, a frequent and dangerous clinical error is the treatment of specific symptoms of a disorder with multiple drugs rather than treating, more specifically, the underlying disorder. For example, it is not uncommon for a psychiatrist to be referred a patient who is taking one type of benzodiazepine for anxiety, a different type of benzodiazepine for insomnia, an analgesic for unspecific somatic complaints, and a subtherapeutic dose of an antidepressant (e.g., 50 mg/day of imipramine) for feelings of sadness. Often, the somatic complaints, insomnia, and anxiety are components of the underlying depression, which is aggravated by the polypharmaceutical approach inherent to symptomatic treatment. In such circumstances, full explanation to the patient of the syndrome of depression, with emphasis on the necessity of adequate doses and duration of treatment with an antidepressant, should precede discontinuation of the benzodiazepine and analgesic medications and the proper administration of

an antidepressant agent. After the decision has been made to initiate psychopharmacologic treatment, the clinician must select the specific drug. Usually, this choice is
made on the basis of the patient's prior history of response to medication, the side
effect profile of the drug chosen, and the patient's most likely response to those
specific side effects.

Choice of Medication

Choice of a medication also involves an understanding of the *pharmacokinetics* of a particular drug as well as a familiarity with the relative benefits of the
available routes of administration of that medication. Most antidepressant and
antipsychotic drugs have sufficiently long half-lives to permit a once-a-day dosing
regimen, which may increase compliance. The choice of a particular medication
may depend on whether that drug is available in injection and liquid forms in
addition to tablet, pill, or capsule forms.

Once a decision has been made as to the need for and the choice of a specific
drug, attention must be paid to issues related to patient information about indications
for and risks and benefits of the medication. A general principle is that the more the
patient understands about his or her illness and the reason that medications have
been chosen to treat the illness, the more compliant the patient will be. The clinician
must also consider the physical, intellectual, and psychological capacities of the
patient and her or his caretakers when selecting a new medication. For example,
impulsive patients with a history of suicide attempts and alcohol abuse may not safely
or reliably be treated with a monoamine oxidase inhibitor because of the need to
follow a strict dietary regimen. In general, the more complicated the instructions, or
the more medications that are prescribed, and the greater number of times per day the
medication is to be taken, the more difficulty the patient will have in complying.

*A major component of the treatment plan should comprise the evaluation of
response and criteria for discontinuation of the medication.* Far too frequently,
medications are discontinued with the assumption of "failure of response to the
medication" without an adequate (i.e., dose, serum level, and duration) drug trial.
Different treatment approaches range from a second trial with a related class of
medication to the use of complementary or different treatment modalities.

Finally, for those patients whose specific target symptoms do respond to somatic
intervention, an end point for treatment must be determined. It is not uncommon that
patients are continued on medications beyond the point that therapeutic benefit is
derived. A common example is the use of benzodiazepines for the treatment of
anxiety; patients may be maintained on this drug for years without the assessment of
its therapeutic benefit by gradual discontinuation.

ANTIPSYCHOTIC DRUGS

Available antipsychotic drugs may be categorized into several classes: the phenothiazines (including their derivatives), the thioxanthenes, the butyrophenones, and
the dibenzoxazepine, dibenzodiazepine, and indole derivatives. The drugs that are
commonly used are shown in Table 18–1.

Table 18–1 **Selected Antipsychotic Drugs and Dosages (see also Table 5–4)**

CLASS/ GENERIC NAME	TRADE NAME	DOSE EQUIVALENT (mg)	*USUAL MAINTENANCE DAILY ORAL DOSE (mg)
Phenothiazine (Aliphatic)			
Chlorpromazine hydrochloride	Thorazine	100	200–600
Piperidine Phenothiazine			
Thioridazine hydrochloride	Mellaril	90–104	200–600
Mesoridazine besylate	Serentil	50–62	150–200
Piperazine Phenothiazine			
Trifluoperazine	Stelazine	2.4–3.2	5–10
Fluphenazine hydrochloride	Prolixin	1.1–1.3	2.5–10
decanoate enanthate		0.61	10 mg/day oral fluphenazine = 12.5–25 mg/2 weeks fluphenazine decanoate
Perphenazine	Trilafon	8.9–9.6	16–24
Thioxanthenes			
Chlorprothixene	Taractan	36–52	75–200
Thiothixene	Navane	3.4–5.4	6–30
Butyrophenones			
Haloperidol	Haldol	1.1–2.1	2–12
Haloperidol decanoate			10 mg/day oral haloperidol = 100–200 mg/4 weeks haloperidol decanoate
Dibenzoxazepine			
Loxapine	Loxitane	10	20–60
Indole derivatives			
Molindone hydrochloride	Moban	5.1–6.9	15–60
Diphenylbutylpiperidine			
Pimozide	Orap	N/A	2–10
Dibenzodiazepine			
Clozapine	Clozaril	50	200–900

Silver JM, Yudofsky SC, Hurowitz G: Psychopharmacology and Electroconvulsive Therapy. In Hales RE, Yudofsky SC, Talbott JA (eds): The American Psychiatric Press Textbook of Psychiatry, 2nd ed. Washington, DC, American Psychiatric Press, 1994
* Dose ranges required for patients varies. Adjustment in doses may be required depending on the patient's clinical status and responsiveness to medication.

Although there are many therapeutic agents available in parenteral, oral, and depot preparations, the choice of a drug in treating psychosis is determined largely by the side effect profile of the specific drug and the ability of the individual patient to tolerate or benefit from those side effects. Clozapine has a unique pharmacologic profile when compared with currently available antipsychotic drugs. It will be discussed in a separate section in this chapter.

Mechanisms of Action

The prevailing theory regarding the mechanism of action of antipsychotic drugs was based on the observation that all of the currently available antipsychotic drugs have a similar action on the dopamine system: the blocking of the binding of dopamine to the postsynaptic dopamine receptor in the brain. The dopamine-2 (D-2) receptor, which is not linked to adenylate cyclase, was believed to be responsible for the action of this class of drugs. The theory that psychosis is a result of an excess of dopamine or the result of abnormal activity of certain dopamine receptors has been confirmed by the observation of increased dopamine concentrations and an increased number of dopamine-2 receptors in the brains of some patients with schizophrenia (see Chapter 4 by Dr. Stoudemire).

There are several dopamine pathways in the brain that are affected by the antipsychotic drugs. The nigrostriatal system is involved in motor activity. A relative deficiency of dopamine after administration of antipsychotics due to the blockage of the dopamine receptor leads to extrapyramidal disorders, such as those seen in Parkinson's disease. As a result of this, antipsychotic drugs have been termed "neuroleptics" because their actions imitate a neurologic illness. Dopamine receptors in the pituitary and hypothalamus (the tuberoinfundibular system) affect prolactin release, appetite, and temperature regulation. Since dopamine inhibits the release of prolactin, the antipsychotic drugs result in an increase in prolactin levels. Dopamine pathways also connect the limbic system, the midbrain tegmentum, septal nuclei, and mesocortical projections. These areas are believed to be involved in thought and emotion and may be responsible for the antipsychotic action of these drugs. Revised "dopamine hypotheses" have focused on these various pathways, which amends the prevailing theory to accommodate new findings, including the discovery of dopamine receptors that are limited to limbic areas.

Indications and Efficacy

The most common use of antipsychotic drugs is in the treatment of acute psychotic exacerbations and in the maintenance of remission of these psychotic symptoms in patients with schizophrenia. Psychotic symptoms include abnormal thought content such as delusions, perceptual abnormalities such as hallucinations, and abnormal thought form such as disorganized speech.

The impressive data on the effectiveness of antipsychotic drugs as maintenance treatment for schizophrenia have been reviewed thoroughly by Davis and Andriukaitis (1986). Without continued treatment with antipsychotic medication after remission of acute psychotic symptoms, there is a relapse rate of approximately 8 to 15% per month for patients with schizophrenia (Davis and Andriukaitis, 1986). Patients maintained on drugs have a relapse rate ranging from 1.5 to 3% per month.

Antipsychotic drugs are effective in ameliorating psychotic symptoms that result from diverse etiologies such as mood (affective) disorders with psychotic features, drug toxicities such as "steroid psychoses" (delirium), and brain disorders such as Huntington's disease or post–head injury. Acute manic symptoms are effectively treated with antipsychotic drugs, with a more rapid response than with lithium. Patients with borderline and schizotypal personality disorders have been treated with antipsychotic drugs. Brief treatment with relatively low-dose antipsychotic drugs may be effective in alleviating the symptoms of somatization, anxiety, and psychotic ideation in these patients. Patients with psychotic or delusional depression may be successfully treated with a combination of antipsychotic and antidepressant drugs, but not with antipsychotic drugs alone.

The sedative side effect of antipsychotic drugs may often lead to their misuse in several clinical situations. These drugs frequently are improperly prescribed as hypnotic or anxiolytic agents. In addition, the antipsychotic drugs are administered to patients who are chronically agitated and violent. Because of the potential long-term risks of these drugs (see section on tardive dyskinesia), antipsychotics are not recommended for the treatment of anxiety or insomnia. Similarly, although these drugs are valuable for acute episodes of agitation and aggression, they should generally not be used for the treatment of chronic aggression and agitation except under special circumstances.

Clinical Use of Antipsychotic Drugs

General Principles

Drug potency refers to the milligram equivalence of drugs, not to the relative efficacy. For example, although haloperidol is more potent than chlorpromazine (2 mg haloperidol = 100 mg chlorpromazine), therapeutically equivalent doses are equally effective (12 mg haloperidol = 600 mg chlorpromazine). These doses are listed in Table 18–1. By convention, the potency of antipsychotic drugs is compared with a standard 100-mg dose of chlorpromazine. As a rule, *the high-potency antipsychotic drugs with an equivalent dose of less than 5 mg have a high degree of extrapyramidal side effects (EPS) and low levels of sedation and autonomic side effects* (e.g., haloperidol, thiothixene, fluphenazine). Low-potency antipsychotic drugs have an equivalent dose of greater than 40 mg (e.g., chlorpromazine and thioridazine). These have a high level of sedation and autonomic side effects and a low degree of EPS. Those antipsychotic drugs with intermediate potency (equivalent dose between 5 mg and 40 mg) have a side effect profile that lies between these two groups (e.g., loxapine).

Treatment with antipsychotic medication must be tailored to the individual patient. Flexible guidelines that are supported by scientific principles and research should be followed. These guidelines are outlined in Table 18–2.

Risks, Side Effects, and Their Management

Extrapyramidal Reactions

Serious side effects of antipsychotic use result from the blockade of the postsynaptic dopamine receptor. A variety of extrapyramidal symptoms may emerge, including acute dystonic reactions, parkinsonian syndrome, akathisia, akinesia, "rabbit syndrome," tardive dyskinesia, neuroleptic-induced catatonia, and the neuroleptic malignant syndrome.

Among the most disturbing and frightening adverse drug reactions that occur with the administration of antipsychotic drugs are *acute dystonic reactions*. This

Table 18–2 **Guidelines for Antipsychotic Drug Therapy**

1. Obtain thorough medical evaluation, including evaluation for tardive dyskinesia.
2. Select drug on the basis of side effect profile, risk/benefit ratio, and history of prior use and response.
3. Inform the patient and family of risk of tardive dyskinesia.
4. Initiate drug therapy at low dose (chlorpromazine [CPZ] equivalent 50 mg orally three times a day).
5. Use prophylactic anticholinergic medication with high-potency antipsychotic drugs or in patients younger than 40 years old.
6. Gradually increase dose (50–100 mg CPZ equivalent every other day) until improvement or usual maximum dose of 600 mg CPZ equivalent is reached.
7. Maintain maximum dose for 2 to 4 weeks.
8. Consider using sedative drugs or beta-blockers for agitation.
9. If response is inadequate, obtain plasma level of drugs.
10. If level is low, increase dose to equivalent of 1000 mg CPZ.
11. Maintain dose for 2 to 4 weeks. If improvement is inadequate, gradually decrease drug and substitute with an antipsychotic from a different class.
12. Monitor patient closely for therapeutic effects and side effects of treatment.
13. Decrease dosage of antipsychotic medications as soon as possible after initial control of psychotic symptoms.

Silver JM, Yudofsky SC, Hurowitz G: Psychopharmacology and Electroconvulsive Therapy. In Hales RE, Yudofsky SC, Talbott JA (eds): The American Psychiatric Press Textbook of Psychiatry, 2nd ed. Washington, DC, American Psychiatric Press, 1994

reaction most frequently occurs within hours or days of the initiation of antipsychotic therapy. *The most common feature of this syndrome includes uncontrollable tightening of the face and neck and spasm and distortions of the head and/or back (opisthotonus).* If the extraocular muscles are involved, an oculogyric crisis may occur, wherein the eyes are elevated and "locked" in this position. Laryngeal involvement may lead to respiratory and ventilatory difficulties.

Intravenous or intramuscular administration of anticholinergic drugs provides rapid treatment of acute dystonia. Table 18–3 lists the drugs and dosages used to treat dystonic reactions. Note that the anticholinergic drug given to reverse the dystonia will wear off after several hours. Since antipsychotic drugs may have long half-lives and duration of action, additional oral anticholinergic drugs should be prescribed for several days after the dystonic reaction has occurred.

The *parkinsonian syndrome* has many of the features of classic idiopathic Parkinson's disease: diminished range of facial expression (masked facies), cogwheel rigidity, slowed movements (bradykinesia), and "pill-rolling" tremor. The onset of this side effect is gradual and may not appear for weeks after neuroleptics have been administered. Drugs used in the treatment of the parkinsonian side effects of antipsychotic agents are listed in Table 18–3.

Akathisia is an extrapyramidal disorder consisting of an unpleasant feeling of restlessness and the inability to sit still. It is a common reaction and most often occurs shortly after the initiation of antipsychotic drugs. Unfortunately, *akathisia is frequently mistaken for an exacerbation of psychotic symptoms, anxiety, or depression.* The patient may pace or may become agitated or angry with the inability to control symptoms associated with akathisia. If the dose of antipsychotic medications

Table 18–3 **Drugs for Treatment of Extrapyramidal Disorders**

GENERIC NAME (TRADE NAME)	(STARTING DOSE)
Anticholinergic Drugs	
Benztropine (Cogentin)	P.O. 0.5 mg t.i.d.
	I.M./I.V. 1 mg
Biperiden (Akineton)	P.O. 2 mg t.i.d.
	I.M./I.V. 2 mg
Diphenhydramine (Benadryl)	P.O. 25 mg q.i.d.
	I.M./I.V. 25 mg
Ethopropazine (Parsidol)	P.O. 50 mg b.i.d.
Orphenadrine (Norflex, Disipal)	P.O. 100 mg b.i.d.
	I.V. 60 mg
Procyclidine (Kemadrine)	P.O. 2.5 mg t.i.d.
Trihexyphenidyl (Artane)	P.O. 1 mg t.i.d.
Dopamine Agonists	
Amantadine (Symmetrel)	P.O. 100 mg b.i.d.
Beta-blockers (Akathisia)	
Propranolol (Inderal)	P.O. 20 mg t.i.d.

Silver JM, Yudofsky SC, Hurowitz G: Psychopharmacology and Electroconvulsive Therapy. In Hales RE, Yudofsky SC, Talbott JA (eds): The American Psychiatric Press Textbook of Psychiatry, 2nd ed. Washington, DC, American Psychiatric Press, 1994

is increased, the restlessness continues or exacerbates. Lowering the dose may improve the symptoms. In the past, anticholinergic drugs were suggested as the first line of therapy, but they often are ineffective. Benzodiazepines, such as diazepam, may be effective. The treatment of choice of akathisia is beta-adrenergic blocking drugs, particularly propranolol.

Akinesia (or the similar term *bradykinesia*) is characterized by diminished spontaneity, few gestures, unspontaneous speech, and apathy. As with the parkinsonian syndrome, this may appear only after several weeks of therapy. This syndrome may be mistaken as depression in patients treated with antipsychotic agents. The anticholinergic drugs in the dose ranges suggested in Table 18–3 are effective in treating akinesia.

The "rabbit syndrome" consists of fine, rapid movements of the lips that mimic the chewing movements of a rabbit. This side effect occurs late in neuroleptic treatment and is treated effectively with anticholinergic drugs. It has been found to be present in approximately 4% of patients receiving neuroleptic therapy (without concomitant anticholinergics) (Yassa and Lal, 1986).

Tardive dyskinesia (TD) is a disorder characterized by involuntary movements of the face, trunk, or extremities. The syndrome is related to exposure to dopamine-receptor blocking agents, most frequently the classic antipsychotic agents (see Table 18–4). The APA Task Force on Tardive Dyskinesia estimates that among patients receiving chronic neuroleptic treatment, 15 to 20% will have some evidence of this condition. The most commonly hypothesized mechanism for the development

Table 18–4 **Clinical Features of Tardive Dyskinesia**

The following abnormal movements may be seen in tardive dyskinesia:

Facial and oral movements

Muscles of facial expression: involuntary movement of forehead, eyebrows, periorbital area, cheeks; involuntary frowning, blinking, smiling, grimacing

Lips and perioral area: involuntary puckering, pouting, smacking

Jaw: involuntary biting, clenching, chewing, mouth opening, lateral movements

Tongue: involuntary protrusion, tremor, choreoathetoid movements (rolling, wormlike movement without displacement from the mouth)

Extremity Movements

Involuntary movements of upper arms, wrists, hands, fingers: choreic movements (i.e., rapid, objectively purposeless, irregular, spontaneous), athetoid movements (i.e., slow, irregular, complex, serpentine). Tremor (i.e., repetitive, regular, rhythmic)

Involuntary movement of lower legs, knees, ankles, toes: lateral knee movement, foot tapping, foot squirming, inversion and eversion of foot

Trunk Movements

Involuntary movement of neck, shoulders, hips: rocking, twisting, squirming, pelvic gyrations

Adapted from National Institute of Mental Health: Abnormal Involuntary Movement Scale. In Guy W: ECDEU Assessment Manual. Rockville, MD, U.S. Department of Health, Education, and Welfare, 1976

---

of TD is that postsynaptic dopamine receptor supersensitivity develops after use of dopamine-receptor blocking drugs. Other hypotheses have also been proposed.

The most significant and consistently documented risk factor for the development of TD is *increasing age of the patient*. Other risk factors may include the dose of antipsychotic medication, the total time on antipsychotics, a history of drug holidays (a greater number of drug-free periods is associated with an increased risk), the time since the first exposure to antipsychotic drugs (including drug holidays), the presence of brain damage, and diagnosis (especially the presence of a mood disorder).

The issue of informed consent with respect to antipsychotic medications and the risk of TD has been extensively reviewed (Munetz and Roth, 1985). It is usually difficult, if not impossible, to obtain informed consent from an acutely psychotic patient. A general guideline is to inform and educate the patient's family about the risks of TD before starting the antipsychotics and to educate the patient gradually about this disorder as soon as possible after agitation and psychosis remit. In many circumstances, true informed consent may be impossible to obtain from an acutely psychotic patient for several weeks. The psychiatrist also needs to be aware that some states legally mandate that informed consent be obtained from patients before the initiation of antipsychotic treatment (e.g., California and New Jersey). All such discussions with patients and their families should be documented in the patients' records. An informed consent that is exclusively in the written form has been shown to be less effective in communicating information to the patient than an oral consent obtained in conjunction with education of the patient (Munetz and Roth, 1985). The psychiatrist must designate adequate time to the provision of informed consent consistent with the confusional state and cognitive capabilities of the patient.

Prevention is the most important aspect of TD management. Periodic assessments must be made to determine the patient's requirement for continuing antipsychotic drug therapy. In addition, every 6 months a reevaluation is required to ascertain the lowest possible dose of antipsychotic drug that still proves to be effective in the treatment of psychotic symptoms.

There is no reliable treatment of TD other than discontinuing the antipsychotic medication. If discontinuation of the antipsychotic drug is possible in light of the severity of the patient's psychotic symptoms, improvement in the TD may be gradual. Worsening of the involuntary movements often initially occurs with discontinuation of neuroleptics. The new neuroleptic clozapine does not appear to cause TD, although it has the major liability of possibly causing agranulocytosis (see below).

Neuroleptic Malignant Syndrome. In rare instances, patients on antipsychotic medications may develop a potentially life-threatening disorder known as neuroleptic malignant syndrome (NMS). While most frequently occurring with the use of high-potency neuroleptics (haloperidol), this condition may emerge after the use of any antipsychotic agent. The patient with NMS becomes severely rigid and occasionally catatonic. There is fever, elevated white blood cell count, tachycardia, abnormal blood pressure fluctuations, tachypnea, and diaphoresis. Creatinine phosphokinase (CPK) levels are elevated due to muscle breakdown, and CPK levels are an excellent parameter to check for the presence of the disorder and response to treatment. A prodrome to neuroleptic malignant syndrome is *neuroleptic-induced catatonia*, wherein the prominent signs are extrapyramidal symptoms and a catatonic behavioral state that may be mistaken for a worsening of the psychosis. Neuroleptic-induced catatonia is best treated with amantadine 100 mg b.i.d. over several weeks.

The key treatment steps after recognition of NMS are discontinuation of all medications, thorough medical evaluation, and physical support, including intravenous fluids, antipyretic agents, and cooling blankets. Several treatments have been suggested to control NMS. These include amantadine, electroconvulsive therapy, and benzodiazepines. As noted above, amantadine appears more useful in the treatment of neuroleptic-induced catatonia than do the anticholinergic drugs. Dantrolene sodium (a direct-acting muscle relaxant) and bromocriptine (a centrally active dopamine agonist) appear to be the most successful agents in the treatment of NMS, but their efficacy over supportive care has not been definitively proven. Because these two agents may treat differing symptoms of NMS and act through separate mechanisms, they also may be useful in combination. Unfortunately, no controlled clinical trials related to the somatic treatment of NMS have yet been conducted.

Anticholinergic Effects

In the treatment of a patient with antipsychotic drugs, anticholinergic side effects may be caused by either the neuroleptic or the anticholinergic drug that has been prescribed to alleviate extrapyramidal side effects. Anticholinergic effects are categorized as peripheral or central. Among the peripheral side effects, the most common are dry mouth, decreased sweating, decreased bronchial secretions, blurred vision (due to inhibition of accommodation), difficulty in urination, and constipation. Central side effects of anticholinergic drugs include impairment in concentration, attention, and memory. In cases of toxicity, anticholinergic delirium—which includes hot, dry skin, dry mucous membranes, dilated pupils, absent bowel sounds, and tachycardia—may appear.

Other Side Effects

Blockade of alpha-adrenergic receptors can result in orthostatic hypotension and dizziness. Mesoridazine, chlorpromazine, thioridazine, and clozapine are the most potent alpha-1 blockers of the antipsychotic drugs. Changes in hormonal function have been reported to occur with neuroleptic treatment. Because of the dopamine blocking effect, prolactin levels increase, which may result in gynecomastia in both men and women. Galactorrhea, although unusual, also may occur. Additional neuroendocrine side effects of neuroleptics mediated by hyperprolactinemia include amenorrhea, weight gain, breast tenderness, and decreased libido.

Sexual dysfunction also may be caused by neuroleptic therapy. In men, difficulty in achieving or maintaining an erection, decreased ability to achieve orgasm, and changes in the quality of orgasm are reported. Thioridazine may cause painful retrograde ejaculation in which semen is ejected into the bladder. Women may experience changes in the quality of orgasm and decreased ability to achieve orgasm with antipsychotic use. Menstrual irregularities also may occur.

Pigmentary changes in the skin and eyes may occur, especially with long-term treatment. Pigment deposition in the lens of the eye does not affect vision. Pigmentary retinopathy, which can lead to irreversible blindness, has been associated specifically with the use of thioridazine. Pigmentary retinopathy has most often been reported with doses above the recommended dosage ceiling for thioridazine (i.e., 800 mg/day). Almost all patients on neuroleptics, especially the aliphatic phenothiazines (e.g., chlorpromazine), become more sensitive to the effects of sunlight, which can lead to severe sunburn. Especially in the summer months, patients should avoid excess sun exposure and use ultraviolet blocking agents, such as sunscreens that contain para-aminobenzoic acid (PABA).

Several of the antipsychotic medications have cardiac effects that can be detected on the electrocardiogram. For example, thioridazine is associated with prolonged QT intervals, and this change is related to plasma level concentration. There have been reports of other arrhythmias and sudden death with antipsychotic agents probably due to their quinidinelike effects.

Increases in liver function enzymes have been rarely associated with antipsychotic treatment. Many cases of this reaction were linked to impurities in the original formulation of chlorpromazine, and the incidence has profoundly decreased over the years. Transient leukopenia and, in rare cases, agranulocytosis have been associated with neuroleptic treatment. These are idiosyncratic reactions that usually occur within the first 3 to 4 weeks after the initiation of treatment with an antipsychotic drug. Clozapine has a special propensity for this side effect.

The antipsychotic drugs have been shown to lower seizure threshold, a phenomenon that has been confirmed in animal models. Special precautions must be taken with the use of antipsychotic agents in those patients with a history of convulsions who are not on anticonvulsant therapy and in those patients with episodic aggression whose dyscontrol may result from "subictal seizures."

Antipsychotic drugs directly affect the hypothalamus and suppress control of temperature regulation. In combination with the alpha-adrenergic receptor and cholinergic receptor blocking effects of antipsychotics, this effect becomes particularly serious in hot, humid weather.

As a general guideline, antipsychotic drugs should be used in pregnant patients only if absolutely necessary, at the minimal dose required, and for the briefest possible time.

The treatment of refractory psychosis had been limited for many years by the fact that all of the available antipsychotic medications were equally effective. The introduction of the atypical neuroleptic clozapine, for use in treatment-resistant schizophrenia, has changed this situation. Clozapine is atypical because it causes significantly less extrapyramidal side effects, does not elevate serum prolactin, and has not been found to date to induce tardive dyskinesia. Significant improvement has been found in up to 30% of patients with schizophrenia who have failed to respond to typical antipsychotic medications.

Unfortunately, the use of clozapine is associated with potentially severe side effects. There is a 2% risk of developing potentially fatal agranulocytosis. For this reason, weekly blood counts are required by the manufacturer for any patient prescribed clozapine. Clozapine treatment has been found to carry a significant risk of seizures. The overall cumulative risk to patients has been estimated to be 10% after almost 4 years of treatment, but the risk is dose related.

ANTIDEPRESSANT DRUGS

The modern era of drug treatment of depression began in the 1950s when iproniazid, a monoamine oxidase inhibitor (MAOI) used for the treatment of tuberculosis, was noted to elevate the mood of these patients. Imipramine, the first of the "tricyclic antidepressants" (TCAs), was developed as a derivative of chlorpromazine with the hope that the drug would be more effective as an antipsychotic agent. Although imipramine did not exhibit antipsychotic efficacy, it was found to be effective in the treatment of depression.

Since that time, many other antidepressant drugs have been approved for use in the United States. Among this group are other derivatives of the TCA family, drugs with related structures (e.g., tetracyclics), drugs of the MAOI family, and atypical antidepressants. For simplicity, the term "cyclic antidepressants" (CyAD) will be employed in this chapter to describe TCAs, tetracyclics, heterocyclic antidepressants, and serotonin specific reuptake inhibitors (SSRIs) fluoxetine, sertraline, and paroxetine. The currently available antidepressants in the United States are listed in Tables 18–5, and 18–6).

Mechanisms of Action

Antidepressant drugs acutely affect the serotonergic and catecholaminergic systems in the central nervous system. The CyAD and SSRIs block the presynaptic

Table 18–5 **Selected Antidepressent Drugs and Dosages**

CLASS/GENERIC NAME	TRADE NAME	DOSE RANGE (mg)
Tertiary Amine Tricyclics		
Imipramine	Tofranil	75–300
	Tofranil PM	
	SK-Pramine	
Amitriptyline	Elavil	75–300
	Endep	
Doxepin	Adapin	75–300
	Sinequan	
Trimipramine	Surmontil	50–200
Secondary Amine Tricyclics		
Desipramine	Norpramin	75–300
	Pertofrane	
Nortriptyline	Aventyl	50–150
	Pamelor	
Protriptyline	Vivactil	10–60
Tetracyclic		
Maprotiline	Ludiomil	150–200
Dibenzoxazepine		
Amoxapine	Asendin	75–400
Triazolopyridine		
Trazodone	Desyrel	200–600
Unicyclic		
Bupropion	Wellbutrin	150–450
Selective Serotonin Reuptake Inhibitors		
Fluoxetine	Prozac	10–40
Sertraline	Zoloft	50–200
Paroxetine	Paxil	10–40

Table 18–6 **Selected Monoamine Oxidase Inhibitors Drugs and Dosages**

CLASS GENERIC NAME	TRADE NAME	USUAL DAILY MAXIMUM ORAL DOSE (mg)
Hydrazines		
Phenelzine	Nardil	90
Isocarboxazid	Marplan	50
Nonhydrazines		
Tranylcypromine	Parnate	60
Pargyline	Eutonyl	150

Silver JM, Yudofsky SC, Hurowitz G: Psychopharmacology and Electroconvulsive Therapy. In Hales RE, Yudofsky SC, Talbott JA (eds): The American Psychiatric Press Textbook of Psychiatry, 2nd ed. Washington, DC, American Psychiatric Press, 1994

reuptake of serotonin (5-HT) and/or norepinephrine (NE) and thereby increase the amount of these neurotransmitters available at the synapse. The MAOIs intensify monoaminergic transmission by blocking the catabolism of several biogenic amines, including NE, 5-HT, tyramine, phenylephrine, and dopamine (DA). It seems that bupropion's main mode of action also involves reuptake inhibition, but in this case it is the reuptake of dopamine (DA) that is affected. Trazodone has mixed effects on the serotonin system, but apparently achieves an antidepressant effect through its antagonism of the 5-HT2 receptor.

These acute effects of antidepressants on neurotransmitters were translated into the catecholamine hypothesis of depression, which postulated that depression was caused by a relative deficiency of catecholaminergic neurotransmitters that was "corrected" by antidepressant drugs (see Chapter 6 by Drs. Marin, Frances, and Widiger). Two major subtypes of depression were hypothesized to prevail. The first was characterized by a deficiency of norepinephrine. For this type of depression, the appropriate medication would be one with primary effects on reuptake inhibition of NE. For the second subtype, depression that was characterized by a lack of serotonin, an antidepressant that blocked the reuptake of 5-HT, was advocated. The relative affinities of the CyAD and SSRIs on the inhibition of presynaptic reuptake of 5-HT or NE are listed in Table 7–12). With further research, investigators discovered that, while the effects on reuptake inhibition are immediate, it is the effect of antidepressants on receptor sensitivity after chronic administration that most clearly parallels the well-known delayed clinical response to these agents.

Monoamine oxidase (MAO), through oxidative deamination, inactivates biogenic amines such as norepinephrine, serotonin, dopamine, and tyramine. Monoamine oxidase inhibitors block this inactivation and thereby increase the amount of these transmitters available for synaptic release. Currently available MAOIs are either hydrazine or nonhydrazine derivatives. The hydrazine derivatives, isocarboxazid and phenelzine, are related to iproniazid. The nonhydrazine derivatives include tranylcypromine and the antihypertensive drug pargyline (Table 18–6) MAO must be regenerated before the activity of the enzyme is reestablished. In practical terms, this means that the effects (including risks of drug and food interaction) of the "irreversible" MAO inhibitors will last until sufficient MAO has been regenerated. For this reason, the clinician must wait 10 to 14 days after discontinuation of these drugs before instituting other antidepressants or permitting certain drugs or foods that may interact adversely with the MAOIs.

Selegiline is a selective MAO-B inhibitor that is approved for use in the treatment of Parkinson's disease. At dosages greater than 20 mg/day, Selegiline is a nonselective MAO inhibitor and possesses antidepressant properties, although it is not used for the treatment of depression in the United States.

Indications and Efficacy

Although the antidepressant drugs have many potential therapeutic uses, the primary approved indication for these drugs is the treatment of depression that corresponds to the diagnosis of major depressive disorder. Approximately 70 to 80% of depressed patients respond to an adequate trial of an antidepressant. Among the other disorders that may respond to antidepressants are panic disorder, obsessive–compulsive disorder, enuresis, chronic pain, migraine headaches, bulimia, and attention-deficit hyperactivity disorder.

Patients with depression that is characterized by the symptoms of oversleeping, overeating, mood reactivity, and prominent anxiety ("atypical depression") may show a preferentially positive response to MAOIs. Monoamine oxidase inhibitors have even been suggested as the treatment of choice in this group of patients.

The role of lithium in the prevention and treatment of episodes of bipolar illness is discussed in detail in a later section. For patients with recurrent unipolar depressions, maintenance CyAD with and without lithium are effective in decreasing the chance of relapse.

Panic disorder responds to drugs from the CyAD (imipramine, desipramine), SSRIs, and MAOI (phenelzine, tranylcypromine) families of antidepressants. The use of SSRIs to treat panic disorder has also been recently explored and they may have efficacy in this condition as well as in depression.

Clinical Use of Antidepressants

The psychiatric history, current symptoms, physical examination, and mental status of patients with depressed mood are major factors in the choice of the appropriate therapeutic modality. Diagnostic factors that may influence the choice of antidepressant drug include a history of manic or hypomanic episodes, the presence of psychosis, the prior course of episodes of depression, and the presence of "atypical" symptoms.

A history of previous episodes of mania or hypomania should alert the clinician to the possible precipitation of these episodes with antidepressants. If hypomania occurs while the patient is on antidepressant therapy, a reduction in dosage should be attempted as a first effort to control these symptoms, or lithium alone should be used. Patients with bipolar disorder may experience more frequent mood cycling and general increases in resistance to treatment when treated chronically with CyAD. Precipitation of hypomania or mania in a depressed patient treated with CyAD or MAOI suggests that the patient has a bipolar mood disorder. Pretreatment with lithium in usual therapeutic doses before the administration of antidepressant drugs should be considered in depressed patients who have experienced previous manic episodes but concurrent treatment with lithium will not guarantee by any means that the patient will not develop hypomania or mania, nor will it ensure that the patient will not have more frequent manic/depressive episodes (increased cycling).

As noted, antidepressants have been shown to decrease the interval between affective episodes and increase "cycling" in bipolar patients. For bipolar patients who develop mixed manic-depressive states or increased cycling on antidepressants, lithium, carbamazepine, or valproate should be started, and the antidepressant drug should be gradually tapered. This effect should also be considered in unipolar depressed patients. Because of the demonstrated efficacy of lithium in the prevention of relapse in unipolar and bipolar patients (see section on lithium), the use of lithium should be considered in patients in whom the interval between episodes has been decreasing.

Patients with delusional (psychotic) depression respond poorly to treatment when antidepressant medications are used as the sole agent. Patients with delusional depression respond better to combined treatment of antidepressants *and* antipsychotics than to either alone but generally show the best response to electroconvulsive therapy.

Psychotherapy is vitally important in the treatment of patients with depression. Studies have demonstrated that the response to the combination of psychotherapy and medication is superior to that of either treatment as the sole modality (Conte et al, 1986).

Treatment of depressed patients with pharmacologic agents must be guided by scientific principles that are tailored to the needs of individual patients. This requires guidelines for initiation of therapy (see Table 18–7) in addition to an overall treatment strategy. As with the antipsychotic drugs, the choice of which antidepressant to use is often dependent on the side effect profile of the drug. In general, drugs with more potent effects on inhibiting norepinephrine reuptake are more stimulating. Thus, desipramine may be poorly tolerated in agitated, depressed patients. Drugs with marked antihistaminic effects and predominantly serotonergic effects (amitriptyline,

---

Table 18–7 Guidelines for Use of Cyclic Antidepressant (CyAD) Drugs*

1. Complete a thorough medical evaluation, especially with regard to cardiovascular and thyroid status.
2. Select drug on the basis of side-effect profile (stimulating effect, sedating effect, anticholinergic effect, and cardiovascular effect) and history of previous response.
3. Inform the patient and family of risks and benefits. Emphasize the expected 2–3 week "delay" in therapeutic response and anticipated side effects and their management.
4. Initiate and increase dose slowly (e.g., for imipramine, start at 25 mg qHs and increase by 25 mg every third day). Fluoxetine is usually given in the morning at 10–20 mg/day and if necessary can be increased to 20–40 mg/day after 3 weeks.
5. Increase dosage until dose equivalent of 150–200 mg imipramine is reached. Stablize at that dose for 1 week. Trazodone and amoxapine have higher therapeutic dose ranges (200–600 mg/day). Fluoxetine (20–40 mg/day) and protriptyline (10–40 mg/day) have a lower therapeutic range.
6. If there is no significant effect after 2 weeks, slowly increase dosage to maximum recommended dose.
7. If there is no significant improvement after 14–21 days, obtain plasma level (if appropriate) and electrocardiogram (if TCA) and adjust dose as needed (e.g., increase by 50 mg per week). An electrocardiogram should be obtained before each dose increase (if TCA) in patients with severe heart disease. Serum levels stabilize on a given dose after 7–10 days. Therapeutic serum levels are best established for imipramine, desipramine, and nortriptyline.
8. A therapeutic trial is defined as a 6-week treatment with antidepressant, with at least 3 weeks with a therapeutic serum level. Then consider an MAOI after a washout period or go to ECT immediately. Reevaluate diagnosis.
9. Elderly and medically ill patient may require lower dose ranges than those noted above.
10. Most of the currently available AD can be given once a day at bedtime; SSRI's and protriptyline should be given early in the day. Bupropion requires multiple daily doses.

* Note special exemptions *especially for fluoxetine.*
MAOI, Monoamine oxidase inhibitor; ECT, electroconvulsive therapy.
Silver JM, Yudofsky SC, Hurowitz G: Psychopharmacology and Electroconvulsive Therapy. In Hales RE, Yudofsky SC, Talbott JA (eds): The American Psychiatric Press Textbook of Psychiatry, 2nd ed. Washington, DC, American Psychiatric Press, 1994

doxepin, trazodone) are sedating. This effect may be advantageous in patients with marked initial insomnia but undesirable in patients with psychomotor retardation. The SSRIs with the exception of paroxetine have few anticholinergic effects and do not result in weight gain, although fluoxetine may be stimulating and cause insomnia, and sertraline and paroxetine may be associated with more gastrointestinal side effects such as nausea and/or diarrhea.

The initial therapeutic response of the depressed patient to medications may be detected as early as the first week with the patient showing improvement in sleep and energy. Mood, however, may not respond for 1 to 4 weeks after medication has been initiated. Of crucial importance is the fact that the patient may have a return of energy while still experiencing the hopelessness that characterizes the depression. Thus, the patient may be at an increased risk of suicide at this time, for she or he may regain energy requisite to complete a suicidal act that was not present before treatment.

A complete trial of antidepressant medication consists of treatment with therapeutic doses of a drug for a total of 6 weeks before concluding that the depression is refractory to standard pharmacotherapy. Once the patient's depressive symptoms have resolved, the dose of the antidepressant and the length of time necessary for continuance on the medication must be determined. Results from a National Institutes of Mental Health (NIMH) collaborative study indicate that antidepressant therapy should not be withdrawn before there have been 4 to 5 symptom-free months (Prien and Kupfer, 1986). After the maintenance phase of treatment, antidepressants should be gradually tapered over several months and discontinued. In patients with chronic depression, longer periods of antidepressant treatment are warranted to protect against recurrence.

For patients who have not responded to an adequate trial of one particular antidepressant, several strategies may be taken in choosing a drug for a subsequent trial. If the patient did not respond to an antidepressant of the "noradrenergic" type (e.g., desipramine), one that is more serotonergic may be tried, although there is no evidence to suggest that switching from one antidepressant to another has any real benefit other than adjustment in side effect profiles. In some patients who have shown an incomplete response to a single antidepressant, the addition of lithium has resulted in prompt and dramatic alleviation of the depressive symptoms. Thyroid hormone supplementation with T_3 preparations also has been reported to possibly potentiate antidepressant effects in tricyclic nonresponders.

Despite concerns over severe reactions that may occur with concomitant treatment with CyAD and MAOIs, the combination may be safely prescribed, provided specific precautions are taken, such as starting the medications together and ensuring that frequent, daily BP monitoring takes place during the "loading" phase of treatment. *Please note that it is extremely hazardous to add the CyAD to established MAOI treatment.* MAOIs cannot be prescribed with SSRIs. For patients on fluoxetine, MAOIs cannot be initiated until 5 weeks after fluoxetine has been discontinued.

Risks, Side Effects, and Their Management

The side effect profile of a specific antidepressant drug in large part determines the selection of a particular drug for an individual patient. In addition, patients have varying reactions to side effects when they occur. For example, for some patients, the almost omnipresent anticholinergic effects (i.e., dry mouth, blurred vision) of most CyAD are intolerable, while other patients note the presence of these side effects without complaint.

The antidepressant drugs vary greatly in their relative potential to produce anticholinergic side effects (see Table 7–12). Because of the anticholinergic effects, patients with prostatic hypertrophy and narrow angle glaucoma must be treated with caution. The precautions and evaluations of these complications are outlined in the section on antipsychotic drugs. Trazodone has anticholinergic effects only in higher doses, and SSRIs are almost devoid of such effects.

Trazodone, trimipramine, amitriptyline, and doxepin are most sedating. If this property is adversely experienced by the patient, a less-sedating antidepressant should be prescribed (e.g., desipramine or protriptyline). Fluoxetine has a generally activating effect and should be given in the morning.

Orthostatic hypotension is the cardiovascular side effect that most commonly results in serious morbidity, especially in the elderly and in patients with congestive heart failure. The symptoms of orthostatic hypotension usually consist of dizziness or lightheadedness when the patient changes from a lying to sitting or sitting to standing position. Although orthostatic hypotension may occur from any CyAD (especially the tertiary CyAD), nortriptyline has been found to cause less orthostatic hypotension than imipramine. Fluoxetine also probably has major advantages in this regard. The MAOIs also may cause significant hypotension.

Carefully controlled studies have demonstrated that some TCAs are potent antiarrhythmic agents and possess quinidine-like properties. Even trazodone has been reported to cause heart block as an idiosyncratic effect in a few patients. The effects of the TCA on the cardiac conduction system are of great clinical importance. Because prolongation of the PR and QRS intervals can occur with TCA use, these drugs should not be used in patients with preexisting heart block, such as second-degree heart block, or markedly prolonged QRS and QT intervals. In such patients, TCA can lead to second-degree or third-degree heart block—a life-threatening condition. Patients with relatively focal, benign, and stable right bundle and left bundle branch blocks may at times be treated with TCA after clearance by cardiology and dosing initiated in the inpatient setting with frequent cardiac monitoring. Information available to date suggests that bupropion and the SSRIs are free of clinically significant effects on the cardiac conductive system.

Sexual dysfunctions associated with CyAD antidepressants include impotence, ejaculatory dysfunction, and decreased interest and enjoyment of sexual activities for both men and women. Trazodone is the only antidepressant that has been associated with priapism, which may be irreversible and require surgical intervention. Sexual dysfunction is a common occurrence in patients treated with MAOIs and most frequently includes anorgasmia and impotence. More recently, delayed ejaculation in men as well as anorgasmia in both men and women have been reported with fluoxetine.

Patients treated with CyAD may experience an undesirable weight gain. This does not appear to relate to improvement of mood, as changes in weight and appetite are not correlated to response to treatment. Treatment of depressed patients with fluoxetine may actually be associated with weight loss.

As with most drugs, allergic and hypersensitivity reactions may occur with antidepressants but are extremely rare and may be connected to those pill forms that contain yellow dye with tartrazine. For more serious skin eruptions, the drug should be discontinued, preferably over several days to reduce the possibility of antidepressant withdrawal symptoms. Tremor is a common side effect of antidepressants, such as imipramine and desipramine, that affect predominantly the noradrenergic system. Dose reduction or changing the type of antidepressant may ultimately be required to alleviate the tremor.

The potential of antidepressants to induce seizures is difficult to assess. Maprotiline has been associated with seizures in both therapeutic and toxic doses, especially at doses above 200 mg/day. Amoxapine and desipramine may have a higher risk of seizures after overdosage than other antidepressant drugs. Amoxapine has dopamine-blocking activity and may cause extrapyramidal symptoms and rarely even tardive dyskinesia with chronic treatment. While there is an increased risk of seizures associated with the use of bupropion, this is low when single dosages do not exceed 150 mg and the total daily dosage is not greater than 450 mg. Patients with obvious risk factors for seizures (patients with epilepsy, head trauma, abnormal EEGs) should not be treated with bupropion.

Because the incidence of suicide and suicide attempts is high in depressed patients, deliberate overdosage with antidepressant drugs is a common occurrence. As many as 10,000 cases of antidepressant overdoses each year are attributed to suicide attempts. It is unfortunate that a population that is at high risk for suicide is trusted with drugs that have a low LD_{50}—a relatively low ceiling for toxic doses. For patients at high suicide risk, clinicians should consider giving only a week's supply of antidepressants. The SSRIs are relatively much less toxic in overdose situations as compared to tricyclics.

The major complications from overdose with CyAD drugs include those that arise from neuropsychiatric impairment, hypotension, cardiac arrhythmias, and seizures. Because most antidepressants have significant anticholinergic activity, anticholinergic delirium often occurs when the CyAD are taken in high doses. Other complications of anticholinergic overdose include agitation, supraventricular arrhythmias, heart block, hallucinations, severe hypertension, and seizures. These drugs also lower the seizure threshold and can result in prolonged seizures.

Because the CyAD are metabolized by the liver, drugs that induce hepatic microsomal enzymes will result in a decrease in plasma levels of the antidepressant drugs. These agents include alcohol, anticonvulsants, barbiturates, chloral hydrate, glutethimide, oral contraceptives, and cigarette smoking. Antipsychotic drugs, methylphenidate, SSRIs, and increasing age are associated with increased plasma levels of the tricyclics.

Most clinical concern regarding the use of the MAOIs stems from the reaction that occurs when ingested tyramine is not metabolized because of the MAOI inactivation of intestinal monoamine oxidase. This reaction has been called the "cheese reaction" because tyramine is present in relatively high concentrations in aged cheese. Tyramine may act as a false transmitter and displace norepinephrine from presynaptic storage granules.

Patients receiving MAOI treatment should be instructed to avoid cheeses (except cottage cheese and cream cheese), alcohol (except clear spirits and white wine), yeast extract, broad beans, smoked or pickled fish, beef or chicken liver, fermented sausage, and stewed bananas (Folks, 1983). In addition, certain general anesthetics and drugs that have sympathomimetic activity—including certain decongestant sympathomimetics such as phenylpropanolamine—should not be taken while a patient is being treated with an MAOI. Ephedrine and pseudoephedrine may be constituents of "over-the-counter" drugs. Local anesthetics that contain epinephrine must not be used. Appetite suppressants must be avoided. Synthetic and natural opioids should be used with caution. Meperidine (Demerol) must be absolutely avoided because of a potentially catastrophic lethal interaction with MAOIs. The fact that SSRIs such as fluoxetine may cause hypertension when used with MAOIs has been previously mentioned.

The tyramine reaction can range from mild to severe. In the most mild form, the patient may complain of sweating, palpitations, and a mild headache. The most severe form manifests as a hypertensive crisis, with severe headache, increases in blood pressure, and possible intracerebral hemorrhage. The severity of this reaction cannot be predicted by MAOI dose, food type or amount ingested, or even prior history of a crisis. For example, a patient may ingest cheese without any reaction at one time but may have a life-threatening hypertensive crisis on a subsequent occasion when he combines the same amount of cheese with the same dose of MAOI. For this reason, patients should be carefully instructed not only about prevention but also about not gaining false confidence if dietary guidelines are broken without immediate consequences.

There is no adequate published study that establishes the optimum treatment of this reaction. Treatment strategies have relied on clinical experience and published case reports. If patients on MAOIs experience a severe or even moderately painful occipital headache, they should immediately seek medical assessment, which will include having their blood pressure monitored. If the blood pressure is severely elevated, a drug with alpha-adrenergic blocking properties, such as intravenous phentolamine (Regitine) 5 mg or intramuscular chlorpromazine 25 to 50 mg, may be administered. Because treatment with phentolamine may be associated with cardiac arrhythmias or severe hypotension, however, this should be done only in an emergency room setting by qualified medical personnel with proper monitoring equipment. It is advisable to have patients on MAOIs carry an identification card or Medic Alert bracelet as notification to emergency medical personnel that the patient is currently taking MAOIs. Patients should always carry lists of prohibited foods and medications and should be told to notify physicians that they are taking an MAOI before accepting a medication or anesthetic. A frequently encountered situation is when the patient has dental procedures performed. In this instance, local anesthetics must be used without vasoconstrictors (e.g., epinephrine). Carrying supplies of nifedipine to take in case of emergency (10 mg sublingually) has also been recommended.

ANXIOLYTICS, SEDATIVES, AND HYPNOTICS

Anxiety disorders are the most frequently diagnosed psychiatric illnesses in the general population, with a 6-month prevalence rate approaching 16% (Reich, 1986). Approximately one-third of the population suffers from insomnia during the course of a year, and 4% of adults use a medically prescribed drug to produce sleep (Mellinger, Balter, and Uhlenhuth, 1985).

Given these figures, it is to be expected that drugs that produce sedation and reduce anxiety historically have been the most widely used drugs. The commonly used anxiolytics and hypnotics and usual dosages are shown in Table 18–8.

Mechanisms of Action

The existence of benzodiazepine receptor-binding sites has been confirmed by positron emission tomography (PET) using radiolabeled benzodiazepines. These

Table 18–8 **Selected Anxiolytic Drugs: Dosages and Half-Lives**

CLASS/GENERIC NAME	TRADE NAME	USUAL DAILY DOSE (mg)	APPROXIMATE ELIMINATION T$\frac{1}{2}$ INCLUDING METABOLITES
Benzodiazepine Anxiolytics			
Alprazolam	Xanax	0.75–1.5, generalized anxiety disorder	12 hours
		2–6, panic disorder	
Chlordiazepoxide	Librium	15–100	1–4 days
	Libritabs		
Clorazepate	Tranxene	15–60	2–4 days
Clonazepam	Klonopin	1–4	1–2 days
Diazepam	Valium	4–40	2–4 days
	Valrelease	15–45	
Halazepam	Paxipam	40–160	2–4 days
Lorazepam	Ativan	2–6	12 hours
Benzodiazepine Hypnotics			
Estazolam	Prosom	1–2	10–24 hours
Quazepam	Doral	7.5–15	3 days
Oxazepam	Serax	30–120	12 hours
Prazepam	Centrax	20–60	2–4 days
Flurazepam	Dalmane	30	3 days
Temazepam	Restoril	30	12 hours
Triazolam	Halcion	0.125–0.25	4–6 hours
Barbiturates			
Phenobarbital		30–120	2–4 days
Amobarbital	Amytal	50–300	1–2 days
Secobarbital	Seconal	100–200	1–2 days
Nonbenzodiazepines/Nonbarbiturates			
Hydroxyzine hydrochloride	Atarax	75–400	Less than 4 hours
Hydroxyzine pamoate	Vistaril	200–400	
Diphenhydramine*	Benadryl	25–50	
Chloral hydrate		750 (sedation)	Less than 12 hours
		500–1000 (hypnotic)	
Azapirone			
Buspirone	Buspar	15–60	2–7 hours

* Diphenhydramine, while an antihistamine, is also a hypnotic and has strong anticholinergic properties.
Silver JM, Yudofsky SC, Hurowitz G: Psychopharmacology and Electroconvulsive Therapy. In Hales RE, Yudofsky SC, Talbott JA (eds): The American Psychiatric Press Textbook of Psychiatry, 2nd ed. Washington, DC, American Psychiatric Press, 1994

receptors are intimately linked with the receptor for gamma-aminobutyric acid (GABA), the major inhibitory neurotransmitter in the brain. Administration of GABA results in an opening of chloride channels and a decrease in neuronal activity.

The mechanism of action of buspirone, a nonbenzodiazepine anxiolytic, remains unclear. The drug has effects on many systems, especially the serotonergic and dopaminergic systems. One primary mode of biological activity is that it serves as a "partial agonist" of the serotonin IA receptor, meaning that its activity depends on whether it is in a cellular milieu that is either hyper- or hypoactivated in regard to serotonin neurotransmission. It is believed that buspirone has a modulation or normalizing effect on serotonin neurotransmission, augmenting deficient serotonin neurotransmission or serving to downregulate overactivated systems. Few of these actions are similar to those of the benzodiazepines, and cross-tolerance does not exist between buspirone and the benzodiazepines.

Indications and Efficacy

Benzodiazepines

The efficacy of the benzodiazepines in the treatment of anxiety, including symptoms of worry, psychic anxiety, and somatic symptoms (gastrointestinal and cardiovascular), has been clearly and repeatedly demonstrated in many well-controlled studies.

Benzodiazepines have been shown effective in the treatment of panic attacks. These include alprazolam (Xanax), diazepam (Valium), lorazepam (Ativan), and clonazepam (Klonopin). Some clinicians have raised concerns about the development of dependency on these drugs when used in the long-term treatment of panic disorder.

Although only a few benzodiazepines have specific FDA-approved indications for the treatment of insomnia, almost all benzodiazepines may be used for this purpose. The three benzodiazepines most commonly used as hypnotics are flurazepam (Dalmane), temazepam (Restoril), and triazolam (Halcion). Each has different pharmacodynamic and pharmacokinetic profiles that importantly influence clinical application.

Buspirone (Buspar)

Double-blind, controlled studies have shown that buspirone is efficacious in the treatment of generalized anxiety, and its efficacy is not statistically different from that of the benzodiazepines provided the drug is given in therapeutic doses (20 to 60 mg/day) and for a sufficient period of time (at least 3 to 4 weeks). It is reported that buspirone, unlike the previously available anxiolytics, is not sedating, has no dangerous interactions with alcohol, has a low dependence liability, and does not impair psychomotor performance. At higher dosages, buspirone may have antidepressant effects. Common side effects include dizziness, nausea, headache, and increased anxiety.

Clinical Use of Anxiolytic and Sedative Drugs

Pharmacotherapy of Generalized Anxiety Disorder

The first step in the treatment of a patient with anxiety is a thorough medical, neurological, and psychiatric evaluation. Many patients with the symptoms of generalized anxiety disorder either have or have had panic disorder. The presence of panic attacks changes the focus of treatment. Medications should be considered as only one component in the treatment of anxiety. Psychotherapy is required to help the patient understand and control the circumstances that surround the anxiety. For most patients, anxiolytic medications are indicated only for relatively short-term use (i.e., 1 to 2 months), although some patients may require more prolonged treatment. The benzodiazepines generally are contraindicated in patients with sleep apnea and patients with a history of alcohol and drug abuse.

Because benzodiazepines frequently cause sedation, may impair performance on tasks that require a high degree of mental alertness, and may lead to dependence, this class of drugs should be used for as brief a period of time as possible in the lowest effective dose (see Table 18–9).

Several clinically important facets of the anxiolytic response to buspirone differentiate it from the benzodiazepines. Buspirone does not interact with other sedating drugs (including alcohol), does not seem to impair mechanical performance such as driving, and is not associated with dependence, tolerance, or withdrawal. It also does not have muscle relaxant or anticonvulsant properties, as do the benzodiazepines. Studies suggest that response to buspirone occurs in approximately 2 weeks, as compared with the more rapid onset associated with benzodiazepines.

Pharmacotherapy of Panic Disorder

Many patients who have the symptoms of generalized anxiety disorder either currently have or have had a history of panic disorder. Anxiety may develop in response to frequent spontaneous panic attacks, termed "anticipatory anxiety." Breier, Charney, and Heninger (1986) have reported that over 80% of patients with panic disorder or agoraphobia with panic attacks have anticipatory or generalized anxiety that is responsive to treatment with benzodiazepines.

Table 18–9 Guidelines for Anxiolytic Treatment with Benzodiazepines

1. Complete a thorough medical evaluation, especially with regard to thyroid status, caffeine intake, and current medications. Include a thorough evaluation of drug and alcohol history. Patients with sleep apnea should not receive benzodiazepines.
2. Evaluate patient for psychodynamic and social factors that may contribute to or precipitate anxiety.
3. Initiate benzodiazepines at a iow dose (e.g., diazepam 2 mg three times a day) and increase every few days until sedation or therapeutic effect is obtained (up to 15 mg three times a day).
4. Caution patient on sedative properties, performance impairment, dependence properties, and drug and alcohol interactions.
5. Set guidelines for duration of expected treatment clearly to the patient in advance.
6. Reevaluate need for medication every month. Avoid refills by telephone.
7. Taper medication as soon as possible, by approximately 10% per week for patients on long-term treatment (greater than 3 months).
8. In patients with chronic anxiety or prone to anxiety and requesting or needing chronic therapy, obtain a psychiatric consultation.

Silver JM, Yudofsky SC, Hurowitz G: Psychopharmacology and Electroconvulsive Therapy. In Hales RE, Yudofsky SC, Talbott JA (eds): The American Psychiatric Press Textbook of Psychiatry, 2nd ed. Washington, DC, American Psychiatric Press, 1994

Drugs from several families of psychotropic medications may be used in the treatment of panic disorder. The benzodiazepines, specifically alprazolam and clonazepam, have been shown effective. These medications should be initiated at relatively low doses (e.g., alprazolam 0.25 mg t.i.d. or clonazepam 0.5 mg b.i.d.) and increased gradually over 1 to 2 weeks. After successful treatment of panic disorder with alprazolam, withdrawal and discontinuation of medication are difficult because of increased panic attacks and occurrence of withdrawal symptoms, including malaise, weakness, insomnia, tachycardia, lightheadedness, and dizziness. Discontinuation of these medications should be extremely slow (10% per 1 week).

Because panic disorder usually requires a prolonged period for successful treatment, benzodiazepines may be associated with an increased risk of dependence. Therefore, we recommend the use of antidepressants be considered as the initial treatment of panic disorder. For most patients, imipramine, desipramine, or nortriptyline should prove effective. A decision as to which of these drugs to choose should be based on the same factors discussed in the section on antidepressant drugs. Monoamine oxidase inhibitors are usually reserved for patients who have not responded to CyAD, although they may be used as a primary treatment. Fluoxetine is an effective treatment but must be started at low dosages (i.e., 2.5 to 5 mg) since patients with panic attacks are highly sensitive to the anxiogenic effects of this drug. The doses, durations, and side effects of antidepressants used for the treatment of panic disorder parallel those described in the previous section for the treatment of depression.

Patients with panic disorder are exceedingly sensitive to a temporary exacerbation or worsening of symptoms in the first weeks of treatment with CyAD or SSRIs. Therefore, doses should be started very low and increased in lower increments. The treatment of panic and other anxiety disorders is discussed in detail in Chapter 8.

Pharmacotherapy of Insomnia

A complete medical, sleep, and psychiatric history is required before administration of drugs to produce sleep. There are multiple causes for insomnia, and the differential diagnosis of sleep disorders must be considered before the prescribing of any hypnotic. Among the common disorders associated with insomnia are depression, psychoses, anxiety, central nervous system disorders, and other medical illnesses associated with pain and discomfort. Stimulants (including caffeine) as well as alcohol may lead to insomnia.

The individual hypnotic benzodiazepines have varying pharmacodynamic and pharmacokinetic profiles that importantly influence their use in clinical practice. For example, flurazepam is rapidly absorbed and metabolized into compounds with a half-life as long as several days and may result in daytime sedation. Triazolam is a benzodiazepine hypnotic with an intermediate rate of absorption and a very short half-life (1.5 to 5 hours). The rapid elimination of this drug may lead to early-morning awakening, rebound insomnia, dissociative reactions, and anterograde amnesia.

Pharmacotherapy of Obsessive–Compulsive Disorder

It appears that the usual antidepressants and anxiolytics are not generally effective in the treatment of obsessive–compulsive disorder. Clomipramine has been extensively studied in the treatment of this disorder and is significantly beneficial compared to other antidepressants. It is the only drug that has been approved for the treatment of obsessive–compulsive disorder. A member of the TCA family, its major side effects are sedation and anticholinergic effects. Fluoxetine is also effective in the treatment of obsessive–compulsive disorder in higher doses (60–80 mg/day).

Risks and Side Effects of Anxiolytic and Hypnotic Drugs

The production of sedation by benzodiazepines may be considered either a therapeutic action or a side effect. Hypnotics are expected and required to produce sedation to be efficacious. However, when the patient complains of sleepiness the following day, this therapeutic action becomes a side effect.

Physical dependence may occur when benzodiazepines are taken in dosages higher than usual or for prolonged periods of time. If precipitously discontinued, severe withdrawal symptoms (hyperpyrexia, seizures, psychosis, and death) may occur. Other symptoms of withdrawal may include tachycardia, increased blood pressure, muscle cramps, anxiety, insomnia, panic attacks, impairment of memory and concentration, and perceptual disturbances. These withdrawal symptoms may begin as soon as the day after discontinuing benzodiazepines and may continue for weeks to months.

As a general principle for all drugs, discontinuation should be accomplished gradually. For patients treated with benzodiazepines for longer than 2 to 3 months, we suggest that the dose be decreased by approximately 5 to 10% a week. Thus, for a patient receiving 4 mg/day of alprazolam, the dose should be tapered by 0.25 mg per week for 16 weeks. The last few dosage levels may be the most difficult to discontinue, and the patient will require increased attention and support from the physician at this time. Clonazepam may be substituted for alprazolam to assist with the discontinuation process. Since clonazepam has a prolonged half-life, tapering can be accomplished with less rebound anxiety than occurs with alprazolam withdrawal.

Buspirone, when administered to subjects who had histories of recreational sedative abuse, showed no abuse potential. Buspirone has almost no abuse potential and is relatively nontoxic in overdose situations.

Overdose

Benzodiazepines are remarkably safe when taken in overdose. Dangerous effects occur when the overdose includes several sedative drugs, especially alcohol. As with most medications, use of anxiolytics during pregnancy or when breastfeeding should be avoided whenever possible.

Drug Interactions

Most sedative drugs, including narcotics and alcohol, potentiate sedation from benzodiazepines. Cimetidine, oral contraceptives, acute alcohol intake, propranolol, and disulfiram inhibit the hepatic metabolism and increase the elimination half-life of benzodiazepines that are metabolized by oxidation, which include diazepam and chlordiazepoxide. However, benzodiazepines such as lorazepam, oxazepam, and temazepam are metabolized by glucuronide conjugation, and therefore their half-life is not affected by liver disease, aging, and medication, all of which affect oxidative capacities in the liver associated with the drugs just cited. Buspirone does *not* appear to interact with alcohol to increase sedation and motor impairment.

Barbiturates

The use of barbiturates for the treatment of anxiety (and insomnia) has been largely supplanted by the much safer benzodiazepines. With barbiturates, potentially fatal respiratory depression can occur at only several times the standard therapeutic dosages. Barbiturates are potent inducers of hepatic microsomal enzymes and therefore interact with many other drugs that are metabolized in the liver.

The clinical use of barbiturates is determined by their respective onsets of action and half-lives. The ultra-short barbiturates thiopental (Pentothal) and methohexital (Brevital) are used primarily as intravenous agents for the induction of general anesthesia. Amobarbital (Amytal), pentobarbital (Nembutal), and secobarbital (Seconal) have been used as sedative agents. Amobarbital is also valuable for the acute management of agitated patients when administered parenterally in doses of approximately 250 mg. Phenobarbital, a long-acting barbiturate, may be used as an anxiolytic agent, although tolerance to this effect occurs after several weeks. The principal clinical application of phenobarbital is as an anticonvulsant drug.

Alcohol Detoxification

Because of the cross-tolerance of benzodiazepines and alcohol, the benzodiazepines are used frequently for the treatment of alcohol withdrawal and detoxification. A relatively simple procedure for treating alcohol withdrawal is the benzodiazepine loading dose technique. This technique takes advantage of the long half-life of benzodiazepines such as diazepam and chlordiazepoxide. Unit doses of 20 mg diazepam (or 100 mg chlordiazepoxide) are administered hourly to patients until there are no signs or symptoms of alcohol withdrawal. Thereafter, no further doses of benzodiazepines are administered. Because of the long half-lives of benzodiazepines, the therapeutic plasma level of the benzodiazepine is maintained during the period of risk for alcohol withdrawal symptoms (see also Chapters 10 by Dr. Swift and 19 by Dr. Dubin).

ANTIMANIC DRUGS

Clinical investigations have conclusively demonstrated that lithium is effective in the prophylaxis of recurrent mood (affective) disorders. For the patient with acute mania, treatment with antipsychotic drugs and electroconvulsive therapy is efficacious. In fact, these treatments elicit responses more rapidly than does lithium carbonate, and they are often administered while awaiting the therapeutic response to lithium. Other classes of drugs with different chemical structures and with apparently different mechanisms of actions have been reported to be effective in the prophylaxis and treatment of mania. Among these are the anticonvulsant drugs carbamazepine (Tegretol) and valproic acid (Depakote), the calcium channel-blocking drug verapamil (Calan and Isoptin), the alpha-adrenergic agonist clonidine (Catapres), the benzodiazepine anticonvulsant clonazepam (Klonopin), and the beta-adrenergic receptor-blocking drug propranolol (Inderal). In this section we will review the clinical use of lithium, carbamazepine and valproic acid for which the efficacy in bipolar disorder is well established (Table 18–10). The other drugs mentioned above are not routinely used to treat bipolar illness and their efficacy is questionable.

Lithium

Mechanism of Action

Despite extensive investigations, lithium's mechanism of action remains unknown, but it may reduce the sensitivity of neurotransmitter receptors (including dopamine, acetylcholine, serotonin, and opiates) as well as reduce receptor density of multiple transmitter systems. The antidepressant efficacy of lithium is most likely due to its ability to enhance serotonergic activity. Antimanic effects may result from effects in supersensitive, dopaminergic receptors or muscarinic–cholinergic enhancing action as well as in down regulating neuronal second messenger systems.

Indications and Efficacy

Lithium, usually administered as the carbonate salt, has been shown efficacious in the treatment of many of the mood disorders. Acute manic episodes respond to treatment with lithium within 7 to 10 days. Because manic episodes have so great a potential for psychosocial disruption, behavioral control is usually desired before lithium becomes effective. Supplemental medication (most often antipsychotic drugs), therefore, is administered on an acute basis. Lithium has been proved effective and is the drug of choice for preventing both manic and depressive episodes in patients with bipolar disorder (Consensus Development Panel, 1985). Patients with less-severe bipolar illness, such as cyclothymia or bipolar II disorder (patients with episodes of major depression punctuated by periods of hypomania), may also exhibit improvement with lithium therapy.

Table 18–10 **Antimanic Drugs**

CLASS/GENERIC NAME	TRADE NAME	USUAL DOSE RANGE (mg/day)	PLASMA LEVELS
Lithium			
Lithium carbonate	Eskalith Lithane Lithonate Lithotabs	600–1800	0.6–1.2 mEq/l
Time-release	Eskalith CR		
Lithium citrate (syrup)	Cibalith-S		
Carbamazepine	Tegretol	800–1200	8–12 µg/ml
Valproic acid	Depakene Depakote	750–1000	50–100 µg/ml

Lithium may be effective in the prevention of future depressive episodes in those patients with recurrent unipolar depressive disorder (Consensus Development Panel, 1985) and as an adjunct to antidepressants in patients partially refractory to treatment with antidepressants alone (discussed in the section on antidepressants). Finally, lithium may be useful in the maintenance of remission of depression after electroconvulsive therapy.

Clinical Use

Before the initiation of treatment, patients should be informed of side effects that occur commonly with lithium treatment, which include nausea, diarrhea, polyuria, polydipsia, thirst, fine hand tremor, and fatigue. These may be transient or, in some patients, may persist with therapeutic lithium levels. Women of childbearing age should have a pregnancy test and be advised that lithium has been reported to cause fetal cardiac defects (Ebstein's anomaly) when taken in the first trimester.

Because of the narrow range between the therapeutic and toxic doses of lithium, the optimum dose for an individual patient cannot be based on the dosage administered but rather should be based on the concentration of lithium in the plasma. Thus, appropriate use of lithium requires familiarity with its pharmacokinetics. Lithium is completely absorbed by the gastrointestinal tract and reaches peak plasma levels in 1 to 2 hours. The elimination half-life is approximately 20 to 24 hours. Steady-state lithium levels are obtained in approximately 5 days.

Therapeutic plasma levels for patients on lithium therapy range from 0.5 to 1.5 mEq/L. Most healthy patients may be conservatively started on a 300 mg b.i.d. dosage of lithium, and this dose may be increased by 300 mg every 3 to 4 days. Larger "loading" doses may be used in acute manic states (e.g., 1200 mg/day in divided doses). Elderly patients are extremely sensitive to the neurotoxic side effects of lithium and generally should be treated with doses of lithium that produce serum levels at the lower end of the therapeutic range. In the healthy patient with no renal function impairment, plasma level determinations are obtained biweekly. Since steady-state plasma levels are not obtained until the patient has been on a constant dose regimen for at least 5 days, this method may slightly underestimate the steady-state level. Lithium levels must consistently be obtained 12 hours after the last lithium dose. After therapeutic lithium levels have been established, levels should be monitored every month for the first 6 months and every 2 to 3 months thereafter. GI side effects can be minimized by having patients take their lithium after meals.

The frequency of lithium dosing needs to be considered individually for each patient. Since lithium has a serum half-life of approximately 24 hours, the administration of lithium as a single daily dose is possible. For example, for the patient receiving a maintenance dose of lithium of 1200 mg/day, a dosing regimen of either 1200 mg once a day or 300 mg four times a day is theoretically possible. In addition, there are slow release formulations available that maintain a higher plasma level throughout the day, while multiple doses with the usual carbonate salt will result in several peak levels throughout the day that rapidly decrease after ingestion of each dose. Both regimens are therapeutically effective and well tolerated by most patients. However, there are specific reasons for choosing differing dose regimens. The multiple-dose regimen will expose the kidney to four peak levels of intermediate concentration, while the single daily dosing regimen will expose the kidney to one higher peak dose. It has been suggested that nephrotoxicity (if indeed it occurs with lithium) is related to the duration of exposure to high lithium levels and not the absolute level of a single peak level. For this reason, single daily dosing with the usual formulation may be preferable. Gastric irritation may be associated with the duration of the peak plasma level, and lithium should always be taken on a full stomach as noted above (see Table 18–11).

Risks, Side Effects, and Their Management

Most of the effects of lithium on the kidney are reversible after discontinuation of the drug. Although permanent morphologic changes in renal structure have been reported, the exact clinical implications of these changes have yet to be established. Renal function tests are required before lithium therapy is initiated and at specified intervals throughout the course of treatment.

The most noticeable effect of lithium on renal function is the vasopressin-resistant impairment in the kidney's ability to concentrate urine. This is nephrogenic diabetes insipidus (NDI), and it may result in polyuria. A majority of patients on lithium therapy may complain of increased frequency of urination. Preventive and management strategies for NDI include decreasing the daily lithium dose and increasing liquid intake. Amiloride 5 mg b.i.d. has been suggested as a treatment for polyuria because of its effect on blunting the inhibitory effect of lithium on water transport in the renal collecting tubule (Battle et al, 1985). This treatment was reported to be effective and did not increase lithium levels. Nevertheless, it is prudent to continue to monitor serum lithium levels when amiloride is combined with lithium.

Lithium nephropathy, characterized by tubular interstitial nephritis, has been reported as a consequence of long-term lithium therapy. Although mild decreases in the glomerular filtration rate (GFR) occur in some patients treated with lithium, there have been no published reports of irreversible renal failure as a result of chronic nontoxic lithium therapy.

In all patients treated with lithium, renal function tests should be monitored, but whether or not lithium has any nephrotoxic effects with long-term use is controversial.

Table 18–11 **Guidelines for Lithium Treatment**

1. Complete a thorough medical evaluation.
2. Complete appropriate medical laboratory evaluations.
3. Inform patient and family of proper use of lithium. Include common side effects, importance of monitoring lithium levels, exact procedures for accurate lithium monitoring, early signs and symptoms ot toxicity, potential long-term side effects, and warnings regarding pregnancy during treatment (if patient is female).
4. Initiate therapy at 300 mg twice a day and increase by 300 mg every 3 to 4 days.
5. Obtain lithium levels (12 hours after last dose) twice a week, until lithium level is approximately 1.0 mEq/L.
6. Treatment of acute manic symptoms may require concomitant therapy with antipsychotic medications.
7. Repeat lithium levels every month for the first 6 months, then every 2 to 3 months.

Silver JM, Yudofsky SC, Hurowitz G: Psychopharmacology and Electroconvulsive Therapy. In Hales RE, Yudofsky SC, Talbott JA (eds): The American Psychiatric Press Textbook of Psychiatry, 2nd ed. Washington, DC, American Psychiatric Press, 1994

Preliminary laboratory evaluations include serum testing for blood urea nitrogen (BUN), creatinine, and electrolytes, and a urinalysis. Some conservative clinicians recommend a 24-hour collection of urine to measure the creatinine clearance. Impairment in concentrating urine may be assessed by the 12-hour fluid deprivation test, wherein the patient first refrains from drinking any fluid for 12 hours. After this time, a urine specimen is collected, and the urine osmolality is measured. A urine specific gravity of less than 1.010 may imply disordered kidney function and may indicate that further specific renal function studies are required.

Hypothyroidism may occur in as many as 20% of patients treated with lithium (Myers et al, 1985). Many patients have an elevation of thyroid antibody titer during lithium treatment. Lithium-induced hypothyroidism may be less likely in patients who do not have antithyroid antibodies present before treatment.

Initial laboratory tests include T3 RU (resin uptake), T4 RIA (radioimmunoassay), T4I (free thyroxine index), and thyroid-stimulating hormone (TSH). TSH is the most sensitive of these tests for detecting hypothyroidism. Because of the association between the presence of antithyroid antibodies and the subsequent development of hypothyroidism, antithyroid antibodies should also be measured before lithium treatment. Thyroid-stimulating hormone should be reassessed after every 6 months of lithium therapy. If laboratory tests indicate the development of hypothyroidism (such as an elevated TSH level), the patient should be evaluated clinically for signs and symptoms of hypothyroidism. In collaboration with the endocrinologist, the psychiatrist should decide on the appropriate treatment, which may include low doses of supplementation of thyroid replacement.

The effects of lithium on calcium metabolism may be related to very rare reports of possible lithium-induced hyperparathyroidism. Hyperparathyroidism is associated with neuropsychiatric symptoms, which include mood changes, anxiety, psychosis, delirium, and dementia.

Lithium therapy may be associated with several types of neurologic dysfunction. Fine resting tremor is a neurologic side effect that may be detected in as many as one-half of patients in lithium treatment. Severe neurotoxic reactions occur with toxic lithium levels, and these symptoms include dysarthria, ataxia, and intention tremor, which also may occur with lithium levels in the "therapeutic range." Complaints of impairment of memory and concentration are relatively infrequent. Elderly patients are much more sensitive to these reactions, and they occur at lower serum levels.

Mitchell and Mackenzie (1982) reported changes in T-wave morphology on the electrocardiogram (flattening or inversion) in 20 to 30% of patients on lithium. Before the initiation of treatment with lithium, all patients should have a complete cardiac evaluation, including history and physical examination pertinent to the cardiovascular system and an electrocardiogram in patients over 40 years old. Clinically significant cardiac side effects with lithium are extremely rare.

Weight gain is a frequent side effect of lithium treatment. Patients with polydipsia may drink fluids with a high caloric content, such as carbonated soft drinks, and thereby gain weight. Weight gain may also be a direct effect of lithium therapy. Possible mechanisms include influences on carbohydrate metabolism, changes in glucose tolerance, or changes in lipid metabolism.

The most frequent dermatologic reaction is skin rash, which is reported in up to 7% of lithium-treated patients. Hair loss and hair thinning have also been reported.

Gastrointestinal difficulties are frequent, especially nausea and diarrhea. While these symptoms may be manifestations of toxicity, they also occur at lithium levels within the therapeutic range. Gastrointestinal symptoms may improve with reducing the dose, changing to a slow-release formulation, or ingesting lithium with meals.

The most frequent hematologic abnormality detected in patients on lithium is leukocytosis (approximately 15,000 white blood cells per mm^3). This change is generally benign and may, in fact, be used to treat several conditions associated with depressed granulocytes. Lithium-induced leukocytosis is readily reversible with discontinuation of lithium therapy. Before initiation of therapy with lithium, a white blood cell count with differential should be obtained and should be repeated at yearly intervals thereafter.

Because of the narrow range between therapeutic and toxic plasma lithium levels, the psychiatrist must allow sufficient time to inform the patient and the family about the signs, symptoms, and treatment of lithium toxicity (see Table 18–12). The patient must be made aware of circumstances that may increase the chances of toxicity, such as drinking insufficient amounts of fluids, becoming overheated with increased perspiration, or ingesting too much medication. The psychiatrist must emphasize the prevention of lithium toxicity through the maintenance of adequate salt and water intake, especially during hot weather and exercise. The signs and symptoms of lithium toxicity can be divided into those which usually occur with lithium levels at 1.5 to 2.0 mEq/L, 2.0 to 2.5 mEq/L, and >2.5 mEq/L; these are listed in Table 18–12. The drug should *not* be given to women who are pregnant or who are likely to become pregnant, due to toxic fetal effects.

Drug Interactions

Diuretics increase lithium levels and should be used with caution when treating lithium-induced diabetes insipidus. Specific nonsteroidal antiinflammatory drugs (NSAIDs) such as indomethacin also can increase the plasma lithium level. Theophylline will increase renal clearance and result in a lower lithium level.

Lithium has been reported to increase the intracellular levels of some antipsychotic drugs and may aggravate the inherent neurotoxicity of these agents as well. Thiazide diuretics raise lithium levels and, if used, warrants close monitoring of lithium levels. Furosemide and spironolactone appear to affect lithium levels minimally.

Anticonvulsant Mood Stabilizers

Evidence from controlled studies indicates that the anticonvulsants carbamazepine, and valproic acid are effective in both the acute treatment and the prophylactic treatment of mania in some patients with bipolar disorder. These findings have largely been confirmed in bipolar patients unresponsive to lithium or in bipolar patients unable to tolerate lithium-induced side effects (Keck et al, 1992). Also, patients with frequent recurrences (including rapid cycling bipolar patients) may respond more favorably to these drugs.

Table 18–12 **Signs and Symptoms of Lithium Toxicity**

Mild to Moderate Intoxication (Lithium Level 1.5–2.0 mEq/L)

Gastrointestinal
  Vomiting
  Abdominal pain
  Dryness of mouth
Neurological
  Ataxia
  Dizziness
  Slurred speech
  Nystagmus
  Lethargy or excitement
  Muscle weakness

Moderate to Severe Intoxication (Lithium Level 2.0–2.5 mEq/L)

Gastrointestinal
  Anorexia
  Persistent nausea and vomiting
Neurological
  Blurred vision
  Muscle fasciculations
  Clonic limb movements
  Hyperactive deep tendon reflexes
  Choreoathetoid movements
  Convulsions
  Delirium
  Syncope
  Electroencephalographic changes
  Stupor
  Coma
  Circulatory failure (lowered blood pressure, cardiac arrhythmias, and conduction abnormalities)

Severe Lithium Intoxication (Lithium Level >2.5 mEq/L)

Generalized convulsions
Oliguria and renal failure
Death

Mechanism of Action

Carbamazepine and valproic acid have multiple effects on the central nervous system that may have a role in the treatment of psychiatric disorders. Of particular interest is the effect of carbamazepine on "limbic kindling" and the hypothesis that this mechanism relates to the pathophysiology of affective disorders. In the process of kindling, repetitive stimuli eventually may lead to either a behavioral or convulsive response. Carbamazepine and valproic acid have been shown to inhibit the development of this response.

Clinical Use

Carbamazepine should be initiated at a dosage of 200 mg twice a day. Dose increments of 200 mg/day every 5 to 7 days should be made until a plasma level of 4 to 12 μg/ml is obtained. Too-rapid increases in dose may lead to dizziness, ataxia, and other adverse reactions. Although the maximum recommended dosage of carbamazepine by the manufacturer is 1200 mg/day, some investigators have administered higher dosages for the treatment of mania. Valproic acid should be initiated at a dosage of 250 mg twice a day. The dose is increased by 250 mg approximately every 5 days until a plasma level between 50 and 100 μg/ml is obtained. Treatment principles for the use of these anticonvulsants are listed in Table 18–13.

Risks, Side Effects, and Their Management

The most serious toxic hematologic side effects of carbamazepine are aplastic anemia, with a prevalence rate of less than 1/50,000 (Hart and Easton, 1982), and leukopenia (total white blood cell count of less than 3,000 cells per mm^3), with a prevalence of approximately 10%. Persistent leukopenia and thrombocytopenia occur in approximately 2% of patients, and "mild anemia" occurs in fewer than 5% of patients.

Hart and Easton (1982) recommend obtaining blood and platelet counts before carbamazepine therapy and complete blood counts every 2 weeks for the first 2 months, and quarterly thereafter (see Table 18–13). Patients with abnormal results on baseline tests should be considered at high risk and require a risk–benefit assessment before treatment is initiated. During therapy, the development of leukopenia necessitates follow-up laboratory evaluations every 2 weeks. If the counts do not return to normal in 2 weeks, the drug dose should be reduced.

Carbamazepine occasionally may result in hepatic toxicity. This is usually a hypersensitivity hepatitis that appears after a latency period of several weeks and is associated with elevations in SGOT (serum glutamic-oxaloacetic transaminase), SGPT (serum glutamate pyruvate transaminase), and LDH (lactic dehydrogenase). Cholestasis is also possible, with increases in bilirubin and alkaline phosphatase.

Table 18–13 **Evaluation and Monitoring of Anticonvulsant Treatment of Bipolar Disorder**

1. Complete medical evaluation (see numbers 7 and 8).
2. Inform patient and family of potential side effects of treatment and of the importance of monitoring serum levels.
3. Initiate carbamazepine (CBZ) at 200 mg twice a day. Initiate valproic acid (VPA) at 250 mg twice a day.
4. Increase CBZ dose by 200 mg or VPA dose by 250 mg every 3–5 days.
5. Obtain serum levels every week until therapeutic levels are obtained (CBZ: 8–12 μg/ml; VPA: 50–100 μg/ml).
6. Monitor levels every month for the first 3 months and every 3 months thereafter.
7. Hematologic monitoring for CBZ: obtain complete blood count and platelet count every 2 weeks for the first 2 months of treatment and every 3 months thereafter.
8. Liver function monitoring (CBZ and VPA): obtain SGOT, SGPT, LDH, and alkaline phosphatase every month for the first 2 months of treatment and every 3 months thereafter.

SGOT, serum glutamic-oxaloacetic transaminase; SGPT, serum glutamate pyruvate transaminase; LHD, lactate dehydrogenase.
Silver JM, Yudofsky SC, Hurowitz G: Psychopharmacology and Electroconvulsive Therapy. In Hales RE, Yudofsky SC, Talbott JA (eds): The American Psychiatric Press Textbook of Psychiatry, 2nd ed. Washington, DC, American Psychiatric Press, 1994

Carbamazepine has anticholinergic activity, which may lead to blurred vision, constipation, and dry mouth. In addition, patients may also complain of dizziness, drowsiness, and ataxia. These symptoms may often occur at therapeutic plasma levels, especially in the early phases of treatment. The development of rashes is also common. Weight gain does not appear to be a side effect of carbamazepine therapy. Concurrent use of the calcium channel blocker verapamil with carbamazepine can result in increases in carbamazepine that leads into the toxic range. For this reason, these drugs should not be used concomitantly.

Carbamazepine is essentially a tricyclic agent and, similar to the CyAD, has quinidinelike side effects.

The side effect that is of most concern with the use of valproic acid is the development of hepatotoxicity. Fortunately, fatal cases of hepatotoxicity have been limited to children who have been treated with multiple anticonvulsants. On occasion, patients will have increases in liver function tests. These changes may normalize if the patient is maintained on VPA, although discontinuing the medication may be necessary. Other common side effects include drowsiness, weight gain, tremors, and alopecia.

PSYCHOSTIMULANTS

The use of psychostimulants such as methylphenidate is primarily limited to treating attention-deficit hyperactivity disorder (ADHD) (see Chapter 16 by Dr. Dulcan). In neurology, psychostimulants such as methylphenidate, dextroamphetamine, and pemoline are used to treat narcolepsy (see Chapter 22 by Dr. Doghramji). Some psychiatric research has suggested that these drugs may be of benefit in depression or as an adjunct to cyclic antidepressants, or they may predict responsiveness to cyclic antidepressants. Their use for these purposes, however, is not generally accepted in psychiatric practice, and psychostimulants are primarily employed in adjunctive polypharmacy regimens in refractory depressions.

Despite the very limited use for psychostimulants in most mood disorders, several clinical situations exist in which they may be of some definite benefit. Some general hospital psychiatrists advocate their use in anergic, apathetic, and withdrawn medical patients, such as those recovered from cerebrovascular stroke or other debilitating medical illnesses. The short-term use of methylphenidate 10 to 40 mg/day or dextroamphetamine 10 to 20 mg/day has been recommended to "activate" such anergic and apathetic patients. The clinical efficacy of such strategies has mostly been reported in short-term uncontrolled studies. More recently, the use of methylphenidate for depression associated with AIDS has also received support (see Chapter 21 by Dr. Moran).

Psychostimulants, however, may cause restlessness, anxiety, agitation, insomnia, and, primarily with amphetamines, paranoid reactions and dependency may occur. In addition, a rebound depression is quite common after the drugs are discontinued in patients who have become dependent on them. For these reasons, the use of psychostimulants is still largely reserved for carefully selected patients.

ELECTROCONVULSIVE THERAPY

Electroconvulsive therapy (ECT) is the use of electrically induced convulsions (i.e., grand mal or motor seizures) to treat psychiatric illnesses such as depression and mania or psychiatric symptoms such as psychosis or catatonia. Although ECT was first used in the late 1930s, the treatment today remains clinically relevant because of its high degree of efficacy, safety, and utility.

Mechanisms of Action

The mechanisms of action of ECT are complex and not completely understood. Nevertheless, ECT has been found to affect many of those transmitters and receptors that have been implicated in depression and its treatment. In studies involving both humans and animals, ECT has been found to affect such brain transmitters as serotonin, gamma-aminobutyric acid (GABA), endogenous opiates and their receptors, and catecholamines, including dopamine, norepinephrine, epinephrine, and their receptors. It also affects a wide variety of other neurotransmitters, neuropeptides, and neuroendocrine pathways.

Indications

ECT is primarily indicated in the treatment of severe depression—particularly depression in which symptoms are intense, prolonged, and accompanied by profound alterations in the patient's level of vegetative functioning, including sleep, appetite, libido, and activity level. As has been demonstrated in previous sections of this chapter, CyAD, SSRIs, and MAOIs are the primary somatic treatments for depression. In patients with major depression with psychotic features, severe obsessional features, or active suicidal ideation, ECT is considered by some investigators and clinicians as the first-line treatment. In general, schizophrenic patients with prominent affective and catatonic symptoms respond the best to ECT, whereas those patients with chronic symptoms often fail to respond. There is no indication that ECT alters the fundamental psychopathology of schizophrenia.

Yudofsky (1981) outlined special clinical situations in which ECT may be advantageous over other treatment approaches and may be the "first line" of treatment. Among these situations are the following:

1. Patients whose severe mood disorders have not responded to adequate psychopharmacologic treatment.
2. Patients with delusional (psychotic) depression (see Chapter 7).
3. Patients who cannot tolerate the side effects of antidepressant or antipsychotic agents.
4. Patients whose acute symptoms are so severe that a rapid and dramatic response is required.
5. Patients with histories of depressive episodes that have responded successfully to previous electroconvulsive treatments.

ECT also may be used in the treatment of acute and chronic manic episodes resistant to medication.

Contraindications

The contraindications to ECT are relatively few. First, patients with clinically significant space occupying cerebral lesions must not receive this treatment because of the risk of brain stem herniation. Second, patients with significant cardiovascular problems that may include recent (within 6 months) myocardial infarction, severe cardiac ischemia, and uncontrolled hypertension are at higher risk for complications. Such patients may or may not be safely given ECT and must be evaluated before treatment by a cardiologist and an anesthesiologist familiar with the potential side effects of ECT. Before the use of muscle relaxants in electroconvulsive therapy technique, degenerative diseases of the spine and other bones comprised a significant risk from ECT. Today, however, adequate anesthetic techniques render ECT generally safe in patients with these disorders. Patients should generally be discontinued from their monoamine oxidase inhibitors for at least 2 weeks before the initiation of ECT to prevent dangerous increases in blood pressure during treatment.

Medical Evaluation Before Treatment

Before receiving ECT, a patient should have a complete medical and neurological examination, complete blood count, blood chemistry analysis, urinalysis, and electrocardiogram. A chest X-ray must be obtained because of the use of positive-pressure respiration during general anesthesia. Electroencephalogram and a computerized tomographic (CT) scan may be required for patients with known or suspected brain disease such as stroke or brain tumors. X-ray of the lumbosacral region of the spine may be obtained if orthopedic problems are suspected.

Because of the high degree of fear and misinformation related to ECT, we encourage that ample time be devoted to discussion of the risks, benefits, and techniques of ECT with both patients and their families.

Technique

In the United States, ECT treatments are generally given on an every-other-day basis (three times a week) for 2 to 3 weeks for a total of 6 to 9 treatments on average. Seizure lengths of between 25 and 60 seconds per treatment are considered adequate for therapeutic purposes. Electrodes may be placed unilaterally on the nondominant cerebral hemisphere (i.e., the electrodes over the right hemisphere for a right-handed individual) or bilaterally over both temples. One technique of inducing seizures at the initial treatment session is to determine the seizure threshold, which is determined by administering relatively low dosages of current at first and increasing the current in a stepwise fashion until a seizure is elicited. For unilateral ECT, subsequent treatments are administered at a dosage of several times the threshold dosage. Bilateral treatments may be administered at minimally suprathreshold dosages. With these parameters, unilateral ECT is associated with fewer cognitive side effects but is not as rapidly efficacious as bilateral stimulation. Some authorities recommend "high charge" ECT, that is, current at two times the minimal amount needed to elicit a seizure. Some evidence suggests that this technique is more effective than the graduated stimulus method that minimizes the amount of electrical charge administered.

Side Effects

For each treatment there is an initial confusional period that lasts for approximately 30 minutes. Memory impairment that occurs with ECT is highly variable. While certain patients report no problems with their memory, others report that their memory "is not as good as it used to be" after receiving ECT. It has been found that patients who experience retrograde amnesia (i.e., diminished ability to recall information that was recently learned before ECT was administered) following bilateral ECT seem to have recovered complete memory function by 6 months after treatment, with little evidence that new learning ability is still deficient at this time. In those patients who do have memory impairment following bilateral ECT, information acquired during the days and weeks before, during, and for several weeks following ECT may be permanently lost.

Electroconvulsive therapy remains an effective if not preferred treatment for those patients with severe depressions that include those with delusional and suicidal features. ECT is only one component of a larger treatment plan that includes psychosocial interventions. The optimum strategy for treatment of a patient after a course of ECT is not clear. While some patients will do well with maintenance with antidepressant medications, other patients may require lithium, either alone or in addition to antidepressants. Finally, since patients who have been previously refractory to or intolerant of antidepressants receive ECT, it can be predicted that they will not respond to these drugs after ECT. Therefore, maintenance ECT, at a frequency of one treatment per month for a period of 6–12 months, may be given to maintain remission in patients who are at extremely high risk for relapse.

CLINICAL PEARLS

- A relatively easy way to remember the differential side effects of the antipsychotic or neuroleptic drugs is that the "low-potency" drugs such as chlorpromazine and thioridazine have relatively *high* anticholineric and orthostatic hypotensive side effects and low extrapyramidal side effects, The "high-potency" drugs such as haloperiodol, thiothixene, and fluphenazine conversely have *low anticholinergic and orthostatic hypotensive side effects* and a high propensity for extrapyramidal side effects. Hence, the side effects in the "high-potency" and "low-potency" drugs vary inversely in this respect.
- Monitoring serum CPK levels is an excellent way to identify the prodrome or the presence of neuroleptic malignant syndrome as well as to monitor the course of the patient's recovery from NMS.
- It is imperative that patients being considered for long-term use with neuroleptic (antipsychotic) agents be given informed consent, that they be monitored frequently for extrapyramidal side effects using structures rating instruments such as the AIMS scale (Abnormal Involuntary Movements Scale), and the informed consent is updated every 6 months. Neuroleptic drugs should always be used in the lowest possible dose, and the need for continued treatment should be periodically documented.
- In respect to the antidepressant drugs, one usually chooses a drug based on its side effect profile, matching the side effects of the drug with the symptoms and physiological vulnerabilities of the patient. For example, patients with severe anxiety, agitation,

and insomnia may benefit more from relatively sedating antidepressants such as imipramine. Alternatively, patients who are more apathetic and anergic may benefit from more "stimulating" drugs such as fluoxetine and desipramine.

- Most antidepressant drugs, with the exception of bupropion, should be given once a day, usually 7 hours before bedtime. Fluoxetine and other SSRIs. as well as tricyclic protriptyline, because of their stimulant properties, are usually best given in the early parts of the day.
- The most common reasons for "refractory" depression are noncompliance with medication and patients being treated with inadequate doses of antidepressants for too brief a period of time.
- Patients who have Parkinson's disease with psychotic symptoms should be considered for treatment with clozapine. This drug not only has very few if any extrapyramidal side effects that could possibly worsen the Parkinson's disease, but some investigators have reported that it actually improves the symptoms of Parkinson's disease.
- The most problematic aspect of treating elderly patients with cyclic antidepressants is the development of orthostatic hypotension. Of the traditional cyclic antidepressants, nortriptyline has the fewest orthostatic side effects, and of the new antidepressants, bupropion and the SSRIs appear to have the definite advantage.
- Of the traditional tricyclic antidepressants, desipramine appears to have the fewest anticholingeric side effects. Of the newer drugs. the SSRIs and bupropion have the advantage over both the older and newer drugs in this respect.
- The benzodiazepines can be best differentiated into two classes. Oxazepam, temazepam, and lorazepam are all primarily metabolized by conjugation, and therefore their half-lives are not affected by aging or liver disease. Practically all of the other drugs, with the exception of clonazepam, are metabolized by way of oxidative mechanisms and therefore may be affected by age, liver disease, or other medications that may affect hepatic enzymatic activity.
- Lorazepam and midazolam are the only two benzodiazepines that may be reliably absorbed by the intramuscular route and are the preferred benzodiazepines to be given intravenously.
- Shorter-acting benzodiazepines such as triazolam and lorazepam may cause anterograde-amnesia.
- In respect to the cardiovascular side effects of the cyclic antidepressants, almost all of them, with the exception of trazodone, the SSRIs, and probably bupropion, have quinidinelike side effects. Carbamazepine also is a tricyclic compound with quinidinelike side effects.
- Electroconvulsive therapy is often the safest and most predictable treatment for certain patients with profound depressions and those who are elderly and medically debilitated who may not be able to tolerate the side effects of the cyclic antidepressants. The primary risk with electroconvulsive therapy is in patients who have expanding intracranial mass lesions, patients who have experienced a recent myocardial infarction, or patients with severe cardiovascular disease in which the hypertension and tachycardia associated with seizure activity may place an excessive demand on the myocardium. These latter side effects can be managed through appropriate autonomic blockade with agents such as labetalol, esmolol, or pretreatment with nifedipine.

ANNOTATED BIBLIOGRAPHY

American Psychiatric Association: Tardive Dyskinesia: A Task Force Report of the American Psychiatric Association. Washington, DC, American Psychiatric Association, 1992

This report reviews current knowledge of assessment, risk factors, prevention, and treatment of tardive dyskinesia.

American Psychiatric Association: The Practice of Electroconvulsive Therapy: Recommendations for Treatment, Training, and Privileging. A Task Force Report of the American Psychiatric Association. Washington, DC, American Psychiatric Association, 1990

This is the state-of-the-art review of the current practice of ECT.

Dubovsky SC: Psychopharmacologic Treatment in Neuropsychiatry. In Yudofsky SC, Hales RE (eds): The American Psychiatric Press Textbook of Neuropsychiatry, 2nd ed., pp 411–438. Washington, DC, American Psychiatric Press, 1992

This is a succinct review of the use of psychopharmacologic agents in patients with neuro-psychiatric disorders.

Guttmacher L: Concise Guide to Somatic Therapies. Washington, DC, American Psychiatric Press, 1988

This is a short but succinct reference for biological therapies in psychiatry.

Hales RE: Psychopharmacologic side effects and drug interactions of importance in the critical care unit. Prob Crit Care 2:134–148, 1988

This is a review of the benefits and risks of using psychopharmacologic drugs in the intensive care unit setting.

Kass FE, Oldham JM, Pardes H: The Columbia University College of Physicians and Surgeons Complete Home Guide to Mental Health. New York, Henry Holt and Co., 1992

Meltzer H (ed): Psychopharmacology: The Third Generation of Progress. New York, Raven Press, 1987

This is a superb and encyclopedic source on clinical psychopharmacology. It covers almost every aspect of clinical psychopharmacology from basic neuropharmacologic mechanisms to practical clinical applications. Excellent as a reference source for special study or complex clinical situations.

Schatzberg AF, Cole JO: Manual of Clinical Psychopharmacology. Washington, DC, American Psychiatric Press, 1989

This is an excellent short guide to practical clinical psychopharmacology that is well referenced and contains excellent tables.

Silver JM, Yudofsky SC, Hurowitz G: Psychopharmacology and Electroconvulsive Therapy. In Hales RE, Yudofsky SC, Talbott JA (eds): The American Psychiatric Press Textbook of Psychiatry, 2nd ed. Washington, DC, American Psychiatric Press, 1994

This is an expanded discussion of many of the basic principles discussed in this chapter.

Stoudemire A, Fogel BS, Gulley LR, Moran MG: Psychopharmacology in the Medical Patient. In Stoudemire A, Fogel BS (eds): Psychiatric Care of the Medical Patient. New York, Oxford University Press, 1993

This is an expanded and detailed discussion of the special modifications that must be made in the use of psychopharmacologic agents in medically ill patients. It deals on a specialty-by-specialty basis with each of the major organ systems and the possible vulnerabilities of medically ill patients to psychopharmacologic agents.

Stoudemire A, Atkinson P: Use of cyclic antidepressants in patients with cardiac conduction disturbances. Gen Hosp Psychiatry 10:389–397, 1988

This review article discusses in depth the special considerations that must be made in choosing psychopharmacologic agents in patients with cardiac conduction disturbances.

Yudofsky SC, Hales RE, Ferguson T: What You Need to Know about Psychiatric Drugs. New York, Grove Weidenfeld, 1991

These books are excellent resources for patient education about psychiatric disorders and treatments.

REFERENCES

American Psychiatric Association: DSM-IV Draft Criteria 3/1/93. Washington, DC, American Psychiatric Association, 1993

American Psychiatric Association: Diagnostic and Statistical Manual of Mental Disorders, 4th ed. Washington, DC, American Psychiatric Association, in press [1994]

Baldessarini RJ: Chemotherapy in Psychiatry: Principles and Practice. Boston, Harvard University Press, 1985

Baldessarini RJ: Drugs and the Treatment of Psychiatric Disorders. In Gilman AG, Goodman LS, Murel F (eds): The pharmacologic Basis Therapeutics, 7th ed, pp 385–445. New York, Macmillan, 1985

Battle DC, VonRiotte AB, Gaviria M, et al: Amelioration of polyuria by amiloride in patients receiving long-term lithium therapy. N Engl J Med 312:408–414, 1985

Breier A, Charney DS, Heninger GR: Agoraphobia with panic attacks: Development, diagnostic stability, and course of illness. Arch Gen Psychiatry 43:1029–1036, 1986

Consensus Development Panel: Mood disorders: Pharmacologic prevention of recurrences. Am J Psychiatry 142:469–476, 1985

Coffey CE: The Clinical Science of Electroconvulsive Therapy. Washington, DC, American Psychiatric Press, 1993

Conte HR, Plutchik R, Wild KV et al: Combined psychotherapy and pharmacotherapy for depression: A systemic analysis of the evidence. Arch Gen Psychiatry 43:471–479, 1986

Davis JM, Andriukaitis S: The natural course of schizophrenia and effective maintenance drug treatment. J Clin Psychopharmacol 6:2S–10S, 1986

Folks DG: Monoamine oxidase inhibitors: Reappraisal of dietary considerations. J Clin Psychopharmacol 3:249–252, 1983

Gelenberg AJ, Kane JM, Keller MB, Lavori P, Rosenbaum JF, Cole K, Lavelle J: Comparison of standard and low serum levels of lithium for maintenance treatment of bipolar disorder. N Engl J Med 321:1489–1493, 1989

Hart RG, Easton JD: Carbamazepine and hematological monitoring. Ann Neurol 11:309–312, 1982

Keck Jr PE, McElroy SL, Nemeroff CB: Anticonvulsants in the treatment of bipolar disorder. J Neuropsychiatry Clin Neurosci 4:395–405, 1992

Mellinger GD, Balter MB, Uhlenhuth EH: Insomnia and its treatment: Prevalence and correlates. Arch Gen Psychiatry 42:225–232, 1985

Mitchell JE, Mackenzie TB: Cardiac effects of lithium therapy in man: A review. J Clin Psychiatry 43:47–51, 1982

Munetz MR, Roth LH: Informing patients about tardive dyskinesia. Arch Gen Psychiatry 42:866–871, 1985

Myers DH, Carter RA, Burns BH et al: A prospective study of the effects of lithium on thyroid function and on the prevalence of antithyroid antibodies. Psychol Med 15:55–61, 1985

National Institute of Mental Health: Abnormal involuntary movement scale. In Guy W (ed): ECDEU Assessment Manual. Rockville, MD, U.S. Department of Health, Education, and Welfare, 1976

Prien RF, Kupfer DJ: Continuation drug therapy for major depressive episodes: How long should it be maintained? Am J Psychiatry 143:18–23, 1986

Reich J: The epidemiology of anxiety. J Nerv Ment Dis 174:129–136, 1986

Silver JM, Yudofsky SC, Hurowitz G: Psychopharmacology and Electroconvulsive Therapy. In Hales RE, Yudofsky SC, Talbott JA (eds): The American Psychiatric Press Textbook of Psychiatry, 2nd ed. Washington, DC, American Psychiatric Press, 1994

Yassa R, Lal S: Prevalence of the rabbit syndrome. Am J Psychiatry 143:656–657, 1986

Yudofsky SC: ECT in general hospital psychiatry: Focus on new indications and technologies. Gen Hosp Psychiatry 3:292–296, 1981

Alan Stoudemire (ed). *Clinical Psychiatry for Medical Students*, Second Edition. Copyright © 1994, 1990 by J. B. Lippincott Company.

19 Psychiatric Emergencies: Recognition and Management

William R. Dubin

Emergency management of psychiatric disorders is one of the unique areas of medicine in which physicians must have a broad knowledge of both medicine and psychiatry. The interplay between physical illness and psychological functioning is dramatic. This chapter's purpose is to provide an introduction to evaluating and treating psychiatric emergencies by highlighting the major syndromes most commonly seen in the emergency department (ED). Topics include the evaluation and treatment of psychosis; violence; suicide; rape; child, spouse, and elder abuse; and legal issues pertaining to emergency psychiatry.

ACUTE PSYCHOSIS: DIFFERENTIATING MENTAL DISEASE DUE TO MEDICAL, NEUROLOGIC AND TOXINS FROM FUNCTIONAL PSYCHIATRIC ILLNESS

The most important decision in evaluating a psychotic patient is to differentiate mental disorders due to medical, neurologic, or toxic causes from a "functional" psychiatric illness. Between 3.5 and 18.4% of patients considered to be primarily psychiatric in nature have undetected medical illness (Dubin and Weiss, 1984). Clinicians often make a premature psychiatric referral in the context of metabolic-, neurologic-, or toxin-induced brain dysfunction because of:

1. *Bias against psychiatric patients or patients with psychiatric symptoms.* Psychiatric patients often make physicians uncomfort-

able or anxious because of their bizarre or disruptive behavior. Physicians may not view such patients with the same urgency or seriousness as they do patients with cardiovascular disease or physical trauma. In a recent report, for example, a homeless street person with undiagnosed severe hypothyroidism was initially treated for psychiatric illness (Shader and Greenblatt, 1987). Too often, initial decisions are based on a single piece of data, symptom, item of past history, or previous diagnosis (Leeman, 1975).

2. *Disordered perceptions.* A common misconception is that delusions, hallucinations, and disorganized thoughts are synonymous with functional psychiatric illness. On the contrary, these symptoms, like pain or headache, are ubiquitous and occur in functional *and* medical illness. Psychotic symptoms may also occur transiently in certain personality disorders during times of emotional crisis.

3. *Violence.* Because violence makes clinicians anxious, they quickly tend to refer any violent or potentially violent patient for psychiatric evaluation. However, 17% of violence that occurs in psychiatric settings results from underlying medical or neurologic illness (Tardiff and Sweillam, 1980). Violence, like disordered perceptions, is etiologically nonspecific.

4. *Self-induced illness.* The least-tolerated patients are those who are believed to create their own disease, such as alcoholics, drug abusers, or suicidal patients (Weissberg, 1979). Consequently, clinicians tend to minimize these patients' symptoms. An example is a patient who presents with a suicide attempt by overdose with antidepressants who initially is fully alert and clinically stable. In patients like this, physicians tend to trivialize the seriousness of the overdose. Yet, half the patients who die from a tricyclic antidepressant overdose present fully alert and stable but have a catastrophic deterioration within 1 hour after admission to the ED (Callahan and Kassel, 1985).

5. *Ageism.* Clinicians often fail to take seriously or follow up the complaints and illnesses of elderly patients, attributing these complaints to old age or hypochondriasis (Goodstein, 1985). This problem may be further exacerbated in the patient with dementia. The term "dementia" is used generically to describe chronic irreversible and progressive deterioration of higher intellectual functioning. But 30 to 40% of all patients who present with symptoms of dementia have potentially treatable and sometimes completely reversible underlying causes for their altered mental status (Dubin, 1984). Premature labeling can preclude the physical, neurological, and laboratory evaluation necessary to determine the etiology of a patient's cognitive dysfunction.

DELIRIUM, DEMENTIA, AND OTHER DISORDERS WITH COGNITIVE IMPAIRMENT

Delirium is commonly encountered in the ED. Delirium specifically refers to a (usually) reversible disturbance of cerebral functioning due to a toxic, neurological, or metabolic disturbance (see Chapter 4 by Dr. Stoudemire). The onset is acute, generally developing over a 6- to 96-hour period, and is characterized by impairment of alertness, thinking, memory, perception, concentration, and attention (Lipowski, 1967). The incidence varies from 5 to 15% (Wise, 1987). The level of consciousness is altered and fluctuates in a sine-wave fashion.

Several common clinical features are highly suggestive of delirium: clouding of consciousness, age over 40 with no previous psychiatric history, disorientation, abnormal vital signs, visual hallucinations, and illusions (Dubin, Weiss, and Zeccardi, 1983; Hall, Popkin, and DeVaul, 1978).

The differential diagnosis of delirium is so extensive that physicians may tend to avoid searching for an etiology (Wise, 1987). For example, an elderly delirious patient may have multiorgan disease (e.g., pulmonary insufficiency, cardiac failure, preexisting brain damage) and may be taking multiple medicines (Wise, 1987). In such a patient, each problem is a potential contributor to the delirium and should be pursued and evaluated independently.

For the sake of differential diagnosis, clinicians should consider two categories of illness severity: *emergent* and *urgent*. Emergent conditions are life threatening; they require immediate attention and are of major concern to the psychiatrist (Table 19–1) (Anderson, 1987). Most other causes of delirium, while not life threatening, require treatment (Table 19–2) (Dubin and Weiss, 1985).

Laboratory studies that will help rule out emergent illnesses include a complete blood count, glucose, serum electrolytes, blood urea nitrogen, chest radiograph, electrocardiogram, arterial blood gases, and a urinary drug screen. Patients who present with an acute behavioral change and/or clouded consciousness unexplained by this laboratory evaluation may require computerized axial tomography followed by a lumbar puncture.

Table 19–1 **Life-Threatening Causes of Delirium (Selected List)**

Meningitis and encephalitis
Hypoglycemia
Hypertensive encephalopathy
Diminished cerebral oxygenation
Anticholinergic intoxication
Intracranial hemorrhage
Wernicke's encephalopathy
Drug or alcohol withdrawal or intoxication

Table 19–2 **Selected Causes of Cognitive Dysfunction**

Cardiac

Arrhythmias
Congestive heart failure
Myocardial infarction

Pulmonary

Chronic Obstructive Pulmonary Disease
Pulmonary emboli

Hepatic

Cirrhosis
Hepatitis
Wilson's Disease

Renal

Worsening of mild nephritis by urinary tract infection
Dehydration with elevation of blood urinary nitrogen (BUN) over 50 mg/dl.

Vascular

Subdural hematoma
Cerebrovascular accident

Endocrine Disease

Thyroid Disease
Cushings Disease
Diabetes
Addison's Disease
Hypoglycemia

Electrolyte Imbalance

Hyponatremia
Hypernatremia
Hypercalcemia

Vitamin Deficiencies

Thiamine
Niacin
Riboflavin
Folate
Ascorbic Acid
Vitamin A
Vitamin B_{12}

Drug Induced

Alcohol
Tranquilizers
Over-the-counter preparations
Any drug used to treat medical illness, e.g. Dilantin, aminophylline, digitalis, steroids

Exogenous Toxins

Carbon monoxide
Bromide
Mercury
Lead

Infections

Tumors

Normal Pressure Hydrocephalus

Depression

Acquired Immune Deficiency Syndrome

At times, extreme agitation can significantly impede the evaluation. In these cases pharmacologic intervention (rapid tranquilization) will be helpful so that the appropriate medical-neurological examination can be completed. This procedure is discussed later under the section about violence.

In addition to medication, psychological support is important. Patients should have a staff member, if available, or a family member with them at all times during the evaluation. This can be reassuring to patients and can reduce mishaps such as pulling out intravenous lines or falling out of bed (Wise, 1987). Delirium is also discussed in Chapter 4.

Functional Psychiatric Illness

The ED physician's task is (1) to differentiate primary metabolic-, neurologic-, or toxin-induced brain dysfunction from functional psychiatric illness and to rule out any life-threatening causes of aberrant behavior; (2) to medically and/or psychiatrically stabilize the patient; and (3) to determine the most appropriate treatment setting (inpatient, outpatient, partial hospital). Ultimately, correctly diagnosing patients with functional psychiatric illness is essential because there are specific treatments for each illness (i.e., lithium for bipolar disorder, antidepressants for depression, antipsychotic medications for schizophrenia). However, for the few hours that the patient is in the ED, the treatment of aberrant behavior, agitation, excitement, and potential violence is the overriding priority. In this setting, the primary interventions include psychotherapy, pharmacotherapy, and at times physical restraints. While psychotropic medication has greatly enhanced our ability to attenuate the behavioral emergency effectively, verbal intervention remains an integral part of successful treatment.

THE EMERGENCY DEPARTMENT INTERVIEW

Treatment is inextricably interwoven with the evaluation process (Dubin and Weiss, 1991). The initial interview not only serves to elicit important diagnostic information, it may be therapeutic in itself. The goal of the interview is to gather information about the present illness, past psychiatric and medical history, family and occupational history, and drug and alcohol use. *The interviewer should not be distracted by the patient's bizarre behavior or verbalizations.* Such behavior often makes physicians feel uncomfortable; as a result, they are indifferent or overtly hostile. This approach may exacerbate the patient's symptoms. A controlled, patient professional composure on the physician's part is reassuring to psychotic patients, who may feel very much out of control. Even the most psychotic patient usually has enough self-awareness to form a rudimentary alliance when addressed with respect and dignity.

Emergency psychiatry work with hostile, uncooperative, or insulting patients can be especially difficult and frustrating. Hanke (1984) presents a thorough and comprehensive review of working with such difficult patients. She notes that the most common negative feelings are various forms of anger, anxiety, and despair. While clinicians may be aware of strong negative feelings, most commonly we express them in an indirect way that we may not recognize. Negative feelings may impede clinical judgment and decision making in the following ways:

1. *Arbitrary inferences*, or jumping to a conclusion based on inadequate or incorrect data ("Nothing will help this patient").
2. *All-or-nothing thinking*, or seeing situations as strictly black and white ("No one talks to me like that").
3. *Personalization*, or taking too much blame or too much credit without an objective reason ("With a little crisis intervention, I solved the patient's problem").

In general, if a clinician has an extremely negative reaction toward a patient, it suggests that the patient has struck an area of emotional vulnerability in the physician. Hanke (1984) suggests five guidelines to help manage negative responses to patients:

1. View the patient's maladaptive behavior as symptomatic of their condition rather than as a personal attack.
2. View negative reactions as overreactions.
3. Find a rational reaction to overreactions by identifying the type of response (i.e., arbitrary inference, all-or-nothing thinking, or personalization).
4. Generate alternate reactions. For example, instead of viewing patients as "a manipulative sociopath," try to see them as pitiful or self-destructive, or as someone's son.
5. Maintain a larger perspective on negative reactions by attributing multiple causes to the negative reaction; for example, the negative feelings come from the patient's profanity (50%), the clinician's fatigue from being on call all night (25%), and the overcrowded waiting area (25%).

While it is difficult to eliminate negative feelings completely, clinicians should try to neutralize them to prevent distorting their clinical judgment in a way that impedes optimum care.

To begin the interview, physicians should introduce themselves and address the patient as "Mr. Smith" or "Ms. Jones." If the patient does not pose an imminent risk, the physician should sit. Standing over the patient may impede rapport by implying domination or intimidation. To establish a friendly atmosphere, it often helps to offer the patient food or a drink (avoid hot liquids) or to offer to call a friend.

One of the major paradoxes in emergency medicine occurs in respect to emergency psychiatry. Most emergency departments focus on rapid intervention and disposition, but in emergency psychiatric interventions *time is a major treatment variable*. The intensity of a patient's symptoms often diminishes in a structured, supportive environment with "tincture of time." Therefore, clinicians must restrain the impulse to "get right to the heart of the matter." The interview should begin with very nonspecific, less-intrusive questions. After the patient begins to show some comfort with the interviewer, the physician can then start to ask about specific details. Questions should be open-ended to avoid simple "yes" or "no" answers. The physician should keep the interview format flexible, without trying to adhere to a predetermined rigid structure.

When interviewing an acutely disturbed agitated patient, the physician often must structure the interview by asking straightforward questions. If the patient begins to ramble, the interviewer should then restructure the interview to help patients to pick up the trend of their thinking. The interviewer should not take a passive role but should be an active, involved participant.

With patients with hallucinations or delusions, it is important not to use simple logic in an attempt to convince them that their perceptions are wrong. This maneuver tends to make patients feel more defensive and misunderstood and may destroy any rapport that may have developed.

Except with the extremely paranoid patient, "laying on of hands" often helps establish rapport. This can be done by asking patients if the interviewer can take their pulse or blood pressure or feel their forehead. Unless there is some reason not to do it, the physician should offer to shake the patient's hand during the introduction.

An important element of the interview is helping patients identify their feelings. The patients' need to protect their integrity and self-control may initially make them reluctant to engage in the interview. If patients are resistant to the idea of talking, it is useful to elicit their feelings about the situation and to try to understand their predicament of being in the hospital and not knowing what will happen.

When a psychotic patient does not respond to questioning, the interviewer should then use whatever data are available to make contact with the patient. This may include noting the patient's words, expressions, appearance, or behavior, as well as the physician's subjective reactions and feelings that are elicited by the patient. Comments should be as specific as possible ("I don't know what Jesus says to you" or "I see you are in a bathrobe. I gather you were brought to the hospital unexpectedly.").

But despite the physician's most empathic and sensitive interventions, some patients will remain mute. Muteness is usually an angry response symbolizing an attempt to control the environment (Robbins and Stern, 1976). While medical and neurologic illnesses have been reported as etiologic for cases of mutism, it is rarely a sign of neurologic disease (Wells, 1980). When patients are mute, the first step is to indicate that appropriate responses are expected. If the patient continues to remain silent, the interviewer then should pause and observe what the silence is communicating. At no time should the clinician indicate a sense of futility by angrily and repeatedly asking questions and getting no reply. If the clinician cannot engage the patient in conversation, she or he should try to gather diagnostic information from the patient's family, friends, or spouse. If time permits, a sodium amytal interview may sometimes lead to dramatic improvement. If muteness persists, admission to a psychiatric unit for evaluation and treatment is indicated.

The most difficult patients for even experienced psychiatrists to interview are the *paranoid* patients. Perry (1976) has outlined an excellent approach to interviewing paranoid patients. If the patient is frightening, physicians should *not* ignore their own fear. Patients can quickly sense this discomfort and may become frightened themselves, leading to an escalation of symptoms. Sometimes clinicians may have to acknowledge their fears by saying to the patient, "The way you're looking makes me feel that you're on the verge of striking out. What can we do to help you feel more in control of things?" If the physician remains professionally confident and in control, patients are usually reassured. The patient's anxiety can be further ameliorated if the interview is conducted with the door open or if additional staff are present.

It is important to be tactful with paranoid patients because they are defensive, irritable, and easily humiliated. Paranoid patients who are angry often begin with a tirade of accusations about being mistreated. The clinician may have to interrupt and say to the patient, "How do you feel I might help you?" With the angry, paranoid patient, the physician should always maintain a professional demeanor by not becoming too friendly, intrusive, or controlling and by avoiding jokes or patronizing reassurance.

Occasionally, paranoid patients can make the interviewer feel defensive and foolish by twisting the meaning of the interviewer's words, making it impossible to sustain any direction in the interview. Under these circumstances, the interviewer should alter the course of the interview by explaining to the patient that he or she is making the interviewer uncomfortable and suggesting that they discuss reasons for doing this. If meaningful contact cannot be made, the interview should be terminated until the situation and the patient's condition permit a more productive interaction, usually after the patient has been medicated (see below).

THE VIOLENT PATIENT

The risk of violence in hospital settings appears to be increasing (Lavoie, Carter, Danzi et al, 1988; Pane, Winiarski, and Salness, 1991). In the emergency departments of teaching hospitals with more than 40,000 patient visits a year, 32% had one verbal threat a day, 18% noted that weapons were displayed at least once each month, and 43% reported a physical attack on a medical staff member at least once a month (Lavoie, Carter, Danzi et al, 1988). Forty-six percent of the hospitals in this study noted that weapons were confiscated at least once each month from patients or visitors. Against this backdrop it becomes increasingly essential that clinicians learn the basic skills for management of aggressive patients. Patients can usually be successfully treated in the ED if the clinician approaches the patient in an objective, systematic manner and understands the dynamics of violence (Dubin, 1981). Simply stated, most patients tend to become violent when they feel helpless or passive (Lion, 1972). Successful interventions often alleviate these feelings and diminish the chances of behavioral dyscontrol.

Usually, a prodromal pattern of behavior precedes overt violence. Fortunately, sudden, unexpected physical assault is rare, and most violence is a predictable culmination of a 30- to 60-minute period of escalation. This prodrome can often be observed in the patient's posture, speech, and motor activity. Most violence is preceded by a period of increasing restlessness and pacing. Hyperactivity itself may be a sign of a psychiatric emergency that requires immediate intervention. Patients who manifest rigid postures by literally "having their back up in the air," those who clench their fists and jaws, and those whose temporal arteries are visibly pulsating are in the early stages of escalation. As part of the prodromal syndrome, patients are often verbally abusive and profane. *The clinician's response to such verbal stridency is central to the outcome of the intervention.* When verbal abuse is personalized and the clinician reacts defensively or angrily, the risk of violence is increased. *It is important to remember that verbal abuse is an attempt by the patient to assert autonomy and diminish feelings of helplessness.*

Treatment of Violence

As with psychotic patients, verbal intervention can be strikingly effective with potentially assaultive patients. Even with patients who appear to be on the verge of total loss of control, appropriate and well-timed verbal interventions can have a positive impact on behavior. Patients are terrified of losing control and welcome therapeutic efforts to restore it and prevent their acting out (Lion and Pasternak, 1973). The agitated, fearful, panicky feeling that is especially common in psychotic patients prior to their assaultiveness can be attenuated by empathic verbal interventions. Talking gives the patient an outlet for the tension that is being generated and is important for ventilating angry, hostile feelings (Lion, 1972).

During the interview, the clinician should focus on the patient's underlying feeling state or affect. Efforts to calm a patient through rationalization and intellectualization are usually not therapeutic and may only increase the patient's frustration and feelings of being misunderstood. Physicians often are reluctant to have patients express their anger, fearing that this will only escalate their loss of emotional control. On the contrary: ventilating angry feelings reduces the agitation. Often the hostile feelings frighten the patient, and by acknowledging these feelings some degree of emotional catharsis can be achieved, diminishing the need for further aggression (Lion, Levenberg, and Strange, 1972).

During the interview, the clinician should stay at least an arm's length from the patient. Never leave potentially violent patients alone, as this could be interpreted as rejection or could permit them to hurt themselves. An interviewer who feels anxious or unsure of how the patient will respond should ask the police, security personnel, or the family to remain nearby to help control the patient if necessary. There is some disagreement as to whether the patient or the interviewer should be closer to the door during the interview; a compromise would be to have both equal distance from the door.

As noted earlier, as part of verbal intervention it can be helpful to offer the patient food or a drink (again, avoiding hot liquids for obvious reasons). Offering food symbolizes friendship and caring and often helps alleviate a patient's angry affect. During the interview, it is also important to observe the patient's behavior; it may suggest that the patient is not as threatening as she or he may sound. When patients have their hands behind their backs or in their pockets or comply with all the interviewer's requests, they are less likely to become violent despite their strident speech.

The ultimate threat comes from patients with weapons. If a patient admits to having a weapon, never immediately ask for it, but explore the fear that led the patient to arm himself or herself. A weapon symbolizes a defense against feelings of helplessness and passivity. An immediate request to give up a weapon may heighten these feelings and further exacerbate the threat. During the interview, if the patient agrees to give up the weapon, the interviewer should *never* accept the weapon directly from the patient. Instead, the patient should be asked to put the weapon on the table or the floor so that the interviewer can pick it up at the end of the interview. If the patient refuses to give up the weapon, the clinician should immediately notify hospital personnel. If the patient actually threatens the interviewer with the weapon, the clinician should avoid exacerbating the patient's feelings of helplessness and shame. Nonthreatening expressions of a desire to help, coupled with an expression of fear, are the response most likely to avert physical harm ("I want to help you, but I'm too frightened to think with a gun pointed at me") (Dubin, Wilson, and Mercer, 1988).

While staff often voice concern about the threat of armed patients, consideration must also be given to weapons, especially guns, carried by police officers and security personnel. Generally, it is preferable to have them disarmed while in the ED. There are several anecdotal reports of patients who have taken guns from police officers in such situations and injured themselves and/or others. In several instances this occurred with patients who were not under the supervision of the police. Table 19–3 summarizes basic techniques in managing the violent patient.

Rapid Tranquilization

While verbal intervention is the mainstay of evaluation and treatment, medication is often necessary. In rapid tranquilization (RT), antipsychotic medication usually in combination with a benzodiazepine is given at 30- to 60-minute intervals; ideally, patients respond significantly within 30 to 90 minutes (Dubin, Weiss, and Dorn, 1986). The target symptoms for RT include *tension, anxiety, restlessness, hyperactivity,* and *motor excitement.* Core psychotic symptoms such as hallucinations, delusions, and disorganized thought are usually not affected by RT and may require 7 to 10 days of appropriate antipsychotic drug treatment to attenuate. *The goal of RT is to calm patients so that they can cooperate in their evaluation, treatment, and disposition.* Occasionally, there is concern that RT will obscure the patient's mental status and that antipsychotic treatment should be withheld until a diagnosis is made. This specious argument can lead to withholding an effective treatment and may prolong the risk of violence. A psychiatric diagnosis is not made on a single mental-status evaluation and, as stated earlier, definitive psychiatric treatment is not the primary task in the ED.

At times, clinicians also withhold medication for fear that it will obscure or worsen underlying medical conditions; instead, they physically restrain patients while they attempt a physical evaluation and laboratory workup. Besides the questionable accuracy of a physical examination done on a restrained, agitated patient, restraints carry significant medical risks (Gutheil and Tardiff, 1984; Johnson, Alvarez, and Freinhar, 1987). With the exception of anticholinergic delirium (which can be worsened by RT due to the anticholinergic properties of some neuroleptics), the safety of RT in medically ill patients has been repeatedly demonstrated (Dubin, Weiss, and Dorn, 1986).

RT is effective across all diagnostic categories regardless of the etiology of the aggression. It is effective in psychosis secondary to functional psychiatric illness such

Table 19–3 **Dos and Don'ts of Treating Violent Patients**

DO	DON'T
Anticipate possible violence from hostile, threatening, agitated, restless, abusive patients or from those who lack control for any reason.	Don't ignore your gut feeling that a patient may be dangerous.
Heed your gut feeling. If you feel frightened or uneasy, discontinue the interview and get help.	Don't see angry, threatening, or restless persons right away.
Summon as many security guards or orderlies as possible at the first sign of violence. Patients who see that you take them seriously often will not act out further. If they do, you will be prepared.	Don't compromise your ability to escape a dangerous situation. Don't sit behind a desk or between a patient and the door.
Ask if the patient is carrying a weapon. These must be surrendered to security personnel. Never see an armed patient.	Don't antagonize the patient by responding angrily or being patronizing.
Offer help, food, medication. Bolster patients by commenting on their strength and self-control.	Don't touch or startle the patient or approach quickly without warning.
If restraint becomes necessary, assign one team member each to the patient's head and to each extremity. Be humane but firm, and do not bargain. Search the patient for drugs and weapons.	Don't try to restrain a patient without sufficient backup.
If the patient refuses oral medication, offer an injection after a few moments. Be prepared to administer it if the patient continues to refuse.	Don't neglect looking for medical causes of violence.
Keep a close eye on patients who are sedated and/or restrained. Restrained patients should never be left alone.	Don't bargain with a violent person about the need for restraints, medication, or psychiatric admission.
Hospitalize patients who state their intention to harm anyone, refuse to answer questions about their intent to harm, are abusing alcohol or drugs, are psychotic, have cognitive impairment, or refuse to cooperate with treatment.	Don't forget medical-legal concerns, such as full documentation of all interventions and the duty to warn and protect. If the patient is transferred, tell the admitting physician about any specific threats and victims.
Warn potential victims of threatened violence and notify the appropriate protection agencies.	Don't overlook family and friends as important sources of information
Follow up on any violent person and document this in the chart.	

(Used with permission from Dwyer B, Weissberg M: Treating violent patients. Psychiatric Times, p. 11, December 1988.)

as schizophrenia or mania, as well as in behavioral syndromes secondary to dementia, delirium, or alcohol and substance abuse or withdrawal (Dubin, Weiss, and Dorn, 1986). However, in substance- and alcohol-abuse patients, RT should be used for behavioral dyscontrol only. Cross-tolerant agents such as benzodiazepines for alcohol withdrawal are preferred for treatment of the withdrawal syndrome itself.

Until recently, the mainstay of rapid tranquilization has been high-potency antipsychotics (i.e., thiothixene, haloperidol, fluphenazine, and loxapine). However, recent reports suggest that high-potency antipsychotic medication combined with a benzodiazepine (usually lorazepam) is more effective than either drug alone (Garza-Treviño, Hollister, Overall et al, 1989; Barbee, Mancuso, Freed et al, 1992). Both medications are drawn up in the same syringe and given intramuscularly. The most common side effect of lorazepam includes sedation and ataxia (Dubin, 1988). The most common side effects of these high-potency neuroleptics are extrapyramidal symptoms, in contrast to the low-potency neuroleptics (e.g., chlorpromazine and thioridazine), whose primary side effects are hypotension and sedation (see Chapter 17 by Drs. Ursano, Silberman, and Diaz).

The dosages used during RT are generally modest, and most patients respond in one to three doses given over 30 to 90 minutes (Table 19–4) (Dubin, Weiss, and Dorn, 1986). While some patients may require higher doses, there are currently no predictive clinical variables for this subgroup. No ceiling doses have been established, and the ultimate number of doses is an empirical decision based on an assessment of the patient's clinical status. During RT, medication is given at 30- to 60-minute intervals; most studies have found 60-minute intervals sufficient. An important caveat is to try to use the minimum dosage over the maximum amount of time clinically feasible.

While RT was conceptualized as an ED procedure, its use has expanded to the intensive care unit (ICU) setting. In the ICU, the delirious agitation and combativeness of patients frequently impedes medical treatment and sometimes can be life threatening. Several studies have clearly demonstrated the efficacy and safety of RT in critically ill delirious patients in the ICU (Dudley, Rowlett, and Loebel, 1979; Adams, 1984; Sos and Cassem, 1980; Tesar, Murray, and Cassem, 1985).

Intravenous (IV) administration of medication is frequently the preferred route of choice in the ICU. Patients for whom IV administration may be useful include those with lowered cardiac output who will not absorb IM medication, those incapable of taking oral medication, and those with extensive tissue damage, such as burn patients. While IV antipsychotic medication is safe and effective, the onset of action is variable. Some investigators used the IV route when a more rapid effect was desired (Clinton et al, 1987), while others found the onset of action variable (i.e., 10 to 40 minutes) (Tesar, Murray, and Cassem, 1985). The incidence of side effects from IV administration appears to be no greater than with other routes of administration. A recent study

Table 19–4 **Rapid Tranquilization of the Violent Patient***

lorazepam (Ativan) 2–4 mg I.M. combined with haloperidol (Haldol) 5 mg
  I.M. or thiothixene (Navane) 5 mg I.M.
RT with an antipsychotic alone
thiothixene (Navane) 10 mg I.M. or 20 mg concentrate
haloperidol (Haldol) 5 mg I.M. or 10 mg concentrate
loxapine (Loxitane) 10 mg I.M. or 25 mg concentrate

* All doses given at 30- to 60-minute intervals. Use half-dose for medically ill or older patients.

suggests that patients who receive IV haloperidol actually have a lower incidence of extrapyramidal symptoms compared to patients receiving oral medication (Menza et al 1987). Goldstein (1987), in an excellent review of RT in the ICU, provides a useful guideline for the IV use of antipsychotics (Table 19–5). One caution: haloperidol is not *specifically* approved for IV use and documentation of the rationale for this maneuver should be made.

Side Effects During RT. Side effects during RT are generally few, mild, and reversible. Most studies have found that fewer than 10% of patients develop extrapyramidal symptoms (muscle rigidity, drooling, dystonias, akathisia, bradykinesia, etc.) within the first 24 hours of RT (Dubin, Weiss, and Dorn, 1986). Extrapyramidal symptoms are not dose related and can occur even after one dose. By far the most common extrapyramidal symptoms are *dystonic reactions*, which are involuntary turning or twisting movements produced by massive and sustained muscle contractions (Mason and Granacher, 1980). They are sudden in onset and can be bizarre in presentation, which often leads to a misdiagnosis of (hysterical) conversion disorder. Dystonia usually involve muscles of the back, neck, and oral area. The back may be extended (opisthotonos) or the head may arch severely backward (retrocollis) or sideways (torticollis) (Hyman and Arana, 1987). The eyes may be pulled upward in a painful manner (occulogyric crisis). At times, patients may complain of thickness of the tongue or difficulty swallowing.

The most serious form of dystonia is laryngospasm. This contraction of the muscles of the larynx can compromise the airway and lead to severe respiratory distress. While it is extremely rare, clinicians should be alert for it.

Table 19–5 **Treatment Guidelines for the Use of Intravenous Haloperidol in the Intensive Care Setting**

STARTING DOSE	
Degree of Agitation	**Dose**
Mild	0.5 to 2.0 mg
Moderate to severe	2.0 to 10 mg

Titration and Maintenance:

Allow 20 to 30 minutes before the next dose.

If agitation is unchanged, administer double dose every 20 to 30 minutes until patient begins to calm.

If patient is calming down, repeat the last dose at the next dosing interval.

Adjust dose and interval to patient's clinical course. Gradually increase the interval between doses until the interval is 8 hours, then begin to decrease the dose.

Once stable for 24 hours, give doses on a regular schedule and supplement with PRN doses.

Once stable for 36 to 48 hours, begin attempts to taper dose.

When agitation is very severe, very high boluses (up to 40 mg) may be required (Tesar, Murray, Cassem, 1985).

* Haloperidol is not specifically approved by the FDA for the intravenous route; careful documentation for the necessity and rationale for its use should be made.
(Used with permission from Goldstein MG: Intensive care unit syndromes. In: Stoudemire A, Fogel BS, eds. Principles of Medical Psychiatry. Orlando: Grune & Stratton, 1987)

A side effect that can be frequently misdiagnosed as a psychotic decompensation is *akathisia*. This Greek word literally means "inability to sit still." Patients feel uncomfortably restless, and pacing is their only relief. They will often say they feel "unable to relax," "tense," "all wound up like a spring," "irritable," or "like jumping out of my skin" or that they have "restless" legs (Van Putten and Marder, 1987). *Severe* akathisia can lead to a psychotic decompensation, and in its most severe manifestation patients have committed suicide and homicide (Van Putten and Marder, 1987). In the ED, akathisia is likely to occur under one of the following scenarios:

1. A patient is being rapidly tranquilized and after two or three doses appears to be worsening behaviorally.
2. A patient responds to RT and then several hours later becomes agitated, with the psychosis appearing to break through.
3. A patient who is known to comply with drug treatment has been taking medication and is brought to the hospital because of an apparent relapse.

The treatment for dystonia and akathisia is the same: benztropine (Cogentin) 2 mg or diphenhydramine (Benadryl) 50 mg IM or IV. These doses can be repeated at 5-minute intervals, up to three doses. Generally, relief occurs within 1 to 3 minutes after injection. While the response is dramatic in most patients, a few may not respond. In these cases, diazepam (Valium) 5 mg IV or IM or lorazepam (Ativan) 2 to 4 mg IV or IM may be helpful. In severely thought-disordered, agitated patients, it may be impossible to differentiate akathisia from psychotic excitement (Van Putten and Marder, 1987). Occasionally, treating the patient first for akathisia will resolve the diagnosis if the patient has a positive response to benztropine or diphenhydramine.

The issue of prophylactic treatment during RT is unresolved (Dubin, Weiss, and Dorn, 1986). In the first 24 hours after RT, the occurrence of extrapyramidal symptoms appears to be low and most patients do not need antiparkinsonian agents. Yet it is clinically appropriate to use prophylactic antiparkinsonian drugs with patients who have a previous history of extrapyramidal symptoms, who are reluctant to take medication for fear of extrapyramidal symptoms, or who are paranoid and in whom extrapyramidal symptoms may lead to noncompliance. If a patient is rapidly tranquilized in the ED and then admitted to the hospital, benztropine or diphenhydramine should be ordered on a PRN ("as needed") basis since dystonia or akathisia can occur *several hours* after medication is given. If a patient is discharged from the ED, they should be given several 2-mg benztropine tablets, informed of the possible extrapyramidal side effects, and told when to take the benztropine.

Of major concern to many clinicians is *neuroleptic malignant syndrome* (NMS) (see also Chapter 18 by Drs. Silver, Hales, and Yudofsky). This *extremely serious*, life-threatening idiosyncratic reaction to neuroleptics causes autonomic instability with hyperthermia, hypertension, and "lead-pipe" rigidity as hallmark symptoms (Mueller, 1985). It is an ill-defined sensitivity reaction that may occur in about 1% of patients on antipsychotic medication. Variables that place patients at risk for NMS are young, chronic, male patients who are dehydrated, malnourished, neurologically impaired and placed in poorly ventilated seclusion rooms or in restraints (Mueller, 1985). To date, there have been no reports of this syndrome occurring with

RT in the ED. There has been a single case report of a gynecology patient developing NMS after an injection of haloperidol 5 mg for sedation before surgery (Konikoff et al, 1984). Another case was recently reported of a psychiatric patient who developed NMS 18 hours after receiving a total of haloperidol 45 mg over 18 hours (O'Brien, 1987). Despite these reports, concern about NMS should not deter the clinician from using an effective treatment such as RT unless the patient has a history of NMS.

Hypotension is a major concern with the use of low-potency antipsychotics such as chlorpromazine. When it occurs, treatment consists of keeping the patient supine or in the reverse Trendelenberg position, administering IV fluids for hypovolemia, and giving only noradrenergic drugs such as levarterenol or metaraminol (Bassuk, Panzarino, and Schoonover, 1984). Mixed α and β or β-adrenergic agonists such as isoproterenol and epinephrine should never be used because they could further reduce blood pressure (Bassuk, Panzarino, and Schoonover, 1984).

The risk of *tardive dyskinesia* (TD) has not been well defined in RT patients. However, since most patients who develop TD have been on antipsychotic medication for long periods of time, it does not appear that a patient is at risk from RT. *Seizures* from antipsychotic medications are rare, with only two reported seizures occurring in patients on low-potency drugs during RT (Hamid and Wertz, 1973; Man and Chen, 1973). Patients in alcohol withdrawal and drug intoxication do not appear to be at higher risk for seizures when treated for extreme agitation with antipsychotic medication (Dubin, Weiss, and Dorn, 1986). There are no reports of sudden death related to RT. The cardiovascular safety of antipsychotic medication has been demonstrated repeatedly, often in patients with severe, unstable cardiovascular illness (Dubin, Weiss, and Dorn, 1986). Other potential side effects generally develop from long-term use and are not of concern in RT.

Physical Restraint

At times, verbal intervention and rapid tranquilization will not be sufficient and additional personnel may be necessary. A show of force often induces compliance. Security personnel should be called in a quiet, nonthreatening manner. Patients should never be threatened with, "Either you cooperate or we are going to call security." The security force should never be presented as a challenge to a patient's masculinity or a threat to her or his passivity. When security guards are present, it is usually sufficient to have them visible, but not threatening; it is rarely necessary to have them in the interview room. The presence of security guards conveys to the patient that his or her impulses are going to be controlled and also allays the staff members' fears. When used in this manner, security guards should be unarmed, and they should should never approach patients while carrying weapons. The risk is too great that the patient may take the weapon if a physical struggle develops.

The ultimate method of behavior control is restraints, which should be used when patients may be harmful to themselves or others or when they remain agitated and noncompliant and violence seems imminent. Patients should not be threatened with restraints, but when they are inevitable maximum force should be used immediately and without belligerence (Bell and Palmer, 1981). Restraints provide a sound means for calming patients who do not respond to medication. Contrary to most clinicians' concerns, restraining a patient does not interfere with the therapeutic alliance; in the end, patients are usually grateful that they were prevented from acting destructively. The procedure for using restraints is outlined in Table 19–6. In all restraint episodes, documentation should clearly outline the behavior requiring restraint, efforts that were made to attenuate the patient's behavior before the use of restraints, the use of all medication, continuous documentation of all efforts to remove the patient from restraints, and monitoring of the patient to prevent injury (5-minute checks of extremities to ensure adequate circulation and adequate hydration and exercise of limbs when appropriate). All clinicians should review and thoroughly understand restraint guidelines (Gutheil and Tardiff, 1984).

The final decision to be made in the ED is which setting (outpatient or inpatient) is most appropriate for continued treatment. Criteria for hospitalization are summarized in Table 19–7 (Dubin and Weiss, 1991). Psychiatric consultation is almost always indicated in this situation.

Table 19–6 **Guidelines for Using Restraints**

At least four, and preferably five, persons should be used to restrain the patient. Leather restraints are the safest and surest type of restraints.
Explain to patients why they are going into restraints.
A staff member should always be visible and reassuring the patient while they are being restrained. This helps alleviate the patient's fear of helplessness.
Patients should be restrained with legs spread-eagled and one arm restrained to one side and the other arm restrained over the patient's head.
Restraints should be placed so that intravenous fluids can be given if necessary.
Raise the patient's head slightly in order to decrease the patient's feelings of vulnerability and reduce the possibility of aspiration.
The restraints should be checked every 5 minutes for safety and comfort.
After the patient is in restraints, the clinician should begin treatment using verbal intervention or RT. Even in restraints, most patients still take antipsychotic medication in concentrated form.
After the patient is under control, one restraint at a time should be removed at 5-minute intervals until the patient has only two restraints on. Both of these remaining restraints should be removed at the same time. It is inadvisable to have only one limb in restraints.

(Adapted from Dubin WR, Weiss KJ: Psychiatric Emergencies. In: Michels R, Cavenar JO, Brodie HK et al (eds): Psychiatry, Vol. 2. Philadelphia, JB Lippincott, 1985.)

Table 19–7 **Criteria for Hospital Admission**

The patient shows no improvement with medication and interview.
The patient improves, but remains so psychotic that they cannot care for their daily needs (i.e., work, housing, grooming, etc).
The patient poses a physical threat.
The patient is having command hallucinations.
The physician is in doubt about the severity of the condition.
The patient is toxic from drugs and/or alcohol or prescribed medication.
The patient is psychotic and has exhausted caregivers or all sources of external support.

THE SUICIDAL PATIENT

Suicide is one of the most dire consequences of mental illness and occurs in all diagnostic psychiatric categories. The annual suicide rate in the United States averages 12.5 suicides per 100,000 population. The suicide rate in users of psychiatric emergency services is ten times greater than that in the general population (Hillard, 1983). Emergency department clinicians are frequently the first to encounter patients who have either completed suicide, attempted suicide, or have suicidal ideation. Important in the evaluation and treatment of these patients is knowing the risk factors for suicide and having the skill to elicit key clinical features that differentiate the truly suicidal patient from the attention-seeker. *Never dismiss any patient as a nonrisk before a thorough evaluation is completed, even if the patient is well known to the ED staff or has a previous history of multiple attempts.*

In assessing patients, a number of risk factors have been enumerated (Dubin and Weiss, 1991). These factors are only guidelines that can help the physician judge the ultimate risk of suicide for each individual patient. One of the most important risk factors is the *lethality of attempt.* For example, someone whose gun misfires during a suicide attempt has made a much more lethal attempt than someone who swallows five aspirin. *In general, the more lethal the attempt, the greater the risk of suicide.* The concept of lethality, however, must also be based on the patient's perspective (Dubin and Weiss, 1985). For example, many patients overdose on benzodiazepines, believing they are fatal; others overdose on aspirin, thinking a household drug must be harmless. The benzodiazepine patient may be the more suicidal of the two, but the aspirin patient is more likely to die of medical complications.

Another important indicator of suicidal risk is the *imminence of possible rescue;* that is, the less imminent the chance of rescue, the greater the risk of suicide

Epidemiological studies have identified other risk factors (Cross and Hirschfeld, 1989). Males exceed females at levels for the risk of suicide. Generally, the suicide rates increase directly with age in the general population and in the white male population. In nonwhites, the peak occurs in the late 20s to early 30s. In white females, the peak suicide rate occurs in the 45 to 54 age range. Whites are twice as likely as nonwhites to commit suicide, though in the 25 to 34 year age group they are equal. Rates for the widowed, divorced, or separated are higher than for those who are married, and rates are highest in Protestants, intermediate in Jews, and lowest in Catholics. Other factors that increase the risk of suicide are (Dubin and Weiss, 1991):

Unemployment
Poor physical health
Past suicide attempts
Depression resistant to treatment
Family history of suicide, especially parent
Psychosis
Alcoholism/drug abuse
Chronic, painful disease
Sudden life changes
Patient living alone
Anniversary of significant loss

Treatment

The ED treatment of the suicidal patient is a complex problem that should generally be managed by a psychiatrist. Suicide attempts, gestures, or thoughts are always tinged with ambivalence about death, and the patient's presence in the ED may be a manifestation of part of the desire to live (Dubin and Weiss, 1991).

It is important to instill hope in the patient. Confront the patient's sense of hopelessness by helping the patient to develop a realistic, concrete approach to their own problems. Emphasize the patient's past successes in dealing with similar situations. Point out that the patient's negative beliefs are a result of a viewpoint that is perhaps distorted and hopeless; they are not necessarily the way things really are. Stress the patient's positive traits and accomplishments. Mobilize the patient's support system by asking family, spouse, parents, and friends to come to the ED; this will enhance the patient's sense of self-esteem and will increase their feeling of being loved.

Approach the suicidal patient in an objective, nonjudgmental, and concerned manner. Avoid reprimanding the patient for the suicide attempt. When evaluating the suicidal patient, phrase questions concerning suicide in the general context of feelings of depression and hopelessness (i.e., How bad do you feel? What do you feel the future has in store for you? If you felt this bad before, can you describe what was happening?). Question the patient specifically about the suicide plan. *It is a myth that asking about specific suicide plans and thoughts will plant the idea of suicide.* Exploring the patient's feelings can be cathartic. Encouraging patients to discuss their feelings and fantasies often dispels the mystique of suicide, and they will begin to consider other alternatives to resolve their conflict.

The central issue in the treatment of suicidal patients is educating them about other solutions to their problems. This is done by listening to the patient and providing guidance, interpretation, and education. Involving significant others when appropriate can increase the patient's feelings of emotional support and control. Using ancillary systems such as social services, job programs, welfare assistance programs, and psychiatric outpatient and inpatient programs can further enhance support. The physician can also increase the patient's feelings of support by making such statements as, "I'm going to help you by giving you medication to relax you, by making an appointment for you, by calling your family, etc." The important phrase is "I'm going to help."

Nonverbal communication (i.e., a patient who comes to the emergency room with a bag packed and expects to be admitted) frequently gives clues to the nature of suicidal intent. Patients who recently made a will or straightened out their financial affairs may not be expecting to live too long. If the patient is in treatment, the treating psychiatrist or therapist should be notified of the suicidal gesture/attempt while the patient is in the ED. Patients can often provide information that will facilitate emergency treatment.

Disposition

Table 19–8 outlines the general indications for hospitalization of suicidal patients (Dubin and Weiss, 1991; Walker, 1983). If the patient is hospitalized, they

Table 19–8 **Indications for Hospitalization of Suicidal Patients**

Psychosis
Intoxication with drugs or alcohol that cannot be evaluated and treated over a period of time in the emergency department.
No change in affect or symptoms despite the intervention of the physician, family, and friends.
Command hallucinations.
Low availability of outpatient resources.
Family exhaustion.
Escalating number of suicide attempts.
Uncertainty about the risk of suicide.

should be continuously observed; a staff member should accompany the patient to the bathroom. The patient should wear a gown, and ties, belts, shoelaces, or stockings should be removed.

Under no circumstances should a suicidal patient be allowed to leave the emergency department until an evaluation by a psychiatrist is completed. If the patient insists on leaving before such an evaluation, they should be detained under the appropriate legal guidelines until a reasonable assessment can be made. The patient's rights are secondary to this potentially life-threatening situation.

State laws permit involuntary commitment of a person who is demonstrably suicidal and refuses voluntary hospitalization. Physicians can be held liable for professional negligence if they fail to identify the suicide risk, do not try to detain a suicidal person, or prescribe medications that are later used by the patient to attempt suicide. *Thorough documentation of the patient's history, examination, and treatment plan are the best protection against charges of negligence.*

When a patient is discharged from the ED, all efforts should be made to have friends or relatives accompany the patient home and spend the next 24 hours with him or her. *Almost without exception, a patient who presents with suicidal ideation or gestures should not be sent home alone.* Patients should be given the name and phone number of the treating ED physician and reassured that they can call at any time. Ideally, the patient should have an outpatient appointment the next day, if outpatient treatment is deemed safe. All efforts should be made to avoid giving medication to patients who are being discharged. However, when clinically determined that medication would be of benefit, not more than three pills should be dispensed in total. Initially definitive drug therapy is the responsibility of the physician who will be involved in the ongoing treatment of the patient.

ACUTE ALCOHOL AND DRUG INTOXICATION AND WITHDRAWAL

Substance-abuse emergencies are a common ED problem. The treatment of substance abuse is complicated because patients often ingest multiple substances. Intoxication and withdrawal states frequently present both a medical and behavioral emergency, requiring close collaboration between the psychiatrist and other ED physicians. Since substance abuse is extensively reviewed in Chapter 10 by Dr. Swift, only highlights pertaining to the ED will be addressed here.

Assessment

Many patients are brought to the ED because of acute alcohol intoxication. Treatment with such patients begins with the initial interview, which can strongly influence the course of treatment. Interviewers should be tolerant and nonthreatening and should accept the intoxicated patient just as they accept insults and rudeness as part of the illness. Food and support will often serve to calm the patient. The availability and presence of security personnel can deter the belligerent patient from violent outbursts and will help reassure the interviewer. The patient will respond in a calmer fashion if placed in a quiet room with minimal stimulation. Intoxicated patients should be prevented from harming themselves or others; physical restraints may be needed.

A physical examination is mandatory to rule out other medical conditions that may accompany alcohol intoxication, such as bleeding, cardiac arrhythmias, pneumonitis, and head injuries. Use caution with stuporous patients. Before letting them sleep it off, rule out head injury or make sure the patient did not overdose with other drugs.

Usually, the preferred disposition is to send patients home with support of family and friends and refer them to an alcohol program the next day. Part of the follow-up includes a referral to Alcoholics Anonymous. No ataxic patient should ever be discharged. Criteria for hospitalizing a patient withdrawing from alcohol are summarized in Table 19–9 (Greenblatt and Shader, 1977).

Table 19–9 **Criteria for Hospitalization of a Patient Withdrawing From Alcohol**

Alcohol withdrawal delirium (Delirium tremens)
Hallucinosis
Seizure in patient with no known seizure disorder
Presence of acute Wernicke's and/or Korsakoff's syndrome (alcohol amnestic disorder)
Fever over 101° F
Head trauma with a period of unconsciousness or altered sensorium
Clouding of sensorium
Presence of major medical illness (e.g., respiratory failure or infection, hepatic decompensation, pancreatitis, gastrointestinal bleeding, severe malnutrition)
Known history of delirium, psychosis, or seizures in previous untreated withdrawal episodes

(Reprinted with permission from Greenblatt DJ, Snader RI. Treatment of the alcohol withdrawal syndrome. In: Snader RI, ed. A manual of psychiatric therapeutics. Boston: Little, Brown, 1977.)

A frequently misdiagnosed syndrome in the ED is the Wernicke-Korsakoff syndrome, which is characterized by ophthalmoplegia, nystagmus, impaired recent memory, peripheral neuritis, and ataxia (Reuler, Girard, and Cooney, 1985). Patients require immediate intervention as many of the neurologic signs are reversible if treated in a timely fashion. Treatment usually begins in the ED with thiamine 100 mg intramuscularly, which should be continued throughout treatment. The patient should be hospitalized and withdrawn from alcohol and should receive vigorous vitamin therapy. (See also Chapter 10 by Dr. Swift.)

Patients in delirium tremens (DTs) or alcohol withdrawal delirium are often referred to psychiatrists because of their extreme agitation and hallucinations. DTs is a serious withdrawal syndrome that occurs 3 to 4 or as late as 10 days after cessation of drinking. Mortality has been reported between 1 and 10%, with hyperthermia and peripheral vascular collapse as the usual causes of death. Symptoms of DTs are similar to those found in delirium, with waxing and waning of symptoms, visual hallucinations, disorientation, gross tremors, and elevated autonomic signs. DTs is a medical emergency requiring immediate, aggressive intervention.

In a comprehensive review of inpatient management of alcohol withdrawal and DTs, Frances and Franklin (1987) note that benzodiazepines are clearly the medication of choice because of their relatively high therapeutic safety index, the option of oral, IM, or IV administration, and their anticonvulsant properties. In contrast, barbiturates, which once were a popular treatment intervention, have fallen into relative disuse because of a high incidence of respiratory depression and a low therapeutic safety index. All benzodiazepines are equally efficacious; special circumstances may favor a particular drug (Frances and Franklin, 1987). The long half-lives of chlorodiazepoxide and diazepam (24 to 36 hours) give an advantage of a smooth induction and gradual decline in blood levels so that there are fewer symptoms on discontinuation of lower dosage. Chlorodiazepoxide gives greater sedation, while diazepam has greater anticonvulsant activity, which may make it more preferable for patients with a history of seizures. In elderly patients or those with liver diseases, lorazepam or oxazepam, which have short half-lives, are preferred. Lorazepam also has the advantage of being the only benzodiazepine other than midazolam that has rapid and complete absorption following IM administration. Relative potencies are as follows: diazepam 10 mg = chlorodiazepoxide 25 mg = lorazepam 1 mg. A standard management regimen for alcohol withdrawal as suggested by Frances and Franklin (1987) is outlined in Table 19–10.

Drug Intoxication and Withdrawal

The evaluation of patients intoxicated or withdrawing from controlled substances can pose one of the more complex problems in the ED. Frequently, patients ingest multiple medications; at other times, they may self-medicate their own withdrawal, thereby presenting a confusing picture. Often, because of the patient's agitated behavior, treatment is necessary before the results of blood screens are available. The most common problem is extreme agitation secondary to intoxication from cocaine, amphetamines, or phencyclidine. Treatment interventions are outlined in

Table 19–10 **Treatment of Alcohol and Substance Intoxication
and Withdrawal States**

Alcohol Withdrawal States (Frances and Franklin, 1987; Hyman and Arana, 1987)	
	Chlorodiazepoxide—25–100 mg po QID on first day; 20% decrease in dose over 5 to 7 days plus 25–50 mg po QID PRN for agitation, tremors, or change in vital signs; or substitute
	Lorazepam 2 mg orally q 2 hr for elderly patients or patients with liver disease
	Thiamine 100 mg po qd
	Folic acid 1 mg po QID
	Multivitamin one per day
	Magnesium sulfate 1 mg IM q 6 hr × 2 days (if status postwithdrawal seizures)
*Extreme agitation	Lorazepam, 2–4 mg IM q 1 hr or rapid tranquilization (See Table 19–4)
Barbiturate Withdrawal	
	Pentobarbital challenge test:
	Give pentobarbital 200 mg po and observe patient for 1 hr. If:
	patient asleep—not barbiturate-dependent
	no effect —repeat 200 mg hourly until nystagmus or drowsiness develops
	nystagmus and/
	or drowsiness—total dosage is starting point for detoxification with 10% reduction each day, tapered over 10 days
Cocaine and Amphetamine Intoxication	
Mild to moderate agitation	Diazepam, 10 mg orally q 8 hr
Severe agitation	Thiothixene, 20 mg concentrate or 10 mg IM
	Haloperidol, 10 mg concentrate or 5 mg IM
Phencyclidine (PCP) Intoxication	
	Ammonium chloride, 2.75 mEq/kg/dose in 60 ml of saline given by nasogastric tube in conjunction with ascorbic acid (2 g/500 ml IV) q 6 hr until urine pH is below 5
Hyperactive, mild agitation, tension, anxiety, excitement	Diazepam, 10–30 mg orally
	Lorazepam, 3–4 mg (0.05 mg/kg) IM may be considered as an alternative in uncooperative patients
Severe agitation and excitement with hallucinations, delusions, bizarre behavior	Haloperidol, 5–10 mg IM q 30–60 min.
Opioid Withdrawal	
	Methadone, 10–20 mg orally, titrated by 10%/day
	Clonidine, 0.1 mg BID or TID may be used as an adjunct to methadone or alone to decrease the hyperadrenergic symptoms
Anticholinergic Delirium	
	Use of phystostigmine has been questioned; should be used with the supervision of a medical consultant in doses of 1–4 mg IM or IV

* Rapid tranquilization in alcohol withdrawal states is for severe agitation and behavioral dyscontrol. The actual treatment of withdrawal is with a cross-tolerant medication.

Table 19–10 (Dubin, Weiss, and Dorn, 1986). The signs and symptoms of intoxication and withdrawal with various drugs are discussed in Chapter 10.

VICTIMS OF VIOLENCE

Rape

Rape is an act of aggression and hostility in which victims are often brutalized; if ED diagnostic and treatment procedures are handled in an insensitive, disrespectful manner, a "second rape" may occur (Goodstein, 1984). Evaluations are often undertaken without offering an explanation to the patient or getting her consent. Multiple questions from clinical personnel, family, and legal staff are often asked in a negative tone and may involve off-color comments by the interviewer. The legal aspects of the case are often delayed and protracted, and newspapers may publish the victim's name and address (25% of the cases). Clinical follow-up for pregnancy, venereal disease, and vaginal infections may be lengthy. This entire process psychologically prolongs the rape.

In approaching the rape victim, it is important to realize that patients have several important psychological, medical, and legal needs. The phenomenon of AIDS has cast another specter over the trauma of rape.

Evaluation and Treatment

Psychological Interventions. The victim's response may vary widely from confusion, guilt, agitation, and terror to some evidence of fear and anxiety. Some patients may display complete calm and even occasionally smile, indicating they are essentially still in a state of emotional shock. Since patients may resent the offer of psychiatric help, immediate psychiatric intervention should be reserved for complicated cases or for dealing with families. However, psychological care begins the moment the patient arrives. The patient should have immediate attention and privacy and should be asked to sign consent forms for examination and future release of medical records. *Police officers should not be present during the history and physical examination, nor should family members and friends.* However, rape patients should never be left alone and a female should be with female victims.

Many patients tend to blame themselves for their handling of the rape encounter. The patient will need support and reassurance that whatever she did was appropriate because it helped her come out of the encounter alive. At times, patients will need to repeat the story continuously. An important task is to listen and to allow the patient to share her feelings of pain, anger, and embarrassment. Patients who are unwilling to talk about the experience and their feelings even after being encouraged to do so should be respected.

Burgess and Holmstrom (1980) describe two phases of psychological reaction to a rape: disorganization and gradual reorganization. In the disorganization phase, emotions may be expressed openly (crying, shaking, and inappropriate smiling) or victims may feel numb and empty and unable to express emotion. Fear and physical symptoms are prominent. The reorganization phase usually begins 2 to 3 weeks after the rape. The victim may change the locks on her doors, move to a new residence, or change her phone number. Nightmares, phobias, and hyperactivity may occur. The victim may resort to maladaptive solutions such as drugs, alcohol, or suicidal or homicidal plans. During the reorganization phase, symptoms gradually diminish and, within months to years, the victim returns to normal functioning.

Before being discharged from the ED, patients should be counseled as to the potential psychological sequelae of the rape and told where they can receive psychological help if necessary (perhaps the name of a psychiatrist and information about Women Organized Against Rape, a local counseling center, or support groups). Patients should not be sent home alone. All efforts should be made to arrange for family or friends to be with her for at least 24 hours after she is discharged to provide continued emotional support.

Medical Interventions. Hanke (1984) outlines the following steps for the treatment of the physical trauma of the rape:

1. Obtain the patient's permission to have needed physical exams done, specimens collected, photographs taken, and releases of information completed.
2. Before doing the physical exam, be sure the patient will agree to it. If the patient is reluctant to allow an exam, reassure her of the need for the exam for her physical safety and legal defense.
3. Obtain specimens from the vaginal pool for the police laboratory to test. Obtain cervical and rectal cultures for gonorrhea and obtain a serology for syphilis.
4. *Establishing that a rape occurred is a legal decision, not a medical diagnosis.* Record the history in the patient's own words, document laboratory work, and save all clothing. Defer the diagnosis of rape.
5. To prevent pregnancy, offer a 5-day course of medroxyprogesterone or diethylstilbestrol. If the patient is taking oral contraceptives or has an intrauterine device, medication is not needed.
6. To protect the patient against venereal disease, penicillin should be given. If the patient is allergic to it, use oral tetracycline or intramuscular streptomycin.

Spouse Abuse

Spouse abuse is generally wife abuse. It is rarely the presenting complaint, and many women will not volunteer information unless asked. Spouse abuse occurs in all social classes and ethnic groups, but the highest incidence is among the poor. Specific recommendations for clinical recognition of wife abuse include the following (Goodstein, 1984):

1. Consider abuse in women who present with injuries to the head, face, back, and arms. Familiar excuses for bruises and lacerations are "I walked into a door" or "I fell off a chair."

2. Suspect abuse if there are chronic injuries or a substantial delay between the time of injury and presentation for treatment.
3. Ask patients wearing sunglasses to remove them, as they may be used to hide black eyes.
4. Ask about abuse in women who come for treatment with strong themes of separation anxiety from the spouse or who have the triad of trauma, depression, and problems with children.
5. Inquire about other violence at home, especially child abuse and incest.

Emergency treatment centers around caring for any acute trauma and ensuring the immediate safety of the woman and her children. If it is not safe for them to go home, they can be referred to emergency shelters for abused women. Hospitalization is not indicated unless trauma requires it or the woman is seriously suicidal or homicidal. ED treatment is difficult because the patient will be distressed by the intensity and range of her feelings, which include loss of control, helplessness, fear, anger, shame, doubts about sanity, and ambivalence about the abuser. It is very unlikely that an abusive cycle can be broken during a single emergency visit, but the first step toward intervention in a dangerous relationship can be taken. Referral to private therapy, a mental health agency, or community service should be made from the ED. If therapy is not possible for the couple, the victim should be encouraged to seek help alone. In an excellent review of the battered-wife syndrome, Goodstein (1984) outlines in depth a variety of psychosocial interventions.

Child Abuse

There are four types of child abuse: *physical abuse, sexual abuse, neglect,* and *emotional abuse.* ED clinicians should be familiar with their state laws; most states require that reports of suspected abuse or neglect be filed immediately. Interviews with family about child abuse should be handled in a nonthreatening, supportive, empathic manner and should involve both the child and the broader family unit. Hanke (1984) suggests leading up to the question of physical abuse by obtaining more general information such as difficulties during pregnancy, labor, or delivery, feeding or sleeping problems, and presence of colic. Other initial questions include whether the child is provocative, is always getting into trouble, has temper tantrums, or gets into fights with siblings and peers. Questions about actual abuse should aim at getting a clear picture of the parent's and child's behavior before, during, and after an episode of abuse.

Parents may become angry or defensive and deny that they have harmed the child or have done anything wrong. The task is not to blame the parents or get them to admit to wrongdoing, but to make sense of the history and physical findings. The interview should focus on how the child's behavior leads the parents to overreact. The clinician should avoid trying to rescue the child from parents. The main focus of the interview is to convince the parents that physical abuse of the child is a family problem that you would like to help them with. When all data point to child abuse as the most likely diagnosis, or there is other evidence to reasonably suspect the diagnosis, it is wise to review the case with a social work consultant and to file a report as specified by state law.

Sexual abuse in children should be suspected in the following situations (Hanke, 1984):

1. Gynecologic symptoms in prepubertal children
2. Pregnancy in a girl under 12 years old
3. Abrupt changes in behavior or school performance
4. Suicidal behavior in a preadolescent girl
5. Vague somatic complaints from the child or the mother
6. Overstimulation between father and daughter (bathing together, wrestling, excessive physical contact).

Sexual abuse is a sensitive topic. The interview should be conducted in a nonjudgmental and empathic but fact-finding manner. The procedure for data collection is the same used in suspected child abuse. ED interventions are directed toward protecting the child and family from further abuse and engaging the family in treatment.

Elder Abuse

Research on domestic violence has focused primarily on child and spouse abuse. Until recently, neglect and abuse of elderly persons has received little attention in the medical literature. Conservatively, there are 1.1 million elderly people who are victims of moderate to severe abuse annually (Bourland, 1990). To intervene and effectively prevent cases of elder abuse, physicians must be aware that the problem exists and that detection of elder abuse requires a high index of suspicion (Jones, Dougherty, Schelble et al, 1988).

The majority of victims of elder abuse are white, widowed women, usually older than 75 years of age, and without the sufficient income to live independently (Bourland, 1990; Jones, Dougherty, Schelble et al, 1988). In addition, victims tend to be more dependent on the care-giver for carrying out the activities of daily living. Abused victims have significantly greater cognitive impairment and are more likely to display such problematic behaviors as incontinence, nocturnal shouting, wandering, or manifestations of paranoia (Bourland, 1990). The abuser more often is a relative and frequently lives in the same household. About 40% of abusers are spouses and about 50% are children or grandchildren (Bourland, 1990). The care-giver is likely to be under great stress. Alcoholism, marital problems, unemployment, financial difficulties, social isolation, drug abuse, a family history of violence, or the presence of mental illness or mental retardation or dementia in the family care-giver are all risk factors for elder abuse and neglect (Bourland, 1990).

Abuse can take various forms and usually falls into one of several categories (Bourland, 1990; Jones, Dougherty, Schelble et al, 1988). Physical abuse is an act of violence that results in bodily harm or mental distress. Such abuse can be detected by signs of physical injury including injuries that are in various stages of healing. Common are lesions consistent with the shape of a weapon or are located in areas normally covered by clothing. Injuries may occur around the mouth, face, or eyes and should raise suspicion of abuse. Alopecia and hemorrhaging at the nape of scalp are findings that strongly suggest hair pulling. Bruises, burns, and human bite marks should also arouse suspicion. Ambulation that appears to be painful or an unusual gait may be symptoms of sexual assault or other hidden injuries.

Physical neglect is the deliberate or unintentional withholding of assistance vital to the performance of activities of daily living. Physical neglect is far more common than physical injury and should be suspected in elderly patients who exhibit signs such as pallor, wasting, dehydration, and decubitus ulcers. Improper care of medical problems, untreated injuries, or poor hygiene may also indicate that no one is attending to the patient's basic needs.

Psychological abuse is repeated verbal abuse and threats of deprivation of property or services resulting in emotional suffering. The care-giver may threaten nursing home placement or withdrawal of financial support or may resort to simple name-calling. When psychological abuse occurs, there may be no physical signs of abuse; however, behavioral findings may include depression, withdrawal, anger, infantile behavior or agitation, or the expression of ambivalent feelings toward family.

In addition to a physical examination, certain studies can be helpful in detecting patients who are suspected victims of elder abuse (Jones, Dougherty, Schelble et al, 1988). These studies include a radiologic screen for fractures or evidence of physical abuse; a metabolic screening for nutritional, electrolyte, and endocrine abnormalities; and a toxicologic and drug level screen to determine over- or undermedication. Hematologic screening for coagulation defect is important when abnormal bleeding or bruising is documented; computed tomography may be necessary if there has been a major change in neurologic status or head trauma.

The intervention when one suspects elder abuse will depend on the type of abuse present, its severity, and the care-giver's interest in improving the home environment. Clinicians must take responsibility for educating themselves about various local community, social, and health services. Unlike abused children, abused elderly persons can refuse protective services. Intervention without the care-giver's consent is protected when there is probable cause of suspected abuse and the elderly victim either consents to intervention or is incapable of giving informed consent. In such instances, the physician should contact the adult protective services division of the local service agency, if the community has one, or the local law enforcement agency. If the patient is discharged from the emergency department, follow-up arrangements should be made immediately with the guarantee of a home visit by a visiting nurse or social worker.

FORENSIC ISSUES: COMPETENCY AND COMMITMENT

Commitment laws vary throughout the United States, and clinicians must be familiar with the commitment laws of their state. There are two types of commitment (Hanke, 1984). In *voluntary commitment*, a patient agrees to be admitted to a psychiatric unit for hospitalization. Generally, patients are admitted to unlocked units. Criteria for release from the unit vary from state to state; some states require the patient to request discharge in writing, after which he or she may be allowed to leave or may be detained for variable periods of time. *Involuntary commitment* is undertaken when a patient is mentally ill and refuses to be admitted voluntarily for treatment. In the broadest sense of the term, most involuntary commitments are allowed when patients either pose a danger to themselves or others or demonstrate a lack of ability to care for themselves to such an extent that without intervention they would be at medical risk for death. The evidence needed to determine or predict dangerous behavior is controversial: some state laws require evidence of an imminent act, while others require that a threatened act or steps toward commission of an act be documented. Some states actually require that suicidal or homicidal acts be committed before involuntary commitment can take place. Since most states require that psychiatric treatment occur in the least restrictive setting, involuntary commitment is viewed as a treatment of last resort when other treatments or approaches have failed.

COMPETENCE

Under the law, all adults are presumed to be competent unless judged by a court to be incompetent (Dubin and Weiss, 1991). However, in a psychiatric emergency, waiting for a court to act is rarely feasible. Therefore, the patient's ability to make decisions regarding treatment and/or hospitalization is based on clinical competence. The main criteria used by clinicians to assess the patient's clinical competence are orientation to time, place, person; awareness of the psychological condition under consideration; understanding the potential benefits and risk of proposed treatment; and understanding the consequences of refusing treatment (Dubin and Weiss, 1991). A patient who is delirious, grossly psychotic, demented, or intoxicated is probably not competent to make decisions. In such cases consent for treatment should be obtained from family members. If the patient is dangerous, consent issues are less important because most state laws permit treatment of dangerous patients against their will. If alternative consent is not available, the clinician can, in good faith, treat a severely psychotic patient. Failure to do so could be considered negligence.

INFORMED CONSENT

There are three basic elements to informed consent: information, competence, and voluntariness (Dubin and Weiss, 1991). A patient cannot be expected to consent to or refuse treatment without having enough information to weigh the risk and benefits. The clinician is responsible for providing this information, including whatever the patient might want to know about the treatment side effects, legally known as material risk. To satisfy the legal requirement for informed consent, the clinician cannot merely recite a list of side effects. Rather, the clinician must discuss all treatment side effects that could reasonably make a difference with the patient about whether to accept of reject treatment. Furthermore, one cannot withhold treatment information for fear that the patient will refuse treatment based on the information. A useful decision tree (Groves and Vaccarino, 1987) outlines an approach for obtaining informed consent (Figure 19–1).

Competence as discussed above is the ability of the patient to understand treatment information and make a decision.

Voluntariness means that the consent to treatment must be given voluntarily, that is, with free will. The concept of free will—the absence of being forced to choose—is practical rather than philosophical. To say "sign this admission paper or I will call the police" is a type of coercion that negates voluntariness. Any treatment given under conditions of a threat could be seen by a court as assault or battery.

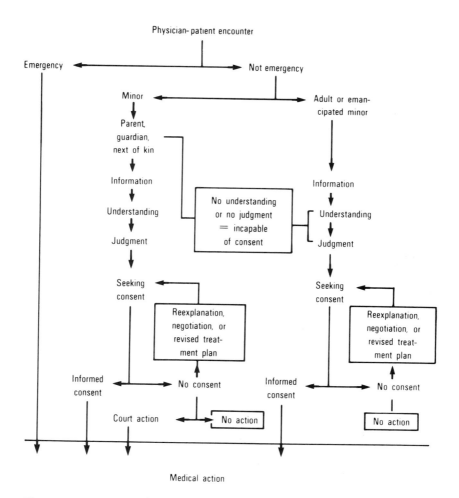

Figure 19–1. *Seeking and obtaining informed consent. (Reproduced with permission from Groves JE, Vacarino JM. Legal aspects of consultation. In: Hackett TP, Cassem NH, eds. Massachusetts General Hospital handbook of general hospital psychiatry, 2nd ed, p 601. Littleton, MA: PSG Publishing Co., 1987)*

Initial consent procedures should become an automatic part of every clinical interaction. At a minimum, there should be documentation that the proposed benefits and the potential risks of treatment were discussed with the patient. Consent should not be set aside except under conditions of manifest danger to the patient or others. Even then, when the emergency subsides, the patient usually retains the right to refuse treatment and be supplied with information about potential risks. To insure that all patients are assessed for competence and that they are provided with sufficient information to give an informed consent, the following procedure should be followed during the initial examination (Dubin and Weiss, 1991):

1. The patient's orientation to time, place, and person should be assessed as well as the patient's understanding of the emergency visit.
2. The patient should be informed of the clinician's role, the clinician's understanding of the clinical situation, and how the assessment for the need for treatment will be conducted.
3. The clinician should explain the clinical findings, what they mean, and what can be done to remedy the situation.
4. The patient should reiterate in their own words the explanation for the situation and then solicit questions or comments.
5. If possible, the treating physician should obtain written consent from the patient.

CLINICAL PEARLS

Suspect a medical, neurologic, or substance-induced mental syndrome if the patient has one of any of the following: clouded consciousness, age over 40 with no previous psychiatric history, disorientation, abnormal vital signs, visual hallucinations, or illusions

- The most common emergent life-threatening illnesses that present as psychiatric emergencies can usually be detected by a complete blood count, glucose, serum electrolytes, blood urea nitrogen, chest radiograph, electrocardiogram, arterial blood gases, and a urinary drug screen.
- The most common drug combination for rapid tranquilization is haloperidol 5 mg with 2 to 4 mg of lorazepam given intramuscularly in the same syringe.
- The target symptoms of rapid tranquilization are tension, anxiety, restlessness, and hyperactivity.
- No patient that presents suicidal should be discharged home alone.
- Head injuries, bruises, lacerations, dehydration, or broken bones should trigger suspicion of spouse abuse, elder abuse, or child abuse.
- When patients are a danger to themselves or others, informed consent can be set aside; however, it should be obtained once the emergency subsides.

ANNOTATED BIBLIOGRAPHY

Dubin WR, Weiss KJ: Handbook of Psychiatric Emergencies. Springhouse, PA, Springhouse Corporation, 1991

This handbook is comprehensive without overwhelming the reader with detail. It is designed in a very practical manner so that information is readily obtainable and usable. The format is designed to lead the reader through the process of evaluation, treatment, and disposition. Each clinical problem is discussed in the following manner: how to identify the problem, interpersonal interventions, pharmacological interventions, educational intervention, disposition, and medical/legal considerations. The key clinical points in each chapter are summarized in attractive charts and graphs.

Dubin WR, Weiss KJ, Dorn JM: Pharmacotherapy of psychiatric emergencies. J Clin Psychopharmacol 6:210–222, 1986

> This article is a comprehensive review of most of the studies in the literature that have addressed drug management of psychiatric emergencies. In addition to this comprehensive review, the authors propose basic guidelines for the drug management of psychiatric emergencies. The extensive, comprehensive bibliography is useful for those who wish to read the literature on rapid tranquilization.

Tardiff KJ: Management and Treatment of the Violent Patient. Washington, DC, American Psychiatric Press, 1989

> This book is a well-written, concise presentation of the principles and clinical issues involved in the management of aggressive patients. This book is easily readable and the information is immediately applicable to most emergency department clinical situations. This book includes an excellent chapter on recognition of potentially aggressive patients, and gives a good overview of interpersonal and pharmacologic interventions for managing aggressive patients.

Van Putten T, Marder SR: Behavioral toxicity of antipsychotic drugs. J Clin Psychiatry 48(9 Suppl):13–19, 1987

> This article presents an excellent discussion of the antipsychotic drug side effects of akathisia and akinesia. Of importance is the excellent discussion of akathisia, which is often misdiagnosed in the treatment of psychiatric emergencies. The discussion is clinically pertinent with excellent clinical examples. The discussion on akinesia is also comprehensive in its clinical description and clinical vignettes. This is an important article for clinicians who will be using antipsychotic drugs in their daily practice.

REFERENCES

Adams F: Neuropsychiatric evaluation and treatment of delirium in the critically ill cancer patient. Cancer Bull 36:156–160, 1984

Anderson WH: The Emergency Room. In Hackett TP, Cassem NH (eds): Massachusetts General Hospital Handbook of General Hospital Psychiatry, 2nd ed. Littleton, MA, PSG Publishing Co., 1987

Barbee JG, Mancuso DM, Freed CR et al: Alprazolam as a neuroleptic adjunct in the emergency treatment of schizophrenia. Am J Psychiatry 149:506–510, 1992

Bassuk EL, Panzarino PJ, Schoonover SC: General Principles of Pharmacologic Management in the Emergency Setting. In Bassuk EL, Birk AW (eds): Emergency Psychiatry: Concepts, Methods, and Practices. New York, Plenum, 1984

Bell CC, Palmer JM: Security procedures in a psychiatric emergency service. J Natl Med Assoc 73:835–842, 1981

Bourland MD: Elder abuse: From definition to prevention. Postgraduate Med 87:139–144, 1990

Burgess AW, Holmstrom LL: Rape trauma syndrome. Am J Psychiatry 137:1336–1347, 1980

Callaham M, Kassel D: Epidemiology of fatal tricyclic depressant ingestion: Implications for management. Ann Emerg Med 14:1–9, 1985

Clinton JE, Sterner S, Stelmachers Z et al: Haloperidol for sedation of disruptive emergency patients. Ann Emerg Med 16:319–322, 1987

Cross CK, Hirschfeld RMA: Epidemiology of Disorders in Adulthood: Suicide. In Michels R et al (eds): Psychiatry, Vol. 3. Philadelphia, JB Lippincott, 1989

Dubin WR: The evaluation and management of the violent patient. Ann Emerg Med 10:481–484, 1981

Dubin WR: Assessment and Management of Psychiatric Manifestations of Organic Brain Disease. In Dubin WR, Hanke H, Nickens HW (eds): Clinics in Emergency Medicine: Psychiatric Emergencies. New York, Churchill Livingstone, 1984

Dubin WR: Rapid tranquilization: Antipsychotics or benzodiazepines. J Clin Psychiatry 49(Suppl):S-11, 1988

Dubin WR, Weiss KJ: Diagnosis of organic brain syndrome: An emergency department dilemma. J Emerg Med 1:393–397, 1984

Dubin WR, Weiss KJ: Psychiatric Emergencies. In Michels R, Cavenar JO, Brodie HK et al (eds): Psychiatry, Vol. 2. Philadelphia, JB Lippincott, 1985

Dubin WR, Weiss KJ: Handbook of Psychiatric Emergencies. Springhouse, PA, Springhouse Corporation, 1991

Dubin WR, Weiss KJ, Dorn JM: Pharmacotherapy of psychiatric emergencies. J Clin Psychopharmacol 6:210–222, 1986

Dubin WR, Weiss KJ, Zeccardi J: OBS: The psychiatric imposter. JAMA 249:60–62, 1983

Dubin WR, Wilson S, Mercer C: Assaults against psychiatrists in outpatient settings. J Clin Psychiatry 49:338–345, 1988

Dudley DL, Rowlett DB, Loebel PJ: Emergency use of intravenous haloperidol. Gen Hosp Psychiatry 1:240–246, 1979

Dwyer B, Weissberg M: Treating Violent Patients. Psychiatric Times, p 11, December 1988

Frances RJ, Franklin JE: Alcohol-induced Organic Mental Disorders. In Hales RE, Yudofsky SC (eds): Textbook of Neuropsychiatry. Washington, DC, American Psychiatric Press, 1987

Garza-Treviño ES, Hollister LE, Overall JE et al: Efficacy of combinations of intramuscular antipsychotics and sedative-hypnotics for control of psychotic agitation. Am J Psychiatry 146:1598–1601, 1989

Goldstein MG: Intensive Care Unit Syndromes. In Stoudemire A, Fogel BS (eds): Principles of Medical Psychiatry. Orlando, Grune and Stratton, 1987

Goodstein RK: Situational Emergencies. In Dubin WR, Hanke N, Nickens HW: Clinics in Emergency Medicine: Psychiatric Emergencies. New York, Churchill Livingston, 1984

Goodstein RK: Common clinical problems of the elderly camouflaged by ageism and atypical presentation. Psych Ann 15:299–312, 1985

Greenblatt DJ, Shader RI: Treatment of the Alcohol Withdrawal Syndrome. In Shader RI (ed): A Manual of Psychiatric Therapeutics. Boston, Little Brown, 1977

Groves JE, Vaccarino JM: Legal Aspects of Consultation. In Hackett TP, Cassem NH (eds): Massachusetts General Hospital Handbook of General Hospital Psychiatry, 2nd ed. Littleton, MA, PSG Publishing Co., 1987

Gutheil T, Tardiff K: Indications and Contraindications for Seclusion and Restraint. In Tardiff K (ed): The Psychiatric Uses of Seclusion and Restraints. Washington, DC, American Psychiatric Press, 1984

Hall RCW, Popkin MK, DeVaul RA et al.: Physical illness presenting as psychiatric disease. Arch Gen Psychiatry 35:1315–1320, 1978

Hamid TA, Wertz WJ: Mesoridazine versus chlorpromazine in acute schizophrenia: A double-blind investigation. Am J Psychiatry 130:689–692, 1973

Hanke N: Handbook of Emergency Psychiatry. Lexington, MA, The Collamore Press, 1984

Hillard JR: Emergency Management of the Suicidal Patient. In Walker JI (ed): Psychiatric Emergencies: Intervention and Resolution. Philadelphia, JB Lippincott, 1983

Hyman SE, Arana GW: Handbook of Psychiatric Drug Therapy. Boston, Little Brown, 1987

Johnson SB, Alvarez WA, Freinhar JP: Rhabdomyolysis in retrospect: Are psychiatric patients predisposed to this little-known syndrome? Int J Psychiatry Med 17:163–171, 1987

Jones J, Dougherty J, Schelble D et al: Emergency department protocol for the diagnosis and evaluation of geriatric abuse. Ann Emerg Med 17:1006–1015, 1988

Konikoff F, Kuritzky A, Jerushalmi Y et al: Neuroleptic malignant syndrome induced by a single injection of haloperidol (letter). Br Med J 289:1228–1229, 1984

Lavoie FW, Carter GL, Danzi DF et al: Emergency department violence in United States teaching hospitals. Ann Emerg Med 17:1127–1233, 1988

Leeman CP: Diagnostic errors in emergency room medicine: Physical illness in patients labeled "psychiatric" and vice-versa. Int J Psychiatry Med 6:533–540, 1975

Lion JR: Evaluation and management of the violent patient. Springfield, IL, Charles C. Thomas, 1972

Lion JR, Levenberg LB, Strange RE: Restraining the violent patient. J Psychiatr Nurs and Ment Health Serv 10:9–11, 1972

Lion JR, Pasternak SA: Countertransference reactions to violent patients. Am J Psychiatry 130:207–210, 1973

Lipowski ZJ: Delirium, clouding of consciousness and confusion. J Nerv Ment Dis 145:227–255, 1967

Man PL, Chen CH: Rapid tranquilization of acutely psychotic patients with intramuscular haloperidol and chlorpromazine. Psychosomatics 14:59–63, 1973

Mason AS, Granacher RP: Clinical Handbook of Antipsychotic Drug Therapy. New York, Brunner/Mazel, 1980

Menza MA, Murray GB, Holmes VF et al: Decreased extrapyramidal symptoms with intravenous haloperidol. J Clin Psychiatry 48:278–280, 1987

Mueller PS: Neuroleptic malignant syndrome. Psychosomatics 26:654–661, 1985

O'Brien PJ: Prevalence of neuroleptic malignant syndrome (letter). Am J Psychiatry 144:1371, 1987

Pane GA, Winiarski AM, Salness KA: Aggression directed toward emergency department staff at a University teaching hospital. Ann Emerg Med. 20:283–286, 1991

Perry S: Acute Psychotic States. In Glick RT, Meyerson AT, Robbins E et al (eds): Psychiatric Emergencies. New York, Grune and Stratton, 1976

Reuler JB, Girard DE, Cooney TG: Wernicke's encephalopathy. NEJM 16:1035–1039, 1985

Robbins E, Stern M: Assessment of Psychiatric Emergencies. In Glick RA, Myerson AT, Robbins E et al (eds): Psychiatric Emergencies. New York, Grune and Stratton, 1976

Salamon I: Violent and Aggressive Behavior. In Glick RA, Myerson AT, Robbins E et al (eds): Psychiatric Emergencies. New York, Grune and Stratton, 1976

Shader RI, Greenblatt DJ: Back to basics—Diagnosis before treatment: Hopelessness, hypothyroidism, aging and lithium. J Clin Psychopharmacol 7:375, 1987

Sos J, Cassem NH: Managing postoperative agitation. Drug Ther 10:103–106, 1980

Swift RM: Alcohol and Drug Abuse in the Medical Setting. In Stoudemire A, Fogel BS (eds): Principles of Medical Psychiatry. Orlando, Grune and Stratton, 1987

Tardiff K, Sweillam A: Assault, suicide, and mental illness. Arch Gen Psychiatry 37:164–169, 1980

Tesar GE, Murray GB, Cassem NH: Use of high-dose intravenous haloperidol in the treatment of agitated cardiac patients. J Clin Psychopharmacol 5:344–347, 1985

Van Putten T, Marder SR: Behavorial toxicity of antipsychotic drugs. J Clin Psychiatry 48(9 Suppl):13–19, 1987

Walker JI: Psychiatric emergencies: Intervention and resolution. Philadelphia, JB Lippincott, 1983

Weissberg MP: Emergency room medical clearance: An educational problem. Am J Psychiatry 136:787–790, 1979

Wells CE, Duncan GW: Neurology for Psychiatrists. Philadelphia, FA Davis, 1980

Wise M: Delirium. In Hales RE, Yudofsky SC (eds): Textbook of Neuropsychiatry. Washington, DC, American Psychiatric Press, 1987

Alan Stoudemire (ed). *Clinical Psychiatry for Medical Students*, Second Edition. Copyright © 1994, 1990 by J. B. Lippincott Company.

20 Psychiatric Aspects of Medical Practice

James L. Levenson

Psychiatric disorders are common in medical patients, although the measured frequency varies depending on the criteria used. A reasonable estimate would be that 25 to 30% of medical outpatients and 40 to 50% of general medical inpatients have diagnosable psychiatric disorders (see Table 20–1). The most common psychiatric syndromes are depression, anxiety, and substance abuse in medical outpatients (Von Korff et al, 1987; Kessler, Cleary, and Burke, 1985) and disorders associated with cognitive impairment (delirium, dementia, etc.), depression, and substance abuse in medical inpatients (Wallen et al, 1987; Fulop et al, 1987). Most physicians underdiagnose and undertreat psychiatric disorders in the medically ill (Jencks, 1985; Cavanaugh, 1983). This is unfortunate because (1) many patients with serious psychiatric illnesses depend on primary care physicians, not mental health professionals, for their mental health care (Schurman, Kramer, and Mitchell, 1985; Shapiro et al, 1984); (2) without recognition and intervention, coincident psychopathology increases medical care utilization and costs (Levenson, Hamer, and Rossiter, 1990; Saravay et al, 1991; Mayou, Hawton, and Feldman, 1988); and (3) there are effective interventions for psychiatric disorders in the medically ill (Levenson, 1992).

The goals of this chapter are to examine the sources and consequences of psychiatric symptoms and disorders specific to medical patients and to understand the physician's corresponding responsibilities and opportunities for treatment. This chapter is grounded in the biopsychological model of illness (see Chapters 1, 2, and 14 of *Human Behavior: An Introduction for Medical Students*, edited by Dr. Stoudemire, and Chapters 1 and 2 of this text). Major psychiatric disorders that are often encountered in the medical setting are also discussed individually elsewhere in

Table 20–1 **Prevalence of Selected Psychiatric Disorders**

	COMMUNITY	PRIMARY CARE PATIENTS	MEDICAL INPATIENTS
All psychiatric disorders			
	15–20%	25–30%	40–50%
Depression			
Depressive symptoms	10–15%	10–30%	20–35%
Major depressive disorder	2–4%	5–10%	5–25%
Anxiety			
Anxiety symptoms	10–20%	12–20%	20–30%
Panic disorder	1–2%	2–15%	—
Cognitive disorders			
	1%	—	15–20%
	5–10% (over 65)		30–50% (over 65)

this book, including delirium, dementia and other disorders with cognitive impairment, (Chapter 4), personality disorders (Chapter 6), mood disorders (Chapter 7), somatoform disorders (Chapter 9), and substance abuse (Chapter 10).

This chapter focuses on special aspects of psychiatry in medical practice not discussed in depth in the earlier chapters. First, *psychological and emotional reactions to physical illness* are discussed, including the management of these reactions in the general medical setting. Second, the nature of *grief and mourning* and the *dying patient* are considered. Third, *drugs and medical disorders that can produce psychiatric symptoms* are reviewed. Finally, guidelines are provided for the evaluation of patients' *competency* and for *obtaining psychiatric consultation*.

Many aspects of this chapter reflect and expound upon topics discussed elsewhere in this volume but are also an extension of areas discussed in the companion text to this volume, *Human Behavior: An Introduction for Medical Students* (Stoudemire, 1994). Specifically, students may wish to consult chapters in that text on psychological reactions to medical illness by Dr. Stephen Green, Dr. Susan Shelton on the doctor–patient relationship, and the biopsychological model in medical care by Drs. Cohen-Cole and Levinson.

COMMON PSYCHOLOGICAL REACTIONS TO MEDICAL ILLNESS AND TREATMENT

Regression and Dependency

Regression, a return to more childlike patterns of behavior and feeling, is a universal human reaction to illness. Sick patients wish to be comforted, cared for, and freed from the responsibilities of adult life. In moderation this is adaptive, as the ill patient must give up some control over their bodies and lives and accept some dependency on others. Regression is problematic when it becomes more extreme. It is difficult to care for a patient who has minimal pain tolerance, cannot tolerate being alone, is infantile, overly needy, whining, and easily upset or frustrated.

Not all patients regress in the same fashion. The varieties of regression are similar to the developmental phases of early childhood. Like young infants, some regressed patients are overdependent and seem to want "feeding" on demand, constantly pushing the nurses' call button in the hospital or, as outpatients, telephoning the physician too much. They let others make decisions, complain petulantly about their care, and avoid sharing responsibility.

Other regressed patients resemble children in the "terrible twos." They have an excessive need to control their medical care in the hospital environment and get into struggles over less-critical elements of their care. They may have tantrums over getting their way and tend to be perfectionistic and intolerant of any irregularities, disarray, or tardiness.

Like many 3- to 4-year-olds, some patients who regress need to feel powerful and admired. They tend to be aggressive and narcissistic, oblivious to the needs of other patients around them. They may be sexually provocative, particularly if the illness has assaulted their sense of self-esteem and power (e.g., acute paraplegia or myocardial infarction).

These developmental descriptions of regression are illustrations that do appear as described, but also appear at milder, more easily tolerated levels. When ill, we all regress more or less along each of these lines: the need to be cared for, the need for control and order, the need for increased self-esteem. Some patients find such regression comfortable (ego-syntonic), particularly if it elicits comforting responses from those around them. Others are very uncomfortable with their regression (ego-dystonic), feeling embarrassed at the unexpected emergence of childlike feelings or actions.

Sources

As noted, moderate regression is adaptive. In the face of illness, adults hope to receive the nurturance, reassurance, and care provided by parents during childhood. Patients who regress behaviorally to an extreme often have preexisting psychopathology, particularly personality disorders. Those who use a narrow range of inflexible defenses become more helpless and regressed when serious illness overwhelms them. Patients who find regression too comfortable have usually received significant secondary gain from previous illnesses. Those who suffered serious deprivation in childhood, with emotionally or physically absent or dysfunctional parents, may experience the care of physicians and nurses as the only nurturing experiences they have ever had. As adults they unconsciously yearn to recreate this experience and so may regress excessively when ill.

Intervention

When regression is marked, physicians and nurses become impatient and angry, especially with those patients whom they feel should not act "childishly" (e.g., patients who are health care professionals). As with other reactions to illness, physicians should avoid scolding or shaming patients (a parallel regression in the physician).

Instead, the physician can explain to the patient that feeling more dependent or needy is part of an expected reaction to illness. Patients who make repeated, unreasonable, or unrealistic demands may require limit-setting. While tolerating some necessary regression, the physician takes steps to mobilize the patient physically and emotionally to participate in treatment and rehabilitation. Psychiatric consultation should be sought if regression is too great or persists too long, creating significant interference in treatment, distress for the patient, or unnecessary invalidism.

Anxiety

Anxiety occurs with the same symptoms in the medically ill as in healthy individuals, but a correct diagnosis is more difficult with coexistence of physical disease because the signs of anxiety may be misinterpreted as those of physical disease, and vice versa. Many somatic pathophysiological events share symptoms with anxiety states, such as tachycardia, diaphoresis, tremor, shortness of breath, or abdominal or chest pain. Panic attacks present with so many prominent somatic symptoms that they are routinely misdiagnosed as a wide variety of physical illnesses. On the other hand, autonomic arousal and anxious agitation in a medically ill patient may be prematurely attributed by the physician to "reactive anxiety," when they also can be signs of a pulmonary embolus or cardiac arrhythmia.

Physicians tend to become desensitized in working with seriously ill patients and may lose sight of the spectrum of normal anxious reactions. For example, having diagnosed diabetes mellitus in an asymptomatic young adult patient, the physician may assume that a diagnosis of "just chemical diabetes" ought not to cause too much anxiety. The physician may not notice that the patient is frightened, or if the physician does notice, she or he may conclude that the patient is responding with pathological anxiety. The patient may be thinking about serious complications (amputations, blindness, and kidney failure) witnessed in relatives with the disease, leading to more anxiety than the physician expected.

Sources

There are many reasons for anxiety in the medically ill patient. Different individuals will react to the same diagnosis, prognosis, treatment, and complications with widely varying concerns. Patients may be very aware of some fears, but simultaneously affected by less-conscious ones. Ideally, the physician explores this with the patient by inquiring about those aspects of the illness that are causing anxiety and by observing the patient's behavior.

Fear of death frequently occurs during the course of an illness, but not necessarily in proportion to the severity of disease. Many other factors may magnify or diminish this fear (e.g., previous losses, religious beliefs, personality, intractable pain, and previous experiences in the medical care system, including witnessing other patients' deaths). While for some patients with minor illness the fear of death can be overwhelming, for others, with major or even terminal illness, it may be less important than other fears.

Fear of abandonment ("separation anxiety") occurs in the medically ill as the fear of being alone. It may occur under the same circumstances that give rise to the fear of death, but here an individual is less concerned about the end of life and more concerned with the thought of being separated from loved ones. For some individuals who are immature, overly dependent, or overwhelmed, being hospitalized may itself precipitate acute separation anxiety. The patient must leave the security of home, family, and friends for the impersonal and anonymous institution of the modern hospital.

Closely related to separation anxiety is the *fear of strangers* ("stranger anxiety"). Visiting a physician when ill requires a patient to answer personal questions and to be physically examined by and put one's trust in (usually) previously unknown physicians and other members of the health care team. As patients become more acutely ill, or face a terminal illness, the fear of abandonment tends to be much greater than the fear of strangers. The sick and dying very rarely wish to be left alone. Residents and interns are often surprised at how anxious some patients become when it comes time for physicians to rotate to a new service each month, not recognizing how important they have become to their patients. What has become routine for the house staff is a repetitive source of anxiety for patients.

The morbidity and disability caused by physical disease produce a number of other fears. *The fear of loss of, or injury to, body parts or bodily functions* includes fear of amputations, blindness, and mutilating scars and is particularly highly charged when directed at the genitalia ("castration anxiety"). *The fear of pain* is universal, but the threshold varies greatly among individuals. Some patients experience intense *fear of loss of control.* They may also fear that they will no longer be able to manage a career, family, or other aspects of their life. Directed inwardly, individuals may be frightened by loss of control over their own bodies, including fear of incontinence or metastasis. Closely related is the *fear of dependency.* Here, it is not so much the loss of control of one's body or life that frightens the patient but having to depend on others. For some this fear of dependency is part of a more general *fear of intimacy.* Certain individuals (particularly schizoid, avoidant, paranoid, and some compulsive personalities) are frightened of getting close to people in any setting. Physical illness is very threatening to them because they must allow physicians and nurses to penetrate the interpersonal barriers they have constructed.

Finally, some patients experience *guilty fears* ("superego anxiety") related to their anticipation that others will feel angry or disappointed by them. This is particularly common with illnesses attributable to patients' habits (smoking, diet, alcohol, etc.) and in situations where patients have not complied with physicians' advice. Some patients may feel their illness is a punishment from God or has some special punitive significance for past "sins."

Consequences

Some degree of anxiety is adaptive during physical illness because it alerts the individual to the presence of danger and the need for action. An appropriate and tolerable amount of anxiety aids patients in getting medical help and adhering to physicians' recommendations. The total absence of anxiety may be maladaptive, promoting a cavalier attitude of minimizing disease and the need for treatment. In most such cases, however, the absence of anxiety is only an apparent one—the patient is often extremely anxious unconsciously and is resorting to defenses like denial (see below) in order not to be overwhelmed by the illness. Too much anxiety is also maladaptive, leading to unnecessary invalidism. Becoming paralyzed with fear of disease progression or relapse, such patients give up functioning occupationally, socially, and/or sexually. In most diseases a modicum of anxiety is expectable and adaptive, but occasionally even a normal amount of anxiety can pose some risk. For example, immediately after an acute myocardial infarction, any anxiety-associated increases in heart rate and blood pressure may be considered dangerous and warrant treatment.

Intervention

First, the physician should explore the particular patient's fears. If the physician wrongly presumes to know why the patient is anxious without asking, then the patient is likely to feel misunderstood. Facile, nonspecific reassurance can undermine the physician–patient relationship, as the patient is likely to feel the physician is out of touch with and not really interested in what they are actually feeling.

Knowing the patient's specific fears leads the physician to appropriate therapeutic interventions. Unrealistic fears can be reduced by cognitive interventions. For example, the patient who is frightened of having intercourse after a heart attack can be reassured that it is unnecessary to give up sex. Fears of closeness can be reduced by taking extra care to respect the patient's privacy. When fears of pain, loss, or injury to body parts are not unrealistic, it is helpful for the physician to emphasize the ways in which medical care can reduce suffering and enhance functioning through rehabilitation. Physicians should tell patients about disease-specific support organizations for patients and families, which provide a continuing antidote for anxiety.

When clarifying the patient's anxieties and intervening in one of these ways is insufficient, the judicious, short-term use of benzodiazepines may be helpful (see Chapters 8 (Drs. Nagy, Krystal, and Charney) and 18 (Drs. Silver, Hales, and Yudofsky). However, drug therapy for anxiety is no substitute for the reassurance and support that can be provided through the doctor–patient relationship. Antianxiety medication is best directed at new symptoms of anxiety that have been precipitated by an identifiable recent stressor (e.g., hospitalization). Drug therapy of anxiety in the medically ill should be time-limited (usually 1 to 3 weeks), because tolerance and dependence may develop with long-term use. If benzodiazepines are abruptly discontinued, significant withdrawal symptoms may occur, including rebound anxiety and insomnia, agitation, psychosis, confusion, and seizures. While benzodiazepines are relatively safe in the medically ill, their most common side effect, sedation, may intensify confusion in delirium and dementia, suppress respiratory drive in severe pulmonary disease, and interfere with optimal participation by patients in their medical care. Sustained use of benzodiazepines or other sedatives will aggravate depression. Antianxiety medication prescribed during a medical hospitalization should not be automatically continued after discharge.

In deciding whether psychiatric consultation and intervention are required, it is important to distinguish normal, expectable anxiety from more serious "pathological" anxiety. Anxiety is usually a symptom of a psychiatric disorder when it remains unrealistic or out of proportion despite the physician's clarification and reassurance, as described above. Other signs that anxiety requires psychiatric intervention are sustained disruption of sleep or gastrointestinal functions, marked autonomic hyper-arousal (tachycardia, tachypnea, sweating), and panic attacks. Psychiatric consultation should also always be requested when anxiety fails to respond to low doses of benzodiazepines, is accompanied by psychosis, or renders patients unable to participate in their medical care (including those who threaten to leave against medical advice).

Depression

In addition to clinical psychiatric depressions, depressed states in the medically ill may include grief, sadness, demoralization, fatigue, exhaustion and psychomotor slowing. The same pitfalls of under-or overdiagnosis described for anxiety also occur with depression. The vegetative signs and symptoms of depression (e.g., anorexia, weight loss, weakness, constipation, insomnia) may be incorrectly attributed to a physical etiology and lead the physician to undertake unnecessary diagnostic evaluations. On the other hand, the physician must also guard against prematurely concluding that somatic symptoms are due to depression, as an occult medical disease (e.g., malignancy) may be missed. Desensitization to illness and suffering may make physicians unaware of, or impatient with and intolerant of, normal reactive depression. Physicians sometimes err in the other direction and regard a serious (and treatable) coexisting psychiatric depression as merely a "normal" response to physical illness.

Sources

Medically ill patients feel sad or depressed about many of the same issues discussed above under anxiety. When a feared event has not yet taken place, patients are anxious; when the loss or injury has already occurred, the patient becomes depressed. Thus, depression may arise secondary to loss of relationships, loss of body parts or functions, loss of control or independence, chronic pain, or guilt. Hospitalization results in separation of the patient from loved ones, which is a potential source for depression, especially for young children and mothers of infants. Medical illness also may reawaken dormant grief and sadness when a patient recalls the parent or sibling who died from the same disease the patient has. Patients who cannot express anger, either because they have always had difficulty doing so or because they are afraid of offending those with whom they are angry (e.g., physicians), are at higher risk for depression.

Another explanation for depression in the medically ill is *learned helplessness*, a behavioral model derived from animal experiments. When repeatedly exposed to painful or other aversive stimuli while being prevented from controlling or escaping from such stimulation, many species become passive, withdrawn, and unmotivated. In patients, the course of physical illness, particularly when there are multiple relapses, relentless progression, and/or treatment failure, may produce a very similar state of helplessness, giving up, and the perception that one has no control over one's fate. Both experimentally and clinically, learned helplessness can be reduced by increasing the subject's sense of control. Physicians may unwittingly add to some patients' helplessness by not actively eliciting patients' participation and preferences in decision making about their health care.

Consequences

In the face of disease and disability, patients frequently feel discouraged, dejected, and helpless and need physicians who are able and willing to listen to such feelings. When feelings of sadness become too great and demoralization or clinical depression occurs, a number of maladaptive consequences may ensue, including poor compliance, poor nutrition and hygiene, and giving up prematurely. If severe, patients may become actively or passively suicidal (e.g., a transplant patient who deliberately misses doses of maintenance immunosuppressive drugs). Recognizing these serious consequences helps the physician to distinguish pathological depression from normal depressive reactions, including grief (see below).

Intervention

As with the anxious patient, the first step for the physician is to listen and understand. Physicians can help patients by encouraging them to openly express sadness and grief related to illness and loss. Physicians should avoid premature or unrealistic reassurance or an overly cheerful attitude as this tends to alienate depressed patients, who feel that their physician is insensitive and either does not understand or does not want to hear about their sadness. Physicians *should* provide specific and realistic reassurance, emphasizing a constructive treatment plan, and mobilize the patient's support system. For patients who seem to be experiencing learned helplessness, enabling them to have a sense of more control over their illness will be helpful. Physicians can accomplish this by encouraging patients to express preferences about their health care, by giving them more control over the hospital and nursing routines, and by emphasizing active steps patients can undertake, rather than just passively accepting what is prescribed by others for them. Patients who are demoralized before beginning or at the start of major treatment (e.g., transplantation, amputation, dialysis, chemotherapy, colostomy) can benefit from speaking with successfully treated patients who have had the same disorder.

Normal depressive reactions to illness must be differentiated from pathological depression, which requires psychiatric consultation and intervention (antidepressants and psychotherapy). Patients experiencing normal degrees of depression retain their abilities to communicate, make decisions, and participate in their own care when encouraged to do so. Depression usually constitutes a psychiatric disorder when depressed mood, hopelessness, worthlessness, withdrawal, and vegetative symptoms (e.g., insomnia, anorexia, fatigue) are persistent *and* out of proportion to coexisting medical illness. Urgent psychiatric referral should always be obtained when the patient is thinking about suicide (see below) or has depression with psychotic symptoms. Psychiatric consultation should also be obtained if less serious depression fails to improve with the physician's support and reassurance and becomes prolonged, if antidepressant medication is needed, or if patients remain too depressed to participate in their own health care and rehabilitation. The treatment of depression is discussed from the biological standpoint in Chapters 7 and 18, and psychotherapy for depression is discussed in Chapter 17 (Drs. Ursano, Silberman, and Diaz).

Assessing Suicide Risk in Medical Patients

All physicians should be able to screen patients for suicide risk in the medical setting. Chapter 19 addresses assessment of suicide in the emergency setting. Suicide is a common preventable cause of death in the medically ill, and patients frequently drop hints to their physicians about suicidal impulses or plans. Chronic illness and chronic pain are risk factors for suicide. The physician's concern should increase when other risk factors are present. These include major mood disorder, alcoholism, schizophrenia, disorders associated with impaired cognition, recent loss of a loved one, divorce, loss of a job, or a family history of suicide.

Whenever patients appear depressed or despondent, physicians should explicitly ask about suicidal feelings and plans. Physicians are sometimes reluctant, fearing that they will "put ideas into the patient's head" or offend the patient. Others simply are not sure how to ask. The great majority of patients who are experiencing suicidal thoughts are relieved to discuss them with a caring physician. The physician should ask gradually and directly, with a series of questions like: "How bad have you been feeling? Have you ever felt bad enough to not go on with life? Have you ever thought of doing something about it? What did you think of doing?" Ominous signs indicative of serious suicide risk include:

1. The motive behind the suicidal wish is entirely self-directed, with no apparent intent to influence someone else.
2. Detailed suicide plans are contemplated over an extended period of time.
3. Lethal means have been considered by and are available to the patient.
4. A suicide attempt was made in an isolated setting where the individual was unlikely to be discovered.
5. The individual is putting affairs in order, i.e., making out a will, reviewing life-insurance coverage, or giving away prized possessions.
6. Hints or direct statements are made about feeling suicidal. Spontaneous statements like "I'm going to kill myself" should never be dismissed as "just talk," but always carefully and thoroughly explored by the primary physician.

The presence of any suicidal ideation, with or without any attempt, is an indication for psychiatric consultation, and it is the physician's responsibility to ensure that it is obtained. Physicians must also guard against unwittingly providing the means for suicide: for significantly depressed patients, physicians should prescribe all medications in carefully monitored, small supplies (usually 1 week at a time).

Denial

Denial is a defense mechanism that reduces anxiety and conflict by blocking conscious awareness of thoughts, feelings, or facts that an individual cannot face. Denial is common in the medically ill, but varies in its timing, strength, and adaptive value. Some patients are aware of what is wrong with them but consciously suppress this knowledge by avoiding thinking about or discussing it. Others cope with the threat of being overwhelmed by their illness by unconsciously repressing it and thereby remain unaware of their illness. Physicians may sometimes misperceive as deniers patients whose lack of awareness stems from not having been sufficiently informed about and/or not understanding the nature of their disease. While denial of physical disease may accompany and be a symptom of a major psychiatric disorder (e.g., schizophrenia), outright denial also occurs in the absence of other significant psychopathology. Marked denial, in which the patient emphatically refuses to accept the existence or significance of obvious symptoms and signs of a disease, may be seen by the physician as an indication that the patient is "crazy," because the patient seems impervious to rational persuasion. In the absence of other evidence of major psychopathology (e.g., paranoid delusions), such denial is not often a sign of psychosis but rather is a defense against overwhelming fear.

Denial also occurs as a direct consequence of disease of the central nervous system, commonly in dementia along with other cognitive deficits and, rarely, as an isolated finding with parietal lobe lesions (anosognosia).

Sources

Denial is a defense mechanism used in the face of intolerable anxiety or unresolved conflict. The medically ill patient, threatened with any of the fears outlined above, may resort to denial. Individuals who deny other life stresses, such as marital or occupational problems, are particularly likely to use denial in the face of clinical illness. Denial is also common in individuals who are threatened by dependency associated with illness, for whom the sick role is inconsistent with their self-image of potency and invulnerability.

To avoid fear and conflict, the patient may deny all or only part of the disease and its consequences. Some will deny that they are ill at all; others will accept the symptoms but deny the particular diagnosis (usually displacing it to a more benign organ system, e.g., interpreting angina as indigestion), the need for treatment, or the need to alter lifestyle.

Consequences

Denial is not always a pathologic defense and may serve several adaptive purposes. When denial occurs as part of the initial shock upon learning of a serious diagnosis or complication, it allows the individual sufficient time to adjust to the bad news and avoid overwhelming, full, immediate awareness. A lesser, continuing degree of denial helps patients function without being overly preoccupied with full consciousness of the morbidity or mortality associated with their diseases.

The adaptive value of denial may vary depending on the nature or stage of illness. For example, myocardial infarction and sudden death may occur when denial prevents an individual with symptoms of coronary artery disease from acknowledging the symptoms and promptly seeking medical care. Those who delay going to the hospital after the acute onset of coronary symptoms have greater morbidity and mortality. Physicians seldom have an opportunity to affect denial at that stage of illness (that is, prior to seeking medical care), except by educating the general public. Moderate denial during hospitalization may be very adaptive, perhaps even reducing morbidity and mortality in some diseases (Levenson et al, 1989). If not excessive, such denial reduces anxiety but does not prevent the patient from accepting and cooperating with medical treatment.

Denial after hospital discharge may also be helpful or harmful. Too little denial may leave the patient flooded with fears of disability and death, resulting in unnecessary invalidism. However, excessive denial may result in the patient's rushing back to full-time work, disregarding the rehabilitation plan, ignoring modifiable risk factors, and adopting a cavalier attitude toward medication or other treatment.

Intervention

When a patient's denial does not preclude cooperation with treatment, the physician should leave it alone. The physician does have an ethical and professional obligation to ensure that the patient has been informed about their own illness and treatment. Following that, if the patient accepts treatment but persists in what seems an irrationally optimistic outlook, the physician should respect the patient's need to use denial to cope. For some the denial is fragile, and the physician must judge whether the defense should be supported and strengthened, or whether the patient would do better by giving up the denial to discuss fears and receive reassurance from the physician. The physician should not support denial by giving the patient false information but rather by encouraging hope and optimism.

When denial is extreme, patients may refuse vital treatment or threaten to leave against medical advice. Here the physician must try to help reduce denial, but not by directly assaulting the patient's defenses. Since such desperate denial of reality usually reflects intense underlying anxiety, trying to scare the patient into cooperating will intensify denial and the impulse to flight. A better strategy for the physician is to avoid directly challenging the patient's claims while simultaneously reinforcing concern for the patient and maximizing the patient's sense of control. Involving family members should be considered, as they may be more successful in convincing the patient that accepting medical care is in their own best interests. Psychiatric consultation is very helpful in cases of extreme or persistent maladaptive denial and should always be obtained if the denial is accompanied by symptoms of a major psychiatric disorder (see also Chapters 5 and 14 in Stoudemire, 1994).

Noncompliance

Noncompliance with medical treatment is a frequent behavioral response to medical illness. It may occur in up to 90% of those receiving short-term medication regimens and probably averages about 50% in the drug treatment of patients with chronic disease (Eraker, Kirscht, and Becker, 1984). Physicians generally underestimate its occurrence, misled both by wishful thinking and by stereotypes of the noncompliant patient. Noncompliance is common in patients who poorly understand their treatment, in those who are hostile to medical care, in those with major psychiatric disorders, and in those who flatly deny their illness. However, noncompliance also occurs in "ideal" patients and is not confined to any socioeconomic or ethnic group. Physicians are also misled because patients overestimate their compliance when asked. They may be embarrassed by their failure to stick to the regimen, frightened of the consequences (including fear of angering their physician), or unconscious of the problem. The physician will be more likely to get accurate information by asking in a friendly, nonjudgmental way without any threats, accusations, or anger. The physician must avoid shaming or infantilizing the patient through scolding or patronizing.

Labeling a patient as "noncompliant" implies that the physician's recommendations are entirely correct, but sometimes our instructions are unnecessary, debatable, or even wrong. Physicians must also avoid concluding noncompliance whenever there is unexplained failure of the patient to respond to the usual treatment. This may be an appropriate time to suspect noncompliance, but the physician should not reach a conclusion without evidence.

A patient is noncompliant when the patient and physician both share the belief that treatment is warranted, but the patient fails to follow through. However, physicians must remember that patients have their own value and belief systems that guide their actions. Scientific principles and the medical literature are not as compelling for most patients as they are for physicians. Religious beliefs, cultural values, and the patient's own theories of causation and treatment, which may be culture-bound or idiosyncratic, all influence patient responses to physicians' recommendations.

Noncompliance is not a monolithic behavior. While some patients are globally noncompliant, others are only with a particular aspect of treatment. Some have difficulty keeping appointments, others with taking medication. Many have difficulty complying with recommended changes in habits or lifestyle, including patterns of work and sleep, smoking, diet, and exercise. Others may follow recommendations coming from one trusted doctor (often a primary care physician), while ignoring the advice of unfamiliar consultants. Some individuals are only intermittently noncompliant (for example, only during periods of depression).

Sources

As suggested above, preexisting beliefs the patient has about diagnosis and treatment are a major source of deviation from the treatment plan. Many ethnic subcultures have their own traditional theories of disease and therapy that may influence how members take medications. Such patients tend to hide this from physicians who are not members of the same ethnic/cultural group, because the patients think their beliefs will not be accepted or because they are embarrassed to acknowledge "old-fashioned," "superstitious" ideas. A similar phenomenon is seen with those who believe various "counterculture" theories of disease like homeopathy or naturopathy and with followers of religions that practice faith-healing. Some patients have deep and powerful beliefs about the right and wrong way to treat their illness, based on past personal or family experience. If a severe side effect has previously occurred with dire consequences or, alternatively, the patient knows someone who did well despite refusing treatment, the physician may find the patient very reluctant to accept treatment.

Noncompliance is more likely to occur when the treatment regimen is too complex (i.e., multiple drugs on different dosage schedules), expensive, inconvenient, or long term, or if it requires alteration of lifestyle. Misunderstanding or lack of knowledge may be the most common source of apparent noncompliance. Physicians widely overestimate patients' understanding of the reasons for treatment, the method and schedule prescribed, and the consequences of not following through. Physicians tend to assume that they are understood by patients, when they are often not. One study showed that "q6 hours" was correctly understood by only 36% of the patient sample (Mazzullo, 1976).

The previously described emotional and defensive reactions to illness (anxiety, depression, denial, and regression) are also major causes of noncompliance. Patients may be frightened by the treatment itself, or simply avoid carrying out the treatment or habit-change because it reminds them of the feared disease. Patients who are depressed may do a poor job of following treatment recommendations because of poor concentration, low motivation, pessimism, or acting out of suicidal feelings. Individuals who need to feel strongly in control of their lives may get into struggles with physicians over compliance as a way of maintaining a sense of power over their lives and disease.

Consequences

Noncompliance results in inadequate treatment, poor follow-up, and failure to reduce risk factors, with consequent increased morbidity and mortality. Noncompliance also causes much frustration and consternation for the physician and strains the doctor–patient relationship. A vicious circle may be established in which the patient, finding that the physician becomes angry over incomplete compliance, volunteers less and less about it. The physician in turn feels increasingly upset that the patient seems to be ignoring instructions and is not being forthright.

Intervention

Trying to scare the patient into compliance is rarely successful. Patients who are noncompliant because they are already frightened will become even more anxious and harder to work with. The physician should inform patients of the consequences of not following recommendations, but preferably by emphasizing the benefits of treatment. Positive reinforcement to motivate behavior is almost always more effective than negative reinforcement or punishment, a truism well established in behavioral psychology. Scolding, shaming, or threatening seldom has a beneficial effect. It is also important to maintain a nonjudgmental, nonpunitive attitude when a patient confesses noncompliance, so that the patient will be open about deviations later in the course of treatment.

Physicians can also enhance compliance by careful attention to treatment recommendations. The regimen should be simplified by minimizing the number of drugs and the number of times per day they need to be taken. Even the most highly motivated patients will have difficulty if they must take one drug q.i.d., one t.i.d, one b.i.d., and one every other day. When a regimen remains necessarily complex, the physician should help the patient determine which aspects of treatment are most important. It is also helpful to implement the complex regimen gradually, adding one drug at a time, and to tailor dosage schedules to the patient's lifestyle. Compliance is also enhanced by incorporating the patient's preferences, which may be based on realistic factors (e.g., differing side effect profiles) or on less-objective beliefs (e.g., the drug that the patient's sister did well on).

Physicians should also exercise some restraint pursuing therapeutic goals. While physicians have an ethical responsibility to maximize patients' health, therapeutic perfectionism fails to recognize that, for a particular patient, other values may counterbalance some aspects of treatment. Physicians also have an ethical responsibility to respect the individual patient's autonomous wishes and not to ignore them in the pursuit of an ideal therapeutic outcome. Compromise with the patient is not only ethically justified, but is also a practical way of enhancing compliance with the most essential aspects of treatment.

Psychiatric consultation is appropriate whenever noncompliance appears linked to a major psychiatric disorder. It may also be very helpful whenever physician and patient are at a standoff, although the physician should not expect the psychiatrist to compel the patient to become compliant. Instead, the psychiatrist helps arbitrate the dispute by eliciting the patient's values and motivation, recognizing psychological factors like anxiety or a personality disorder that may be interfering, and repairing misunderstandings in the patient's relationship with the primary physician (see also Cohen-Cole and Levinson, in Stoudemire, 1994).

Discharges Against Medical Advice

Leaving the hospital against medical advice (AMA) might be viewed as a drastic extension of noncompliance. Approximately 1% of all general hospital discharges are AMA. Patients who leave AMA have many different motives. Some are patients whose psychological reactions to illness are so intense that they try to flee (e.g., a patient phobic about undergoing general anesthesia who leaves AMA the night before surgery). Some patients are angry, feeling mistreated, misinformed, ignored, or insulted by medical or nursing staff members. Such perceptions may conform to actual experience, may be distortions arising from a patient's disordered personality, or more often may be both. Any patient who suddenly, and for no apparent reason, wishes to leave during the first few days of hospitalization may be dependent on alcohol or other substances. Agitation and irritability may reflect early withdrawal symptoms, and the patient may wish to leave the hospital to gain access to the abused substance and avoid further withdrawal. Another segment of potential AMA discharges are patients who are delirious or demented. If the physician has not recognized that the patient has a neurologic syndrome, the patient's attempt to leave the hospital may be misperceived as rationally motivated, when instead it results from the patient's confusion and misperception of reality.

The direct consequence of AMA discharges is the disruption or cessation of medical care. Such discharges are rarely if ever amicable, leaving patients, physicians, and other hospital staff resentful, hurt, and indignant. Rather than approaching the widening breach in the relationship as something to be repaired, physicians and staff may respond in a legalistic and bureaucratic manner. Patients may in turn become more upset, feeling further misunderstood and not cared for.

When a patient first expresses the intention of leaving the hospital AMA, the physician should not coerce, threaten, or try to scare the patient into remaining. The first step is to try to restore the alliance by listening to the patient's grievances, giving them legitimate consideration, and trying to work out compromises. Suspected withdrawal syndromes should be appropriately treated. If the patient still wishes to leave, the physician should calmly explain the potential consequences, emphasizing the benefits further hospitalization can offer.

If these initial steps do not lead to constructive negotiations, psychiatric consultation is indicated. The actual AMA form used by many hospitals should not be overvalued: while it serves an administrative purpose, it is unnecessary and is insufficient to protect against future lawsuits. Rather, the physician's ethical and legal obligation in such a situation is to ensure that the patient is making an informed choice. The patient's reasons for leaving and the physician's concerns that have been communicated to the patient should be documented in the patient's chart. If it appears that the patient is incapable of understanding the need for continued treatment due to mental illness or severe medical illness or both, this too should be documented and the possibility of involuntary medical treatment should be considered.

Doctor-Shopping

Physicians commonly encounter patients who appear to be shopping around for medical care, either visiting a succession of doctors or several simultaneously for the same complaints. Some are patients with strong psychological motivations for staying in the sick role (e.g., hypochondriacs). Others may be seeking a particular diagnosis, treatment approach, or personality style in their physician and will continue searching until they find it. A few are unconsciously gratified by frustrating and defeating the efforts of physicians (e.g., factitious disorder, a variant of which is called the Munchausen's syndrome). Of course, there are also those who shop around because they have received bad medical care elsewhere and/or have an illness that has defied correct diagnosis. Certain medical and psychiatric diagnoses are notorious for eluding diagnosis, and it is not unusual for the patient to have visited many physicians before being correctly diagnosed. Panic disorder is typically misdiagnosed as various medical illnesses because of the prominent somatic symptoms; myasthenia gravis, in its early stages, is often mistaken for "stress" or depression because routine physical and laboratory examinations are normal.

On first seeing a patient who appears to have been doctor-shopping, the physician should carefully and objectively consider the chief complaint and previous evaluation and treatment. The physician should not pursue extensive diagnostic evaluation or aggressive treatment solely because of strong pressure from the patient to "do something!" There is neither an ethical nor a legal obligation to duplicate workups when they are not clinically indicated. Were the patient's evaluation and treatment elsewhere adequate? Were they optimal? What led the patient to change physicians? Some patients are shopping around not because they want more procedures, but because they are looking for a physician who will spend adequate time listening to them.

In all cases, one should temper enthusiasm with moderation. The physician should not tell the patient that "there is nothing wrong," nor should the physician be overconfident. Do not promise that you will "certainly find out what is wrong and take care of it." This is particularly important for patients who have visited several good physicians and are still frustrated. Acknowledging the limitations of medicine is often better than promising too much. Psychiatric consultation is indicated if the physician suspects underlying primary psychopathology, such as depression or panic disorder.

The physician must recognize that many doctor-shoppers may refuse psychiatric consultation, particularly those who are receiving substantial secondary gain by staying in the sick role. Doctor shopping is also discussed in the context of the somatoform disorders in Chapter 9.

NORMAL AND PATHOLOGICAL GRIEF

Normal Grief

Grief is the psychological response to loss. We are most familiar with grief following the death of a loved one, but analogous reactions follow other losses (e.g., body parts or functions, independence, affection). Grief, and the mourning process through which it is resolved, follow a typical course with recognizable manifestations (Fig. 20–1) (Brown and Stoudemire, 1983). Psychological symptoms of grief begin with an initial state of shock and disbelief, followed by painful dejection, despair,

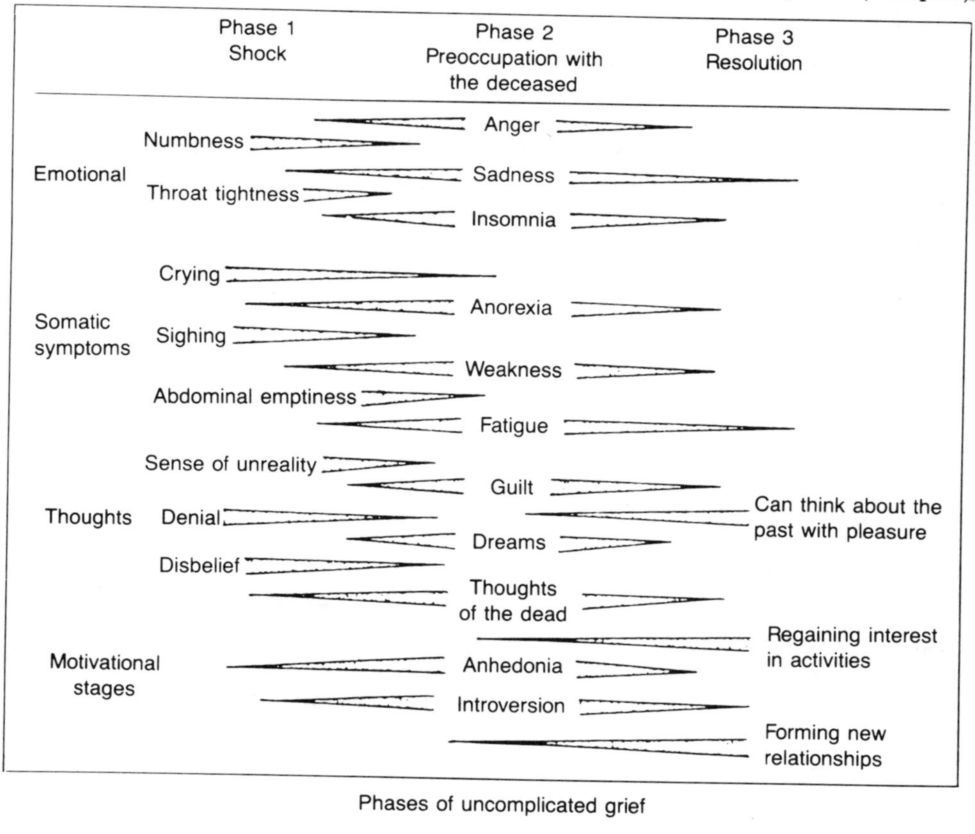

Phases of uncomplicated grief

Figure 20–1. *Phases of grief. (Reproduced with permission from Brown JT, Stoudemire A. Normal and pathological grief. JAMA 250:378, 1983)*

helplessness, protest, and anger. Social dysfunction occurs with loss of interest in life's activities, social withdrawal, apathy, and inertia. While some individuals retreat into silent sadness, others are affectively very demonstrative and cry. Somatic symptoms accompanying grief include insomnia; anorexia and weight loss; tightness in the throat, chest or abdomen; and fatigue.

The initial phase of shock and numbness lasts days and is followed by a period of preoccupation with the deceased. During the day, thoughts focus on recalling the life of the deceased and on one's own relationship with the deceased. Anger, jealousy, and resentment about the lost loved one may resurface, along with guilt over unresolved conflicts and regret over missed opportunities. The living experience self-blame, wishing they had acted or felt differently in the past, ruminating over why they have been the ones to survive, and wondering if they should have done something more during the terminal illness. Sleep is delayed by these obsessive thoughts and is often interrupted by dreams about the deceased. Fleeting hallucinations may occur in which the dead seem to appear at one's bedside or in a crowd, or in which the deceased's voice calls out, usually the name of the living.

The length and intensity of the phases of shock and preoccupation are affected by the suddenness of the death. When there has been no warning, the period of shock and disbelief is prolonged and intense; when death has been long expected, much of the mourning process may occur while the loved one is still alive, leaving an anticlimactic feeling after the death. In normal grief, the intensity of symptoms gradually abates, so that by 1 month after the death, the mourner should be able to adequately sleep, eat, and function at work and at home. Crying and feelings of longing and emptiness do not disappear but are less intrusive. By 6 to 12 months most normal life activities will have been resumed. For major losses, the grieving process continues throughout life, with the reappearance of the symptoms of grief on anniversaries of the death or other significant dates (family holidays, wedding anniversaries, birthdays). "Normal" reactions demonstrate a wide range of variability, and there is not a "right way" to mourn applicable to everyone (e.g., not all must "get out" their feelings of grief in verbal form).

Distinguishing Grief from Depression

Many of the psychological, social, and vegetative symptoms of depression also occur in grief (Table 20–2). Distinguishing them is important for physicians, for the indicated interventions are quite different. As noted, in normal grief severe symptoms should abate after several months, while in depression symptoms persist longer. While wishes to join the deceased are normal in acute grief, frank suicidal ideation (especially with a plan) is not and suggests a major depression. Transient hallucinatory experiences occur with grief, but not the more sustained psychotic symptoms (e.g., delusions of decay, nihilism, or guilt) indicative of a psychotic depression. Crying and intense feelings of sadness and loneliness occur in both grief and depression, but in grief they occur as "pangs" interspersed with periods of more normal feeling; in depression they are more continuous. Self-reproach is experienced in both, but not equivalently. In grief, self-blame is focused on the deceased, e.g., what one could have done differently. The depressed are primarily negative about themselves, feeling

Table 20–2 **Distinguishing Grief from Major Depression***

	GRIEF	MAJOR DEPRESSION
Time course	Severe symptoms ≥1–2 months	Longer
Suicidal ideation	Usually not present	Often present
Psychotic symptoms	Only transient visions or voice of the deceased	May have sustained depressive delusions
Emotional symptoms	Pangs interspersed with normal feelings	Continuous pervasive depressed mood
Self-blame	Related to decreased	Focused on self
Response to support and ventilation	Improvement over time	No change or worsening

* It should be noted that depressive *symptoms* are a pervasive part of the grief response and that a clear delineation— grief *vs* depression is not always possible.

worthless, guilty, and helpless, not just in regard to the deceased. Finally, grief and depression respond differently to intervention. The grieving welcome emotional support from others, congregate with them, and feel better after ventilating their feelings. Those who have major depression tend to withdraw from reassurance and feel worse when encouraged to ventilate.

Pathological Grief

In some individuals, grief and mourning do not follow the normal course. Grieving may become too intense or last too long; be absent, delayed, or distorted; or result in chronic complications. Risk factors for pathological grief in the mourner include sudden or terrible deaths, an ambivalent relationship with or excessive dependency on the deceased, traumatic losses earlier in life, social isolation, and actual or imagined responsibility for "causing" the death. Grief that is too intense or prolonged exceeds the descriptions given of normal grief and can lead to an inability to function occupationally or socially for months. *Absent or delayed grief* occurs when the feelings of loss would be too overwhelming and so are repressed and denied. Such avoidance or repression of affect tends to result in the later onset of much more prolonged and distorted grief and in a higher risk for developing a major depression, especially at later significant anniversaries. Physicians should be careful not to assume that grief is absent just because the individual is quiet and not affectively demonstrative. This may be a matter of personal or cultural style; what counts is the individual's internal experience of grief.

Distorted grief occurs when any one facet of grieving becomes disproportionate in magnitude or duration. "Survival guilt" refers to the feeling that one does not deserve to have outlived the deceased and is especially common in those who have shared a traumatic experience with the deceased (e.g., same organ transplant program, airplane crash, or concentration camp). It is normal in moderation, but can become so pronounced that the survivors remain too guilty to ever return to full lives.

Some degree of identification with the deceased is also normal. Grief is partly resolved through intensification of traits shared with or admired in the deceased and the treasuring of special inherited possessions. When conscious or unconscious identification is too strong, it leads to a variety of maladaptive outcomes. The living may abdicate personal life or identity to pursue the interests of the deceased. Through a process of conversion, mourners may develop symptoms identical to those of the loved one's illness. When denial of the loss is very pronounced, there may be an attempt to maintain the deceased's room and belongings entirely unchanged.

Prolonged pathological grief results in chronic complications, including major depression, substance dependency, hypochondriasis, and increased morbidity and mortality from physical disease.

The Physician's Role

Physicians are in a critically important position to identify and help manage grief, especially if they have long-established relationships with patients and their families. During the acute phase of shock following a death, the physician can help the family accept the reality of the loss and provide a calm and reassuring presence that facilitates both the release of emotion and the planning necessary by those grieving. The physician must sit down, not stand, when talking with anyone experiencing acute grief; otherwise, the physician will be perceived as too busy or uncomfortable or eager to leave. Patients frequently seek out their personal physicians when they are acutely suffering from grief, often focusing on the somatic manifestations. The physician can explain the normal symptoms and process of grief and mourning, reassuring patients that they are not "losing their minds" (a common fear, especially if vivid nightmares or fleeting hallucinatory phenomena have been experienced). Family members who wish to should be allowed (but never pressured) to see the body of the deceased in the hospital, after the physician prepares them for any distortion of appearance due to the fatal disease, accident, or treatment.

The physician's role in the management of grief has expanded in importance in recent years. The physician should address resuscitation status, advance directives, and related treatment issues with patients who are competent and with their families when the patients no longer are. Besides the medical, ethical, and legal reasons for doing so, there are psychological benefits in making patients and families feel heard, respected, and able to contribute to terminal care. Discussion regarding the patient's wishes, e.g., organ donation, is another vital responsibility of physicians that may provide a source of hope and meaning in the face of senselessness and despair.

Physicians should resist the temptation to sedate the individual suffering from acute grief, since this tends to delay and prolong the mourning process. Antidepressants should not be prescribed for acute grief but rather reserved for a possible subsequent major depression. If insomnia is severe and not spontaneously improving after several days, a brief course of a benzodiazepine hypnotic may be prescribed, but extended use will be more harmful than beneficial.

THE DYING PATIENT

Helping dying patients is a major responsibility of the physician. Elizabeth Kubler-Ross drew professional attention to this long-neglected subject 20 years ago and described five sequential stages that characterize the typical response to impending death: denial, anger, bargaining, depression, and acceptance (Kubler-Ross, 1969). As we have learned more, there does not appear to be a unique or correct order. Individual patients will experience each of these reactions (and others) in varying degrees, combinations, and sequences. How a patient copes with the knowledge that she or he has a fatal illness generally reflects the style used to cope with other life stresses. A compulsive patient may become obsessed with statistical prognostic information, while a histrionic one exhibits dramatic emotional outbursts. Usual coping styles may become exaggerated or markedly change. Some variability in patients' psychological responses to dying derives from the nature of the illness (e.g., acute vs. chronic, occult vs. easily visible) and beliefs about the illness (e.g., viewing the illness as a punishment).

Cultural and religious background profoundly influence how patients respond when they learn they are dying. Knowing this background is important for the physician, but it can also be misleading, as the prospect of death may produce abrupt changes in the patient: an agnostic may become deeply religious; a lifelong skeptic of medicine may become obsessed with medical progress; patients who have been very distant from their families may seek to reunite; and those who have been close may begin to withdraw from their relationships in anticipation of ultimate separation. Most patients take comfort through some form of sustaining hope, including hopes for miraculous cures, new medical discoveries, the resolution of personal conflicts or alienated relationships before death, leaving a legacy, or something as simple as enough improvement to briefly leave the hospital and walk in the garden.

Physicians' Reactions to the Dying Patient

Physicians' reactions are also important in the management and support of the dying patient. Many physicians, as do most people, have an aversion to death. The dying patient may make the physician feel like a failure, since treatment has been ineffective and it appears that there is nothing more to offer the patient. This is especially likely to occur with younger patients because it is harder for the physician to resort to fatalistic rationalizations (e.g., "she lived a full life" or "he died due to the inevitable progression of old age"). Even experienced physicians feel sad if the dying patient has become well known to them. Sadness in the physician is also likely if the physician is reminded of a personal loss in his or her own life. Sadness, helplessness, and a feeling of failure in the physician may interfere with optimal care in a number of ways. The physician may avoid the patient, spending little or no time with them while on rounds, which the physician rationalizes as not wanting to disturb the patient. Avoidance is particularly unfortunate because most patients have a fear of dying alone and because the physician is less available to provide specific comfort-care measures. The secure belief that the physician's attention will continue unceasingly until death is a benefit to patients often underestimated by physicians. Support through human contact often is most meaningful and invaluable to the patient precisely when techno-logical treatment options have been exhausted.

Some physicians take an overly cheerful approach, trying thereby to instill hope. When this is excessive it alienates patients, who contrast their fate with that of the seemingly happy physician, creating a gulf between them. Believing that they ought to be truthful, some physicians are overly blunt, announcing to the patient, "Nothing more can be done; we have done everything we can think of." This robs patients of hope. It is possible to be truthful without being so disheartening. Other physicians have difficulty accepting that further treatment is useless and resort to excessive heroics, needlessly prolonging death. Finally, many well-meaning physicians, sensing a patient's need to talk about dying, may prematurely refer the patient to a psychiatrist, social worker, or chaplain. At best, the patient will take this as a sign that the physician is uncomfortable discussing these issues; at worst, the patient may worry that the physician thinks there is something wrong with how the patient is reacting, or that the feelings are too unimportant for the physician's attention. Most patients prefer talking about death and dying directly with their primary physician.

Intervention

How to inform a patient of a grave diagnosis and prognosis is part of the art of medicine. The physician must gauge how much to tell and at what rate, taking into account the patient's intellectual abilities and emotional and physical state. The questions the patient asks are an indicator of whether the physician is going too fast or too slow. Important information may require repetition within the same session and over several visits. Shock induced by the initial pronouncement may interfere with the patient's registering other needed information. Physicians must balance their truth-telling obligation with some respect for different patients who want to know more or less about the details of a grave prognosis.

Another important responsibility for the physician is to discuss the patient's preferences and values regarding future treatment decisions, particularly those in-volving the termination of aggressive treatment. This should not be raised too quickly after the patient has been first told of a serious diagnosis, both because the patient may be too overwhelmed to participate meaningfully in such a discussion and because the patient may misinterpret the discussion as a sign that the physician is ready to give up. However, physicians tend to err in delaying such discussion until the patient's illness has progressed to the point when it can no longer be avoided. Unfortunately, by then the patient may no longer be competent, the physician will feel less certain that the patient's preferences have not been unduly influenced by physical discomfort, family pressure, or financial worries. This problem is avoidable by initiating discussion before the final stages of illness. Physicians should also allow the patient the oppor-tunity to include family members in the discussion.

In the face of serious illness, physicians feel better "doing something." Anticipat-ing a patient's inevitable and impending death, physicians should focus on what can be done. Quality of life during the process of dying can be significantly improved through adequate pain control (which even now is often underprescribed), attention to bowel and bladder function, hygiene, and other comfort measures. For some patients comfort is the primary goal, while other patients may be willing to sacrifice some comfort for greater mobility and the chance to even briefly leave the hospital. Physicians should encourage patients to make wills and put their affairs in order, help mobilize the patient's support system, and discuss options like hospice.

Patients with grave illnesses often have questions about what to tell their children. Most children do not develop a firm concept of the finality of death until between ages 8 and 11, but children, like adults, vary in the intellectual and emotional maturity necessary to comprehend death. Patients and families should be urged to gauge their answers by the nature of their children's questions. Questions spontaneously asked by a child of any age should be answered truthfully in language the child can understand. The adult should indicate his or her continued availability for further questions and comfort. Should children attend funerals? If the child wishes to go this should be respected and supported. If the child appears very reluctant or refuses, this too should be respected. When in doubt, it is probably helpful for the child to attend, as funerals are rituals that have evolved in our cultures to help us collectively deal with death.

As noted, psychiatric consultation should not be sought prematurely as a substitute for direct conversation between patient and physician. Psychiatric consultation is indicated for the terminally ill patient when suicidal ideation appears, for assistance with management of intractable pain, and for the emergence of major unresolved emotional conflict.

The fundamental fear of dying patients is usually not the fear of death itself, but the fear of being abandoned or deserted by others, including their physician, and dying alone. Perhaps the most reassuring comment that a physician can make to a patient with a terminal illness is, "No matter what happens or how bad things get, we're in this thing together and I'll stick by you no matter what happens. You don't have to worry about suffering alone. As long as you are ill, I'll be here to help you with whatever comes, including making sure you'll be comfortable and kept out of pain." Issues related to death and dying are discussed in the companion text to this volume on human behavior, particularly in the chapter on adult development by Drs. Wolman and Thompson (in Stoudemire, 1994).

DRUGS THAT CAUSE PSYCHIATRIC SYMPTOMS

Drugs used to treat medical illnesses frequently cause psychiatric symptoms or side effects through a variety of mechanisms. Most drugs at toxic levels produce signs of central nervous system disturbance, including drugs that are normally benign with few side effects, such as aspirin. Certain medications frequently cause psychiatric symptoms even at therapeutic drug levels (e.g., L-dopa). This may occur via a direct effect of the drug on the central nervous system (e.g., lidocaine), a metabolic effect of the drug (e.g., hypokalemia caused by thiazide diuretics), or drug interactions. Some drugs may precipitate an underlying psychiatric disorder in vulnerable patients, such as reserpine-induced depression or sympathomimetic-induced panic attacks. Physicians must be vigilant for the possibility of psychiatric side effects induced by medications the patient may be taking without the doctor's knowledge. This is particularly true if the patient is doing this surreptitiously and is embarrassed to tell the physician (e.g., the excessive use of over-the-counter nasal decongestants or inhalers).

Table 20–3 shows many of the drugs that can cause psychiatric symptoms. Most of those shown can cause a wide variety of symptoms, influenced by the patient's

Table 20–3 **Drugs That May Cause Psychiatric Symptoms***

Depression

*Antihypertensives (especially reserpine, methyldopa, beta-blockers, clonidine)
Amphotericin B
*Corticosteroids
Anticonvulsants
*Sedative-hypnotics
Oral contraceptives
Antipsychotics
Metoclopramide

Indomethacin (and other nonsteroidal anti-inflammatory drugs)
Antineoplastic drugs
  Procarbazine
  Tamoxifen
  Vinblastine
  Asparaginase
Ethionamide
Acetazolamide

Mania

*Corticosteroids
Sympathomimetics (esp. nonprescription decongestants and bronchodilators)
Isoniazid

Dopamine agonists
Antidepressants
Zidovudine (AZT)
Stimulants

Anxiety

*Sympathomimetics
*Theophylline
*Caffeine

Stimulants
Antidepressants
*Sedative-hypnotics (withdrawal)

Psychosis (Hallucinations or Delusions)

*Anticholinergics
Antihistamines (cimetidine, ranitidine, diphenhydramine, etc)
Antiarrhythmics (esp. lidocaine, tocainide, mexiletine, quinidine)
*Dopamine agonists
  L-dopa
  Bromocriptine
  Amantadine
*Corticosteroids
Digitalis
Antidepressants
Opiates
  Meperidine
  Pentazocine
Antimalarials
Anticonvulsants
Beta-blockers

Antiviral drugs
  Acyclovir
  Vidarabine
  Interferon
  Zidovudine (AZT)
  Podophyllin
Antineoplastic drugs
  Asparaginase
  Methotrexate
  Vincristine
  Cytarabine
  Fluorouracil
Disulfiram
Sympathomimetics
Metrizamide
Methysergide
Baclofen
Cycloserine
Cyclosporine

* Denotes especially "high-risk" drugs for causing symptoms in question.

premorbid psychopathology and personality style, metabolic status, and preexisting central nervous system pathology. When the effect on the brain is mild to moderate, most of the listed drugs can cause anxiety, depression, sleep disorders (insomnia, hypersomnia, nightmares), and sexual dysfunction. When severe, psychosis (schizophreniform, manic, or depressive), delirium, or dementia may occur, sometimes resulting in seizures and coma (see also Chapter 4).

MEDICAL DISORDERS THAT CAUSE PSYCHIATRIC SYMPTOMS

Many medical disorders produce psychiatric symptoms as part of their pathophysiology, sometimes as the initial presentation of the disease. Here we focus on psychiatric symptoms that are a consequence of the disease process itself through either direct effects on the central nervous system or derangement in metabolism or homeostatic regulatory mechanisms. Some diseases cause a wide range of different neuropsychiatric symptoms in different individuals, largely determined by which areas of the brain have been affected by the disease. These disorders are listed in Table 20–4. Table 20–5 shows diseases that commonly cause specific psychiatric symptoms. While most of these also can cause a range of symptoms, they typically present with the indicated psychiatric syndromes. Symptoms and signs in other organ systems serve as clinical clues to help the clinician suspect a particular cause, but psychiatric symptoms may precede the onset of other clinical signs in most disorders.

When a patient presents with unexplained psychiatric symptoms, certain clues should heighten the physician's suspicions that an underlying medical disorder may be responsible. An underlying medical disorder as etiology should be considered whenever: (1) psychiatric symptoms increase and decrease in concert with prominent physical symptoms; (2) when the "vegetative symptoms" of an apparent psychiatric disorder are disproportionately greater than the psychological symptoms (e.g., a patient with a 50-lb. weight loss and only mild depressive ideation is unlikely to have major affective disorder as the explanation for the weight loss); (3) when significant cognitive abnormalities are present in the mental status examination, particularly changes in level of consciousness, attention, and memory; (4) when the age of onset or course of psychiatric illness is very atypical (e.g., new onset of "schizophrenia" in an

Table 20–4 **Medical Disorders Causing a Wide Range of Psychiatric Symptoms**

Traumatic Brain Injury
Stroke
Systemic Lupus Erythematosus and other forms of Cerebral Vasculitis
Brain Tumor (Primary or Metastatic)
Encephalitis (Acute or Chronic)
AIDS/HIV Encephalopathy
Infectious Endocarditis

Table 20–5 **Psychiatric Presentation of Selected Medical Disorders**

	PSYCHIATRIC PRESENTATION	CLINICAL CLUES	SCREENING DIAGNOSTIC EVALUATION
Endocrine Disorders			
Hypothyroidism	Retarded depression (± psychosis)	Weight gain, fatigue, cold intolerance, hoarseness, bradycardia, constipation, hair loss	Free T$_4$, TSH
Hyperthyroidism	Anxiety, panic attacks, agitated depression (often retarded in the elderly)	Tremor, tachycardia, heat intolerance	Free T$_4$, T$_3$-RIA, TSH
Hyperadrenalism (Cushing's)	Depression or mania	Hypertension, diabetes, hirsutism, moon facies, weight gain	Dexamethasone suppression test
Hypoadrenalism (Addison's)	Depression	Postural hypotension, nausea, vomiting, skin pigmentation, weight loss	Cosyntropin stimulation test
Pheochromocytoma	Panic attacks	Labile hypertension, headache, sweating, nausea, palpitations	24-hour urinary catecholamines and metanephrines
Metabolic Disorders			
Hypoglycemia	Anxiety, panic attacks	Sweating, tachycardia, headache	Blood glucose during symptoms
Hypokalemia	Depression	Weakness, EKG changes	Serum K$^+$
Hyponatremia	Depression, psychosis	Weakness, nausea, vomiting, seizures	Serum Na$^+$
Hypercalcemia	Retarded depression	Weakness, nausea, confusion	Serum Ca^{++}
Hypocalcemia	Anxiety	Tremor, tetany, paresthesias	Serum CA^{++}
Hypermagnesemia	Retarded depression	Hypotension, nausea, vomiting	Serum Mg^{++}
Hypomagnesemia	Anxiety, psychosis	Tremor, tetany	Serum MG^{++}, Ca^{++}
Hypophosphatemia	Depression	Weakness, paresthesias	Serum PO$_4$$^{--}$
Vitamin B$_{12}$ deficiency	Psychosis, dementia	Megaloblastic anemia, peripheral neuropathy, myelopathy (but may occur in absence of these)	Serum B$_{12}$
Hepatic encephalopathy	Confusion, psychosis	Asterixis, jaundice	Liver function tests, serum NH$_3$
Uremia	Depression, dementia	Anemia, nausea, edema	BUN, creatinine
Porphyria (acute intermittent)	Psychosis	Episodic abdominal pain with nausea and vomiting, constipation, neuropathy	Blood and urine porphyrin screen
Lead poisoning	Personality change, depression	Colic, anemia, peripheral neuropathy	Serum FEP*

Neurologic Disorders

Disorder	Psychiatric symptoms	Clinical features	Diagnostic tests
Normal pressure hydrocephalus	Depression, dementia	Gait apraxia, urinary incontinence	CT or MRI scan
Multiple sclerosis	Depression	Multiple intermittent neurological symptoms over time	Neurological evaluation, MRI, CSF (oligoclonal bands)
Huntington's disease	Personality disorder, psychosis	Movement disorder, family history	Neurological exam
Parkinsonism	Depression, dementia	Bradykinesia, tremor, rigidity	Neurological exam
Wilson's disease	Psychosis	Movement disorder, liver disease, Kayser-Fleischer rings	Slit-lamp exam, serum ceruloplasmin

Neoplastic Disorders

Disorder	Psychiatric symptoms	Clinical features	Diagnostic tests
Pancreatic cancer	Depression	Weight loss, abdominal pain	Abdominal CT or MRI scan
Paraneoplastic limbic encephalitis (usually associated with small-cell carcinoma of the lung)	Psychosis, dementia	Seizures, fluctuating course	EEG, lumbar puncture

Infectious Diseases

Disorder	Psychiatric symptoms	Clinical features	Diagnostic tests
Infectious mononucleosis	Depression	Lymphadenopathy, hepatosplenomegaly, sore throat, malaise	CBC, Monospot
Viral hepatitis	Depression	Anorexia, fatigue, jaundice, malaise, hepatomegaly	Liver function tests, serologies
Encephalitis	Psychosis	Fever, seizures	EEG, lumbar puncture
Whipple's disease	Depression, dementia	Diarrhea, weight loss, arthritis, lymphadenopathy	Malabsorption studies, small bowel biopsy

*FEP, free erythrocyte protoporphyrin

85-year-old patient); and (5) whenever there are objective findings of central nervous system disease (e.g., pathological reflexes, abnormal EEG or CT or MRI scan, or changes in spinal fluid). As with drug-induced psychiatric symptoms, medical illnesses may cause mild to moderate changes in affect, personality, sleep, or sexual function, which can be easily missed or misattributed. When severe, medical illnesses produce psychosis, delirium, or dementia, which are less likely to be missed but whose nature or causation may still be misinterpreted (see Chapters 1 and 4).

The physician should also keep in mind those diseases that do not produce psychopathology per se but may be mistaken for it. Recurrent pulmonary emboli may be misdiagnosed as anxiety or panic attacks because of episodic autonomic arousal. Early myasthenia gravis is often mistaken for depression or a conversion disorder because the clinician finds a normal examination in a patient who complains of weakness and fatigue whenever they work too hard. Multiple sclerosis may be misdiagnosed as conversion disorder because the pattern of the patient's symptoms seems changing and inconsistent and does not conform to simple neuroanatomical localization.

COMPETENCY

When a patient refuses diagnostic procedures or treatment, or seems unable to make medical care decisions, physicians often question whether the patient is competent. Strictly speaking, "competency" is a legal concept and is determined by the court; physicians, including psychiatrists, render opinions about competency based on their clinical assessment of the patient's mental status. What physicians must decide is whether the patient appears to have the capacity to participate in rational and reasoned decision making (President's Commission, 1982). Are limited intelligence, a psychiatric disorder, or a medical disease preventing the patient from thinking rationally about medical care? Most determinations of this kind are made by clinicians at bedside; frequency and the need for timely resolution make it impractical to seek judicial action on every case.

While psychiatric consultation is often requested to help determine if the patient is competent, primary physicians can determine this themselves in most cases. Does the physician actually suspect impaired mental capacity, or do the patient and the physician simply disagree? The test of whether a patient possesses the capacity to participate in health care decision making is a simple, functional one: does the patient understand the particular decision at hand? First, the physician must ensure that the patient has been fully informed. Then, the following questions should be asked, taking into account that patients will answer in their own language, not in "medically correct" terms: (1) Can the patient describe what the physician believes is wrong with the patient? (2) Does the patient understand the diagnostic procedure or treatment proposed and the reasons for it? (3) Does the patient understand any alternative procedures or treatments that may exist? (4) Does the patient understand the risks and benefits of each course of action, including the consequences of refusing treatment? If the answer is "yes" to all of these questions, the patient possesses the capacity for decision making. To be viewed as competent, the patient does not necessarily have to have a good reason for disagreeing with the physician, but the patient must be able to demonstrate an understanding of the physician's advised plan.

Since this clinical competency test focuses on particular proposed treatments, it is possible that some patients may be judged able to make some but not all decisions, or that their ability varies over time. Others may be so mentally impaired that it is obvious that they entirely lack decision-making capacity.

Some patients will give answers that demonstrate their ability to understand what the physician has said, but they will persist on an irrational course based on psychotic delusional thinking. This too may be grounds for a determination of incompetence and indicates the need for psychiatric consultation. Psychiatric consultation is also helpful if the primary physician remains unsure of the patient's level of understanding, if there is disagreement among the physicians caring for the patient, or if legal action is considered likely.

If the physician determines that the patient does not possess sufficient capacity, a surrogate decision-maker will be required. If the surrogate is a family member, as it is in most circumstances, this does not necessitate going to court. A court-appointed guardian should be sought when the family members remain intractably divided over health care decisions, when they appear unable to act in the best interests of the impaired patient, or when the treatment is controversial (see also Chapter 19, by Dr. Dubin, Fig. 19-1).

PSYCHIATRIC CONSULTATION

From the other parts of this chapter, it is evident that there are many reasons for a physician to seek psychiatric consultation. Unfortunately, some physicians are reluctant to do so or do not ask for psychiatric assistance very effectively. Some physicians fear that seeing a psychiatrist will upset the patient, who may feel that the physician thinks he or she is crazy. Other physicians approach patients with the belief that all medical pathology should be absolutely ruled out before considering psychological explanations for symptoms. It is certainly reasonable to avoid prematurely concluding that a patient's symptoms are psychogenic, but the relentless pursuit of an organic etiology is costly, exposes patients to unnecessary risks, reinforces a disregard for psychological factors by the patient, and neglects treatable psychiatric disorders.

Some physicians hesitate to obtain psychiatric consultation simply because they are unsure how to tell the patient. It is a mistake to ask for consultation without telling the patient, since this makes it more likely that the patient will misunderstand the physician's intentions. If not told, patients may well wonder if their physician thinks them mentally ill or may believe that their physician is frustrated and wants to transfer their care to someone else. Several studies have demonstrated that when patients are informed by physicians of the purpose of a psychiatric consultation, the great majority have little difficulty accepting it.

The physician should explain that the psychiatrist is a consultant who will advise the patient and the physician, and that the physician is still the primary doctor committed to helping the patient recover. The specific purpose for the consultation should be explained in terms the patient can understand (e.g., "Besides having heart failure, your spirits seem very low. I'd like to have our psychiatrist see if there is anything we can do to help you feel better emotionally as well as physically").

The physician should always formulate a specific question or problem for which the consultant's help is desired (see Table 20–6). If the physician is unsure if psychiatric consultation would be helpful, the physician should discuss this with the consultant. Occasionally, the physician may anticipate problems in persuading the patient to see a psychiatrist. Here, too, discussion with the consultant ahead of time will be helpful. With careful explanation and a respectful approach, a skilled psychiatric consultant can persuade the great majority of patients who initially refuse consultation to agree to be interviewed.

When the patient has unexplained symptoms, physicians should avoid "either/or" thinking (that is, considering the symptoms as either physical or psychological). Otherwise, the physician may be misled into thinking too narrowly about causation. Physicians should never diagnose by exclusion (i.e., conclude that symptoms must be psychogenic because physical and laboratory examinations have revealed only "normal" results). A medical disease may still be present. Psychiatric diagnoses should be made on the basis of positive criteria, not solely on the absence of identifiable physical pathology. In evaluating symptoms of unclear causation, when the physician suspects the possibility of psychogenic origin, psychiatric consultation should not be delayed until the end of hospitalization. Such delays are unfortunate because they leave little time for psychiatrists to do their job, they reinforce the patient's (possibly false) belief that the symptoms are physical, they promote unnecessary diagnostic testing, and they leave the patient with the implied message that the physician is at the end of their rope and is giving up the patient to the care of a psychiatrist.

Even when symptoms clearly appear to be due to conversion, hypochondriasis, or malingering, the physician should never tell the patient, "There's nothing wrong" or "It's all in your head." Patients experience such remarks as humiliating and insulting, and consequently the doctor–patient relationship is seriously strained. Instead, patients can be reassured that extensive diagnostic testing has not turned up any grave or malignant etiology for their illness, and that it appears they have a physical symptom exacerbated by stress for which help is available.

Table 20–6 **Common Indications for Psychiatric Consultation**

Suicidal ideation or behavior.
Verbal threats or dangerous behavior.
Psychosis (hallucinations, delusions, thought disorder).
Need for psychiatric medication or change of dose.
Psychiatric disorder in need of treatment.
Psychiatric disorder complicating medical illness.
Psychiatric symptoms thought to be caused by medical illness.
Psychiatric symptoms thought to be due to medication.
Competency evaluations.
Noncompliance, AMA discharges.
Significant problems in doctor–patient relationship (or nurse–patient relationship).
Evaluation of cognitive dysfunction (delirium, dementia).

ANNOTATED BIBLIOGRAPHY

Drugs that cause psychiatric symptoms. The Medical Letter 31:113–118, 1989

Drugs that cause sexual dysfunction. The Medical Letter 29:65–70, 1987

These two articles provide concise tabular summaries, updated regularly.

Cassem NH (ed): Massachusetts General Hospital Handbook of General Hospital Psychiatry, 3rd ed. St. Louis, Mosby Year Book, 1991

This compact handbook provides a ready and portable reference for managing the most common psychiatric disorders encountered in general hospital patients.

Stoudemire A, Fogel BS (eds): Psychiatric Care of the Medical Patient. New York, Oxford University Press, 1993

This is a definitive reference source for dealing with the psychiatric problems of the medically ill. Each major subspecialty is covered in terms of biological, psychological, and sociologic factors relevant to medical illness that may affect psychiatric functioning. It contains detailed discussions of diagnostic and psychopharmacologic treatment issues in treating the medically ill patient with psychiatric disturbances.

REFERENCES

Brown JT, Stoudemire GA: Normal and pathological grief. JAMA, 250:378–382, 1983

Cavanaugh SC: The prevalence of emotional and cognitive dysfunction in a general medical population: Using the MMSE, GHQ, and BDI. Gen Hosp Psychiatry 5:15–24, 1983

Eraker SA, Kirscht JP, Becker MH: Understanding and improving patient compliance. Ann Intern Med 100:258–268, 1984

Fulop G, Strain JJ, Vita J et al: Impact of psychiatric comorbidity on length of hospital stay for medical/surgical patients: A preliminary report. Am J Psychiatry 144:878–882, 1987

Jencks SF: Recognition of mental distress and diagnosis of mental disorder in primary care. JAMA 253:1903–1907, 1985

Kessler LG, Cleary PD, Burke JD: Psychiatric disorders in primary care. Arch Gen Psychiatry 42:583–587, 1985

Kubler-Ross E: On Death and Dying. London, Macmillan, 1969

Levenson JL: Psychosocial interventions in chronic medical illness: An overview of outcome research. Gen Hosp Psychiatry, 14S:43–49, 1992

Levenson JL, Hamer RM, Rossiter LF: Relation of psychopathology in general medical inpatients to use and cost of services. Am J Psychiatry 147:1498–1503, 1990

Levenson JL, Mishra A, Hamer R, Hastillo A: Denial and medical outcome in unstable angina. Psychosom Med 51:27–35, 1989

Mayou R, Hawton K, Feldman E: What happens to medical patients with psychiatric disorder? J Psychosom Res 32:541–549, 1988

Mazzullo J: Methods of Improving Patient Compliance. In Lasagna L (ed): Patient Compliance. Mount Kisco, NY, Futura Publishing, 1976

President's Commission for the Study of Ethical Problems in Medicine and Biomedical and Behavioral Research: Making Health Care Decisions: A Report on the Ethical and Legal Implications of Informed Consent in the Patient-practitioner Relationship. Washington, DC, U.S. Government Printing Office, 1982

Saravay SM, Steinberg MD, Weinschel B et al: Psychological comorbidity and length of stay in the general hospital. Am J Psychiatry 148:324–329, 1991

Schurman RA, Kramer PD, Mitchell JB: The hidden mental health network: Treatment of mental illness by nonpsychiatrist physicians. Arch Gen Psychiatry 42:89–94, 1985

Shapiro S, Skinner EA, Kessler LG et al: Utilization of health and mental health services: Three epidemiologic catchment area sites. Arch Gen Psychiatry 41:971–978, 1984

Stoudemire A (ed.): Human Behavior: An Introduction for Medical Students, 2nd ed. Philadelphia, J. B. Lippincott, 1994

Von Korff M, Shapiro S, Burke JD et al: Anxiety and depression in a primary care clinic. Arch Gen Psychiatry 44:152–156, 1987

Wallen J, Pincus HA, Goldman HH, Marcus SE: Psychiatric consultations in short-term general hospitals. Arch Gen Psychiatry 44:163–168, 1987

Alan Stoudemire (ed). *Clinical Psychiatry for Medical Students*, Second Edition. Copyright © 1994, 1990 by J. B. Lippincott Company.

21 Psychiatric Aspects of Acquired Immune Deficiency Syndrome

Michael G. Moran

At the turn of the century, the saying "By knowing syphilis, one knows medicine" was common in medical circles. As we approach the new century, the disease that includes more of medicine than any other, demands more of the physician than any other, and taxes our society more than any other is surely acquired immune deficiency syndrome (AIDS). By knowing AIDS, one will know much of medicine, including psychiatry. This syndrome is a psychological malignancy: the patient's defenses and coping mechanisms are attacked and eroded by repeated assaults on livelihood, relationships, sense of integrated identity, and, in the end, on sanity and the very ability to think. AIDS presents myriad psychiatric pictures and complications. A patient can appear angry, inhibited, depressed, manic, psychotic, or demented as a result of AIDS and its sequelae.

The broad scope of this syndrome confronts physicians with their limitations, sometimes in a brutal way. Diagnostic efforts can seem endless and futile. Avenues of treatment may appear few in number and without substance. But there are certain principles that can help the physician conduct a thorough search for treatable causes of the psychological dilemmas and psychiatric complications of AIDS. This chapter seeks to introduce the medical student to current approaches and techniques in the psychiatric management of these patients. An outline of the most common complications of the illness and the complications of treatment is given. A section is included on how and when a psychiatric consultation may be helpful. Following the chapter is a brief list of the current review literature on the psychiatric aspects of AIDS for students with a special interest in this area.

EPIDEMIOLOGY AND DEMOGRAPHICS OF INFECTION WITH HUMAN IMMUNODEFICIENCY VIRUS (HIV)

Human immunodeficiency virus (HIV), the causative agent of AIDS, is transmitted chiefly through the exchange of body fluids (Table 21–1). The most common routes of exchange are male homosexual intercourse, especially anal intercourse; use of contaminated needles during the intravenous administration of drugs; and administration of contaminated blood and blood products. An infected pregnant woman can also transmit the virus to her unborn fetus.

The virus is lymphotropic and neurotropic. It attacks the T4 lymphocyte and causes a time-dependent and progressive destruction of that cell. The clinical results are the development of severe, often life-threatening infections with organisms against which the T4 lymphocyte usually defends or helps defend. The clinical results of the neurotropism are seen in almost all levels of the neuraxis, but cerebral involvement is the most common.

Subacute encephalitis or subcortical dementia are the most common neuropsychiatric presentations. Heightened susceptibility to deliria from a variety of causes may then ensue. It should be noted that primary CNS infection with HIV may occur before overt systemic signs of immunosuppression appear. This is a critical factor that will be discussed in more detail later in this chapter.

Worldwide, homosexual and bisexual men account for about 65% of all AIDS cases; for heterosexual intravenous drug users, about 17%; and for women, about 11%. Most of the women are intravenous drug users and the rest are prostitutes or sexual partners of men at risk. Hemophiliacs and other recipients of blood and blood products constitute less than 5% of AIDS patients (Centers for Disease Control, 1988).

The prevalence of "triply diagnosed" patients (with AIDS, chronic mental illness, and drug use) is increasing (Graham, and Cates, 1992). Parenteral drug abuse appears

Table 21–1 **High-Risk and Low-Risk Behavior Concerning HIV Contagion**

High-Risk Behavior
Sharing drug needles and syringes.
Anal sex, with or without a condom.
Vaginal or oral sex with someone who shoots drugs or engages in anal sex.
Sex with strangers (a pickup or a prostitute) or with individuals with a history of multiple indiscriminately chosen sexual partners.
Unprotected sex (without a condom) with an infected person.
Safe Behavior
Not having sex (abstinence).
Sex with one mutually faithful, uninfected partner.
Not shooting drugs.

(Adapted from: U.S. Department of Health and Human Services. Understanding AIDS. Public Health Service, 1988.)

to be a more common risk factor for acquiring HIV than does homosexual behavior, at least among psychiatrically hospitalized patients (Volavka et al, 1991).

PSYCHIATRIC ASPECTS OF AIDS: THE CLINICAL PICTURE

AIDS-Related Impairment of Cognition

After infection with HIV, the clinical presentations are shaped by the target systems of the virus's attack (the immune system and the nervous system, especially the brain) and by the psychiatric reactions to the diagnosis of the illness and to its immunologic and neurologic complications. The psychiatric problems resulting primarily from immune dysfunction are chiefly deliria that stem from severe infections, their metabolic complications, and the measures used to treat them. The psychiatric problems that arise from the *neurotropism* of the virus can be seen as a species of dementia. The dementia then renders the patient more susceptible to the insults that cause the aforementioned deliria, and some of the causes of the deliria, if they are prolonged, can add to or produce a picture of dementia. Less-common manifestations of neurologic complications of AIDS include a vacuolar myelopathy, similar to that of cobalamin deficiency; cranial nerve syndromes, often caused by localizations of systemic infections; and Landry-Guillain-Barré syndrome. All told, central nervous system disease occurs in *at least* 40% of AIDS patients, and is the initial symptom of the syndrome in at least 10% (see Table 21–2).

To further complicate this picture, sequelae of the immune deficiency, namely certain neoplasms, can occur in the central nervous system and cause neurologic disease; examples are Kaposi's sarcoma and lymphomas of various types including

Table 21–2 **Neuropsychiatric Complications of HIV Infection**

Delirium
    Infectious causes: viral (incl. HIV), mycobacterial, parasitic, bacterial
    Metabolic: volume depletion, electrolyte disturbances
    Medications: CNS depressants and anticholinergics
    Intracranial mass lesions: hematoma, neoplasm
Dementia
    Sequelae of chronic deliria; see above
    HIV infection of the brain
        Subcortical dementia is most common
        No specific treatment
        May present initially as aseptic meningitis
Vacuolar myelopathy
    Resembles cobalamin deficiency
    Mechanism is unknown
Peripheral nervous system involvement
    Local infections or neoplasms
    HIV polyneuropathy

lymphomas involving the central nervous system. Other psychiatric symptoms are best characterized as psychological and are associated with the meanings of the events already catalogued here. These are discussed in a later section.

Delirium in AIDS

Delirium, or acute confusional state, is caused in AIDS by many potential factors; accurate diagnosis requires meticulous and careful clinical investigative work. It occurs in about one-third of hospitalized patients with AIDS. Sometimes no specific etiology is found and empiric treatment must be instituted in any case. More often, more than one candidate can be found as a cause for the delirium. Intracranial and systemic infections (often presenting as a diffuse encephalopathy), electrolyte and volume abnormalities, hypoxemia, and medication side effects are the chief offenders (Glatt, Chirgwin, and Landesman, 1988). The delirious patient may be only mildly disoriented and agitated, in which case a careful mental status exam may be the key to detecting the disorder. The spectrum of delirium can range, however, to combativeness and psychosis, with hallucinations and visual illusions. Misdiagnosis of the patient as "schizophrenic" or "manic" in this setting can result in improper treatment. Undiagnosed delirium is a cause of significant morbidity and mortality. Once delirium is suspected, a search for the infectious agent or metabolic derangement should begin. Some of the most common infectious causes of delirium are discussed below.

Pneumocystis carinii pneumonia (PCP) affects more than 80% of patients. It is the initial opportunistic infection in 60%. Progressive dyspnea with chest pain, fatigue, and fever constitute the clinical picture. Hypoxemia from the pneumonia can be severe, and when cerebral functioning is already marginal because of an intracranial infection or dementia, delirium can result.

Systemic infections can be caused by viruses (probably including HIV), fungi, parasites, and bacteria (including *Mycobacterium* species). Sites of entry into the systemic circulation include focal infections, such as pneumonia, as well as less localized sites such as erosions of the gastrointestinal tract and skin. In such settings, delirium can accompany fever, seeding of the bloodstream with the infectious agent(s), and the metabolic and fluid derangements caused by diarrhea, nausea and vomiting, and decreased ability or desire to eat and drink. These infections are diagnosed by blood culture as well as by examination and culture of the appropriate body fluid.

Toxoplasma gondii causes a focal encephalitis characterized by a picture ranging from mild headache and fever to seizures, neurologic deficits, delirium, and coma (Glatt, Chirgwin, and Landesman, 1988). Extracerebral involvement is unusual. CT and MRI scans may show the characteristic but nonspecific constellation of multiple lesions in the cortical and subcortical regions, enhancing with contrast (Pitchenik, Fischl, and Walls, 1983).

Cryptococcal meningitis is most often unimpressive in AIDS patients in its first stages. It may resemble depression, with lethargy, fatigue, and irritability. A devastating and rapidly progressive illness with meningitic signs, severe delirium, and eventual extraneural involvement is uncommon. CT scan is not helpful in making the diagnosis (Wheelan et al, 1983).

Infections with mycobacteria, especially *Mycobacterium avium-intracellulare* (MAC), are common in AIDS patients. *M. tuberculosis* infections are usually reactivations of earlier acquired disease and are most common in patients with a high background prevalence of the illness. Atypical presentations of *M. tuberculosis* infection are common, and bronchoscopy with biopsy of lung tissue, or biopsy of other tissue suspected of involvement, may be necessary for diagnosis. Intermediate-strength purified protein derivative (IPPD) tuberculin skin tests are too insensitive to be reliably helpful, and late in the course of the illness the patient may not be able to mount the inflammatory immune response that gives the positive reaction.

M. avium-intracellulare is an infective complex that is usually found in immunocompromised hosts. The presentation is generally that of a chronic pulmonary infection that responds poorly to antibiotics, even when in vitro sensitivity has been demonstrated. In AIDS patients, the infection can be disseminated widely, affecting the lungs, liver, bone marrow, and lymph nodes. Biopsy of these tissues yields the diagnosis, as can culture of the blood. A "wasting syndrome" is associated with *M. avium-intracellulare* infections in AIDS patients and consists of malaise, weakness, diarrhea, fatigue, weight loss, and fever (Hawkins et al, 1986). When the fever or diarrhea are severe, delirium can result, even without primary central nervous system infection. The prognosis for patients with *M. avium-intracellulare* infections is poor; there is no effective therapy at this time.

Cytomegalovirus is commonly a disseminated illness in the AIDS patient. The organism probably causes a subacute encephalopathy with associated delirium but can also cause colitis with diarrhea, adrenalitis, and retinitis.

HIV itself produces an acute encephalopathy very similar to that supposedly seen with CMV. Altered mentation, varying alertness, apathy, depressive affect, and decreased mental and verbal acuity and spontaneity are seen. The syndrome can progress and result in paranoid ideation, impulsive behavior, and psychotic symptoms of hallucinations and illusions. Delirium with prominent psychotic symptoms can be the initial presentation of AIDS (Thomas and Szabadi, 1987). Only autopsy reveals the diagnosis with certainty. Other viruses that can cause acute meningitis and possibly encephalopathic presentations include several in the herpes group: Epstein-Barr virus, varicella zoster, and herpes simplex. The latter commonly presents as an intracerebral mass lesion in patients without AIDS; in AIDS patients, such a picture is unusual. A more diffuse encephalopathic syndrome, or widespread mucocutaneous lesions without CNS involvement, can be seen.

Fluid, electrolyte, and oxygenation abnormalities can have profoundly adverse effects on AIDS patients who are already suffering cerebral compromise. Sedating and anticholinergic medications (among others), at doses normally tolerated well by other patients, may induce confusion, disorientation, and psychotic symptoms in severely ill AIDS patients. The door toward diagnosing these problems is opened by a high index of suspicion. Careful attention to variations in mental status, laboratory values, and the list of medications the patient is taking is essential for uncovering the cause(s) of delirium.

Dementia in AIDS

Dementia can result from the chronic sequelae of most of the causes of delirium: severe electrolyte imbalance, hypoxemia, or meningitis, to name a few.

However, cerebral infection with HIV probably causes a large proportion of cases of dementia seen in AIDS patients. The exact percentage of patients who become demented is hard to estimate, but studies suggest that over one-third of patients with debilitating dementia had evidence of active HIV infection at autopsy. The virus has been recovered even from patients who have neurologic symptoms and signs but do not have AIDS or any evidence of immune deficiency. Early detection of subtle HIV-induced neuropsychological impairment requires sophisticated testing. Subjective complaints and neurological signs do not correlate reliably with subtle deficits. Even mild atrophy on brain CT, diffuse EEG slowing, and nonspecific hyperdensities on brain MRI are usually unreliable indices (Perry, 1990). One patient had a rapidly progressive dementing syndrome with motor deficits, hallucinations, and paranoia but no clinical manifestations of immune compromise (Beckett, Summergrad, and Manschreck, 1987).

The neuropathologic picture is rather distinct, as is the early clinical presentation: *subcortical dementia.* Subcortical and white-matter changes dominate in these cases; gray matter is relatively spared. Macrophages, lymphocytes, and perivascular collections of multinucleated giant cells further characterize the microscopic appearance. Inclusion bodies are present in those infected with cytomegalovirus. CMV can cause dementia in AIDS patients, too, but is probably less common as a true etiology for the dementia and occurs after CNS infection with HIV.

Clinical features of subcortical dementia (of any origin) include mental slowness, apathy, impaired cognition, and depressive affect (see Chapter 4 by Dr. Stoudemire for a general description of subcortical dementias). The bedside mental status examination is not sensitive enough to detect impairment early in the course. In rapidly progressive or in advanced cases, disorganization and delirium may be evident. The cortical dementias, of which Alzheimer's disease may be said to be the prototype, cause more debilitating intellectual deficits, and the affected patients are more likely to show amnesia, agnosia, and aphasia. Motor abnormalities (dysarthria, ataxic gait, abnormal involuntary movements, and leg weakness) are more common with subcortical dementia.

Rapid deterioration is the rule. Progressive slowing of mentation brings on muteness and severe confusion, interfering with the accurate communication of needs. There may be periods of severe agitation if the patient becomes delirious; hallucinations and sensory illusions can occur. With advancement of the motor deficits, truncal ataxia can appear, as can spastic weakness, paraplegia, and quadriparesis.

The diagnosis of subcortical dementia is a clinical exercise; HIV dementia itself can be diagnosed definitively only at autopsy. The virus can be grown from the cerebrospinal fluid (CSF) of a fraction of the patients. The CSF is often normal, but may reveal a slight mononuclear pleocytosis and a mild elevation of protein. As mentioned earlier, the MRI and CT scans can be abnormal even before there are clinical manifestations of the dementia. Atrophy and ventricular enlargement can occur early in the course of the illness (Grant et al, 1987). Small white-matter lesions are better revealed by MRI than by CT scan. There are as yet no known scan features that are pathognomonic for HIV brain infection.

The previously discussed neuropsychiatric factors can undermine patients' capacity to modulate and manage their own affective states and adaptive responses to the news of the diagnosis and the evidence of illness progression. For example, delirious or demented patients may be relatively disinhibited and may be more likely to impulsively self-treat with alcohol or other drugs, further impairing their efforts at adapting appropriately to psychological insults. In vitro and in vivo evidence of immune suppression as a result of substance use, coupled with coexistent psychiatric illness, makes substance use especially destructive in patients with a lethal communicable disease (Flavin and Frances, 1987).

Psychological Aspects of AIDS

Early Phases

Even when free of HIV infection, members of groups at high risk for contracting AIDS face considerable anxiety and interpersonal tension because of the threat of the disease. Pressure, which at times can seem to these persons unreasonable and coercive, may be exerted by others in an attempt to change the lifestyles and sexual behavior of the members of the risk group. Persons at little risk for the disease also have psychological reactions to AIDS that powerfully determine their behavior, sometimes with phobias or unnecessary discrimination toward persons with AIDS. Psychosocial characteristics that raise the risk for a severe psychological reaction to infection include past psychiatric history, positive family psychiatric history, high school education or less, and low support from one's spouse, family, or friends (Dew, Ragni, and Nimorwicz, 1990). Other events with powerful meaning and serious impact include the inherent personal and vocational losses, debilitation, probability of isolation, sense of loss of control, and potential for loss of self-esteem seen in persons with AIDS (indeed, in most chronic, debilitating illnesses). Medical personnel need to be acutely aware of their attitudes about AIDS and the persons in the groups at highest risk in order to give the best medical care to affected patients.

The *psychological* reactions to the *meanings* of the illness form an important part of the clinical presentation. The psychological "malignancy" of the syndrome exerts powerful effects on the patient, care-givers, and family and other intimates in the patient's life (Walcott, Fawzy, and Pasnau, 1986). Members of high-risk groups may respond to the risk of infection by changing their behavior (either toward reducing or increasing their risk), changing their mood and self-image, and altering their view of their lifestyle. Fear of the illness and its effects may be so intense that these feelings either are acted on destructively or are projected onto others, with resultant near-paranoia. Some persons who are not in high-risk groups can foster such projections by baiting and criticizing risk-group members, especially homosexual men. The fear of contracting an incurable illness that is associated with wasting, misery, and ostracism is a nightmare in itself. In a setting fueled by prejudicial fantasies and minimal factual information, irrational thought predominates. The crucial role of the physician as a provider of information, an educator, and a role model can help stem the destructive effects of phobic behavior and discrimination.

The Decision to Be Tested: A Painful Dilemma

Counseling for AIDS testing, for those persons who wish to know their serologic status, is described at length in a superb review (Perry and Markowitz, 1988). Pretest counseling involves giving information about the test, its usefulness, and its limitations and assessing the patient's strengths and psychological vulnerabilities. Making such an assessment allows the physician to figure the risk-benefit ratio for the test (as should be done for any medical procedure). The complexity of the decision to test, and its potential for adverse consequences, are well examined in the case illustrations of the paper mentioned.

Patients' abilities to use their own coping capacities and outside support can best be assessed before the test results are given. The physician must systematically seek to understand why patients want the test now, what they expect the result to be, how they plan to react to positive or negative results, whom they plan to tell, and how they expect them to react. After this assessment, patients usually can better tolerate the interviewer's questions about their current state of health, including specific questions about symptoms of HIV infection.

Lastly, recommendations can be made to patients about how to use the strengths and resources already available to them, regardless of the test results (Perry and Markowitz, 1988).

Posttest counseling includes reducing the stress of those who are seropositive and explaining methods to prevent transmission. This is also the time to arrange proper follow-up care. The first 6 months after learning of positive test results is a high-risk period for deliberate self-harming behavior (Gala et al, 1992). A past psychiatric history, or past self-harming behavior in any context, raises the likelihood of other such incidents.

The test results for HIV seropositivity are powerful information: the patient discovers whether he or she has a lethal illness. It comes as no surprise that such information could powerfully affect his or her risk-taking behavior. The prospect of a positive result can make some members of risk groups avoid obtaining test results: in one study of homosexual men who were offered the chance to be tested, only 67% elected to do so. Those found to be seronegative decreased risk-taking behavior by a significantly smaller margin than the seropositive patients did (Fox et al, 1987). In another study, over 2,000 homosexual men were tested for HIV, then asked by mail if they wanted their results. Among the responders, there was no difference between those who chose to learn the result and those who refused. However, there was a significant difference between those who responded and those who did not: the latter group tended to be younger, nonwhite, and less educated. The group that refused to learn the results said they declined because they felt the test was not predictive of the development of AIDS or they were concerned about the worry that a positive result would cause them (Lyter et al, 1987).

Most discussions on AIDS prevention emphasize that giving information, especially about modes of infection, is the way to modify the high-risk activities of certain groups. The nationwide mailing of the Department of Health and Human Services pamphlet "Understanding AIDS" in 1988 is an example of this kind of logic and intervention. Health-related behaviors have been shown to be related to possession of clear, consistent information. But other important factors impinge on such behavior. Peer-group opinions and support also play a major role in maintaining or altering health-related behavior (Klein et al, 1987). When the risk behaviors of a group of homosexual male physicians and college students were studied, the authors concluded that such multifactorial determinants of behavior were at work, and that precise intervention was necessary if behaviors were to be changed. The authors suggested that programs for older, well-educated homosexual men should be designed so as to increase the sense of control over outcome (that is, to promote the notion that changing habits is *effective*). For young, well-educated men, programs aimed at appealing to peer-group norms were thought most likely to succeed (Klein et al, 1987).

This summary of the study is not meant to serve as a comprehensive list of interventions for groups at risk. For example, no mention is made here (nor was any made in the study) of intervention with drug users or prostitutes. The point is that in order to make a substantive change in the intended audience, the intervention will probably need to be tailored specifically to each group. Information, no matter how clearly presented, is usually not enough to change behavior.

Being in a high-risk group can itself be associated with severe psychological distress in the current setting of the AIDS epidemic. Symptoms are usually dominated by anxiety and can include panic attacks. Vigilant self-observation, when fostered by fear about a physical illness, can result in inordinate preoccupation with physical signs and symptoms. When these symptoms become severe enough, they can interfere with social and work functioning (Faulstich, 1987).

"Malignant" Progression of Psychological Symptoms

Once diagnosed, the psychological developments in AIDS patients closely resemble the sequence seen in terminal cancer patients. Many patients are filled with denial and disavowal at the news of their seropositivity or clinical immune deficiency. Anger, despair, and expressed or enacted hopelessness and helplessness are common. As mentioned before, an antecedent personality disorder, especially coupled with substance use, can render the patient prone to living out fantasized solutions to his or her situation or wishes for revenge and restitution. Some of the sense of being endangered and invaded (by the virus) is projected; care-givers are seen as the problem, or at least as inadequate. News reports that suggest slow progress with experimental treatments and minimal attention by the medical establishment to the concerns of affected persons and their associated high-risk groups promote these externalizations. The patient may feel and act overtly hostile to family members, physicians, and other intimates (Faulstich, 1987). If the patient acquired or suspects acquisition of the disease from a lover, that relationship can obviously come under the intense burdens of guilt, fault-finding, and desire for revenge. Other individuals find in the crisis an opportunity for increased emotional intimacy and work together against a common enemy. Such a response is usually founded on the earlier presence of a solid and loving relationship. Ironically, AIDS patients appear to be less suicidal than HIV-positive patients. The brain dysfunction in AIDS-related CNS disorders may reduce suicidality among AIDS patients (McKegney, and O'Dowd, 1992).

Reports suggest that both homicidal and suicidal impulses can lead to sexually risky behavior among distressed infected persons. Alcohol, serving as an anxiolytic, may facilitate the living out of "love suicide" fantasies, in which the uninfected person tries to acquire HIV infection and the infected person tries to infect others. Intravenous drug users with the same conscious and unconscious wishes (to spread the infection or to commit suicide) may display the same kind of behavior by knowingly using and trading contaminated needles. Anecdotal reports suggest that similar behavior occurred in epidemics of polio, tuberculosis, and syphilis (Flavin, Franklin, and Frances, 1986).

Existential Issues

The existential issues of *worth, control,* and *lovability* are paramount in the psychological picture of this illness. Every attentive physician will be able to see the patient striving to regulate her or his feelings of being worthless, out of control, and unlovable. As the patient's ability to function at work or in other settings is eroded, they may become desperate to find a way to prove their worth or demand a show of being valued from others. This may take the form of seeming entitled and demanding with medical care-givers and others.

Chronic, debilitating physical illness is the prototype of an attack on control of one's life. AIDS patients lose their ability to control their bodies (even bowel and bladder function), their place of residence (through repeated hospitalizations), and their sensorium and level of awareness (because of delirium); usually, these relentlessly worsen. The patient's reactions to such loss of control can include what may appear to be a childish attempt to control others, or to fight medical care.

The illness severely strains the patient's sense of being lovable. As mentioned, the strain usually invades intimate relationships. The partners must struggle with questions of sexual intimacy and how to handle the new risk imposed by the disease. If one partner is uninfected and gives any evidence of withdrawal or unavailability in the relationship amid the many medical and psychological crises that ensue, the patient will probably feel unloved. Family and friends who are frightened by the fear of easy contagion or who reject the patient's lifestyle (most often seen with male homosexual patients) may also withdraw. Usually, the patient is at some level aware of the feelings of these others, and major disruptions in the family can ensue. Feeling unloved, the angry and hurt patient may retaliate in an attempt to make others feel the same way. Such actions may serve only to further the avoidant and angry feelings and behavior of family and other loved ones. In other families, such intense evidence of feeling on both sides may provide the opportunity for reviewing the situation of the illness and for allowing appropriate planning and support for the future. Such a scenario is uncommon in the early phases of the illness, where denial, disavowal, and projection of feelings dominate.

As with any patient faced with a virtually inevitable and fatal outcome, death and the meaning of ending one's life become issues with which to reckon. Most patients affected with AIDS are young men, usually healthy before the occurrence of the illness. For them especially, contemplating death is a horror, so out of alignment with "expectable" concerns at their stage in the life cycle. After working through these issues to some extent, other fears often become apparent: many patients are less afraid of death per se than they are of suffocating, being alone as they die, or being left in agonizing pain. The latter is actually less common in the final stages of AIDS. But, as we have seen, *Pneumocystis carinii* pneumonia and interpersonal strife are real, and may lend extra credence to the chances of an isolated or suffocating death.

TREATMENT OF NEUROPSYCHIATRIC AND PSYCHOLOGICAL ASPECTS OF AIDS

In this section, treatment issues will be presented, dealing with the problems arising from neuropsychiatric sequelae (chiefly, delirium and dementia) and from psychological sequelae of AIDS. See Chapter 4 for a systematic overview of the treatment of delirium and dementia.

Treatment and Prevention of Delirium and Dementia

Specific medical treatment of the different infectious and metabolic complications of AIDS, the most common antecedents to delirium, is beyond the scope of this chapter, but details of a working approach are presented. Preventive quarantine, in an effort to isolate the patient from potential carriers of superinfecting pathogens, is bound to fail; as mentioned before, most infections are reactivations of a previously acquired organism. Similarly, most AIDS patients with opportunistic infections do not represent an infectious threat to others. The only exceptions are infections due to *M. tuberculosis*, herpes, and perhaps salmonella (Glatt, Chirgwin, and Landesman, 1988). Thus, the delirium caused by infections and the accompanying fever, bacteremia, and viremia generally cannot be treated by prophylaxis, but rather requires specific treatment of the infection once clinically evident, and by supportive measures.

Persistence of the delirium in spite of what seems to be appropriate treatment should alert the physician to another cause of infection or a separate cause for the delirium, such as a medication, volume depletion, or an intracranial mass. An acute change in sensorium or the appearance of new neurologic signs should prompt the consideration of a complete system review and new physical examination. Rarely, CT and MRI scans might be useful when routine laboratory procedures or bedside examinations show no cause for the new delirium, but the scans are rarely diagnostic.

P. carinii pneumonia responds to appropriate antimicrobial treatment in 60 to 80% of the cases. The infection, and the potential for the associated delirium, recurs in 65% of patients after 18 months. Toxoplasmosis and cryptococcosis are also rarely cured; relapse is the rule. Thus, previous history of pulmonary or disseminated infection with either of these agents should prompt investigation for their presence in the setting of a new delirium.

M. avium-intracellulare infections are not cured in HIV patients by current methods. *M. tuberculosis* may be somewhat more likely to invade the central nervous system and can do so despite appropriate therapy.

The other common causes of delirium are sometimes forestalled with meticulous maintenance and supportive care. Avoiding *medications* with psychotropic activity—especially sedative-hypnotics, anxiolytics, and drugs with high anticholinergic side effects—is an important cautionary step. If necessary, low starting doses (for example, half the dose for a young, otherwise healthy person) should be the rule. The nursing staff should be alerted to early signs of toxicity, such as sedation, confusion, or, in the case of anticholinergic drugs, dry mouth and urinary retention. However, central nervous system side effects can occur without these peripheral signs.

Vital signs can help track *volume status* and *oxygenation*. Patients with diarrhea who have impeded access to fluid replenishment, or who are too demented to ask for fluids, are at greatest risk for hypotension and accompanying cerebral dysfunction. Falls are also then more likely. Patients with pneumonia or antecedent lung disease might require arterial blood gases or saturation monitors to follow oxygenation status. Bedridden patients need close nursing attention to help avoid bedsores, another site for entry of infectious pathogens.

Those cases characterized by severe agitation or psychotic symptoms may require the addition of a high-potency neuroleptic, such as haloperidol, in low doses. The physician must remember that the AIDS patient has an increased susceptibility to extrapyramidal side effects and probably neuroleptic malignant syndrome because of the preexistent brain disease (see also Chapter 18 by Drs. Silver, Hales, and Yudofsky).

Many principles that apply to HIV-associated infections (Glatt, Chirgwin, and Landesman, 1988) are useful in the clinical management of delirium:

1. Most of the infections are incurable and require long-term suppressive therapy. Likewise, delirium may be chronic in many patients, requiring symptomatic, long-term treatment. A thorough search for reversible infectious, metabolic, and drug-induced causes can allow specific treatment of the delirium. The essential points here are the need for a high index of suspicion for the causes listed, careful elimination and treatment of the specific causes when possible, and judicious use of a neuroleptic in selected cases. The section on treatment will discuss the use of neuroleptics. (See Chapter 4 for further details on the diagnosis and treatment of delirium.)

2. These patients rarely have just one infection. Similarly, the causes of delirium are often multiple. The physician's search for etiology should be thorough, and vigilance for changes in mental status should be maintained throughout the care of the patient. Clinical "failure" in the treatment of delirium may result not from clinical error, but from a second cause.

3. Certain infections occur at their observed frequency in AIDS patients because of the prevalence of asymptomatic infection in the local population (e.g., histoplasmosis and cryptococcosis). Likewise, behavior that antedates the HIV infection, seen in the groups at highest risk for AIDS, may play a role in the susceptibility of AIDS patients for delirium. Examples of such behaviors include habitual alcohol or drug use preceding the onset of AIDS. If these behaviors are repeated after the cerebral compromise (from whatever specific etiology) is present in a case of AIDS, the patient is much less likely to tolerate the CNS effects of such behavior than before the HIV infection began. In the setting of depression and hopelessness, self-destructive or suicidal behavior

can then occur because of decreased impulse control (Flavin, Franklin, and Frances, 1986).

To the extent that dementia is caused, in any one patient, by factors that show up early as delirium and are reversible, dementia might be forestalled or prevented. If caused by HIV, there is no current treatment. Whatever the cause, dementia in AIDS is generally managed through supportive measures. Here again, nursing care and meticulous attention to metabolic parameters and medications is preeminent. Cognitive deficits can be symptomatically improved by use of stimulants, such as methylphenidate or dextroamphetamine. Doses generally have to be individualized. Improvement usually takes the form of more organized thinking, improved memory, and more spontaneity and animation (Angrist et al, 1992).

Treatment of the psychological problems associated with AIDS can rarely be divorced from the nonpsychological or purely physiologically oriented treatments, for several reasons. First, symptoms of brain dysfunction from medical and neurologic causes can masquerade as functional psychiatric disorders. An approach that arbitrarily separates the patient into two camps, mind and body, will fail in managing the illness. Second, the psychological reactions, if not addressed, will affect the patient's ability to care for herself or himself and to participate in medical treatment. Third, the psychological effects of the illness extend to the care-givers. If physicians are unaware of or deny the ways they can be affected by working with these patients, appropriate care of the patient will be impossible.

The treatment of *depression* in the AIDS patient is complex and filled with pitfalls. First, the presentation is rarely that of a classic vegetative depression: anger, self-criticism, projection of self-hatred, and preoccupation with somatic symptoms are rather common. In addition, as with any chronic or wasting disease, the absolute diagnosis *or* exclusion of depression is often impossible. The clinician, however, must maintain a high index of suspicion for depression and must be ready to deal with this treatable illness: indeed, mood disorder is a common reason for psychiatric referral of AIDS patients (Seth et al, 1991). Treatment includes psychotherapy, mobilization of the family and other supports, and antidepressants with low (desipramine) or no (fluoxetine or sertraline) anticholinergic effects. Antidepressants must be used carefully because of their anticholinergic, sedating, and hypotensive effects. Studies are in progress to systematically evaluate these drugs in AIDS patients. A number of reports have advocated the use of psychostimulants such as methylphenidate 10 to 40 mg/day given in divided doses early in the day as a treatment of depression in AIDS patients.

TREATMENT DECISIONS
IN IRREVERSIBLE ILLNESS

Early in the course of the illness, soon after diagnosis, involvement of the support system of the patient (family, lover, friends) can be helpful. If this seems impossible, *support groups*, most readily available for homosexual men, are valuable resources. The physician's willingness to discuss the need for referral and support is in itself a supportive act and can help pave the way for a useful experience working with the referral agency or specialist. Since substance use has such an augmenting effect on destructive behavior in this population, the physician should try to help the patient pay special attention to such behavior and obtain appropriate *counseling* and perhaps *disulfiram treatment*.

Emphasis on legal needs is also an important aspect of the counseling at this point. Attention to putting the patient's affairs in order, such as drawing up a will, may be too much for the patient in the acute setting, but dealing with such issues should not be inordinately delayed. Other considerations include designating a close *friend* or *relative* who could serve as legal guardian. Establishing individualized, clear-cut criteria for the timing of need for *hospice care*, or decisions about remaining at home for treatment should be considered. Consultation with *social services* can help in making the appropriate referrals.

In making decisions about major treatment and resuscitative efforts, the physician can be a help and guide for the distressed patient and family. Most patients want the physician to spare them the risk of unnecessary and potentially harmful procedures and drugs. However, such wishes may be obscured by a more overtly expressed and persistent fantasy about cure. If the physician has her or his own fantasies about "rescuing" the patient, the combination can yield a fruitless and futile zeal for treatment. At some point in the course of the illness, a frank discussion with the patient, and perhaps with family or lovers, should focus on these issues. A treatment approach aimed at aggressive palliation of discomfort and symptoms, rather than at unattainable symbols of "cure," is usually experienced as reassuring and supportive (Cassem, 1987; Wachter et al, 1988).

In addition, AIDS patients may be frightening: they have a severe infectious disease, and even education about the level of risk of contagion may not stem associated fears in medical personnel. In addition, the patient may be hostile because of low self-esteem and fears of dying and be out of control because of delirium.

Most AIDS patients are male homosexuals, intravenous drug users, or prostitutes. If the physician is shocked, offended, or disgusted by such persons and is not in control of those feelings, many reactions could occur. In an attempt to disavow such feelings, the physician may adopt an intense therapeutic zeal, aimed at giving "the best" to a hated patient. This could result in "working everything up," a futile and destructive approach in the context of end-stage irreversible illness (see the earlier discussion). In a less-subtle form, hostility toward the patient may take the form of unnecessary intramuscular injections, invasive procedures, or restraints. Among nursing staff, these reactions may appear in a nurse's slowness to respond to the patient's calls, restrictions on visitation, and "forgetting" to take vital signs. Being aware of one's attitudes toward these patients, informal discussions with colleagues, and in-service training sessions can be helpful.

Physicians' Reactions to AIDS Patients

In order to render the best care, physicians must be aware of their own reactions to this devastating illness. Many of these patients were young men, healthy and active before contracting the disease. Overidentifying with the patient is a common and hazardous response that can contribute to rescue fantasies, doomed to fail in this context. The intense investment of time and emotional energy by physicians and staff can leave them vulnerable to repeated assaults on their self-esteem when the patient dies (O'Dowd and McKegney, 1990). In addition, the wish to avoid the illness can impede taking a history (such as for needed family planning and sexual practices [Coverdale and Aruffo, 1992]). Anger at patients who fail to reduce their high-risk behaviors can interfere with proper follow-up and counseling (Carlson, Greeman, and McClellan, 1989).

ROLE OF THE PSYCHIATRIST

The *psychiatrist* can assist in the treatment in several ways: in those situations where the primary physician needs help constructing and implementing a differential diagnostic approach to delirium and dementia; when the patient manifests a major psychiatric illness, such as depression or delirium; as a referral source for psychotherapy for patients or family members; when psychiatric hospitalization is required for psychotic or suicidal patients; and to help manage the reactions of support staff in their dealings with AIDS patients.

Many patients experience referral to a psychiatrist as a rejection or as a criticism by the primary physician. They may feel the primary doctor is saying, "It's all in your head." An open discussion with the patient about the importance of the care for his or her psychological state can reduce these concerns. The primary care physician's unbiased attitude toward psychiatric care is essential. One approach that may be used is to speak of the referral as being helpful *to the primary care physician* in further helping the patient. It is important to arrange a follow-up visit with the primary care physician soon after the psychiatric appointment. Sometimes the patient will refuse to see the psychiatrist. The primary care physician may then elect to proceed with the consultation through personal discussions of the case with the psychiatrist.

CLINICAL PEARLS

- Neuropsychiatric complications of AIDS can be the *first* presentation of the illness. They can also masquerade as functional psychological problems. Persons in high-risk groups and those who appear to be depressed, confused, disoriented, psychotic, or merely easily fatigued should be elevaluated for active HIV infection, dementia, and delirium, as well as functional psychological illness.
- Heterosexuals (outside the high-risk groups of drug users, prostitutes, and hemophiliacs) are at high risk for HIV infection, albeit at an undetermined level. HIV testing, when otherwise clinically indicated, should not be deferred merely becuase the person is heterosexual. Careful counseling and informed consent are required for HIV testing.
- Vigilance in diagnostic and therapeutic zeal must be tempered at some point in the illness with a consideration for what fate awaits the patient after treatment of the acute problem. Physicians treating AIDS patients need to acquaint themselves thoroughly with various strategies for dealing with irreversible illness.
- Some reports suggest that depression in patients with HIV infection responds to psychostimulants such as methylphenidate.

- About 4% of AIDS patients seen for psychiatric consultation demonstrate violent behavior. Most are demented or delirious (Travin, Lee, and Bluestone, 1990).
- Physicians should educate themselves about local laws that address HIV testing, confidentiality of testing results, and duty to protect third parties (Haimowitz, 1989).

ANNOTATED BIBLIOGRAPHY

Cassem NH: Treatment Decisions in Irreversible illness. In Hackett TP, Cassem NH (eds): Massachusetts General Hospital Handbook of General Hospital Psychiatry, 2nd ed. Littleton, MA, PSG Publishing Co., 1987

> This is a useful and detailed exploration of the issues facing any physician treating a terminally ill patient.

Dickens BM: Legal limits of AIDS confidentiality. JAMA 259:3449–3451, 1988

> This article gives a sense of the legal complexities that any physician may encounter when treating an AIDS patient. Especially instructive is the introduction to the multiple layers of laws concerning confidentiality.

Emanuel EJ: Do physicians have an obligation to treat patients with AIDS? N Engl J Med 318:1686–1690, 1988

> This is a thought-provoking examination of a question for every physician.

Ruark JE, Raffin TA, the Stanford University Medical Center Committee on Ethics: Initiating and withdrawing life support. N Engl J Med 318:25–30, 1988

> This thoughtful, scholarly review presents Stanford's approach to the difficult problem of initiating and withdrawing life support.

Wolcott DL, Fawzy F, Pasnau RO: Acquired immune deficiency syndrome (AIDS) and consultation–liaison psychiatry. Gen Hosp Psychiatry 7:280–292, 1986

> The authors give a concise summary of the major neuropsychiatric and psychological issues.

REFERENCES

Angrist B, d'Hollosy M, Sanfilipo M et al: Central nervous system stimulants as symptomatic treatments for AIDS-related neuropsychiatric impairment. J Clin Psychopharmacol 12(4):268–272, 1992

Beckett A, Summergrad P, Manschreck T et al: Symptomatic HIV infection of the CNS in a patient without clinical evidence of immune deficiency. Am J Psychiatry 144:1342–1344, 1987

Carlson GA, Greeman M, McClellan TA: Management of HIV-positive psychiatric patients who fail to reduce high-risk behaviors. Hosp Community Psychiatry 40(5):511–514, 1989

Cassem NH: Treatment Decisions in Irreversible Illness. In Hackett TP, Cassem NH (eds.): Massachusetts General Hospital Handbook of General Hospital Psychiatry, 2nd ed. Littleton, MA, PSG Publishing Co., 1987

Centers for Disease Control: Update, acquired immune deficiency syndrome (AIDS) worldwide. MMWR 34:286–295, 1988

Centers for Disease Control: Revision of the case definition of acquired immune deficiency syndrome. MMWR 36:1S–15S, 1987

Coverdale JH, Aruffo JF: AIDS and family planning counseling of psychiatrically ill women in community mental health clinics. Community Ment Health J 28(1):13–20, 1992

Dew MA, Ragni MV, Nimorwicz P: Infection with human immunodeficiency virus and vulnerability to psychiatric distress: A study of men with hemophilia. Arch Gen Psychiatry 47(8):737–744, 1990

Faulstich ME: Psychiatric aspects of AIDS. Am J Psychiatry 144:551–556, 1987

Flavin DK, Frances RJ: Risk-taking behavior, substance abuse disorders, and the acquired immune deficiency syndrome. Adv Alcohol Subst Abuse 6(3):23–32, 1987

Flavin DK, Franklin JE, Frances RJ: The acquired immune deficiency syndrome (AIDS) and suicidal behavior in alcohol-dependent homosexual men. Am J Psychiatry 143:1440–1442, 1986

Fox R, Odaka NJ, Brookmeyer R et al: Effect of HIV antibody disclosure on subsequent sexual activity in homosexual men. AIDS 1(4):241–246, 1987

Gala C, Pergami A, Catalan J et al: Risk of deliberate self-harm and factors associated with suicidal behavior among asymptomatic individuals with human immunodeficiency virus infection. Acta Psychiatr Scand 86(1):70–75, 1992

Glatt AE, Chirgwin K, Landesman SH: Treatment of infections associated with human immunodeficiency virus. N Engl J Med 318:1439–1448, 1988

Goedert JJ, Biggar RJ, Weiss SH et al: Three-year incidence of AIDS in five cohorts of HTLV-III risk group members. Science 231:992–995, 1986

Graham LL, Cates JA: How to reduce the risk of HIV infection for the seriously mentally ill. J Psychosoc Nurs Ment Health Serv 6:9–13, 1992

Grant I, Atkinson JH, Hesselink JR et al: Evidence for early central nervous system involvement in the acquired immune deficiency syndrome (AIDS) and other human immunodeficiency virus (HIV) infections: Studies with neuropsychologic testing and magnetic resonance imaging. Ann Intern Med 107(6):828–836, 1987

Haimowitz S: HIV and the mentally ill: An approach to the legal issues. Hosp Community Psychiatry 40(7):732–736, 1989

Hawkins CC, Gold JWM, Whimbey E et al: *Mycobacterium avium* complex infections in patients with the acquired immunodeficiency syndrome. Ann Intern Med 105:184–188, 1986

Klein DE, Sullivan G, Wolcott DL et al: Changes in AIDS risk behaviors among homosexual male physicians and university students. Am J Psychiatry 144:742–747, 1987

Lyter DW, Valdiserri RO, Kingsley LA, Amoroso WP, Rinaldo CR Jr.: The HIV antibody test: Why gay and bisexual men want or do not want to know their results. Public Health Rep 102(5):468–474, 1987

McKegney FP, O'Dowd MA: Suicidality and HIV status. Am J Psychiatry 149(3):396–398, 1992

Moran MG, Dubester SN: Connective Tissue Diseases. In Stoudemire A, Fogel BS (eds): Psychiatric Care of the Medical Patient, ch. 33, pp 739–756. New York, Oxford University Press, 1994

O'Dowd MA, McKegney FP: AIDS patients compared with others seen in psychiatric consultation. Gen Hosp Psychiatry 12(1):50–55, 1990

Perry SW: Organic mental disorders caused by HIV: Update on early diagnosis and treatment. Am J Psychiatry 147(6):696–710, 1990.

Perry SW, Markowitz JC: Counseling for HIV testing. Hosp Commun Psychiatry 39(7):731–739, 1988

Pitchenik AE, Fischl MA, Walls KW: Evaluation of cerebral-mass lesions in acquired immunodeficiency syndrome. N Engl J Med 308:1099, 1983

Seth R, Granville-Grossman K, Goldmeier D et al: Psychiatric illnesses in patients with HIV infection and AIDS. Br J Psychiatry 159:347–350, 1991

Thomas CS, Szabadi E: Paranoid psychosis as the first presentation of a fulminating lethal case of AIDS. Br J Psychiatry 151:693–695, 1987

Travin S, Lee HK, Bluestone H: Prevalence and characteristics of violent patients in a general hospital. NY State J Med 90(12):591–595, 1990

Volavka J, Convit A, Czobor P et al: HIV seroprevalence and risk behaviors in psychiatric inpatients. Psychiatry Res 2:109–114, 1991

Wachter RM, Cooke M, Hopewell PC et al: Attitude of medical residents regarding intensive care for patients with the acquired immunodeficiency syndrome. Arch Intern Med 148(1):149–152, 1988

Wheelan MA, Kricheff II, Handler M et al: Acquired immunodeficiency syndrome: Cerebral computed tomographic manifestations. Radiology 149:477–484, 1983

Wolcott DL, Fawzy F, Pasnau RO: Acquired immune deficiency syndrome (AIDS) and consultation–liaison psychiatry. Gen Hosp Psychiatry 7:280–292, 1986

Alan Stoudemire (ed). *Clinical Psychiatry for Medical Students*, Second Edition. Copyright © 1994, 1990 by J. B. Lippincott Company.

22 The Evaluation and Management of Sleep Disorders

Karl Doghramji

THE SCOPE AND CONSEQUENCES OF SLEEP DISORDERS

Sleep difficulties are among the most frequently encountered problems in clinical medicine (Institute of Medicine, 1979). For example, in one study, 80% of the medical patients of a general hospital who received psychiatric consultation complained of disturbed sleep (Berlin et al, 1984). This is due, no doubt, to the sheer preponderance of such complaints in the general population as a whole; 35% of all adults express sleep-related complaints over the course of a year and half (17% of the population) consider their difficulty to be a serious one (Mellinger et al, 1985).

Despite the ubiquity of sleep disturbances, scientists and physicians are only now beginning to understand the debilitation, misery, and suffering they cause. We now know, for example, that insomniacs have an increased risk for the development of emotional disturbances, most notably depressive and anxiety disorders (Tan et al, 1984). In fact, the risk for depression increases with time if insomnia is left untreated (Ford and Kamerow, 1989). Sleep disorders also seem to adversely affect proper mental functioning; 53% of chronic insomniacs complain of memory difficulties and patients with obstructive sleep apnea syndrome have significant impairments in performance on complex motor tasks (Findley et al, 1986). It is not surprising, therefore, that inadequate sleep is associated with decreased work efficiency and impaired industrial productivity (Johnson and Spinweber, 1983) as well as an increased risk of traffic accidents (Mitler et al, 1988). Finally, sleep disorders seem to enhance the propensity for cardiovascular disease (Partinen et al, 1982) and increase the risk of death (Wingard and Berkman, 1983). Physicians should, therefore, be familiar with the techniques for the diagnosis and management of sleep disorders.

NORMAL HUMAN SLEEP

Sleep Stages and Architecture

Owing to the milestone discovery of rapid eye movement (REM) sleep by Aesrinsky and Kleitman in 1953, we now know that sleep is not simply the absence of wakefulness, but a complex behavioral, physiological, and psychological state that is the product of active and coordinated brain processes. One manifestation of these changes is the stages of sleep, which repeat in cyclical fashion throughout the night, forming a pattern widely known as sleep architecture.

Proper characterization of sleep stages necessitates the simultaneous monitoring of the numerous physiologic parameters, a process known as polysomnography. Minimally required are the electroencephalogram (EEG), electrooculogram (EOG), and electromyogram (EMG) of skeletal muscle, usually the submentalis. EEG patterns for the sleep of a young adult are depicted in Figure 22–1. The EEG of individuals who are awake and attentive exhibits a pattern of low voltage and mixed ("random") frequencies. However, during relaxed wakefulness or drowsiness, the EEG reveals a preponderance of rhythmic alpha activity (8 to 12 cps). The transition from wakefulness to stage 1 sleep is marked by the disappearance of rhythmic alpha and the establishment of relatively low voltage and mixed frequency pattern with the prevalence of theta (3 to 7 cps) activity.

During stage 2, two characteristic waveforms are noted: sleep spindles (12 to 14 cps activity lasting 0.5 to 1.5 seconds) and K complexes (negative sharp waves followed by a slower positive component lasting 0.5 seconds or greater). Low-voltage mixed-frequency activity persists in the background. Sleep spindles are synchronized waveforms, i.e., have a uniform oscillatory pattern resulting from the simultaneous activation of a large number of neurons by one or more synchronizing pacemakers located in the thalamus. Spindles are found in all mammals and are identical in all species. They develop before the age of three months in man and may be slower to develop in mental retardation. The significance of K complexes is unknown; they may occur spontaneously or in response to environmental noise.

During stages 3 and 4, high-amplitude slow delta activity (less than 2 cps) dominates the record. During stage 3 sleep, 20 to 50% of the tracing is comprised of delta waves, whereas during stage 4 sleep more than 50% of the record is comprised of delta waves. Stages 3 and 4 sleep are collectively referred to as *delta sleep, deep sleep*, and *slow wave sleep*. Well-formed delta waves are not seen until two to six months after birth. The emergence of delta sleep is a reflection of maturation in brain structure and function.

Although the eyes are still (other than occasional eye blinks) during relaxed wakefulness, involuntary ocular activity occurs just prior to the onset of stage 1 sleep (Fig. 22–2). On the EOG, this is noted as slow ("rolling") eye movements. These usually persist during the initial portions of stage 1. Eye movements are absent during

Awake – low voltage – random, fast

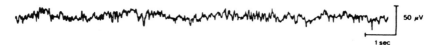

50 μV

1 sec

Drowsy – 8 to 12 cps – alpha waves

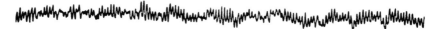

Stage 1 – 3 to 7 cps – theta waves

Theta Waves

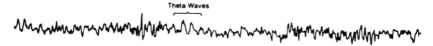

Stage 2 – 12 to 14 cps – sleep spindles and K complexes

Sleep Spindle

K Complex –

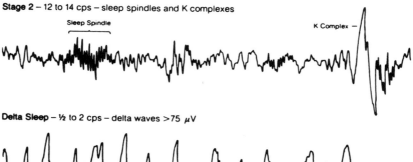

Delta Sleep – ½ to 2 cps – delta waves >75 μV

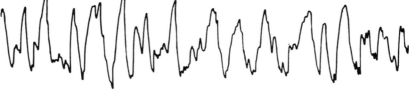

REM Sleep – low voltage – random, fast with sawtooth waves

Sawtooth Waves   Sawtooth Waves

Figure 22–1. *EEG patterns of human sleep. (Reproduced with permission from Hauri JP: Current Concepts: Sleep Disorders, p 5. Kalamazoo, the Upjohn Company, 1992)*

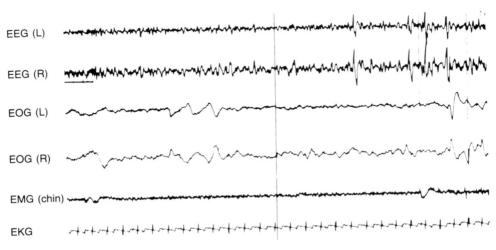

Figure 22–2. *Patient in Stage 1 sleep, the "drowsy" state. In the second line, the underlined section shows some ragged-looking alpha rhythm. Toward the right side of the record, about 20 seconds later, taller, lower-frequency brain-wave patterns are seen as the patient is falling asleep. The eye movement traces show some slow eye movements; the chin muscle activity has calmed down. (Reprinted with permission from Regestein QR, Rechs JR: Sound Sleep, pp 31–33. New York, Simon & Schuster, 1980)*

stages 2, 3, and 4 (Fig. 22–3). During wakefulness, the EMG reveals phasic (episodic) bursts of activity. However, as individuals wind down prior to sleep, EMG tone (amplitude) gradually diminishes and continues to do so as sleep progresses through the various stages. Stages 1 through 4 are collectively referred to as non-REM (NREM) sleep, and constitute approximately 75% of total sleep time in adults.

During REM sleep, the EEG again displays low-voltage mixed frequencies. However, characteristic rapid eye movements are noted on the EOG and the EMG displays the lowest amplitude of the night, a reflection of skeletal muscle atonia mediated through active CNS inhibition (Fig. 22–4).

Sleep is typically entered through stage 1, and an orderly progression from stages 1 through 4 occurs within 45 minutes of falling asleep. Within 90 minutes, the first REM period occurs. This NREM-REM pattern, referred to as a sleep cycle, lasts approximately 90 minutes and recurs continuously throughout the night (Fig. 22–5). Although this cycle is present at birth, each cycle lasts 50 to 60 minutes in neonates.

Delta sleep is most prominent in the first third of the night and virtually disappears during the last third of the night. Greater periods of prior sleep deprivation result in longer periods of delta sleep in the beginning of the night on subsequent nights. In contrast, REM sleep periods, although initially brief in duration, lengthen with each subsequent sleep cycle such that REM sleep is most prominent in the last third of the night. This pattern is relatively independent of prior sleep deprivation and is thought to be controlled by a circadian oscillator in the brain, one which also controls body temperature, the concentration of plasma cortisol, and other biologic cycles.

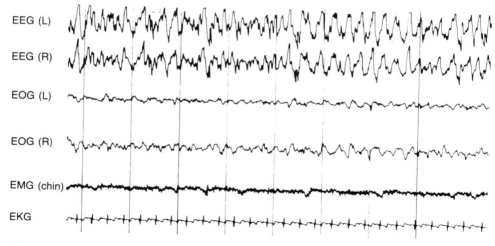

Figure 22–3. *Stage 4 sleep or slow-wave sleep. This deepest stage of sleep is marked by giant slow brain waves, as seen in the top two tracings, especially easy to pick out on the right side of the figure. (Reprinted with permission from Regestein QR, Rechs JR: Sound Sleep, pp 31–33. New York, Simon & Schuster, 1980)*

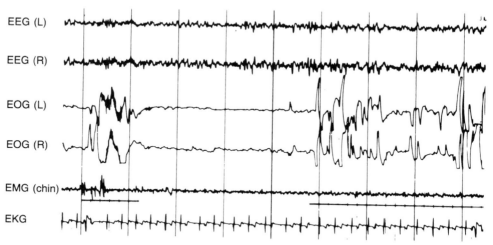

Figure 22–4. *Rapid Eye Movement or dreaming sleep. Here the top two lines resemble those seen in Stage 1 sleep. The muscle line, however, is as thin as it gets, showing the least muscle activity level of the night. Where the muscle trace is underlined on the left, however, there is a burst of muscle activity, and you will notice some noisy widening of the lines tracing eye movements, especially of the left eye, third line from the top. These indicate a muscle twitch that involved areas under the chin and around the left eye. The patient awoke less than a minute later and said she had dreamed that it was hard to breathe. (Reprinted with permission from Regestein QR, Rechs JR: Sound Sleep, pp 31–33. New York, Simon & Schuster, 1980)*

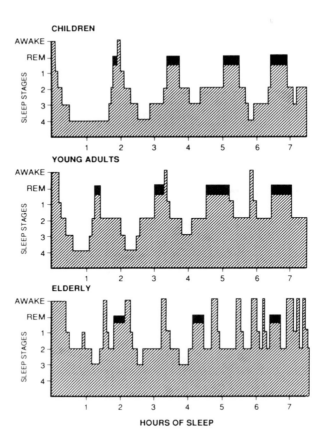

Figure 22–5. *Normal sleep cycles. REM sleep (darkened area) occurs cyclically throughout the night at intervals of approximately 90 minutes in all age groups. REM sleep shows little variation in the different age groups, whereas Stage 4 sleep decreases with age. In addition, the elderly have frequent awakenings and a marked increase in total wake time. (Reprinted with permission from Kales A, Kales JD: Sleep disorders: Recent findings in the diagnosis and treatment of disturbed sleep. N Engl J Med 290:487–499, 1974)*

The percentage distribution of sleep stages in a young adult is outlined in Table 22–1. Many factors alter these percentages. For example, conditions that produce sleep disruption, such as disease states and environmental noise, cause an increase in the proportion of stage 1 sleep and a decrease in delta sleep. Age also has profound effects on sleep. Delta sleep is maximal in children and diminishes markedly with age, especially during adolescence. Seniors may have little or no delta sleep. The loss of delta sleep with age may be a consequence of the diminution in cortical synaptic activity. In contrast, stage 1 sleep increases with age. With aging, there is a

Table 22–1 **Percentage of Sleep Stages in a Young Adult**

NREM	75	REM	25
Stage 1	5		
Stage 2	45		
Stages 3 and 4	25		

general tendency toward sleep fragmentation, characterized by an increase in the frequency of awakenings and brief arousals.

Sleep Depth

The arousal threshold is lowest for stage 1 sleep, i.e., the volume of environmental sound needed to awaken a sleeper from this stage is the lowest. The arousal threshold is highest for delta sleep (hence the synonym "deep" sleep) and variable for REM. Delta sleep also appears to be the most refreshing, and deprivation of this sleep stage often results in daytime sleepiness despite adequate length of sleep. The sense of unrefreshing sleep reported by the elderly is often related to low percentages of delta sleep.

Sleep Needs

Although the precise function of sleep is unknown, Rechtschaffen and his colleagues (1989) recently demonstrated that the lack of sleep leads to serious physical harm and even death in laboratory animals. One day of sleeplessness in humans has minimal effects on cognitive function the following day. However, with greater deprivation of sleep, performance on tasks is impaired. Therefore, adequate time spent asleep is desirable. Nevertheless, the need for sleep is highly variable from person to person. Although the average nightly sleep duration is approximately eight hours, children obtain about ten hours and the elderly less than seven hours. Sleep lengths vary even within similar age groups, with some individuals requiring as little as three hours of nightly sleep. The most prudent answer to the question of "How much sleep do I need?" is that amount of sleep that results in optimal daytime alertness and a sense of mental efficiency and well-being.

When discussing sleep needs, consideration should also be given to the need for optimal sleep quality, as this also contributes to daytime alertness. Sleep quality refers to the integrity of the sleep architectural pattern. Impairments in sleep quality appear polysomnographically as an increase in the number of arousals (brief awakenings and stage changes), awakenings, and body movements; an increase in the shallow stages of sleep (1 and 2); a decrease in deep (delta) sleep; and a decrease in the number of well-formed sleep cycles.

Sleep Deprivation and Rebound

On the first night following total sleep deprivation, a rebound of delta sleep is noted first, i.e., delta sleep is recovered at the expense of other sleep stages. REM rebound occurs later during the night or on subsequent nights. These and other findings are the bases for the belief of many sleep researchers that delta sleep is related to the maintenance of important biological functions. Additionally, selective deprivation of either delta or REM sleep for long periods of time also results in a subsequent rebound in the proportion of that particular sleep stage. For example, REM rebound is often seen following the abrupt discontinuation of drugs that suppress REM activity, such as certain antidepressant agents, and is often experienced as vivid dreaming and nightmares.

Cognitive and Behavioral Aspects of Sleep

Cognitive mental processes seem to be at a low level during stage 1 sleep as sleepers who are awakened from it usually report experiencing thought fragments or vague images. Most individuals awakened from delta sleep report no mental activity at all. In contrast, most sleepers report dreams when awakened from REM sleep. Dreaming also occurs during REM sleep in laboratory animals. Dreaming is only one facet of a host of complex biological processes that are activated during REM sleep and that affect almost every bodily function. These produce, among other things, rapid eye movements, bursts of tachycardia, penile tumescence, and peripheral skeletal muscle atonia. The observation of a highly active mind superimposed upon a picture of a motionless paralyzed body led earlier researchers to refer to REM sleep as "paradoxical" sleep.

The onset of sleep is characterized by a reduced responsiveness to environmental stimuli. Individuals asked to respond to sound or light have an increased reaction time as they approach sleep and no longer react following established sleep. Consequently, sleep-deprived automobile drivers tend to react sluggishly to traffic hazards and are more vulnerable to traffic accidents. Nevertheless, responsiveness to important stimuli is typically maintained during normal sleep, as in the case of a sleeping mother's selective sensitivity to her baby's crying. Sleep also produces retrograde amnesia; memory for events just prior to the onset of sleep is lost if ensuing sleep lasts for more than a few minutes. This is the basis for not recollecting the moment of sleep onset or the events that occur during brief awakenings during the course of the night.

POLYSOMNOGRAPHY

Polysomnography is typically performed in specialized facilities called sleep disorders centers and laboratories. Many are staffed by physicians specializing in sleep disorders medicine. In preparation for polysomnography, patients are introduced to their sleeping quarters during their initial office-based evaluation and provisions are made for special needs. On the night of the test, they arrive at the laboratory well in advance of the study time to acclimate to the new environment. Studies are conducted in noise-free and private rooms and comfort is maximized by making rooms aesthetically pleasing. Contrary to their commonly expressed concerns, most patients experience their sleep in the laboratory to be the same as, and at times even better than, their sleep at home.

As noted above, characterization of sleep stages requires, at the minimum, the EEG, EOG and EMG of the submentalis. However, a typical clinical polysomnogram also includes monitors for airflow at the nose and mouth, respiratory effort strain gauges placed around the chest and abdomen, and noninvasive oxygen saturation monitors that function by introducing a beam of light through the skin. Other parameters include the electrocardiogram and EMG of the anterior tibialis muscles, which are intended to detect periodic leg movements. Finally, patients' gross body movements are continuously monitored by audiovisual means.

The most commonly employed form of polysomnography, referred to as the nocturnal polysomnogram (NPSG), is conducted during the typical sleeping hours of the patient and identifies pathological processes during sleep. Another form is the multiple sleep latency test (MSLT). This test provides an objective measure of daytime somnolence. Objectively derived assessments of the severity of daytime somnolence are of great clinical importance since sleepy patients often cannot accurately estimate the severity of their own sleepiness. For example, patients who are so sleepy that they regularly succumb to involuntary sleep attacks—sleep episodes that strike without warning—will often deny feeling sleepy. The procedure is appropriately performed in any disease state that is associated with daytime somnolence. It is also necessary to definitively establish the diagnosis of narcolepsy. During the MSLT, patients are monitored polysomnographically during brief naps that are allowed at two-hour intervals throughout the day. The speed of falling asleep during naps, referred to as the sleep latency, is an indicator of the severity of daytime sleepiness. An average sleep latency less than ten minutes indicates a significant degree of daytime sleepiness, and one less than five minutes indicates a susceptibility to sleep attacks. Additional specialized forms of polysomnography include the maintenance of wakefulness test (MWT), nocturnal penile tumescence monitoring, and gastroesophageal pH monitoring.

SPECIFIC SLEEP DISORDERS

The disorders listed below adhere to the nomenclature of the International Classification of Sleep Disorders (Diagnostic Classification Steering Committee, 1990). (DSM-IV also has a nomenclature for sleep disorders.)

Inadequate Sleep Hygiene

Many individuals unknowingly engage in habitual behaviors that harm sleep. Insomniacs, for example, often compensate for lost sleep by delaying their morning awakening time or by napping, which actually have the effect of further fragmenting nocturnal sleep. Instead, insomniacs should be advised to adhere to a regular awakening time regardless of the amount of sleep and to avoid naps. Other sleep hygiene measures are outlined in Table 22–2. These measures, in written form, are often helpful when given to patients for home use.

Insufficient Sleep Syndrome

Persons affected with this disorder voluntarily curtail their time in bed, usually in response to social and occupational demands. Although sleep reduction may be as little as one hour per night, over long periods of time such a pattern may lead to

Table 22–2 **Sleep Hygiene Measures**

1. Sleep as much as needed to feel alert during the day, but not more. Curtailing the time in bed seems to solidify sleep; excessive time spent in bed seems to fragment sleep.
2. Establish a regular awakening time in the morning that you can adhere to every day, including weekends and vacations. Such regularity strengthens circadian cycling.
3. Exercise performed regularly (but not too close to bedtime) probably deepens sleep.
4. Excessive noise may disturb sleep; insulate your room against loud noises.
5. Excessive warmth disturbs sleep. Keep the room temperature at a comfortable level.
6. A light snack prior to bedtime may improve sleep, although a large meal and excessive fluids close to bedtime may have the opposite effect.
7. Caffeinated beverages disturb sleep, even though you may not be aware of their effect.
8. Alcoholic beverages, which may assist in falling asleep, can significantly fragment sleep.
9. If you feel angry and frustrated because you cannot fall asleep, don't try harder to fall asleep. Instead, leave the bedroom and do something not very stimulating, like reading a boring book.
10. The chronic use of tobacco disturbs sleep.

daytime hypersomnolence and result in impairment. Sleep logs usually reveal extended bedtime hours on weekends and holidays, during which individuals often awaken spontaneously in the morning. Treatment with stimulant agents is rarely warranted, as no degree of accruing chronic sleep debt can be overcome by stimulant agents. Instead, sufferers, usually younger adults, should be urged to extend bedtimes on a daily basis.

Adjustment Sleep Disorder

This common disorder is caused by acute emotional stressors such as a job loss or a hospitalization. The result is an insomnia, typically a difficulty in falling asleep, mediated through tension and anxiety. Symptoms usually remit shortly following the abatement of the stressors. Treatment is warranted if daytime sleepiness and fatigue interfere with functioning or if the disorder lasts for more than a few weeks. Treatment modalities are similar to those outlined for psychophysiologic insomnia (see below).

Psychophysiologic Insomnia

Although insomnia may be *initiated* by a wide variety of stressors and conditions, it may persist well beyond the resolution of these factors due to the emergence of *perpetuating* factors such as conditioned arousal at bedtime. Patients develop anticipatory anxiety over the prospect of another night of sleeplessness followed by another day of fatigue. Anxiety typically increases as bedtime approaches and reaches maximum intensity following retiring. Sufferers often spend hours in bed awake focused upon and brooding over their sleeplessness which, in turn, aggravates their insomnia even further. Persistent psychophysiological insomnia often complicates other insomnia disorders.

The diagnosis of psychophysiologic insomnia is supported by a history of difficulty in falling asleep selectively related to the patient's own bedroom. Patients also report approaching bedtimes at home with intense anxiety and dread. Although they may have "hard-driving" personalities, psychiatric evaluations usually do not uncover diagnosable psychopathology.

During the clinical examination patients may appear tense. Personality inventories such as the MMPI reveal patterns consistent with somatization of tension. Although polysomnography is not usually necessary to confirm the diagnosis, it can be useful in ruling out other sleep disorders.

Treatment directed toward the reduction of tension through EMG biofeedback training is usually effective within a few weeks. During this treatment, the EMG tension of skeletal muscle, typically the temporalis, is monitored electronically and translated into an auditory tone to the patient. The heightened awareness of muscle tension gives the patient direct feedback while engaging in progressive relaxation exercises. These methods are then practiced at home prior to bedtime. This is usually supplemented by cognitive psychotherapy, which strives to identify and dispel thoughts that are tension producing and that have a negative effect upon sleep, such as the preoccupation with unpleasant work experiences or examinations at school. (See Chapter 17 by Drs. Ursano, Silberman, and Diaz.) During sessions, patients' fears regarding sleeplessness can be overcome by reassurance and by suggestions that they deal with anxiety-producing thoughts during sessions and at times other than bedtime.

Stimulus control therapy, introduced by Bootzin, Epstein, and Wood (1991), is also effective and strives to interrupt the learned association between the bedroom setting and tension. The most salient features of stimulus control therapy are to ask patients to use the bed only for sleep (not for reading or watching television) and to not stay in bed trying to sleep for more than ten minutes at a time, but to go into another room and to return to bed only after feeling sleepy. Patients repeat this maneuver as many times as necessary without extending their time in bed beyond their usual arising time. They are also urged to avoid napping. Compliance with these measures is monitored by sleep logs. Other forms of therapy include insight-oriented psychotherapy, which strives to enhance patients' awareness of ongoing psychological conflicts that stem from prior years and that contribute to sleeplessness through the production of anxiety. Hypnotic agents are also highly effective for this type of insomnia, where they can afford patients with a few nights' sleep and, by so doing, diminish concerns regarding the potential for relentless insomnia that are at the heart of the disorder. Hypnotic agents can be gradually discontinued after a brief period of nightly treatment. Finally, sleep hygiene measures should be closely adhered to during and after the termination of treatment, regardless of type.

Sleep Apnea Syndromes

The two types of sleep apnea syndrome are obstructive sleep apnea syndrome (OSA) and central sleep apnea syndrome (CSA). Their prevalence has been estimated at 1 to 3% of the population (Lavie, 1983). In OSA, the pharyngeal walls collapse repetitively during sleep causing intermittent sleep-related upper airway obstruction and cessation in ventilation (apneas). In CSA, cessation of ventilation is related to a concomitant loss of inspiratory effort. Isolated cases of pure CSA are rare; instead, CSA usually coexists with OSA, in which case the latter is considered to be the primary pathological entity.

Upper airway closure in OSA is thought to occur because of a failure of the genioglossus and other upper airway dilator muscles. Apneas are accompanied by cyclic asphyxia (hypoxemia, hypercarbia, and acidosis) which, in turn, often results in cardiac arrhythmias. Pulmonary and systemic hypertension are evident during apneas. Cardiac output falls during apneas and rises to normal levels following their termination.

Apneas are terminated by arousals, which are sudden generalized activations of the brain that result in transient disruptions of sleep. Arousals also lead to profound sleep fragmentation and poor sleep quality, which are thought to be responsible for the daytime hypersomnolence and emotional consequences of the disorder, discussed further below.

The major presenting symptoms of OSA are summarized in Table 22–3. Snoring is a source of embarrassment and may place significant strain on interpersonal relationships as spouses resort to sleeping in separate beds or bedrooms. Since patients are unaware of their own snoring, bedpartners and family members must be questioned in this regard during the evaluation of OSA. Naps, although frequent, are usually not refreshing. Less commonly, patients complain of repeated awakenings during the course of the night. Many adopt unusual positions during sleep such as sitting up in bed or kneeling at the bedside, usually in association with severe hypoxemia. Sleepwalking and nocturnal vocalizations are common, as are profuse sweating, sleep-related enuresis, and gastroesophageal reflux. Many patients awaken in the morning with frontal headaches, possibly as a result of episodic asphyxia and consequent cerebral vasodilatation, and with mouth dryness, resulting possibly from the continuous flapping of the upper airways during snoring. Most patients are obese at the time of presentation and report gaining weight gradually over the years, often despite heroic attempts to curb this process through diet and exercise. However, normal weight does not preclude the diagnosis.

Associated clinical features include systemic hypertension. This usually decreases or resolves following successful treatment. Cardiovascular diseases are common. Inhibited sexual desire, impotence, and ejaculatory impairment are reported by nearly a third of patients. If left untreated, the illness is associated with increased mortality (He et al, 1988).

Table 22–3 **Major Symptoms of Obstructive Sleep Apnea Syndrome**

Loud snoring
Reports of prolonged pauses in respiration during sleep
Daytime hypersomnolence
Disturbed, nonrefreshing sleep
Weight gain

Depression is common and often accompanied by marked irritability, agitation, heightened anxiety and occasionally aggressiveness leading to violent outbursts (Doghramji, 1993). Spouses are often alarmed by sudden changes in personality as the condition escalates in severity. Many patients misuse alcohol to control anxiety and stimulants to stay awake.

OSA sufferers demonstrate deficits in attention, motor efficiency, and graphomotor ability (Greenberg et al, 1987) as well as in concentration, complex problem solving, and short-term recall (Findley et al, 1986) in proportion to the severity of the hypoxemia. OSA patients have been found to hit a greater number of road obstacles than controls when operating driving simulators (Findley et al, 1989) and are known to have a high rate of auto accidents (Findley et al, 1988).

In a recent study by Kales and colleagues (1985), 66% of patients reported a deterioration in interpersonal relationships, and 64% reported marital discord that they attributed to the disorder; 84% reported occupational impairment, 62% had fallen asleep on the job, and 13% had left their jobs because of the condition. Many also reported academic difficulties secondary to sleepiness.

The male to female ratio is ten to one yet the prevalence increases among females following menopause. The onset of symptoms is usually in the third decade of life to middle age and the prevalence increases dramatically with age and ranges from 31 to 67% in elderly men (Smallwood et al, 1983). Nevertheless, OSA has been identified in children.

Factors that predispose individuals to OSA are summarized in Table 22–4. Sedating pharmacologic agents, including alcohol and benzodiazepine anxiolytic agents such as diazepam and alprazolam, tend to increase the duration and frequency of apneas. Therefore, they are contraindicated for untreated patients.

If the disorder is suspected following a thorough office-based evaluation, the diagnosis can be conclusively established only by nocturnal polysomnography. This reveals obstructive apneas, defined as cessations in air flow through the nares or mouth lasting ten seconds or greater with the concomitant resumption of inspiratory efforts. It also reveals obstructive hypopneas in which air flow diminishes yet does not

Table 22–4 **Predisposing Factors for Obstructive Sleep Apnea Syndrome**

Nasal obstruction
Large uvula
Low-lying soft palate
Retrognathia, micrognathia, and other craniofacial abnormalities
Excessive and redundant pharyngeal tissue
Pharyngeal masses such as tumors or cysts
Macroglossia
Tonsilar hypertrophy
Vocal cord paralysis
Obesity
Hypothyroidism
Acromegaly

completely cease. By convention, the syndrome is defined by the occurrence of five or more breathing abnormalities (apneas and hypopneas) per hour of sleep.

The most established management options, in order of frequency of use, are continuous positive airway pressure (CPAP) applied via a nasal mask, uvulopalato-pharyngoplasty surgery (UPP), and tracheostomy. Weight loss is also recommended as it may lead to diminution of severity in some patients, although it cannot be relied upon as the sole treatment measure as results are unpredictable. Patients must also be urged to refrain from using alcohol, hypnotics, and other CNS depressant agents as these can exacerbate the condition.

CPAP is an ambulatory device that introduces room air at a high flow rate into the upper airway via a nasal mask. The optimum pressure required to eliminate apneas is determined through polysomnography with a variable pressure device, following which patients utilize CPAP continuously at home while asleep. Its main drawbacks are upper airway irritation that can often be adequately managed with humidification, discomfort at the mask site, and increased rates of noncompliance following the first year of continued use (Nino-Murcia et al, 1989).

Concurrent depression and psychosocial and marital difficulties can be addressed by psychotherapy. If psychiatric symptoms are severe, they should be treated aggressively since they can also impact upon the effectiveness of the management of the OSA by causing noncompliance. Antidepressants that are alerting, such as protriptyline, fluoxetine, sertraline, or paroxetine, are presumably best suited to manage depression, which is often accompanied by daytime hypersomnolence. Chronic anxiety, which may complicate the picture, should not be managed with benzodiazepines; instead, the nonbenzodiazepine buspirone, which does not appear to aggravate OSA, is often effective as are behavioral techniques.

If CSA is diagnosed, an attempt should be made to uncover underlying conditions. Although many cases of CSA are idiopathic, it can also be seen in congestive heart failure, nasal obstruction, certain neurological disorders, and following trips to high altitudes. Treatment is directed at the specific abnormality if one is uncovered. However, treatment of the idiopathic variety is often inadequate. Acetazolamide, protriptyline, clomipramine, medroxyprogesterone, and oxygen have been met with variable results. Diaphragmatic pacing or mechanical ventilation must be considered in refractory cases. Regardless of the approach chosen, monitoring the course of treatment with polysomnography is essential, as some treatments such as oxygen may actually exacerbate the condition. CNS depressants such as hypnotic agents and alcohol may have a similar effect and must therefore be avoided.

Narcolepsy

Narcolepsy is a lifelong condition that affects more than 250,000 Americans. It is idiopathic yet thought to be related to neurochemical abnormalities in the brain. Its peak age of onset is the second decade. A genetic basis for the disorder has long been suspected since a familial pattern has been noted in certain breeds of narcoleptic dogs. More recently, clarification of human narcolepsy genetics has been provided by the near 100% association between narcolepsy and the HLA-DR2 antigen, which is governed by the major histocompatibility complex (MHC). In contrast, the incidence of HLA-DR2 in the general population is only 20 to 35%. Narcoleptics also have a high incidence of HLA-DQw1 (Aldrich, 1992).

The five major symptoms of narcolepsy, summarized in Table 22–5, include

1. Persistent daytime sleepiness, the most common presenting complaint. It is usually accompanied by daytime naps that, unlike the case of OSA, are brief (typically 15 minutes) and result in increased alertness. Naps are often accompanied by vivid dreams.
2. Cataplexy, an abrupt paralysis or paresis of skeletal muscles that usually follows emotional experiences such as anger, surprise, laughter, or physical exercise. It may be generalized, in which case the patient typically collapses, or isolated to an individual muscle group resulting in transient loss of function. The episode typically lasts a few minutes, during which the patient is awake. Following its termination the patient typically regains function without any residual impairment. Although cataplexy is the pathognomonic symptom of narcolepsy, it can only be elicited in up to 50% of interviews. Cataplexy should not be confused with its near-homonym catalepsy, or waxy flexibility, an unrelated phenomenon noted in schizophrenia of the catatonic type. It is also not an epileptic phenomenon.
3. Hypnagogic (or hypnopompic) hallucinations, which are vivid and often frightening dreams that occur shortly after falling asleep (or upon awakening).
4. Sleep paralysis, a transient global paralysis of voluntary muscles that usually occurs shortly after falling asleep and lasts a few seconds or minutes. Cataplexy, hypnagogic hallucinations, and sleep paralysis are thought to be manifestations of an underlying aberration in the control of the timing of REM sleep which, in turn, results in "attacks" of REM sleep during wakefulness. These, in turn, result in the occurrence of the physical and cognitive manifestations of REM sleep while individuals are awake.
5. Disturbed and restless sleep, characterized by numerous awakenings and arousals.

Narcoleptics develop significant psychosocial impairments such as job loss and interpersonal difficulties as a result of daytime hypersomnolence. They are also

Table 22–5 **Major Symptoms of Narcolepsy**

Persistent daytime sleepiness
Cataplexy
Hypnagogic or hypnopompic hallucinations
Sleep paralysis
Restless and disturbed sleep

susceptible to auto accidents and to sustaining injuries as a result of falling asleep in inappropriate situations. Many develop depression, anxiety, and substance-use difficulties.

Other than the obvious behavioral manifestations of excessive daytime sleepiness (yawning, drooping eyelids, psychomotor retardation), physical examination is typically unrevealing in narcolepsy. If the diagnosis is suspected, it must be confirmed by an NPSG followed by an MSLT. The former is performed to ensure adequate nocturnal sleep and the lack of intrinsic sleep disorders. The NPSG often reveals a very short REM latency and sleep fragmentation caused by numerous awakenings and arousals. The average MSLT sleep latency in narcoleptics is usually less than ten minutes and often less than five minutes. Additionally, the MSLT reveals REM episodes during at least two naps, an abnormal phenomenon that is highly diagnostic for the disorder.

Treatment of narcolepsy is directed at daytime somnolence, REM-related aberrations, and psychosocial consequences. In milder cases, excessive sleepiness can be managed with conservative measures such as spending an adequate time in bed, taking two or three daily naps, and avoiding alcohol and other sedating substances. Even in more severe cases, judiciously timed naps may minimize the dosage of medication required to control symptoms. Commonly utilized medications for excessive sleepiness include pemoline 18.75 to 112.5 mg/day, methylphenidate 5 to 60 mg/day, and dextroamphetamine 5 to 60 mg/day. In refractory cases, mazindol 3 to 6 mg/day, a tricyclic compound with anorexic properties, may be utilized. Tolerance may be minimized by prescribing the lowest effective dose and asking patients to take regular drug holidays on days when their need for alertness is lowest.

The REM-related symptoms of cataplexy—hypnagogic hallucinations and sleep paralysis—can be controlled with REM-suppressant medications such as the tricyclic antidepressants protriptyline 5 to 30 mg/day, imipramine 50 to 200 mg/day, or nortriptyline 50 to 100 mg/day. Many narcoleptics also require emotional support. Education also plays a key role in management as peers, parents, teachers, and patients themselves may confuse the effects of drowsiness with laziness or lack of motivation.

Idiopathic Hypersomnolence

This is a lifelong and incurable disorder that has a variable age of onset. Its mode of acquisition, whether acquired or inherited, is unclear. The most prominent symptom is unrelenting daytime somnolence. Patients spend lengthy periods of time sleeping at night only to awaken feeling more sleepy. They take frequent and lengthy daytime naps. However, unlike narcoleptics, they awaken from these feeling unrefreshed. Additionally, naps are rarely accompanied by dreams. As a result of their chronic debilitation patients experience lifelong impairment in relationships and employment. In fact, many cannot support themselves financially. Many suffer from depression.

Polysomnography reveals long nocturnal sleep without evidence of other sleep pathology. The MSLT reveals pathologically short sleep latencies without REM periods. Treatment principles are similar to those outlined for narcolepsy. However, treatment is often unsatisfactory.

Periodic Limb Movement Disorder (Nocturnal Myoclonus)

Also referred to as nocturnal myoclonus, this disorder is characterized by the repetitive (usually every 20 to 40 seconds) twitching or kicking of the lower extremities during sleep. Patients usually present with the complaint of unrelenting insomnia, most often characterized by repeated awakenings following sleep onset. A minority complain of chronic daytime hypersomnolence. In either case, they are unaware of the movements and the brief arousals that follow and have no lasting sensation in the extremities. The disorder is more common in middle and older age. Although often idiopathic, the disorder can be seen in association with drug withdrawal states, sleep apnea syndrome, narcolepsy, chronic renal and hepatic failure, as well as during treatment with certain medications such as tricyclic antidepressants. Movements are often exacerbated by stress.

Bedpartners should be questioned for kicking or jerking movements on the part of the patient. Other factors and conditions related to the disorder should be searched for via a thorough history, physical examination, and blood tests. Polysomnography confirms the diagnosis.

Treatment of the idiopathic syndrome is indicated if symptoms interfere with daytime functioning or psychological well-being. Agents which have been shown to have clinical efficacy in methodologically sound clinical trials include baclofen 20 to 40 mg, triazolam 0.125 to 0.25 mg, clonazepam 0.5 to 1.0 mg, and carbidopa 25 mg with levodopa 100 mg. Since the disorder is usually chronic in course, long-term treatment may be necessary; weekly drug holidays may be effective in minimizing tolerance.

Restless Legs Syndrome

The hallmark of this disorder, also referred to as Ekbom's disease, is a "creeping" sensation in the lower extremities and irresistible leg kicks that affect patients upon reclining prior to falling asleep. Unlike the previous disorder, patients are all too aware of these phenomena and resort to moving the affected extremity by stretching, kicking, or walking to relieve symptoms. As a result, they complain of intense difficulty in falling asleep. Many patients are depressed, irritable, and angry. Psychosocial impairment such as job loss and relationship difficulties is quite common.

The disorder is more common in later age and is exacerbated by pregnancy, fatigue, environmental temperature extremes, the intake of caffeinated beverages and tricyclic antidepressants, and drug withdrawal states. Akathisia from neuroleptics or fluoxetine should also be considered (see Chapter 18). It is usually idiopathic, yet has been noted in association with a variety of medical disorders including pernicious anemia (B_{12} deficiency), iron deficiency, uremia, leukemia, rheumatoid arthritis, and fibromyositis (or fibromyalgia—a syndrome of nonspecific "aches and pains" without evidence of immunologic dysfunction).

Polysomnography almost always reveals periodic leg muscle bursts during quiet wakefulness and sleep, the latter associated with arousals and awakenings. The syndrome should be distinguished from nocturnal leg cramps that involve pain in the deep muscles of the lower extremities whose occurrence is independent of sleep. The treatment of the disorder is essentially the same as periodic limb movement disorder.

Drug-Related Sleep Disorders

Recreational, over-the-counter, and prescription drugs can cause disturbed sleep and excessive daytime somnolence, as summarized in Tables 22–6 and 22–7. It should be noted that, although the agents listed in Table 22–6 are associated with insomnia following short-term use, their cessation following long-term administration at high dosages often results in withdrawal symptoms including sleepiness, lassitude, and irritability. Similarly, the cessation of agents associated with daytime sleepiness (Table 22–7) can, after prolonged use, result in insomnia. It should also be noted that although caffeine has a half-life in plasma of three to seven hours, its absorption from the gastrointestinal tract can be erratic and there are wide variations in individual sensitivity to it. Therefore, even caffeinated beverages consumed early in the day can still negatively affect sleep quality at night.

Table 22–6 **Pharmacologic Agents That Can Cause Insomnia**

Monoamine oxidase inhibitors
Anticancer agents
Steroids
Decongestants
Bronchodilators
Weight loss agents
Thyroid preparations
Xanthine derivatives (caffeine, theophylline, etc.)
Nicotine
Stimulants (cocaine, ephedrine, methylphenidate, amphetamines, etc.)

Table 22–7 **Pharmacologic Agents That Can Cause Excessive Daytime Sleepiness**

Alcohol
Antihypertensive agents
Sedative-hypnotic agents
Anxiolytic agents
Antipsychotic agents
Certain tricyclic antidepressants
Opioids and other analgesic agents
Cannabis

Circadian Rhythm Sleep Disorders

This group of disorders features a disturbance in the coordination between internal and environmental circadian rhythms involving the sleep-wake cycle. Thus, patients typically present with complaints of insomnia, excessive daytime somnolence, or both. These conditions are commonly associated with peptic ulcer disease, gastritis, irritability and depression. Patients often misuse alcohol and hypnotic agents to promote sleep and stimulants to stay awake (Segawa et al, 1987).

One of the most common disorders in this group is *time zone change (jet lag) syndrome*, caused by rapid travel across time zones resulting in a mismatch between the sleep schedules of the body and that of the new environment. Eastward flight results in more severe symptoms than westward travel. The severity of symptoms is also related to the number of time zones crossed; travel across more than two to three times zones surpasses the adaptive capabilities of the body. This often leads to a desynchronization between internal body rhythms as well, such as those of temperature, sleep, and hormone secretion. When coupled with the curtailment of sleep length and the disturbance of sleep quality caused by any new environment, this leads to the symptoms of the disorder.

Jet lag countermeasures include the utilization of short-acting hypnotic agents for brief periods of time following arrival in the new locale. A safer and more effective method, however, is simply to maximize exposure to daylight in the new locale, which has the effect of resetting circadian rhythms with one another and with the environment. Individuals should also be urged to gradually shift their sleep/wake schedules prior to travel to coincide approximately with those of their destination.

Another circadian rhythm sleep disorder is *shift work sleep disorder*. Most problematic is variable shift work in which shifts are changed frequently; sleep times typically must be changed accordingly. This often leads to poor sleep quality immediately following the new shift, which is followed by a period of adaptation. The severity of symptoms is proportional to the frequency with which shifts are changed, the magnitude of each change, as well as the frequency of counterclockwise (phase-advancing) changes. However, even fixed-shift workers who must sleep during the day experience difficulties since daytime noise and light often interfere with the quality of their sleep and since they often change their sleep times for social or family events.

One-quarter of the work force is involved in variable shift work, and this proportion is climbing at a rate of 3% per year (Gordon et al, 1986). The elderly are more profoundly affected by rapidly changing shifts. Shift work is also associated with impaired job productivity and performance (Mitler et al, 1988). Job productivity seems to be at its lowest during time periods when individuals are naturally more sleepy, i.e., early morning (circa 2 to 7 A.M.) and midafternoon (circa 2 to 5 P.M.).

Shift workers should be advised to maximize their exposure to sunlight at times when they should be awake and to ensure that the bedroom is as dark and quiet as possible when they are asleep, which is often during the day. Bright artificial light emanating from especially constructed boxes, when administered at critical times, can enhance adaptation of internal rhythms to the new shift (Czeisler et al, 1990). If symptoms are not responsive to conventional countermeasures, it may be necessary to devise more rational shift schedules.

In *delayed sleep phase syndrome*, individuals fall asleep later than normal evening bedtime hours and awaken later than desired, often extending their bedtimes well into the afternoon. Thus, they typically complain of both insomnia and daytime sleepiness. Sufferers are usually young adults who present for treatment because of diminished school performance resulting from daytime sleepiness or missed morning classes. Prior history reveals a tendency for individuals to be night owls, preferring to work and play well into the night. They can be distinguished from people who stay up late by choice because of social or occupational needs in that they cannot fall asleep earlier even if they were to try.

Attempts to advance the sleep/wake cycle by retiring earlier are uniformly unsuccessful. Instead, delaying bedtimes even further by increments of three hours per day are often successful, a process referred to as chronotherapy (Weitzman et al, 1981). More recently, Rosenthal and his colleagues (1990) demonstrated that bright light therapy, when administered for a duration of two hours early in the morning, resulted in an advance of biological rhythms on subsequent nights and progressively earlier sleep times.

In *advanced sleep phase syndrome*, sleep/wake times are advanced in relationship to socially desired schedules. The disorder is more common in the elderly and is responsive to treatment with bright lights when administered in the evening.

Parasomnias

Patients present with complaints regarding disturbing events that occur during sleep or that are aggravated by sleep. Clinical aspects of the most common parasomnias are summarized in Table 22–8.

Medical/Psychiatric Sleep Disorders

There is a close association between disturbed sleep and psychiatric disorders, most notably depression (see Chapter 7 by Drs. Risby, Risch, and Stoudemire). For example, 90% of patients affected with major depression demonstrate clinical evidence of sleep disturbance (Reynolds and Kupfer, 1987). In fact, interrupted sleep, often characterized by early morning awakenings, is regarded as a hallmark symptom of major depression. Conversely, a majority of chronic insomniacs (between 60 and 69%) are affected by at least one major psychiatric disorder, most commonly mood disorders, which includes depression (Jacobs et al, 1988; Tan et al, 1984). Therefore, it is imperative that physicians keep a high index of suspicion for underlying psychopathology with an emphasis on affective disturbances whenever confronted with the complaint of insomnia. This is also true for patients assessed as having a "routine" or "primary" insomnia, who often suffer from undetected depression. Symptomatic management of the insomnia in such patients with, for example, hypnotic agents alone, can lead to treatment failure since the underlying disorder, in this case depression, remains unaddressed.

Depression has profound and predictable effects upon objectively monitored sleep as well. Polysomnographic patterns of patients with major depression in the

Table 22–8 **Parasomnias**

PARASOMNIA	CLINICAL FEATURES	POLYSOMNOGRAPHIC FINDINGS	TREATMENT
Sleepwalking	Ambulation in sleep Age affected: Prepubertal children Difficulty in arousal during episode Amnesia for the episode Episodes occur in first third of night	Sleepwalking out of delta sleep	Prevention: Removal of sharp objects, floor mattresses, etc. Reassurance of parents, psychiatric evaluation for adults.
Sleep Terror	Sudden, intense scream during sleep with evidence of intense fear Other features similar to sleepwalking	Sleep terror beginning during delta sleep	Stress reduction Psychiatric evaluation for adults
Nightmares	Sudden awakening with intense fear Recall of frightening dream content Full alertness upon awakening Usually occur in latter half of night Frequent nightmares can be indicative of psychiatric conditions	Abrupt awakening from REM Tachycardia and tachypnea during episode	Psychotherapy Hypnosis
REM Sleep Behavior Disorder	Violent or injurious behavior during sleep Body movement associated with dreams Dreams are enacted while they occur Neurologic evaluations with MRI of the brain and evoked potentials may reveal structural lesions; most cases idiopathic	Excessive EMG tone or phasic twitching in REM Body movements or complex behaviors during REM	Clonazepam Protective measures Psychotherapy
Sleep Bruxism	Tooth grinding or clenching during sleep Tooth wear and jaw discomfort	Bursts of jaw EMG activity	Dental examination Mouth guards Relaxation training Psychotherapy

acute phase of the illness are summarized in Table 22–9. Many of these patterns are so characteristic that they can be utilized diagnostically with a high degree of accuracy.

In contrast, in certain depressive conditions such as bipolar mood disorder and seasonal affective disorder, sleep is uninterrupted, yet patients complain of unrelenting daytime sleepiness. Hypersomnia is also characteristic of the sleep of younger depressives.

Mania, in the acute phase, is associated with a decrease in total sleep time. Therefore, decreased sleep in a depressed bipolar patient can herald an impending switch into mania and signals the need for close observation. Some researchers have presented evidence indicating that decreased sleep may itself be a precipitant and not just a consequence of mania; thus, situational stressors such as a relationship failure that result in an adjustment sleep disorder can precipitate a manic episode in a depressed bipolar patient (Wehr et al, 1987).

Sleep in other psychiatric disorders has been extensively studied but is of greater interest to researchers than clinicians. Almost any disorder, however, that is associated with psychic activation or anxiety can produce sleep loss and fragmentation. In addition, many medical and neurologic conditions also cause sleep disturbances. For a review of these disorders as well as strategies for management, readers are referred to Moran and Stoudemire (1992).

THE CLINICAL APPROACH TO SLEEP-RELATED COMPLAINTS

Most sleep-disordered patients present for clinical attention with the complaints of insomnia and excessive daytime sleepiness. An important dictum is that insomnia and sleepiness are not disorders in and of themselves, but are *symptomatic manifestations* of a host of underlying sleep disorders. Therefore, the physician confronted with these complaints should strive to identify the underlying disorder(s) prior to treatment. Following their identification, specific treatment can be instituted with confidence. Table 22–10 lists the most common sleep disorders and their most probable presenting complaints.

The diagnostic process, summarized in Table 22–11, begins with a thorough history with particular attention directed toward the hallmark symptoms of the major sleep disorders outlined above. In most cases it is beneficial to also interview the bedpartner, who is more likely than the patient to be aware of unusual events during

---

Table 22–9 **Polysomnographic Findings in Major Depression**

Increased sleep latency and frequency of awakenings during sleep
Diminished proportion, and absolute amount, of delta sleep
Shift of delta sleep activity from the first to the second sleep cycle
Shortened REM latency
Increased frequency of rapid eye movements in the first half of the night
Increased REM sleep time in the first half of the night

Table 22–10 **The Most Commonly Encountered Sleep Disorders**

DISORDER	PRIMARY PRESENTING COMPLAINT	
	Insomnia	EDS
Inadequate Sleep Hygiene	*	*
Insufficient Sleep Syndrome		*
Adjustment Sleep Disorder	*	
Psychophysiologic Insomnia	*	
Obstructive Sleep Apnea Syndrome		*
Central Sleep Apnea Syndrome	*	
Narcolepsy		*
Idiopathic Hypersomnolence		*
Periodic Limb Movement Disorder	*	*
Restless Legs Syndrome	*	
Drug-dependent Sleep Disorders	*	*
Circadian Rhythm Sleep Disorders	*	*
Parasomnias		
Medical/Psychiatric Sleep Disorders	*	*

EDS: Excessive daytime sleepiness

Table 22–11 **The Clinical Evaluation of Sleep Disorders**

Patient Interview
    Chief complaint: insomnia, EDS, or parasomnia?
    History of present illness
    Sleep/wake habit history
    Sleep hygiene history: meal and exercise times, ambient noise, light
      and temperature, etc.
    Pattern of consumption of recreational substances (especially caffeine
      and alcohol) and medications
    General medical, psychiatric, and surgical history
Sleep Diary
Psychological inventories
Bed partner interview
Physical and mental status examination
Serum laboratory tests
Polysomnography

sleep. If the presenting symptom is daytime sleepiness, its severity should be carefully evaluated. Patients almost invariably misjudge the extent of sleepiness; therefore, direct questioning regarding how sleepy an individual feels is often not helpful. The propensity for falling asleep is more accurate a measure; in severe cases, individuals fall asleep while actively engaged in complex tasks such as speaking, writing, or even eating. They may also experience sleep attacks, whose occurrence mandates rapid clinical intervention. Milder levels of daytime sleepiness result in falling asleep in passive situations such as while reading or watching television. If the history is positive for naps, the possibility that they are related to narcolepsy should be examined by determining whether they are refreshing, brief in duration, or accompanied by dreams. The timing of naps should also be determined as this may alert the physician to the possibility of circadian rhythm disorders.

If the presenting symptom is that of insomnia, its duration should be determined. Disorders causing acute insomnia are usually transient in nature and are more likely to resolve with conservative intervention and treatment with hypnotic agents. On the other hand, chronic and unrelenting insomnia, i.e., that which lasts more than a few months, usually requires a more careful investigation and more complex treatments. A determination should also be made as to whether the patient's difficulty is in falling asleep or maintaining sleep. The former may be related to circadian rhythm disorders or chronic psychophysiologic insomnia, and the latter is more consistent with major depression, central sleep apnea syndrome, and periodic limb movement disorder, among others.

Sleeping habits should be carefully reviewed including the patient's usual bedtime, times spent awake in bed prior to and following the onset of sleep, and final morning awakening and arising times. Sleep logs completed daily over two weeks prior to the evaluation are often more revealing and accurate in this regard. The history should also include the pattern of drug, medication, and recreational substance use as well as potential sleep hygiene difficulties.

Most intrinsic disorders of sleep do not exhibit diagnostic signs on physical examination. However, when symptoms are unremitting and severe, a physical examination should be performed to assess the potential for contributory medical and neurological illnesses. A thorough psychiatric history and mental status examination are also important. Finally, serum laboratory tests including thyroid function studies should be considered if not performed within six months prior to the evaluation.

The above office-based diagnostic process is occasionally inconclusive. In fact, studies with insomnia patients have shown that it is insufficient in arriving at the proper diagnosis in 50% of cases (Jacobs et al, 1988). When the diagnosis is in doubt, polysomnography is recommended. Polysomnography is also warranted when seemingly adequate treatment of the *presumed* disorder does not result in the alleviation of symptoms. Polysomnography should always be performed when the office-based evaluation raises the possibility of intrinsic sleep disorders such as obstructive sleep apnea syndrome or narcolepsy; their presence and severity must be established prior to management.

HYPNOTIC AGENTS

A wide array of compounds have been utilized for their sleep-promoting qualities over the years. Alcohol may be one of the most widely utilized agents by insomniacs because it enhances sleepiness and decreases sleep latency. However, it is a poor choice inasmuch as it alters sleep architecture and often results in further daytime somnolence. Patients also report unrefreshing and disturbed sleep during use and frequent nocturnal awakenings following discontinuation (Kay and Samiuddin,

1988). As noted above, alcohol can also result in further impairment in sleep-related respiration in patients with obstructive sleep apnea syndrome, a disorder commonly seen in insomniacs. Antihistamines and over-the-counter products cannot be whole-heartedly recommended either, since they have unpredictable effects on sleep and since they can cause adverse systemic effects due to their anticholinergic, sym-pathomimetic, and other properties. Although barbiturates and barbiturate-like drugs (chloral hydrate and glutethimide, among others) were utilized as hypnotics in the past, they also can no longer be recommended since they have a far greater potential for significant sedation and even death in overdoses when compared to the ben-zodiazepines.

Recently introduced hypnotic agents have proven to be far safer and more efficacious than previously available agents. Hypnotic agents can be distinguished on the basis of elimination half-life, a measure of the rate of drug disappearance from the plasma after distribution equilibrium has been attained. Those with a longer half-life include flurazepam (Dalmane) and quazepam (Doral). Those with an intermediate half-life include estazolam (ProSom) and temazepam (Restoril). Presently, the only short half-life hypnotics available for clinical use in the United States are triazolam (Halcion) and zolpidem (Ambien). All of these agents fall within the benzodiazepine class of compounds, with the exception of zolpidem, an imidazopyridine. Nevertheless, its mode of action at the cellular level is similar to that of the benzodiazepine hypnotics. (Benzodiazepines are also discussed in Chapters 8 and 18.)

There are many factors influencing the decision as to which benzodiazepine to use in an individual clinical situation. The propensity for residual daytime somnolence is one such factor. Benzodiazepines with greater elimination half-lives tend to be associated with a greater potential for daytime carryover effect and sleepiness on the day following administration. Lipophilicity also affects the propensity for daytime somnolence. Agents that are more lipophilic have a higher brain clearance rate and a more rapid redistribution from brain and blood into adipose tissue and other inactive storage sites. In effect, therefore, lipophilicity diminishes duration of action (Green-blatt, 1991). The most lipophilic hypnotic agent of the benzodiazepine class is qua-zepam. This may, in part, be responsible for its minimal tendency for daytime som-nolence after single-dose nocturnal administration (Dement, 1991). Higher dosages also contribute to daytime somnolence, as do longer periods of continued use.

A second factor influencing the choice of hypnotics is the propensity for toler-ance and rebound insomnia, the latter referring to a transient sleep disturbance (relative to baseline sleep) that occurs with abrupt discontinuation of the medication. Rebound can be controlled by gradually tapering when discontinuing the drug. It may occur, however, if patients discontinue the medication on their own accord. Tolerance and rebound tend to be more likely with the short, and possibly with the intermediate, elimination half-life benzodiazepine agents (Roth and Roehrs, 1992). They can be minimized by utilizing the medication at the lowest effective dose and for brief periods of time. Zolpidem promises to have less of a propensity for residual daytime carryover effects (Balkin et al, 1992) as well as for tolerance (Sanger and Zivkovic, 1992).

Hypnotic agents can be utilized in a wide array of disorders including adjust-ment sleep disorder, psychophysiologic insomnia, periodic limb movement disorder, time zone change (jet lag) syndrome and shift work sleep disorder, and even as adjunctive treatments in the insomnia of depression. However, as discussed above, hypnotic agents alone are inappropriate for the treatment of the insomnia of depression. *Regardless of the disorder, however, hypnotic agents should be utilized for brief periods of time and at the lowest effective doses.* During the course of treatment, physicians should carefully monitor patients for adverse effects, such as daytime somnolence, memory difficulties and performance decrements, and habituation and tolerance. Hypnotics are contraindicated in patients suspected of having obstructive sleep apnea syndrome and other sleep-related breathing disorders, in pregnant women and heavy alcohol users, and should be utilized with caution in any chronic disorder.

Antidepressant agents such as trazodone and doxepin are, occasionally, utilized in low doses as hypnotic agents, taking advantage of their sedating qualities. Unfortunately, this practice has not been subjected to rigorous clinical trials. Additionally, antidepressants pose a greater risk for medically serious adverse effects than do the sedative/hypnotic agents. Therefore, this practice cannot be routinely recommended at the present time on a routine basis unless they are used in the context of treating sleep disturbance associated with depression or anxiety.

CONCLUSION

Sleep-related complaints such as insomnia and excessive daytime sleepiness can no longer be regarded as disorders in and of themselves, as they are now known to represent symptoms of a variety of underlying conditions. Thus, their evaluation should include the physician's systematic assessment of the specific sleep-related complaint, guided by a knowledge of the many possible pathological entities. Once the diagnosis is established, treatment can be conducted with confidence. This approach is the most gratifying not only for physicians, but patients as well.

Dedicated to the memory of Dr. German Nino-Murcia; physician, scholar, and friend.

CLINICAL PEARLS

The first task in the management of sleep-related complaints such as insomnia, disturbed sleep, and daytime somnolence is to establish the diagnosis. Symptomatic management is often complicated by treatment failure and can even harm the patient.

- Depression is often overlooked in sleep-disordered patients. This is especially true for insomniacs who are not consciously aware of their depressed feelings. Therefore, the clinician should carefully search for the core symptoms of depression during the routine evaluation of insomnia.
- The patient's bed partner or another household member should be interviewed whenever possible. This can be especially helpful when the patient's clinical interview and examination are inconclusive. The bed partner can provide invaluable ancillary infor-

mation about the patient's sleep such as the presence of snoring, breathing pauses, and unusual body positions or movements.
- Paper-and-pencil inventories are often helpful in the evaluation of sleep-related complaints. These include two-week logs for sleep/wake habits, the Minnesota Multiphasic Personality Inventory (MMPI), and the Beck Depression Inventory (BDI).
- The vast majority of sleep-disordered patients benefit from advice regarding sleep hygiene measures. In some cases, nothing more needs to be done. Tips on improving sleep can be given to patients in written form and compliance can be assessed during follow-up visits.
- Prior to treatment with hypnotic agents, it is important to rule out the possibility of sleep-related breathing disorders such as obstructive sleep apnea syndrome. Hypnotic agents can increase the frequency and length of breathing abnormalities during sleep.
- Excessive daytime sleepiness is often the product of three potential factors: (1) alterations in sleep quality by various sleep disorders, poor sleep hygiene, medications, and medical illnesses; (2) acute and chronic prior restriction in sleep length; and (3) improper timing of sleep.
- Important guidelines for treatment with hypnotic agents include the utilization of the lowest effective dose; regular monitoring for adverse effects such as daytime somnolence and decrements in daytime performance; limiting the duration of treatment to prevent the development of tolerance; and gradually tapering the dosage during the discontinuation phase.

ANNOTATED BIBLIOGRAPHY

Bootzin RR, Epstein D, Wood JM: Stimulus Control Instructions. In Hauri PJ (ed): Case Studies in Insomnia, pp 19–28. New York, Plenum, 1991

> This chapter reviews instructions to patients regarding stimulus control therapy. The textbook also provides a thorough summary of behavioral and psychiatric treatment strategies for the insomniac patient.

Consensus Development Conference Statement: Drugs and insomnia: The use of medications to promote sleep. JAMA 251:2410–2414, 1984

> Outlines the consensus of experts in the field regarding critical questions confronting physicians who wish to utilize hypnotic agents.

Diagnostic Classification Steering Committee, Thorpy MJ (ed) International Classification of Sleep Disorders: Diagnostic and Coding Manual. Rochester, American Sleep Disorders Association, 1990

> This is the most comprehensive and up-to-date listing of disease entities in sleep disorders as well as their diagnostic criteria.

Greenblatt DJ: Benzodiazepine hypnotics: Sorting the pharmacokinetic facts. J Clin Psychiatry 52(Suppl 9):4–10, 1991

> Provides some pharmacokinetic considerations that may be of assistance in the selection of a hypnotic agent.

He J, Kryger MH, Zorick FJ et al: Mortality and apnea index in obstructive sleep apnea. Chest 94:9–14, 1988

> Reviews data regarding the mortality of obstructive sleep apnea patients and how this is affected by various treatment options.

Kryger MH, Roth T, Dement WC (eds): Principles and Practice of Sleep Medicine. Philadelphia, WB Saunders, 1989

> The most comprehensive reference textbook for the physician and scientist interested in sleep and its disorders.

Mitler MM, Carskadon MA, Czeisler CA et al: Catastrophes, sleep, and public policy: Consensus report. Sleep 11:100–109, 1988

> Reviews data regarding the impact of sleep disorders and daytime sleepiness on health, safety, and industrial productivity.

Moran MG, Stoudemire A: Sleep disorders in the medically ill patient. J Clin Psychiatry 53(Suppl 6):29–36, 1992

> Summarizes the effects of miscellaneous medical conditions on sleep and outlines strategies in the management of altered sleep in these populations.

Reynolds CF, Kupfer DJ: Sleep research in affective illness: State of the art circa 1987. Sleep 10:199–215, 1987

> Reviews major findings in the sleep of depressed patients.

Tan TL, Kales JD, Kales A et al: Biopsychobehavioral correlates of insomnia, IV: Diagnosis based on DSM-III. Am J Psychiatry 141:357–362, 1984

> Presents data regarding psychiatric conditions that are associated with chronic insomnia.

REFERENCES

Aldrich MS. Narcolepsy. Neurology 42 (Suppl 6):34–43, 1992

Balkin TJ, O'Donnell VM, Wesensten N et al: Comparison of the daytime sleep and performance effects of zolpidem versus triazolam. Psychopharmacology 107:83–88, 1992

Berlin RM, Litovitz GL, Diaz MA et al: Sleep disorders in a psychiatric consultation service. Am J Psychiatry 141:582–584, 1984

Bootzin RR, Epstein D, Wood JM: Stimulus Control Instructions. In Hauri PJ (ed): Case Studies in Insomnia, pp 19–28. New York, Plenum, 1991

Consensus Development Conference Statement: Drugs and insomnia: The use of medications to promote sleep. JAMA 251:2410–2414, 1984

Czeisler CA, Johnson MP, Duffy JR et al: Exposure to bright light and darkness to treat physiologic maladaptation to night work. N Eng J Med 322:1253–1259, 1990

Dement WC: Objective measurements of daytime sleepiness and performance comparing quazepam with flurazepam in two adult populations using the multiple sleep latency test. J Clin Psychiatry 52(Suppl 9):31–37, 1991

Diagnostic Classification Steering Committee, Thorpy MJ (ed): International Classification of Sleep Disorders: Diagnostic and Coding Manual. Rochester, American Sleep Disorders Association, 1990

Doghramji K: Emotional aspects of sleep disorders: The case of sleep apnea syndrome. New Directions for Mental Health Services, 57:39–50, 1993

Findley LJ, Barth JT, Powers ME et al: Cognitive impairment in patients with obstructive sleep apnea and associated hypoxemia. Chest 90:686–690, 1986

Findley L, Unverzagt M, Suratt P: Automobile accidents involving patients with obstructive sleep apnea. Am Rev Resp Disease 138:337–340, 1988

Findley LJ, Fabrizio MJ, Knight H et al: Driving simulator performance in patients with sleep apnea. Am Rev Resp Disease 140:529–530, 1989

Ford DE, Kamerow DB: Epidemiologic study of sleep disturbances and psychiatric disorders. JAMA 262:1479–1484, 1989

Gordon NP, Cleary PD, Parker CE et al: The prevalence and health impact of shiftwork. Am J Public Health 76:1225–1228, 1986

Greenberg GD, Watson RK, Deptula D: Neuropsychological dysfunction in sleep apnea. Sleep 10:254–262, 1987

Greenblatt DJ: Benzodiazepine hypnotics: Sorting the pharmacokinetic facts. J Clin Psychiatry 52(Suppl 9):4–10, 1991

He J, Kryger MH, Zorick FJ et al: Mortality and apnea index in obstructive sleep apnea. Chest 94:9–14, 1988

Institute of Medicine: Sleeping Pills, Insomnia, and Medical Practice. Washington, DC, National Academy of Sciences, 1979

Jacobs EA, Reynolds CF, Kupfer DJ et al: The role of polysomnography in the differential diagnosis of chronic insomnia. Am J Psychiatry 145:346–349, 1988

Johnson LC, Spinweber CL: Good and poor sleepers differ in navy performance. Military Medicine, 148:727–731, 1983

Kales A, Caldwell AB, Cadieux RJ et al: Severe obstructive sleep apnea-II: Associated psychopathology and psychosocial consequences. J Chronic Dis 38:427–434, 1985

Kay DC, Samiuddin Z: Sleep Disorders Associated with Drug Abuse and Drugs of Abuse. In Williams RL, Karacan I, Moore CA (eds): Sleep Disorders: Diagnosis and Treatment, pp 315–372. New York, John Wiley and Sons, 1988

Kryger MH, Roth T, Dement WC (eds): Principles and Practice of Sleep Medicine. Philadelphia, WB Saunders, 1989

Lavie P: Sleep apnea in industrial workers. Sleep 6:127–135, 1983

Mellinger GD, Balter MB, Uhlenhuth EH: Insomnia and its treatment. Arch Gen Psychiatry 42:225–232, 1985

Mitler MM, Carskadon MA, Czeisler CA et al: Catastrophes, sleep, and public policy: Consensus report. Sleep 11:100–109, 1988

Moran MG, Stoudemire A: Sleep disorders in the medically ill patient. J Clin Psychiatry 53(Suppl 6):29–36, 1992

Nino-Murcia G, McCann CC, Bliwise DL et al: Compliance and side effects in sleep apnea patients treated with nasal continuous positive airway pressure. Western J Medicine 150:165–169, 1989

Partinen M, Putkonen PTS, Kaprio J et al: Sleep disorders in relation to coronary heart disease. Acta Med Scand Suppl 660:69–83, 1982

Rechtshaffen A, Bergmann BM, Everson CA et al: Sleep deprivation in the rat: X. Integration and discussion of the findings. Sleep 12:68–87, 1989

Reynolds CF, Kupfer DJ: Sleep research in affective illness: State of the art circa 1987. Sleep 10:199–215, 1987

Rosenthal NE, Joseph-Vanderpool JR, Levendosky AA et al: Phase-shifting effects of bright morning light as treatment for delayed sleep phase syndrome. Sleep 13:354–361, 1990

Roth T, Roehrs TA: Issues in the use of benzodiazepine therapy. J Clin Psychiatry 53(Suppl 6):14–18, 1992

Sanger DJ, Zivkovic B: Differential development of tolerance to the depressant effects of benzodiazepine and non-benzodiazepine agonists at the omega (BZ) modulatory sites of GABA receptors. Neuropharmacology 31:693–700, 1992

Segawa K, Nakazawa S, Tsukamoto Y et al: Peptic ulcer is prevalent among shift workers. Digestive Diseases Sciences 32:449–453, 1987

Smallwood RG, Vitiello MV, Giblin EC et al: Sleep apnea: Relationship to age, sex, and Alzheimer's dementia. Sleep 6:16–22, 1983

Tan TL, Kales JD, Kales A et al: Biopsychobehavioral correlates of insomnia, IV: Diagnosis based on DSM-III. Am J Psychiatry 141:357–362, 1984

Wehr TA, Sack DA, Rosenthal NE: Sleep reduction as a final common pathway in the genesis of mania. Am J Psychiatry 144:201–204, 1987

Weitzman ED, Czeisler CA, Coleman RM et al: Delayed sleep phase syndrome. A chronobiological disorder with sleep-onset insomnia. Arch Gen Psychiatry 38:737–746, 1981

Wingard DL, Berkman LF: Mortality risk associated with sleeping patterns among adults. Sleep 6:102–107, 1983

Alan Stoudemire (ed). *Clinical Psychiatry for Medical Students*, Second Edition. Copyright © 1994, 1990 by J. B. Lippincott Company.

23 Basic Principles of Pain Management

Richard J. Goldberg

The control of pain is a principal concern of both patients and physicians. While most pain management is successfully undertaken by the patient's primary physician, a number of problems in pain management may require multidisciplinary involvement, including input from such specialists as anesthesiologists, neurosurgeons, and psychiatrists. This chapter addresses principles of severe pain management that are practically useful to both general physicians and psychiatrists who are consultants in this area. The major focus is on the proper use of narcotic analgesics. Additional issues that are addressed include advocacy for proper medical diagnosis; psychosocial problems that complicate pain management; the role of anxiety and depression in pain; and the psychiatrist's role in chronic pain syndromes.

Pain is a private experience. There is no questionnaire, blood test, or technology that can objectively quantify the amount of pain that someone feels. Pain is a complex product with contributions from personality, memory, fantasy, and cultural traditions in the context of neurophysiologic processes. Pain serves an important signaling function in the organism and often leads to recognition of some underlying disease that can be medically or surgically treated. However, despite the available technology, pain often remains inadequately treated, at times because of underlying patient or physician attitudes and sometimes because of medical or psychosocial misunderstandings.

ADVOCACY FOR PROPER DIAGNOSIS

Proper evaluation of the patient with pain includes a review of medical, diagnostic, and management issues pertinent to the pain complaint. For example, a careful review of history and physical examination in an elderly somatizing patient may lead to recognition of the need for evaluation of possible hip fracture. The history and physical examination of patients with low back pain syndromes must always be reviewed carefully with attention to the results of electromyography, nerve conduction studies, myelogram, and computerized tomography (CT) scan or magnetic resonance imaging (MRI) findings. Pain in patients with a history of malignancy should be carefully evaluated with a high index of suspicion that the pain complaint, presumed to require psychological management, is actually associated with cancer progression or cancer treatment (Foley, 1985a).

Patients with a known or presumed history of drug abuse are at special risk for having a medical basis for their pain overlooked, because the medical team often assumes that these patients' pain complaints are simply drug-seeking behaviors. Similarly, patients with chronic schizophrenia or mental retardation may not be able to communicate pain complaints in a way that leads to proper medical diagnostic evaluation, and the psychiatrist should be especially careful before taking a symptomatic treatment approach in these populations. The drug abuser who gets into a motor vehicle accident and is admitted to an orthopedic unit may have complaints of foot pain that are dismissed as drug-seeking behavior but that actually represent early symptoms of a compartment syndrome from an excessively tight cast.

Patients who are suspected of not having "real" pain are often given placebos (usually as saline injections) before the psychiatrist is consulted. A positive response to placebo is often misinterpreted as evidence that the pain has no physiologic basis. Such an interpretation is unwarranted, because 30 to 40% of the population are placebo responders, even in the presence of severe disease (Beecher, 1955). Therefore, rather than having any diagnostic value, placebo use itself is symptomatic of a problem in pain management that is more likely the result of inadequate diagnosis, inadequate use of analgesics, or some psychosocial management issue.

THE PROPER USE OF NARCOTIC ANALGESICS

Dose and Frequency

Non-narcotic analgesics generally do not play a central role in the treatment of *severe* pain in the medically ill. In addition to their use in mild or moderate pain and their specific anti-inflammatory properties, they provide an important and often underutilized adjunctive role in treating severe pain (Moertel, 1980) (see Table 23–1).

The most common cause of problems in acute pain management is the underuse of narcotic analgesics (Marks and Sachar, 1973). In addition to inadequate doses, narcotics are often prescribed in time intervals that extend beyond the effective half-life of the drug. For example, it is not unusual to find patients on a schedule of meperidine given every *4 to 6 hours*, when this drug *actually requires administration every 3 to 4 hours*. When patients start to complain of severe pain at 3 hours after the last dose, they are often thought of as "addicted" to or excessively preoccupied with medication. In fact, such patients may only be expressing the fact that their pain has re-emerged because their dose time has gone beyond the effective

Table 23–1 **Commonly Prescribed Nonnarcotic Analgesics**

DRUG	USUAL ORAL DOSE (milligrams)	COMMENT
Aspirin	600 q3–4h	Gastric distress, GI bleeding
Acetaminophen	650 q3–4h	Useful with aspirin allergy, bleeding diathesis; overdose can cause severe hepatic toxicity; no significant anti-inflammatory effect
Ibuprofen	400 q4–6h; do not exceed 3200/d	Does affect bleeding time but probably less than aspirin; anti-inflammatory response similar to aspirin; gastric distress less than aspirin; useful in arthritides
Indomethacin	25 q8h; do not exceed 150–200/d	As analgesic, probably not superior to aspirin; useful in arthritides; can cause corneal deposits and retinal disturbance; may aggravate depression
Naproxen	250 q6–8h; do not exceed 1250/d	Similar to ibuprofen; may cause less GI upset
Sulindac	150 q12h; do not exceed 400/d	Similar to ibuprofen and naproxen; needs to be taken only two times a day
Piroxicam	20 qd	Long half-life, requires single daily dose

Note: Patients vary in their pharmacokinetic and pharmacodynamic responses to aspirin and the NSAIDs. Dosages should be individualized. In the case of aspirin, salicylate levels may aid in determining optimal dosage.
(Used with permission from Houpt JL: Chronic Pain Management. In Stoudemire A, Fogel BS (eds): Principles of Medical Psychiatry. Orlando, Grune & Stratton, 1987)

duration of the narcotic. Table 23–2 lists usual dose ranges for commonly prescribed analgesics, and Table 23–3 lists the average duration of analgesic activity.

When dealing with an acute pain management problem, look first at the dose and frequency of delivered analgesic. It is important to look directly at the drug administration record, not at orders or progress notes, to confirm what has actually been given to the patient and on what schedule. Ask patients to rate on a scale of 0 to 10 (where 0 represents no pain and 10 represents the most severe pain they have experienced) their level of pain within the first hour after their dose of narcotic and also at the time just before they are due to receive their next dose. If relief is inadequate in the first hour after their dose, the amount prescribed may be too low. If the first-hour pain relief is adequate but pain re-emerges before the next dose, then the duration between doses may be too long. Narcotics should be given on a schedule corresponding to their analgesic half-life. Regarding dose amount, there is no rule that a "typical" order such as 75 mg of meperidine is the correct dose for everyone having acute pain. Some patients may require 150 mg to achieve the same effect. Patients and providers are often fearful about creating addiction by providing regular narcotic doses. This fear is largely unwarranted. In a large review of over 11,000 Medicare inpatients who received narcotics, only four cases of iatrogenic narcotic addiction were documented (Porter and Jick, 1980).

Another issue in the timing of narcotic doses pertains to special procedures. It is important to note whether the patient's pain problem is the result of an intermittent

Table 23–2 **Usual Dose Ranges of Commonly Prescribed Narcotics***

AGENT	USUAL DOSE RANGE (MILLIGRAMS)	COMMENT
Codeine	30–60 PO q.4–6 hr.	Usually combined with an NSAID
Oxycodone	5–10 PO q.4–6 hr.	Comes as tablets with 5 mg oxycodone plus aspirin or acetaminophen
Pentazocine	25–50 PO q.4–6 hr.	Mixed agonist-antagonist; may cause psychotic symptoms†
Butorphanol	1–4 IM q.3 hr.	Mixed agonist-antagonist; less respiratory depression
Meperidine	50–100 SC or IM q.2–3 hr. 50–100 PO q.3–4 hr.	Rapid onset of action; has a psychotoxic metabolite
Morphine	2–8 SC or IM q.4 hr. 5–30 PO q.4 .	Sedating; may lower blood pressure
Hydromorphone	1–2 SC or IM q.3 hr. 2–4 IV q.3 hr. 2–8 PO q.4 hr.	
Methadone	5–20 PO q.6–8 hr.	Long half-life; lower dose in renal failure

Note:
* Commonly used dose ranges are *not* equianalgesic. Higher or lower doses may be appropriate for particular patients, depending upon severity of pain, duration of treatment, tolerance, body weight, pharmacokinetics, drug interactions, and use of adjuncts.
† Mixed agonist-antagonists must not be given together with other narcotics.
(Used with permission from Goldberg RJ: Acute Pain Management. In Stoudemire A, Fogel BS (eds): Psychiatric Care of the Medical Patient. New York, Oxford University Press, 1993

procedure such as debridement, dressing changes, or physical therapy. In such instances, the most important intervention may be to ensure that the patient receives an adequate narcotic dose prior to such an intervention.

The use of narcotic doses that are higher than what is considered standard often raises concerns about respiratory depression, especially if the patient is also on

Table 23–3 **Analgesic Duration (with Oral Dosing)**

ANALGESIC	DURATION OF ACTION
Morphine	4–7 hours
Meperidine	3–5 hours
Methadone	4–6 hours
Hydromorphone	4–6 hours
Pentazocine	4–7 hours
Codeine	4–7 hours
Propoxyphene	4–7 hours
Oxycodone	4–6 hours

(Used with permission from Goldberg RJ: Acute Pain Management. In Stoudemire A, Fogel BS (eds): Psychiatric Care of the Medical Patient. New York, Oxford University Press, 1993 benzodiazepines. Patients develop tolerance to the respiratory depressant effects of narcotics fairly rapidly and can tolerate huge doses if the drug is increased gradually. It is true that patients who have not had a chance to develop tolerance to the respiratory depressant effects of narcotics are at risk for acute respiratory depression, especially if parenteral narcotics are combined with parenteral benzodiazepines. Fortunately, respiratory depression can be reversed by naloxone. When it is necessary to use naloxone, it is best administered in a dilute solution (0.4 mg in 10 ml of saline) slowly given intravenously, titrated against the patient's respiratory rate (Foley, 1985b). Patients receiving this treatment must be closely followed with frequent respiratory rate checks because naloxone has a short half-life, and patients may have to be redosed if taking the longer-acting narcotics such as methadone.

Constipation is an additional dose-dependent effect of narcotics. Uncomfortable and disturbing to patients, constipation can progress to functional ileus if not recognized and addressed by the proper use of diet and cathartics (Twycross and Lack, 1984).

Fixed Versus "As Needed" Dose Schedules

Acute pain management is often inadequate because of inconsistent scheduling of doses. Severe continuous pain is better treated on a fixed rather than "as needed" (p.r.n.) schedule for the following reasons (Goldberg and Tull, 1983): scheduled doses based on the half-life of the narcotic prevent the re-emergence of pain; the dose required to treat re-emergent pain is often larger than what is needed to prevent its recurrence on a fixed schedule; patients on a p.r.n. schedule are in a dependent position requiring them to ask for medication, which can create preoccupation with and delays in administration; and elderly and cognitively impaired patients may have difficulty in initiating appropriate requests for medication.

Route of Narcotic Administration

Oral analgesic administration is preferred when possible because it avoids the discomforts and potential complications of repeated injections and makes the patient less dependent on others for care. The use of parenteral narcotics is warranted when oral medications fail to provide adequate relief, when the patient is no longer able to swallow, or in the case of acute, severe pain requiring immediate relief, such as in trauma, burn, heart attack, or postoperative conditions.

The intravenous (IV) route is best reserved for acute situations, including trauma, burn, heart attack patients, severely cachectic patients who cannot tolerate intramuscular injections, or patients with bleeding disorders or low platelet counts for whom intramuscular injections are contraindicated. Unfortunately, the IV bolus route is associated with a short duration of analgesia because of rapid tissue uptake and elimination. As a result, larger and more frequent doses are needed to treat breakthrough pain, with the potential for a higher incidence of respiratory depression, sedation, nausea, and vomiting. Some of these disadvantages of IV bolus narcotic administration can be avoided by the use of a continuous opioid infusion. An intravenous narcotic drip may be rate controlled by medical and nursing staff or in some cases by patients themselves (White, 1988).

Patient-controlled analgesia (PCA) provides improved titration of analgesic drugs, minimizing individual pharmacokinetic and pharmacodynamic differences. This method also decreases patient anxiety resulting from delays in receiving medication and the slow onset of action from oral or intramuscular routes. In settings in which patient-controlled analgesia is not considered appropriate or available, an intravenous morphine drip may be established (Portenoy, 1986; Goldberg, 1993). When an intravenous route is selected, morphine or Dilaudid seems to be tolerated better than meperidine, which is associated with delirium and psychosis after multiple IV doses because of the accumulation of toxic metabolites. One unfortunate drawback of continuous IV infusion of opiates is the relatively rapid development of tolerance.

Fentanyl is now available in a controlled release transdermal formulation (Abromowicz, 1992). Fentanyl levels are not detectable for a few hours, then gradually increase over 12 to 24 hours, remaining constant until 72 hours. Dosage must be individualized. On average, patches are replaced every 72 hours, providing an effective and convenient alternative to other parenteral routes.

Conversions Among Different Narcotics

Learning to convert to equianalgesic doses among narcotics is a fundamental skill for managing pain problems. To begin, there are several situations in which improper narcotic conversion creates the apparent need for psychiatric consultation. Typically, *this occurs when a patient is changed from a parenteral to an oral narcotic following surgery and is noted to have a dramatic increase in pain and agitation, which actually represent iatrogenic narcotic abstinence.* A successful switch from parenteral to oral narcotics must take into account differences in efficacy due to limited gastrointestinal absorption and first-pass hepatic metabolism. For example, for patients on regular scheduled morphine, the oral to parenteral ratio is approximately 3:1; in the case of meperidine, the oral to parenteral ratio is approximately 4:1. In practical terms, examples of equianalgesic conversions from inpatient parenteral narcotics to outpatient oral narcotics would be 75 mg meperidine IM q.3h. = 60 mg morphine PO q.3h. = approximately four Percocet tablets PO q.3h. (see Table 23–4).

In treating a patient who is having pain control problems, the clinician must always review the record and determine how much and which medications the patient has been receiving. Difficult pain problems often are associated with the use of multiple medications. It is not unusual to find a patient who is receiving injections of meperidine and oral acetaminophen with codeine along with other "p.r.n." narcotics. In order to make sense of the total amount of narcotic that a patient is receiving, it is often helpful to convert all the various analgesics to a single standard. The concept of "oral morphine equivalents" (OME) is useful for this purpose (Goldberg et al, 1986) (see Table 23–4). However, there are some limitations in the data used to generate such conversions. Much of the information is derived from pain relief studies in cancer patients, whose acute pain needs and analgesic metabolism may be different from those of noncancer patients. In addition, figures are often derived from single-dose

Table 23–4 **Analgesic Equivalencies: Conversion to Oral Morphine Equivalents (OMEs)**

One mg of oral	*Is equivalent to*
Morphine	1 mg p.o. morphine
Meperidine	0.2 mg p.o. morphine
Methadone	3 mg p.o. morphine
Dilaudid	8 mg p.o. morphine
Pentazocine	1/3 mg p.o. morphine
Codeine	1/3 mg p.o. morphine
Propoxyphene	0.15 mg p.o. morphine
Oxycodone	2 mg p.o. morphine
One mg of i.m.	
Keterolac	20 mg p.o. morphine
Morphine	6 mg p.o. morphine
Meperidine	0.8 mg p.o. morphine
Methadone	6 mg p.o. morphine
Dilaudid	40 mg p.o. morphine
Pentazocine	1.5 mg p.o. morphine
One tab-cap oral	
Darvocet N 50	10 mg p.o. morphine
Darvocet N 100	20 mg p.o. morphine
Darvon cpd.	10 mg p.o. morphine
Percocet	15 mg p.o. morphine
Percodan	15 mg p.o. morphine
Tylox	18 mg p.o. morphine
Wygesic	20 mg p.o. morphine
Vicodin	13 mg p.o. morphine
ASA + 1.2 g codeine	15 mg p.o. morphine
ASA + 1 g codeine	25 mg p.o. morphine
APAP + 1.2 g codeine	15 mg p.o. morphine
APAP + 1 g codeine	25 mg p.o. morphine
One tab-cap oral	
ASA (325 mg)	5 mg p.o. morphine
APAP (325 mg)	5 mg p.o. morphine
Indocin (50 mg)	10 mg p.o. morphine
Mg. Salicylate (1000 mg)	10 mg p.o. morphine
Vistaril (25 mg)	2 mg p.o. morphine

(Used with permission from Goldberg RJ, Mor V, Wiemann M et al: Analgesic use in terminal cancer patients: Report from The National Hospice Study. J Chronic Dis 39:37–45, 1986)

experiments that overlook the kinetic changes that take place following repeated dosing. Finally, standard conversions do not acknowledge probable differences in pain relief associated with age, sex, race, or quality of pain. Nevertheless, the use of a conversion table can be extremely helpful in the clinical setting in order to condense a variety of medication approaches into a single agent that can simplify treatment.

When evaluating the use of multiple narcotics, always be alert for the inappropriate combination of narcotic agonists and mixed narcotic agonist/antagonists. Specifically, pentazocine is a mixed narcotic agonist/antagonist that, if prescribed for a patient who is on narcotics, can precipitate symptoms of narcotic withdrawal.

The Phenomenon of Tolerance

Any patient who is exposed to continuous doses of narcotics for at least 5 to 7 days will develop tolerance. The tolerant patient is one who notices a shortened duration of analgesic effect and an eventual decrease in pain relief. Tolerance, of course, needs to be differentiated from loss of pain control due to new or advancing disease. Following these considerations, the clinician should determine whether the patient is developing tolerance. Nursing staffs often get anxious continuing narcotics for extended times, even in patients who are having repeated surgical procedures. As a result, there may be an attempt to decrease the dose for such patients just at the time when tolerance warrants an increase in dosage.

The need to adjust the narcotic dose upward because of associated tolerance is demonstrated clearly in the case of the narcotic-addicted patient who requires pain treatment. Patients on methadone maintenance or illicit narcotics may be under-treated because of a lack of understanding of tolerance, and such patients need to be treated with an analgesic dose 50% greater than normal. Generally, the physician or staff is reluctant to be seen as supporting the patient's "habit"; therefore, addicted patients are often given too little analgesic, whereas the pharmacology of addiction actually necessitates a greater dose.

In situations involving pain treatment in the narcotic addict, it is often helpful to keep the management of the addiction separate from the management of the pain. For example, the patient's underlying narcotic addiction can be managed with methadone. Most street addicts can be adequately managed on an oral dose of methadone between 20 and 40 mg/day (or an I.M. dose between 10 and 20 mg/day). With methadone used for maintenance of the underlying addiction, the pain can then be treated as a separate issue, using a different narcotic at doses 50% greater than normal.

Recognizing Narcotic Withdrawal

The recognition and management of narcotic withdrawal are two skills funda-mental to solving some pain management problems. This is because unrecognized narcotic withdrawal may be mistaken for other psychiatric problems.

When narcotics are taken on a regular basis for approximately 3 to 4 weeks, physical dependence will develop. Physical dependence is a condition that is associ-ated with withdrawal symptoms after an abrupt discontinuation or significant de-crease in dosage. Withdrawal symptoms occur more rapidly and more intensively with drugs that have shorter half-lives. Withdrawal symptoms mostly represent nor-adrenergic hyperreactivity and include abdominal pain, diarrhea, muscle aching, yawning, rhinorrhea, and lacrimation.

Narcotic abstinence should always be considered in the evaluation of pain patients who show marked anxiety, agitation, or other autonomic symptoms. One problematic situation occurs when a pain patient with a previous narcotic addiction complains of withdrawal symptoms and requests increased narcotic medication.

Clinicians must learn to sort out objectively a true abstinence syndrome. Street addicts will often complain of withdrawal symptoms as a way of obtaining more narcotics in the medical setting. Such claims are important to listen to but should be regarded skeptically. The naive clinician may inadvertently overdose the patient, because the actual narcotic amount the patient is taking is often much less than what is claimed. As a general rule, it is prudent never to treat a street addict's subjective complaints of withdrawal. Objective withdrawal symptoms should be used as a basis for providing narcotic coverage.

Managing Narcotic Withdrawal

There are several options available for decreasing or discontinuing narcotics in physically dependent patients:

1. Patients can be withdrawn from narcotics by weaning slowly to minimize the development of withdrawal symptoms. Bedtime doses should be decreased last in order to minimize sleep disruption. In general, decreasing the total daily dose between 10 and 25% each day can be attempted.

2. Another technique for narcotic withdrawal involves the use of methadone. With this technique, the narcotic-dependent patient is put on an equivalent dose of oral methadone (see Table 23–4). Because of the relatively long half-life of methadone, its withdrawal symptoms are less intense but more prolonged. With this technique, the withdrawal process may take up to 30 days, and many drug-dependent individuals require months before feeling free of abstinence symptoms.

3. The use of clonidine combined with naltrexone (Stine and Kosten, 1992) may allow for the most rapid narcotic withdrawal process. Clonidine is an alpha-2 adrenergic agonist that diminishes withdrawal symptoms by replacing opiate-mediated inhibition with alpha-2 adrenergic–mediated inhibition, primarily in the locus coeruleus. The disadvantage of using clonidine is the development of sedation and orthostatic hypertension. However, the technique of clonidine detoxification allows for the immediate discontinuation of all opiates. While the specifics of procedure are well described in more detail by Gold et al (1980), a sample withdrawal regimen is shown in Table 23–5.

Non-narcotic Analgesics

While this chapter addresses issues of severe pain and the proper use of narcotic analgesics, the adjunctive use of non-narcotics should not be overlooked.

Among the non-narcotics, the nonsteroidal anti-inflammatory agents (NSAIDs) are the best known. These control pain via inhibition of prostaglandin synthetase

Table 23–5 **Example of Inpatient Clonidine Withdrawal Regimens for 70-kg Man**

I.

Day 1: 0.4 mg P.O. test dose in morning. Repeat 0.4 mg P.O. at bedtime if no significant side effects

Day 2–10: 0.5 mg every morning
0.2 mg every afternoon
0.5 mg every evening

Day 11–14: Taper dose on a daily basis by 50% of the previous dose. Stop on day 14.

II. For moderate to severe opioid dependence

Day 1: 0.3 mg P.O. q.3h. when awake

2: 0.2 mg P.O. q.6h. when awake

3: 0.2 mg P.O. q.8h. when awake

4: 0.1 mg P.O. q.12h

5: Discontinue medication

Hypotension, sedation, and dry mouth are the major side effects.

(Used with permission from Clonidine (Catapres) in detoxification. In Gelenberg AJ (ed): Biological Therapies in Psychiatry, Vol 8, pp 13, 16. Littleton, MA, PSG Publishing Co, Inc, 1985)

function, and therefore provide an alternate and synergistic site of action to the centrally acting narcotics.

The major side effect of the NSAIDs is upper gastrointestinal bleeding, which can be a serious problem, especially in the elderly.

Keterolac (Toradol) is the first member of the NSAID group available for IM injection (Abromowicz, 1990). Peak analgesic effect is in 45 to 90 minutes, with a plasma elimination half-life of 4 to 6 hours in young adults and 5 to 9 hours in the elderly. The primary route of excretion is renal. In acute settings, 30 mg of keterolac IM is about equivalent to 12 mg of morphine IM. With continued use, 30 mg of keterolac is equivalent to about 9 mg of IM morphine.

Anxiolytics may be effective adjuncts in pain management. It is important to consider the potential augmentation of respiratory depression and additive sedative effects associated with benzodiazepines.

Antidepressants are often useful adjuncts in pain management for several reasons. They have a physiologic effect on increasing pain threshold through serotonergic augmenting effects. In addition, they can provide symptomatic relief of symptoms that commonly accompany pain, such as insomnia, fatigue, or discouragement. Antidepressants appear to have differential efficacy in terms of analgesic properties (Max et al, 1992). Whether or not one can actually diagnose a major mood disorder according to DSM-IV criteria is not the issue (Goldberg, 1988). The use of psychiatric diagnostic criteria is problematic in medically ill patients because it is difficult to determine whether the patient's symptoms are due to psychiatric disorder or whether they are a direct effect of the patient's medical illness. Therefore, antidepressants are often used in pain patients on a "target symptom basis" (Goldberg and Cullen, 1986).

With the exception of methotrimeprazine, the neuroleptic medications have little specific analgesic activity and are mostly used for their antiemetic and anxiolytic properties in conjunction with narcotics (Foley, 1985b). (For further discussion of other agents used in analgesic augmentation such as hydroxyzine, stimulants, and steroids, see Goldberg, 1993.)

PSYCHOSOCIAL CONCERNS IN PAIN MANAGEMENT

When psychiatric consultation is requested to address a pain management problem, the consultant should always review the medical evaluation and the adequacy of the analgesic regimen. Many pain problems will be solved on this fairly straightforward medical basis. However, it is often psychosocial issues that account for the inadequate treatment or unresolved pain.

The Role of Anxiety and Depression

Since pain is the product of an interaction between physical and psychosocial dimensions, as well as between peripheral and central neural systems, both significant anxiety and depression can adversely influence pain management (Ward et al, 1982). The consultant often confronts a situation involving the "chicken or the egg" dilemma in which it can be difficult to sort out whether the pain is the cause of the anxiety/ depression or vice versa. It is usually not productive to try to definitively sort out this dilemma. Instead, the consultant should identify signs and symptoms of significant anxiety/depression and explain to the patient (and staff) that anxiety/depression and pain often coexist in a feedback loop in which they reinforce each other. The clinical strategy is to intervene in both areas. Treat the physical basis for the pain as aggressively as possible, and simultaneously address the anxiety/depression.

A thorough history of the anxiety/depression symptoms should reveal to what extent they may have antedated the pain problem. Obviously, there are patients who have pre-existing psychiatric conditions that may augment pain and interfere in management. The treatment of anxiety/depression symptoms in pain patients depends on how they are conceptualized and which of the following interventions the clinician is willing to consider.

Nondrug Treatments

Symptoms of pain, anxiety, and distress can often be addressed without additional medication use. Such approaches can be especially helpful to patients who are concerned about their use of medications and those who wish to play a more active role in their own management. Techniques to consider include relaxation therapy, self-hypnosis, and guided imagery (Goldberg and Tull, 1983). Such self-regulatory techniques are often overlooked because many clinicians are not trained in their use and because they take more time than prescribing medication.

Psychosocial Issues

Pain patients often feel that no one believes their pain is real, that people are not listening to them, that the staff sees them as drug addicts, and that some serious medical issues may have been overlooked. Patients also may feel that no one has addressed their fears, questions, and concerns about their illness and treatment. Therefore, engaging the trust of pain patients may be problematic because of their skepticism or outright hostility. They may begin the interview with a comment such as, "And what are you doing here?" or "Now, I suppose they think I'm crazy." Even if not greeted this way, the consultant needs to ask the patient, "What is your understanding about why I have been asked to see you?" Generally, starting with a review of the medical history is more effective than plunging into a review of psychiatric symptoms or history. During the course of the evaluation, the following issues generally should be covered:

1. What is the patient's understanding of the underlying medical disorder causing the pain? This question helps to elicit medical issues that the patient feels have been overlooked, as well as distortions in understanding that can lead to fears and exaggerated pain behaviors. Clarification is always important.

2. Are there any problems in the medical treatment system? Are there too many providers, all with different ideas about what needs to be done, writing contradictory or inconsistent orders? Are there issues involving the nursing staff causing delays in medication or biases against the patient, leading to a sense of isolation?

3. Is there a problem in the way the patient expresses pain? Individual, family, and cultural issues in pain behavior need to be taken into account (Fabrega and Tyma, 1976).

4. Are there family issues relevant to the pain problem? Do family members disagree with the management approach; are they undermining the program in some way? Is it necessary to meet with the patient and family together to get clues about what is going wrong? Are there new or ongoing stresses between the patient and family (or other close relationships) that may be leading to distress, thus augmenting the pain behaviors?

5. Are there legal issues pending or other issues of obvious secondary gain?

6. Are there significant psychological issues that may influence pain experience? For example, could the patient be "confusing" the situation with someone else's? It is not unusual for patients to assume that their experience will duplicate that of someone with similar symptoms. Does the patient have some morbid fear based on some private psychological associations? This material can be

elicited by asking such questions as, "Do you know anyone else who has been through something like this?" Of course, this area can be difficult to uncover and address.

CHRONIC PAIN

This chapter has addressed issues typically encountered in acute pain management problems. Issues pertinent to chronic pain syndromes often require different strategies (Roy, Tunks, 1982; Wall and Melzack, 1984). In addressing a pain problem, the consultant should always try to determine, "Does this presumed acute pain management problem actually represent a chronic pain syndrome?" It is not unusual for a psychiatric consultation to be requested for a patient whose pain problem has exhausted other providers. Such situations are common with low back pain patients admitted for a myelogram that is read as questionable or negative or with chronic abdominal pain patients with multiple surgeries and "million-dollar" workups. Medical patients and providers are used to thinking of pain in terms of an acute paradigm (i.e., "What can be done now?"). They often overlook the broader picture and can miss the fact that what they are dealing with is better conceptualized as a chronic pain syndrome. Instead of more diagnostic testing or battles over dose or drug, a shift in management philosophy is required.

The chronic pain management philosophy is multidimensional; it addresses diagnosis, of course, but also integrates physical rehabilitations, weight loss, exercise, and group or individual therapy with a focus on resuming more adaptive, normal behaviors. The treatment team does not reinforce maladaptive pain behaviors, including ongoing discussions of pain. The possibility of secondary gain should always be considered. Sometimes financial issues surrounding a lawsuit or disability claim complicate pain management. At other times, interventions with the family to change their view and their toleration of the patient's pain behaviors are necessary. The shift from an acute to a chronic paradigm is difficult but often extremely rewarding. Unfortunately, it usually requires the presence of a multidisciplinary chronic pain program, because it is difficult if not impossible to create and coordinate these resources independently. Finally, when evaluating patients with chronic pain, physicians should always be alert for concurrent or underlying psychiatric diagnoses (Katon, Egan, and Miller, 1985; Benjamin et al, 1988). Detailed discussion of the management of chronic pain may be found elsewhere (Portenoy, 1993).

ANNOTATED BIBLIOGRAPHY

Bonica JJ, Ventafridda V (eds): Advances in Pain Research and Therapy, Vols. 2–5. New York, Raven Press, 1979

Goldberg RJ: Acute Pain Management. In Stoudemire A, Fogel BS (eds): Psychiatric Care of the Medical Patient. New York, Oxford University Press, 1993

> This chapter provides a comprehensive and thoroughly referenced review of acute pain management issues. Some of the supplementary topics include prevention and management of narcotic-induced constipation, allergic and idiosyncratic reactions to narcotics, a more

detailed review of the pharmacology of narcotics augmentation, as well as more details on the use of clonidine and narcotic withdrawal.

Goldberg RJ, Tull RM: Pain. In The Psychosocial Dimensions of Cancer. New York, The Free Press, 1983

This chapter focuses on the treatment of pain in cancer patients. Aside from an overview of the psychopharmacologic aspects of pain management treatment, the chapter addresses some of the psychosocial and attitudinal issues that often interfere with pain management. Other chapters in this volume would be of interest in relation to pain management, including Chapter 4 (Medical Disorders Masquerading as Psychiatric Symptoms) and Chapter 5 (Psychiatric Aspects of Medication). Since the experience of pain is a combination of psychological and physiological events, it also may be worth reviewing the key clinical issues that influence the patient's pain experience, presented in Chapters 1, 2, and 3 of this volume.

Graber RF: Easy-to-miss causes of pain. Patient Care 89–115, 1984

This article reviews a number of treatable causes of pain that are frequently misdiagnosed: postherpetic neuralgia, atypical facial pain, reflex sympathetic dystrophy and causalgia, the myofascial syndrome, temporomandibular joint syndrome, and diabetic neuropathy.

Levine J: Pain and analgesia: The outlook for more rational treatment. Ann Intern Med 100:269–276, 1984

This article reviews recent advances that have been made in research on the physiology of pain, especially research focusing on the primary afferent nociceptor and endogenous analgesia systems. These advances have shed new light on the mechanisms of action of some long-used methods of managing pain, have led to the development of several methods, and have suggested new lines of investigation that may lead to more rational treatment of pain.

Watkins LR, Mayer DJ: Organization of endogenous opiate and nonopiate control systems. Science 216:1185–1192, 1982

This article presents data demonstrating that opiate and nonopiate analgesia systems can be selectively activated by different environmental manipulations and describes the neural circuitry involved. Both neural and hormonal pathways and both opiate and nonopiate substances play roles in the complex modulation of pain transmission. The existence and description of these modulatory mechanisms have important clinical implications for the treatment of pain.

REFERENCES

Abromowicz M (ed): Transdermal fentanyl. The Medical Letter 34:95–98, 1992

Beecher HK: The powerful placebo. JAMA 159:1602–1606, 1955

Benjamin S, Barnes D, Berger S et al: The relationship of chronic pain, mental illness and organic disorders. Pain 32:185–195, 1988

Fabrega H, Tyma S: Language and cultural influences in the description of pain. Br J Med Psychol 49:349–371, 1976

Foley KM: The treatment of cancer pain. N Engl J Med 313:84–95, 1985a

Foley, KM: Non-narcotic and Narcotic Analgesics: Applications. In Foley KM (ed): Management of Cancer Pain, pp 135–148. Syllabus of postgraduate course. New York: Memorial Sloan Kettering Cancer Center, 1985b

Gold MS, Pottash AC, Sweeney DR et al: Opiate withdrawal using clonidine. JAMA 243:343–346, 1980

Goldberg RJ: Depression in primary care: DSM-III diagnoses and other depressive syndromes. J Gen Intern Med 3:491–497, 1988

Goldberg RJ: Acute Pain Management. In Stoudemire A, Fogel BS (eds): Psychiatric Care of the Medical Patient, Oxford University Press, New York, 1993

Goldberg RJ, Cullen LO: Use of psychotropics in cancer patients. Psychosomatics 27:687–700, 1986

Goldberg RJ, Tull RK: The Psychosocial Dimensions of Cancer. New York, Free Press, 1983

Hendler NH, Long DM, Wise NT: Diagnosis and Treatment of Chronic Pain. Littleton, MA, John Wright and Sons, 1982

Katon W, Egan K, Miller D: Chronic pain: Lifetime psychiatric diagnoses and family history. Am J Psychiatry 142:1156–1160, 1985

Marks RM, Sachar EJ: Undertreatment of medical inpatients with narcotic analgesics. Ann Intern Med 78:173–181, 1973

Max MB, Lynch SA, Muir J et al: Effects of desipramine, amitriptyline, and fluoxetine on pain in diabetic neuropathy. N Eng J Med 326:1250–1256, 1992

Moertel CG: Treatment of cancer pain with orally administered medications. JAMA 244:2448–2450, 1980

Porter J, Jick H: Addiction rare in patients treated with narcotics. N Engl J Med 302:123, 1980

Portenoy RK: Continuous infusion of opioid drugs in the treatment of cancer pain: Guidelines for use. J Pain Sympt Management 1:223–228, 1986

Portenoy RK: Chronic pain management. In Stoudemire A, Fogel BS (eds.): Psychiatric Care of the Medical Patient. New York, Oxford university Press, 1993

Roy R, Tunks E: Chronic Pain: Psychosocial Factors in Rehabilitation. Rehabilitation Medicine Library, Williams & Wilkins, Baltimore, 1982

Stine SM, Kosten TR: Use of drug combinations in treatment of opioid withdrawal. J Clin Psychopharm 12:203–209, 1992

Twycross RG, Lack SA: Therapeutics in Terminal Cancer. London, Pitman Publishing, 1984

Wall PD, Melzack R (eds): Textbook of Pain. Edinburgh, Churchill Livingstone, 1984

Ward NG, Bloom VL, Dworkin S et al: Psychobiological markers in coexisting pain and depression: Toward a unified theory. J Clin Psychiatry 43:8, 32–39, 1982

White PF: Use of patient-controlled analgesia for management of acute pain. JAMA 259:243–247, 1988

Alan Stoudemire (ed). *Clinical Psychiatry for Medical Students*, Second Edition. Copyright © 1994, 1990 by J. B. Lippincott Company.

24 Behavioral Medicine Strategies for Medical Patients

Michael G. Goldstein, Laurie Ruggiero, Barrie J. Guise, and David B. Abrams

It is now well established that lifestyle factors significantly contribute to more than half of the annual deaths in the United States (USDHEW, 1979). Behavioral medicine is the interdisciplinary field concerned with the application of behavioral principles and strategies to the modification of lifestyle patterns for the prevention of disease and enhancement of health.

It has become increasingly apparent that physicians have the opportunity to play a very important role in the area of prevention and health promotion (Mullen and Katayama, 1985; Orleans et al, 1985). In this chapter, we define the physician's role in risk factor reduction, describe the barriers to physician involvement in this area, and provide a basic approach to risk factor reduction in the medical setting using two primary examples, smoking and obesity. Finally, we will use case histories of the assessment and treatment of these health risk factors.

THE PHYSICIAN'S ROLE IN RISK FACTOR REDUCTION

Physicians have the potential to play a very important role in the reduction of risk factors for disease. Over 75% of the population contact a doctor at least once each year, and more than 95% contact a physician at least once every five years. Thus, physicians have the opportunity to intervene with the vast majority of individuals who are at risk for disease.

Moreover, patients view their physicians as having considerable influence with respect to their preventive behavior. For example, smokers report that if they were asked by their physician to quit, 75% would give it a try (Louis Harris and Associates, 1978). Finally, physicians can be quite effective when they act to modify their patients' risk factors. Several smoking cessation strategies have been shown to be effective when used by physicians in the primary care setting (Kottke et al, 1988). *Studies have also demonstrated that physician-delivered patient education and counseling can lead to improvement in patients' adherence to treatment regimens* (Inui, Yourtee, and Williamson, 1976; Mullen, Green, and Persinger, 1985). Although a majority of physicians feel that they have an important role to play in health promotion, physicians are reluctant to engage in interventions to reduce risk factors for disease (Mullen and Katayama, 1985; Orleans et al, 1985; Schwartz et al, 1991). Indeed, patient surveys indicate that only a relatively small percentage (27 to 50%) of smokers are advised to quit smoking by their physician (Anda et al, 1987), and only 10% of a sample of family physicians give advice about nutrition to more than 80% of their patients (Kottke et al, 1984). The barriers to physician involvement in risk factor reduction are discussed in the next section.

Barriers to Physician Involvement in Risk Factor Reduction

The barriers to physician involvement in counseling about risk factor reduction, listed in Table 24–1, fall within two domains: physician barriers and practice/organizational barriers. Although physicians are fairly well informed about the importance of health promotion and risk factor reduction, their *knowledge* of patient education and behavioral change interventions, materials, and resources is quite limited (Kottke et al, 1987; Orleans et al, 1985).

Lack of skills is a second important barrier to physician involvement in health promotion interventions (Kottke et al, 1987; Orleans et al, 1985). Skills required for effective health promotion and risk factor reduction include interviewing and assessment skills to enable the physician to make an accurate "diagnosis" of risk or educational need; patient education and counseling skills to enable the physician to intervene to help the patient reduce risk; and skills to help the patient maintain healthy behavior or prevent relapse.

Medical education has neglected training in patient education and counseling skills, although it has been recognized that training in such skills is needed (Preventive Health Care Committee, 1985). Attitudes and beliefs also play an important role in physicians' reluctance to provide health promotion interventions. Because of the deficits in knowledge and skills, physicians lack the confidence to successfully intervene with their patients to reduce or change risk factors (Kottke et al, 1987; Orleans et al, 1985). Physicians' self-perception of the ineffectiveness of such efforts is fueled by the low rates of successful behavior change among patients they try to help. An emphasis on final outcomes, such as smoking abstinence, leads to further frustration, because even the most effective physicians achieve one-year abstinence rates of only 10 to 20% among their smoking patients.

Table 24–1 **Barriers to Physician Involvement in Risk Factor Reduction**

PHYSICIAN BARRIERS

Knowledge Deficit
Importance of risk factor reduction to health care
Effectiveness of physician intervention
Intervention methods
Resources for patients—materials and referrals

Skill Deficit
Interviewing/assessment/diagnostic skills
Patient education skills
Behavioral counseling skills
Maintenance/relapse prevention skills

Beliefs and Attitudes
Patients don't want to change or can't change
Perceived ineffectiveness in helping patients change
Lack of confidence in helping patients change
Emphasis on final outcomes
Disease-oriented biomedical approach
Paternalistic, directive style
Moralistic view of behavioral problems
Poor personal health habits
Dearth of role models practicing preventive care
Lack of commitment to risk factor reduction

ORGANIZATION BARRIERS

Limited use of reminder systems, tracking logs
Little or no reimbursement for preventive services
Poor coordination with self-help and behavioral treatment programs
Limited involvement of office staff in health promotion activities

---

The medical education process contributes to the development of attitudes that are not conducive to a preventive approach to patient care. Traditionally, physician training has emphasized a biomedical model, which is oriented toward diagnosis and treatment of diseases, rather than a systems model, which embraces prevention and health promotion (Engel, 1977); see also Chapter 1 by Drs. Yates, Kathol, and Carter and 2 by Dr. Stoudemire. As a result, many physicians continue to view health promotion activities as outside their role or as unchallenging and uninteresting (Nutting, 1986). Moreover, traditional medical training promotes a paternalistic and directive style that is less likely to lead to change in patient behavior than a collaborative and patient-centered style that involves the patient in the process of change. The dearth of role models in academia and the community who espouse and practice health promotion reinforces the attitude that prevention and health are not as important as more traditional forms of medical intervention. These and other negative attitudes and beliefs listed in Table 24–1 contribute to a lack of commitment to become more involved in risk factor reduction and health promotion activities. The *organizational barriers* that interfere with physician involvement in risk factor reduction are also listed in Table 24–1. Deficits in primary care physicians' knowledge, skills, and attitudes about health promotion interventions and systems/organizational barriers interact to limit the effective use of counseling for risk factor reduction in primary care.

A MODEL FOR RISK FACTOR REDUCTION IN THE MEDICAL SETTING

In this section we describe a model for risk factor reduction in the medical setting that is adapted from models of patient education developed and described by Grueninger, Goldstein, and Duffy (1989)* and Ockene and colleagues (1988). After describing the model, a practical step-by-step approach to risk factor assessment and intervention is outlined.

Grueninger and colleagues (1989) identify five levels of the patient education process (see Fig. 24–1): (1) cognitive (knowledge, concepts, and awareness about risk factors); (2) attitudinal (beliefs, intentions, and readiness for change); (3) instrumental (instrumental skills); (4) behavioral (coping behavior and skills); and (5) social (social support). At each level there is an opportunity for both assessment and intervention. *Assessment* involves gathering data to identify barriers and resources that may impede or facilitate patient education and behavior change. For example, assessment at the cognitive level might include asking the patient about his specific knowledge of risk factors and about his understanding of the relationship between risk factors and illness. *Intervention* involves providing the patient with the necessary information, skills, and support to help him overcome barriers and utilize resources. Thus, intervention at the cognitive level might include creating the individual's risk factors profile and informing the patient about his risk factors and what can be done to alter risk. This model also features a "patient-centered" approach to patient education and counseling, which emphasizes the importance of *tailoring the treatment plan* to each patient's specific needs (Grueninger, Goldstein, and Duffy, 1989; Ockene et al, 1988). Presently, most physicians do not have the knowledge and skills to effectively assess and intervene at each of the levels, especially the instrumental and behavioral levels. Although it may not be appropriate for the physician to intervene at each of these levels, knowledge of the assessment and intervention strategies used by others will help the physician to make appropriate referrals to those professionals who have these skills.

Identification of each patient's *stage of change*, a concept developed by Prochaska and DiClemente (1986), is an important element of patient assessment when counseling patients about lifestyle change. These investigators found that individuals making lifestyle changes, such as giving up smoking, move through predictable stages of change (see Fig. 24–2). The five stages are precontemplation, contemplation, preparation, action, and maintenance.

Precontemplation is a stage of unawareness or denial of the problem or condition. This individual has no intention to change this problem behavior in the foresee-

---

* The authors who contributed to the development of the model of patient education described by Grueninger, Goldstein, and Duffy are too numerous to list here. Readers are referred to the work by Grueninger, Goldstein, and Duffy for a complete list of references and acknowledgments.

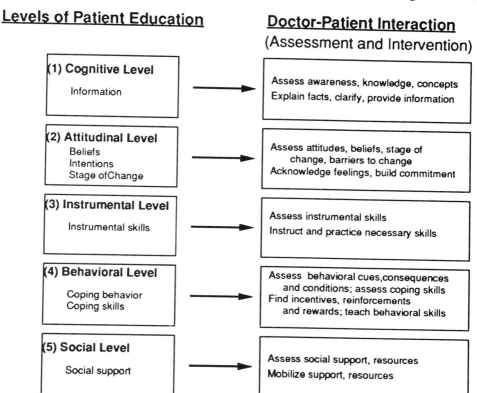

Figure 24–1. *Interactive Patient Education Model. (Adapted from Grueninger, Duffy, Goldstein. In press)*

able future. *Contemplation* is a stage of ambivalence, when pros and cons for change are weighed without definite commitment to taking action. *Preparation* is a stage in which the individual is aware that a behavior is problematic and intends to take action to change this behavior in the next month. In addition, individuals who are prepared for action report having made some changes in the problem behavior in the past year. Individuals who have reached the *action* phase have made a commitment to change and are actively attempting to change their behavior. *Maintenance* is the stage that is reached when the individual has successfully made a change but still needs to monitor behavior to prevent slips or relapses.

Prochaska and DiClemente (1986) found that individuals may take several years to move through the stages of change; moreover, they may cycle repeatedly through the stages (see Fig. 24–2). Ten specific processes of change have been identified. These include cognitive, affective, and behavioral strategies and experiences that facilitate change (see Table 24–2). They also learned that individuals in a given stage respond best to specific change strategies (see Table 24–3). For example, conscious-

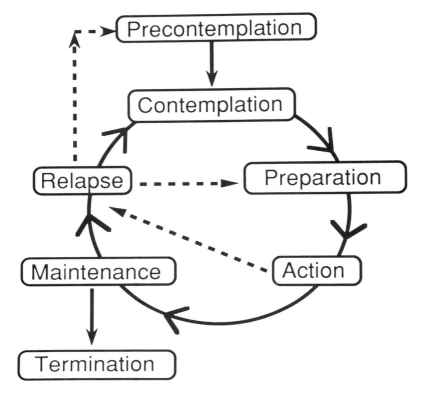

Figure 24–2. *Self-Change Model. (Adapted from Prochaska, DiClemente, 1986)*

ness-raising is most useful for individuals in the contemplation stage, while behavioral strategies are most effective when provided to individuals in the action stage. Knowledge of these findings might help physicians to feel less frustrated when their patients return without having made a recommended change in their behavior. It is unrealistic to expect precontemplators, who are not fully aware of the nature of their problem, to take definitive action. It is especially frustrating, and is not very useful, to provide precontemplators and contemplators with instructions to take action when they have not yet made a commitment to change. Moreover, because most individuals taking action are likely to relapse at least once, a relapse should be viewed as an opportunity for learning rather than as a failure.

An alternative to focusing exclusively on final outcomes is to focus on how to help individuals move more rapidly through the change process. Clinicians adopting this strategy can pick those interventions that are most likely to move the patient to the next stage. For example, for contemplators, helping the individual to recognize the benefits of change and offering personal support may facilitate movement to the action stage. Intermediate outcomes (i.e., movement to the next stage) become the goal of intervention. Further examples of the application of this patient-centered

Table 24–2 **Titles, Definitions, and Representative Interventions of the Processes of Change**

PROCESS	DEFINITIONS: INTERVENTION
Consciousness raising	Increasing information about self and problem: observations, confrontations, interpretations, bibliotherapy
Self-reevaluation	Assessing how one feels and thinks about oneself with respect to a problem: value clarification, imagery, corrective emotional experience
Self-liberation	Choosing and commiting to act or believe in ability to change: decision-making therapy, New Year's resolutions, logotherapy techniques, commitment enhancing techniques
Counterconditioning	Substituting alternatives for problem behaviors: relaxation, desensitization, assertion, positive self-statements
Stimulus control	Avoiding or countering stimuli that elicit problem behaviors: restructuring one's environment (e.g., removing alcohol or fattening foods), avoiding high-risk cues, fading techniques
Reinforcement management	Rewarding one's self or being rewarded by others for making changes: contingency contracts, overt and covert reinforcement, self-reward
Helping relationships	Being open and trusting about problems with someone who cares: therapeutic alliance, social support, self-help groups
Dramatic relief	Experiencing and expressing feelings about one's problems and solutions: psychodrama, grieving losses, role playing
Environmental reevaluation	Assessing how one's problem affects physical environment: empathy training, documentaries
Social liberation	Increasing alternatives for nonproblem behaviors available in society: advocating for rights of repressed, empowering, policy interventions

approach can be found in the sections on the management of smoking and obesity later in this chapter.

A PATIENT-CENTERED APPROACH TO RISK FACTOR INTERVENTION

The step-by-step strategy for risk factor intervention that follows integrates aspects of the model of patient education described by Grueninger, Goldstein, and Duffy (in press), the Prochaska and DiClemente model of stages of change, and a strategy for brief physician counseling developed by the National Cancer Institute known as the "Four As" (Glynn and Manley, 1989). The patient education and counseling process is transformed into a rather simple sequence of specific tasks. The five tasks are: Address the Agenda, Assess, Advise, Assist, and Arrange Follow-up (listed in Table 24–4).

Table 24–3 **Stages of Change in Which Particular Processes of Change Are Emphasized**

PRECONTEMPLATION	CONTEMPLATION	PREPARATION	ACTION	MAINTENANCE
Consciousness raising				
Dramatic relief				
Environmental reevaluation				
	Self-reevaluation			
		Self-liberation		
			Reinforcement management	
			Helping relationships	
			Counterconditioning	
			Stimulus control	

Copyright 1991 by the American Psychological Asssociation. Reprinted by permission from: Prochaska JO, DiClemente CC, Norcross JC: In search of how people change: Applications to addictive behaviors. Am Psychologist 47:1102–1104, 1991.

Table 24–4 **A Patient-Centered Approach to Risk Factor Intervention: The Five A's**

ADDRESS THE AGENDA
- Attend to patient's agenda
- Express desire to talk about risk factors

ASSESS
- Assess knowledge, beliefs, concerns, feelings
- Assess previous experience with change
- Assess stage of change

ADVISE
- Provide personalized information and advice

ASSIST
- Provide support
- Negotiate an intervention plan
- Identify potential barriers and resources

ARRANGE FOLLOW-UP

Adapted from Glynn and Manley, 1989; Grueninger, Goldstein, and Duffy, 1989; Levenkron, Greenland, and Bowley, 1987; and Ockene, 1987

At the start of the counseling session, the physician begins by setting the agenda—bringing up the issue of risk factor assessment or reduction. Of course, it is important that the physician make sure that the patient's agenda has been addressed and his concerns have been answered. Then the physician involves the patient in the process by assessing his level of awareness of risk and his stage of change. If the physician determines that the patient is not in the preparation or action stage, an attempt is made to increase the patient's awareness and build commitment for change. Personalized information, such as providing the patient with specific feedback about the relationship between a risk factor and the patient's health, is most likely to be effective in moving the patient toward action. If the patient is ready for action, the next task is the negotiation of an intervention plan with the patient. During this phase, the patient's resources are used as much as possible and potential implementation problems are solved.

Table 24–5 describes the approach in more detail, delineating specific "skills" for each of the five tasks. Sample physician statements are provided for initiating dialogue with the patient. Clearly, there is more to each of these skills than just asking these questions and making these statements. Information should be provided using language that is at the patient's level of comprehension, checking frequently to ensure that the information is understood. Clarification of the patient's knowledge, beliefs, and feelings requires skill in interviewing. The physician also needs to know how to manage feelings when they are expressed by the patient. Development of rapport and establishment of a trusting therapeutic relationship will facilitate the process of change, especially when the physician is attempting to increase the patient's commitment.

When negotiating intervention plans to help patients change their risk-related behavior, the physician can choose from a variety of options. These options range from simple advice and provision of educational materials to face-to-face counseling by the physician and referral to a formal behavioral medicine treatment

Table 24–5 **A Patient-Centered Approach to Risk Factor Intervention: The Five A's (Expanded)**

ADDRESS THE AGENDA
- Attend to patient's agenda
- Express desire to talk about risk factors
  "I'd like to talk to you about _____"
- Define problem
  "You have _____"
  "This means _____"

ASSESS
- Assess and clarify patient's knowledge, beliefs and concerns
  "What do you know about _____?"
- Assess and clarify patient's feelings about risk and change in behavior
  "How do you feel about _____?"
- Assess patient's previous experience with change
  "What have you tried in the past?"
- Assess stage of change and clarify patient's goals
  "Are you willing to _____ (e.g., stop smoking, change your diet) now?"
  "Are you considering changing _____ in the next few weeks?"
- Assess pros and cons for change
  "What reasons do you have for wanting (and not wanting) to change?"

ADVISE
- Provide personalized information regarding risk and benefits of change
- Provide physiologic feedback when available
  "Your test results (physical findings, etc.) indicate that _____ is affecting your health"
- Tell patient that you strongly advise change

ASSIST
- Provide support, understanding, praise, and reinforcement
  "I can help you by _____"
  "It's often difficult to change _____"
  "It's great that you're considering _____"
- Describe intervention options
- Negotiate an intervention plan—match intervention to stage of change
  For Precontemplators and Contemplators:
  Review patient's pros and cons for change: reinforce pros; express willingness to help patient address cons
  Provide more information, feedback
  Address feelings
  Encourage to consider change
  For patients in Preparation and Action stages:
  Negotiate selection among options
  Solve problems with implementation
  "What problems might arise with _____?"
  Provide resources (e.g., written materials)
  Identify additional resources
  "What (or who) might help you with _____?"
  Teach skills/recommend specific strategies
  Consider a written contract/prescription
  Refer, when appropriate

ARRANGE FOLLOW-UP
- Reaffirm plan
  "Now, what are you going to do?"
- Arrange follow-up appointment or call
  "I'd like to see you again on _____"

Adapted from Glynn and Manley, 1989; Grueninger, Goldstein, and Duffy, 1989; Levenkron, Greenland, and Bowley, 1987; and Ockene, 1987 program. How does one choose among the various options? Careful assessment of the patient can help to provide the answer to this question.

Patient characteristics that predict decreased likelihood of response to minimal interventions include being in an early stage of change (e.g., precontemplation), poor motivation, repeated failures during previous attempts to change, high levels of psychological dependence on the targeted risk behavior, poor social support, and high levels of physical dependence on the targeted risk behavior when appropriate (e.g., nicotine dependence when smoking is the targeted risk factor). When one or several of these patient characteristics is present, it is likely that these patients will require a more intensive intervention or one that combines several modalities (e.g., behavioral, pharmacological, and social interventions). For other patients, a stepwise approach to treatment is reasonable, starting with a minimal intervention (e.g., provision of self-help materials) and moving to more intensive treatments if the minimal interventions are not effective.

As noted in the section of this chapter on the barriers to physician involvement in patient behavior change, most physicians don't feel they have the skills to engage in effective counseling in the area of risk factor reduction. Thus, most physicians are unlikely to provide face-to-face counseling to patients themselves. However, skills can be taught in this area if sufficient time and faculty effort are allocated to training (Levenkron, Greenland, and Bowley, 1987; Ockene et al, 1988). It must also be recognized that even minimal physician-delivered counseling interventions can be quite effective, especially in the area of smoking cessation (Kottke, Battista, De-Friesse, and Brekke, 1988; Schwartz, 1987).

We have described a generic patient-centered approach to risk factor intervention, which stresses the importance of developing an understanding of the patient's readiness to engage in behavior change and also the need to build commitment in patients who were not yet ready to take action. In the next section, we describe some specific behavioral strategies that can be used to provide assistance to those patients who are ready to change their risk-associated behaviors. Case examples illustrate the approach to obese patients and patients who smoke.

ASSESSMENT AND TREATMENT OF OBESITY

Patient Assessment

In deciding when to intervene and at what level, several dimensions of patient characteristics are important: (1) severity of obesity (e.g., Body Mass Index [BMI]); (2) biological factors and medical risk status; (3) behavioral factors including eating and exercise habits; (4) psychological status (e.g., depression); (5) sociocultural-environmental factors, including support from friends, family, and the work environment; and (6) stage of readiness for changing eating and exercise habits to lose weight (see also Fig. 24–1).

Biobehavioral factors must be evaluated to help determine which program might be best for a particular patient. A review of the patient's personal and familial weight history, eating habits, and previous attempts to lose weight (with a focus on what went wrong) can be helpful. Patients may report eating in response to psychological events (such as stress, depression, or social anxiety). They may reveal fatigue, dizziness, or cravings for protein, carbohydrates, or sugar that could reflect biochemical imbalances (e.g., hypoglycemia). They may have an underlying eating disorder such as bulimia.

Interpersonal and sociocultural-environmental factors should also be evaluated. The educational level, economic situation, and living environment of the patient may make it more difficult to change lifestyle. Social support (or lack of it) can also play a crucial role. Sometimes spouses, parents, or family are unaware of their power to support and sustain change; alternatively, they can unwittingly sabotage treatment efforts because of their own lifestyle habits or values. An assessment of the patient's environment often reveals a need to involve other members of the family in lifestyle change efforts.

Patients should be prepared for treatment by ensuring appropriate goals and expectations. One major barrier to successful weight loss is unrealistic expectations about the speed and ease of weight loss. Patients should be discouraged from seeking rapid weight loss or "fad diets." One drawback of all fad diets is that patients eventually feel deprived and must stop the diet. This is when they typically return to their prior eating habits and regain weight.

A Step-Care Model of Treatment

Brownell and Wadden (1991) have proposed a step-care approach to weight loss that is perhaps the most rational and cost-effective way to proceed. The challenge to the physician is to determine which type of treatment is most appropriate for a particular patient (see Fig. 24–3). Since cost, risk, and invasiveness increase with each step, it should be recommended that the patient begin at the lowest step not yet given a fair test. More costly and risky procedures should be reserved for those patients who have not responded to basic strategies.

In general, mildly to moderately obese individuals should be encouraged to seek treatment in low-cost self-help or commercial programs. However, repeated unsuccessful efforts to lose weight can lead to adverse psychological effects, making each future attempt more difficult (Brownell and Wadden, 1991). Therefore, those who have tried and failed to lose weight on several occasions by these methods and those who are moderately to morbidly obese should be strongly encouraged to seek an intermediate level of care, such as a hospital-based behavior modification program.

The basic philosophy of behavior modification is that in order to lose weight and keep it off, a person must gradually replace old maladaptive eating behaviors and exercise habits with new health-promoting ones that can be maintained for a lifetime. Components typically are taught to slow down their eating, to use alternative skills in managing moods (e.g., relaxation training), to use social support (assertiveness), to apply problem-solving skills to increase activity level, and to change their ways of thinking about food (cognitive restructuring). (For more details about clinical techniques, see Abrams, 1984.)

Severely overweight patients and those who have failed with a variety of conventional treatments might be appropriate candidates for a very-low-calorie diet (VLCD)

Classification Decision ➝ Stepped-Care Decision ➝ Matching Decision

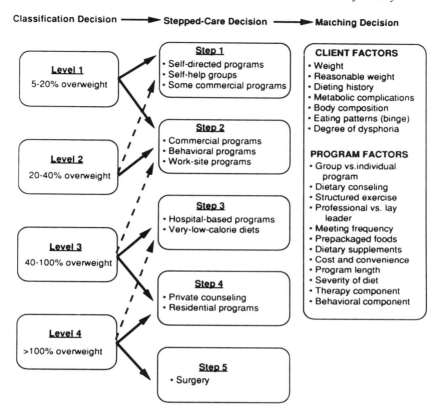

Figure 24–3. *A Step-Care Model for the Treatment of Obesity.* **Classification Decision** divides individuals according to percent overweight into four levels. Each level dictates which of the five steps would be reasonable in the second stage (**Stepped Care Decision**). This indicates that the least intensive, costly, and risky approach will be used from among alternative treatments. **Matching Decision** helps determine final selection of a program based on a combination of client and program variables. **Dashed lines with arrows** show the lowest level of treatment beneficial; however, more intensive treatment is usually necessary for people at the specified weight level. (© 1991 by the Association for Advancement of Behavior Therapy. Reprinted with permission from Brownell KD, Wadden TA: The heterogeneity of obesity: fitting treatments to individuals. Behavior Therapy 22:1622, 1991.)

or gastroplasty surgery. These options are most appropriate when obesity poses a definite and sometimes imminent hazard to health, because maximal interventions also carry a significant degree of risk in the form of side effects and/or complications. Behavior modification programs are now being combined with VLCDs and with gastroplasty to increase adherence/compliance and to improve the maintenance of weight loss (Brownell and Wadden, 1991; Wadden and Stunkard, 1986).

Maintenance of weight loss is the key problem, because long-term results (more than one year) have demonstrated that as many as 75% regain the weight lost in programs (Jeffrey, 1987). The most recent well-controlled maintenance study (Perri, McAllister, Gange, and Nezu, 1988) suggests that involvement in an ongoing intensive maintenance program—which includes continued contact, training in behavioral problem-solving skills, social influence, and exercise—helps patients to maintain weight losses for at least 18 months after completion of an initial treatment program. As a result of findings like these, researchers have suggested that many obese individuals may need to remain in continuous care for their obesity. Furthermore, it has been suggested that obesity should be viewed as a chronic health problem like hypertension or diabetes and should be followed medically in a similar manner (Perri, Sears, and Clark, in press; Wing, 1992). By applying the approach outlined in this chapter, physicians can play a very important and unique role in the ongoing management of obese patients.

A CASE STUDY

A 46-year-old woman weighing 80% over ideal body weight presents to her physician because she is "feeling lousy" with fatigue and frequent headaches. The physician's examination reveals that she has a total cholesterol of 310 and a fasting blood sugar of 210. A dialogue that reflects a patient-centered approach to management follows.

Doctor: Mrs. Jones, you've told me that you're fatigued and have frequent headaches. I think your symptoms are related to several factors. First, your blood sugar is elevated. In addition, your total cholesterol is 310. Both your blood sugar level and your cholesterol level need to come down, or else you stand an increased risk of heart attack, stroke, and the many complications of diabetes. Your weight is an important influence on your blood sugar and cholesterol. Therefore, the best way to reduce your risk is to lose weight and to eat fewer fatty foods. I can help you to select the best means of weight loss. Would you consider trying to lose weight in the next month?

Mrs. Jones: If you think it would be a good idea.

Doctor: It would be a great idea if you're ready to give it a try. What do you know about weight loss?

Mrs. Jones: Weight loss? I'm constantly on a diet. I know so much about weight loss I could write a book. I've been on everything. I've done Weight Watchers, the Scarsdale Diet, all-protein diets.... You name it, I've done it.

Doctor: I'm glad you're interested in losing weight. How many times have you been on a medically supervised diet using such principles as behavior modification and calorie counting?

Mrs. Jones: Well, my previous doctor told me that I should try to lose weight by sticking to 1200 calories per day, but then I just went off. It didn't last much more than a week or two.

Doctor: So you've never really been closely supervised. I have some ideas that may help you, but they involve a strong commitment on your part. Do you want to hear more today?

Mrs. Jones: If you recommend a program, then I'll do my best.

Doctor: Very well, then. Here is my advice. Number one, with respect to your weight, losing 1 to 2 pounds per week over the next 3 months is a reasonable goal. Keep in mind that losing weight is often quite challenging, so don't be discouraged if you don't lose as fast as you might like. Research has shown that even a 10-pound weight loss can have positive health benefits for someone like you. Number two, because your cholesterol is high, you need to reduce your intake of fatty foods. Number three, I recommend that you increase your activity level and even get into a formal exercise program. Given your current weight, your low activity level, and the amount of experience you have had at commercially available programs, I recommend that you go to a professionally led behavior modification program. They will do a thorough assessment of your eating and exercise habits and come up with a treatment program that is tailored for you. They will also be able to help you make dietary changes to reduce your intake of fats. In addition, I can give you this table, which lists foods high and low in fat content. Finally, I will let them know you are able to start an exercise program. You need to begin very modestly and gradually build up. If you like to walk or swim, either one would be fine for you. How do you feel about these options?

Mrs. Jones: Fine. I'm happy to give it a shot.

Doctor: What problems do you see that might arise with your attempt to follow through on this plan?

Mrs. Jones: The main thing, Doctor, is my work. This is a very busy time of year, and it's hard for me to get away from the office. If I can't get an appointment time at the clinic that's suitable, that might get in the way of my following through. Also, trying to exercise when you're real busy at work is just not realistic.

Doctor: I'm glad you are aware of the possible problems you might run into. What might help you to overcome these obstacles and stick to a lifestyle change program that is really essential for your health at this time?

Mrs. Jones: Well, I can ask my boss to let me come in a little earlier so that I can leave and make an afternoon appointment.

Doctor: That sounds like a good idea. Also, be sure to get in touch with me if you have any other questions or need clarification about this plan. So, once again, what exactly are you going to do?

Mrs. Jones: I'll give the behavioral medicine clinic a call to set up an appointment as soon as possible. Changing the amount of fat I eat shouldn't be that hard, at least not when I'm home. Exercising will be tougher, but I guess I could walk in the evening after I get home from the office, maybe a mile at first and build up from there.

Doctor: That sounds like an excellent plan. I'd like to see you again in 3 months and check how much you have improved your cholesterol and blood sugar level. Let's aim for a 1 to 2 pound weight loss per week by then.

In this case, the physician was quickly able to determine that the patient was at the preparation stage. The appropriate intervention for this type of patient, given the severity of her medical problems and her previous experience, was at the intermediate level.

ASSESSMENT AND TREATMENT OF SMOKING

Patient Assessment for Smoking Cessation

It is helpful to assess patient characteristics before deciding on the appropriate level of intervention. Five major characteristics need to be evaluated. These are (1) stage of change or motivation, (2) degree of physiological addiction, (3) degree of psychological dependence, (4) history of attempts to quit, and (5) degree of positive social support and negative support (e.g., another smoker in the household).

If the patient is in the precontemplation or contemplation stage and not strongly motivated to change, then motivating her or him becomes the first priority before deciding on treatment options. Assuming an individual is ready for action, the rule of thumb is that smokers should receive a more intensive (maximal) treatment program if they (1) are physiologically addicted (smoke more than 25 cigarettes per day, usually smoke within 30 minutes of awakening during the morning, and report having withdrawal symptoms during previous quit attempts); (2) are psychologically dependent (smoke for stress management, or to help cope with social interactions); (3) have associated psychiatric illness; or (4) have tried to quit on their own and failed.

Smokers who meet the criteria for physiological addiction may benefit from the use of nicotine replacement strategies (e.g., nicotine transdermal patches, nicotine chewing gum) as an adjunct to behavioral treatment (Brown et al, 1993; Fiore et al, 1992). In contrast, first-time quitters and those individuals who are less biologically addicted and less psychosocially dependent are candidates for minimal levels of treatment, such as self-help or other brief interventions (Abrams and Wilson, 1986; Abrams et al, 1991).

A review of the patient's previous attempts to quit can be revealing (Best, 1976). They may show, for example, that the patient was unable to quit even though he or she cut down (suggesting biological addiction), or that she or he quit for a period but slipped back into smoking when stressed, angry, or depressed (suggesting psychological dependence). If the patient relapsed in a social situation, then social anxiety or lack of assertiveness may be a problem that needs correcting before the next quit attempt. Moreover, recent evidence suggests that a sizeable proportion of smokers also suffer from a past or present psychiatric disorder (e.g., major depressive episode, alcohol or other psychoactive substance-use disorder, anxiety disorders) and also that a majority of individuals with severe psychiatric disorders, such as schizophrenia, smoke (Brown et al, 1993). Relapse to smoking may be precipitated by an exacerbation or reemergence of psychiatric symptoms in these patients.

A Step-Care Model of Treatment

By exploring the patient's status and history on biopsychosocial dimensions, one can decide how to move him or her in a stepwise fashion through three possible levels of treatment: (1) minimal interventions (self-help, physician counseling, commercial programs, hypnosis), (2) intermediate interventions (professionally led programs that feature behavior modification), and (3) maximal interventions (behavior modification plus pharmacological treatments and specialized programs that address psychiatric co-morbidity, including other substance abuse).

Minimal Interventions Several studies suggest the potential power of brief intervention in physicians' offices. Strategies that increase the likelihood of success include face-to-face interventions, the combination of physician and nonphysician counselors, multiple sessions, and multiple intervention modalities (Kottke et al, 1988). Studies have demonstrated that physician interventions are particularly effective in patients with smoking-related illnesses or in those "at risk" for smoking-related disease (Schwartz, 1987). Physician advice is improved when follow-up is provided (Wilson et al, 1982). Other simple strategies that physicians can use in the office are listed in Table 24–6. The use of nicotine replacement strategies is described in the section on maximal interventions. Nicotine replacement without adjunctive behavioral treatment is unlikely to lead to success in smoking cessation. However, recent studies performed in the primary care setting have demonstrated the effectiveness of nicotine transdermal patches when brief counseling and several follow-up visits were also provided (Fiore et al, 1992).

Other minimal interventions are listed in Table 24–6. Generally, it is the lighter, less-dependent smokers who are highly motivated to quit and who have excellent social support for quitting that are the preferred candidates for brief or minimal interventions.

Intermediate Interventions If minimal interventions have been attempted without success, or if the individual is more physiologically or psychologically dependent on cigarettes, then formal behavioral treatment programs of several weeks' duration should be considered. These programs teach skills for quitting as well as for managing acute withdrawal and maintenance/preventing relapse (Lichtenstein, 1982; Abrams et al, 1991; Brown et al, 1993).

Behavioral approaches to quitting include nicotine fading, stimulus control, aversive techniques, cognitive approaches to deal with urges and craving, and relaxation training. Nicotine fading involves switching to a brand of cigarettes with lower nicotine and reducing the number of cigarettes smoked per day on a systematic basis over a period of three to five weeks (Foxx and Brown, 1979). Gradual reduction of nicotine is designed to minimize withdrawal symptoms. Stimulus control involves rearranging the environment and self to make smoking more and more difficult (remove all ashtrays, smoke only in one room of the house, buy packs instead of cartons). Although aversive strategies are unlikely to be widely accepted by consumers, they have yielded some of the most successful outcomes. Most current programs include a variety of techniques rather than one strategy. Reviews of the behavioral literature indicate that at a one-year follow-up, the average participant in

Table 24–6 **A Step-Care Model for the Treatment of Smoking**

I. Minimal Interventions
Self-help programs
Physician counseling
  Advice
  Provide quitting materials (e.g., self-help manuals)
  Contracts
  Set quit date
  Follow-up visits or calls
  Nicotine transdermal patches (with brief behavioral counseling and follow-up)
Commercial programs
Hypnosis/acupuncture
II. Intermediate interventions
Professionally led programs
  Nicotine fading
  Aversive techniques
  Behavior modification
    Self-monitoring of smoking behavior
    Goal setting and self-reinforcement
    Stimulus control
    Coping skills
      Cognitive restructuring
      Assertiveness training
      Problem solving
      Relaxation training
      Relapse-prevention training
III. Maximal interventions
Combined behavior modification/pharmacotherapy
  Nicotine resin complex
  Nicotine transdermal patches
  Clonidine
  Antidepressants
Outpatient treatment programs that address psychiatric co-morbidity
Inpatient treatment programs

the typical behavioral program has a 20 to 40% chance of being abstinent (Schwartz, 1987; Brown et al, 1993).

Maximal Interventions Programs that add nicotine replacement strategies or other pharmacologic procedures (e.g., clonidine) to behavior modification should be considered for the chronic and more "difficult to treat" heavy smoker who has tried to quit repeatedly without success (Fagerstrom, 1978; Abrams et al, 1991; Brown et al, 1993). Nicotine replacement may help to alleviate withdrawal symptoms and facilitate cessation (Hughes, Higgins and Hatsukami, 1990; Fiore et al, 1992). Once cessation has been achieved and maintained, gradual withdrawal from the agent can then be dealt with separately. Use of nicotine replacement without a behavioral treatment program that addresses psychosocial factors may reduce efficacy (Abrams and Wilson, 1986; Abrams et al, 1991; Brown et al, 1993; Fiore et al, 1992), because simply using a pharmacological agent to reduce withdrawal is considered an incomplete treatment of a multifactorial habit. Individuals with a past or present psychiatric disorder may require more intensive treatment to help them quit smoking, especially if they continue to have signs or symptoms of the disorder. Patients abusing alcohol or other psychoactive drugs are unlikely to successfully quit smoking until they stop abusing other drugs (Brown et al, 1993). A past history of depression may dispose an individual to experience depressive symptoms or a full-blown depression when they quit smoking (Brown et al, 1993). Therefore, outpatient or inpatient programs that address both smoking cessation and psychiatric co-morbidity may be needed by smokers with these disorders.

Maintenance Strategies Behavioral techniques for maintenance and prevention of relapse are of recent origin and hold much promise, because 60% of those who quit smoking will relapse within the first three months of quitting (Marlatt and Gordon, 1985). Techniques for relapse prevention include a detailed analysis of "high-risk situations." These are people, places, or emotional states that the smoker feels are most likely to precipitate a return to smoking. Individuals are taught how to cope with these situations using rehearsal and other techniques to resist temptation. If they should have a slip back into smoking (one or two cigarettes), then they are provided with techniques to prevent the slip from becoming a full-blown relapse. Additional support and follow-up (e.g., telephone hot lines) are usually provided during the critical three to six months after quitting when people are most vulnerable to relapse.

In summary, even a small amount of physician time can have a large impact on helping patients become motivated for quitting smoking and then quit and resist relapse. A step-care plan can be adopted with every smoker in the office practice and in the hospital. Those who are not yet ready to quit are targeted for systematic counseling, education, and follow-up. More time and effort are placed on high-risk individuals and those who are willing to take action. Beyond physician advice (which can be very effective), self-help and comprehensive formal programs can be used. Helping patients to quit smoking can have a large impact on chronic disease and disability in the United States over the next decades. (Nicotine addiction is also discussed in Chapter 10).

A CASE STUDY

Ms. Williams is a 37-year-old, hard-working lawyer with two small children. She visits her physician complaining of productive cough and fever for 3 days. After obtaining a history, performing a physical exam, and obtaining a chest X-ray, the physician returns to the examining room to tell the patient the chest X-ray is negative and that she has bronchitis. He also notices from her chart that she has been a chronic smoker. The dialogue that follows reflects a patient-centered approach to smoking cessation.

Doctor: Your chest X-ray looks normal. I think you have bronchitis. I will discuss the treatment of your bronchitis with you, but first I'd like to talk with you about smoking. Are you still smoking?

Ms. Williams: Yes, I'm ashamed to say.

Doctor: Have you thought about giving it up?

Ms. Williams: Yes, I'd like to quit, but smoking really helps me to relax and concentrate at work, and I have this big case coming up. I couldn't possibly try to quit till it's over.

Doctor: Hmm, it seems like you depend on cigarettes to help you deal with stress at work. Your work sounds pretty stressful right now. What reasons do you have for wanting to quit?

Ms. Williams: Well, I know it's not good for my health, especially since I keep getting bronchitis. Also, my father smoked and he died of a heart attack. My husband is not a smoker and he and the kids have been after me to quit, too.

Doctor: You've mentioned some good reasons for quitting. I think your infections would decrease if you quit, and your risk of developing heart disease will decrease dramatically when you quit. I know I've told you about the effects of passive smoke on your children's health as well as the important influence you have on your kids as a role model. I'm glad you're willing to consider quitting, but it sounds like quitting now would be hard on you. I'd like to help you to quit when your case is over, though.

Ms. Williams: That would be fine. My case will be over in 2 months.

Doctor: Why don't you schedule an appointment with me in 2 months, then.

Ms. Williams: OK.

In this case, the physician (1) raised the issue of smoking and allowed the patient to express her ideas and feelings about quitting, (2) explored her reasons for quitting as well as her reasons for continuing to smoke, and (3) recognized that the patient was contemplating quitting, but also that she was not ready for action. Therefore, the physician elected to reinforce the patient's reasons for quitting, personalize her risk, offer to help her quit, and ask her to schedule a follow-up appointment after her court case was over. It is likely that the physician helped to accelerate the patient's movement from the contemplation stage to the preparation or action stage with these interventions. If she returns in two months, or when she returns for any future visit, the physician can continue to build commitment, complete further assessment, and begin to suggest specific smoking cessation strategies.

ANNOTATED BIBLIOGRAPHY

Abrams DB, Emmons KM, Niaura RS et al: Tobacco Dependence: An Integration of Individual and Public Health Perspectives. In Nathan PE, Langenbucher JW, McCrady BS, Frankenstein W (eds): Annual Review of Addictions Research and Treatment, Vol. 1. New York, Pergamon Press, 1991

    A comprehensive review of factors contributing to the development of tobacco dependence, with a description of the full range of potential interventions to prevent and treat tobacco dependence.

Brown RA, Goldstein MG, Niaura R, Emmons KM, Abrams DB: Nicotine Dependence: Assessment and Management. In Stoudemire A, Fogel BS (eds): Psychiatric Care of the Medical Patient. New York, Oxford University Press, 1993

A detailed review of the assessment and management of nicotine dependence, with an emphasis on the role of the physician.

Clark MM, Ruggiero L, Pera V, Goldstein MG, Abrams DB: Assessment, Classification, and Treatment of Obesity: A Behavioral Medicine Perspective. In Stoudemire A, Fogel BS (eds): Psychiatric Care of the Medical Patient. New York, Oxford University Press, 1993

A detailed review aimed at the medical practitioner.

Coates TJ, Polonsky WH: Behavior Therapy. In Michels R (ed): Psychiatry. Philadelphia, JB Lippincott, 1986

Provides a description of the principles and techniques used in behavior therapy with case examples.

Grueninger UJ, Duffy FD, Goldstein MG: Patient Education in the Medical Encounter: An Interactive Approach. In Lipkin M Jr, Lazare A, Putnam S (eds): The Medical Interview. Boston, Springer-Verlag, *in press*

Describes a comprehensive model for patient education and counseling in the medical setting as well as a practical patient-centered strategy for physician-delivered counseling.

Prochaska JO, DiClemente CC: Towards a Comprehensive Model of Change. In Miller WR, Heather N (eds): Treating Addictive Disorders: Processes of Change. New York, Plenum Press, 1986

Description of a comprehensive model of behavioral change that includes an explanation of the stages and processes of change.

Russell ML: Behavioral Counseling in Medicine: Strategies for Modifying At-Risk Behavior. New York, Oxford University Press, 1986

A practical primer for physicians in behavioral counseling techniques.

Sheridan DP, Winogrond IR (eds): The Preventive Approach to Patient Care. New York, Elsevier, 1987

A text on the theory and practice of preventive medicine, using a life-cycle approach.

REFERENCES

Abrams DB: Current Status and Clinical Developments in the Behavioral Treatment of Obesity. In Franks CJ (ed): New Developments in Behavior Therapy: From Research to Clinical Application. New York, Haworth Press, 1984

Abrams DB, Emmons KM, Niaura RS et al: Tobacco Dependence: An Integration of Individual and Public Health Perspectives. In Nathan PE, Langenbucher JW, McGrady BS, Frankenstein W (eds): Annual Review of Addictions Research and Treatment, Vol. 1. New York, Pergamon Press, 1991

Abrams DB, Wilson GT: Habit Disorders: Alcohol and Tobacco Dependence. Frances AJ and Hales RE (eds.). American Psychiatric Association, Annual Review Vol. 5. Washington, DC, American Psychiatric Press, 1986

Anda RF, Remington PL, Sienko DG et al: Are physicians advising smokers to quit? The patient's perspective. JAMA 257:1916–1919, 1987

Best JA: Tailoring smoking withdrawal procedures to personality and motivational differences. J Consult Clin Psychol 4:1–8, 1976

Brown RA, Goldstein MG, Niaura R, Emmons KM, Abrams DB: Nicotine Dependence: Assessment and Management. In Stoudemire A, Fogel BS (eds): Psychiatric Care of the Medical Patient. New York, Oxford University Press, 1993

Brownell KD, Wadden TA: The heterogeneity of obesity: Fitting treatment to individuals. Behav Ther 22:153–177, 1991

Engel GL: The need for a new medical model: A challenge for biomedicine. Science 196:129–136, 1977

Fagerstrom KO: Measuring degree of physical dependence to tobacco smoking with reference to individualization of treatment. Addict Behav 3:235–241, 1978

Fiore MC, Jorenby DE, Baker TB, Kenford SL: Tobacco dependence and the nicotine patch: Clinical guidelines for effective use. JAMA 268:2687–2694, 1992

Foxx RM, Brown RA: Nicotine fading and self-monitoring for cigarette abstinence as controlled smoking. J Appl Behav Anal 12:111–125, 1979

Glynn T, Manley M: How to Help Your Patients Stop Smoking: The National Cancer Institute Manual for Physicians. Bethesda, MD, National Institutes of Health, 1989

Grueninger UJ, Duffy FD, Goldstein MG: Patient Education in the Medical Encounter: An Interactive Approach. In Lipkin M Jr, Lazare A, Putnam S (eds): The Medical Interview. New York, Springer-Verlag, in press

Grueninger UJ, Goldstein MG, Duffy FD: Patient education in hypertension: Five essential steps. J Hypertension 7(Suppl 3):593–598, 1989

Hughes JR, Higgins ST, Hatsukami DK: Effects of Abstinence from Tobacco. In Kozlowski LT, Annis HM, Lappell HD et al (eds): Recent Advances in Alcohol and Drug Problems, Ch 10, pp 317–398. New York, Plenum Press, 1990

Inui TS, Yourtee EL, Williamson JW: Improved outcome in hypertension after physician tutorials: A controlled trial. Ann Intern Med 84:646–651, 1976

Jeffrey RW: Behavioral treatment of obesity. Ann Behav Med 9(1):20–24, 1987

Kottke TE, Battista RN, DeFriesse GH, Brekke ML: Attributes of successful smoking cessation interventions in medical practice: A meta-analysis of 39 controlled trials. JAMA 259:2882–2889, 1988

Kottke TE, Blackburn H, Brekke ML, Solberg LI: The systematic practice of preventive cardiology. Am J Cardiol 59:690–694, 1987

Kottke TE, Foels JK, Hill C et al: Nutrition counseling in private practice: Attitudes and activities of family physicians. Prev Med 13:219–225, 1984

Levenkron JC, Greenland P, Bowley N: Using patient instructors to teach behavioral counseling skills. J Med Educ 65:665–672, 1987

Lichtenstein E: The smoking problem: A behavioral perspective. J Consult Clin Psychol 50:804–819, 1982

Louis Harris and Associates, Inc: Health Maintenance. Newport Beach, CA, Pacific Mutual Life Insurance Co, 1978

Marlatt GA, Gordon JR: Relapse Prevention. New York, Guilford Press, 1985

Mullen PD, Green LW, Persinger GS: Clinical trials of patient education for chronic conditions: A comparative meta-analysis of intervention types. Prev Med 14:751–783, 1985

Mullen PD, Katayama CK: Health promotion in private practice: An analysis. Fam Commun Health 8:79–87, 1985

Nutting PA: Health promotion in primary medical care: Problems and potential. Prev Med 15:537–548, 1986

Ockene JK: Physician-delivered intervention for smoking cessation: Strategies for increasing effectiveness. Prev Med 16:723–737, 1987

Ockene JK, Quirk ME, Goldberg RJ et al: A residents training program for the development of smoking intervention skills. Arch Intern Med 148:1039–1045, 1988

Orleans CT, George LK, Houpt JL, Brodie KH: Health promotion in primary care: A survey of US family practitioners. Prev Med 14:636–647, 1985

Perri MG, McAllister PA, Gange JJ, Nezu AM: Effects of four maintenance programs on the long-term management of obesity. J Consult Clin Psychol 56:529–534, 1988

Perri MG, Sears SF, Clark JE: Strategies for improving the maintenance of weight loss: Toward a continuous care model of obesity management. Diabetes Care, in press

Preventive Health Care Committee, Society for Research and Education in Primary Care Internal Medicine: Preventive medicine in general internal medicine residency training. Ann Intern Med 102:859–861, 1985

Prochaska JO, DiClemente CC: Towards a Comprehensive Model of Change. In Miller WR, Heather N (eds): Treating Addictive Disorders: Processes of Change. New York, Plenum Press, 1986

Schwartz JL: Review and Evaluation of Smoking Cessation Methods. The United States and Canada, 1978–1985. US Department of Health and Human Services, Public Health Service, National Institute of Health, National Cancer Institute, Division of Cancer Prevention and Control. Bethesda, MD, NIH Publication No. 87–2940, 1987

Schwartz JS, Lewis CE, Clancy C, Kinosian MS, Radany MH, Koplan JP: Internists' practices in health promotion and disease prevention: A survey. Ann Intern Med 114:46–53, 1991

US Department of Health, Education, and Welfare, Public Health Service: Healthy People: The Surgeon General's Report on Health Promotion and Disease Prevention. Washington, DC, Government Printing Office, 1979

Wadden TA, Stunkard AJ: Controlled trial of very low calorie diet, behavior therapy, and their combination in the treatment of obesity. J Consult Clin Psychol 54:482–488, 1986

Wilson D, Wood G, Johnston N et al: Randomized clinical trial of supportive follow-up for smokers in family practice. Can Med Assoc J 126:127–129, 1982

Wing RR: Behavior treatment of severe obesity. Am J Clin Nutr 55:5455–5515, 1992

Index

A

Abandonment, fear of, 583–584
Abnormal Involuntary Movements Scale, 459
Achievement tests, 85, 87
   purposes of, 85
Acquired immune deficiency syndrome. *See* AIDS
Acute dystonic reaction, 164, 512–513
Acute stress disorder, 265
   characteristics of, 265
Adaptive behavior, tests of, 85, 87
   purposes of, 85
Adjustment disorder, 198–199
   with anxiety, 233–234
   characteristics of, 198–199
   with depressed mood, 199
Adolescents. *See* Child and adolescent disorders; Medically ill child and adolescent
Adoption studies, of personality disorders, 176
Advanced sleep phase syndrome, 646
Affect
   meaning of, 27
   in schizophrenia, 150
Ageism, in emergencies, 548
Aging
   and cognition, 340
   See also Geriatric patients
Agoraphobia, 234, 236
   behavior therapy for, 241
   characteristics of, 236–237

with and without panic disorder, 236
   See also Panic disorder
AIDS
   clinical management, 620–622
   delirium in, 612, 613–614, 620–622
   dementia in, 122–123, 612, 614–616, 622
   high risk behaviors, 611
   HIV virus in, 611
   infections in, 613–614
   peripheral nervous system involvement, 612–613
   physicians' reactions to, 623–624
   psychiatrist, role in, 624
   psychological reactions to, 616–619, 622
   testing for, 616–617
   treatment decisions, 622–623
   vascular myelopathy in, 612
Akathisia, 164, 513–514, 560
Akinesia, 514
Alcohol, and brain chemistry, 309
Alcoholics Anonymous (AA), 320, 499, 566
Alcoholism
   acute intoxication, 317
   alcohol withdrawal, 317–318
   assessment, case example, 3–6, 43–46
   coexisting disorders, 43–44, 307, 318
   definition of, 307
   drug-assisted detoxification, 318, 532, 567
   emergency treatment of intoxication/withdrawal, 566, 568
   and fetal alcohol syndrome, 316
   genetic factors in, 310
   geriatric patients, 346–348